Developmental Challenges and Societal Issues for Individuals With Intellectual Disabilities

Rejani Thudalikunnil Gopalan
Mahatma Gandhi Medical College and Hospital, India

A volume in the Advances in Medical Diagnosis, Treatment, and Care (AMDTC) Book Series

IGI Global
DISSEMINATOR OF KNOWLEDGE

Published in the United States of America by
IGI Global
Medical Information Science Reference (an imprint of IGI Global)
701 E. Chocolate Avenue
Hershey PA, USA 17033
Tel: 717-533-8845
Fax: 717-533-8661
E-mail: cust@igi-global.com
Web site: http://www.igi-global.com

Library of Congress Cataloging-in-Publication Data

Names: Gopalan, Rejani Thudalikunnil, 1974- editor.
Title: Developmental challenges and societal issues for individuals with intellectual disabilities / Rejani Thudalikunnil Gopalan, editor.
Description: Hershey, PA : Medical Information Science Reference, [2020] | Includes bibliographical references and index. | Summary: ""This book explores the effects of disabilities in intellectual functioning. It also examines the causes, treatment, and rehabilitation of such limitations in adaptive behavior"--Provided by publisher"-- Provided by publisher.
Identifiers: LCCN 2019027029 (print) | ISBN 9781799812234 (hardcover) | ISBN 9781799812241 (ebook)
Subjects: MESH: Intellectual Disability--psychology | Child | Adolescent | Disabled Children--psychology | Sociological Factors
Classification: LCC HV894 (print) | LCC HV894 (ebook) | NLM WS 107 | DDC 362.3085--dc23
LC record available at https://lccn.loc.gov/2019027029
LC ebook record available at https://lccn.loc.gov/2019027030

This book is published in the IGI Global book series Advances in Medical Diagnosis, Treatment, and Care (AMDTC) (ISSN: 2475-6628; eISSN: 2475-6636)

British Cataloguing in Publication Data
A Cataloguing in Publication record for this book is available from the British Library.

Advances in Medical Diagnosis, Treatment, and Care (AMDTC) Book Series

ISSN:2475-6628
EISSN:2475-6636

Mission

Advancements in medicine have prolonged the life expectancy of individuals all over the world. Once life-threatening conditions have become significantly easier to treat and even cure in many cases. Continued research in the medical field will further improve the quality of life, longevity, and wellbeing of individuals.

The **Advances in Medical Diagnosis, Treatment, and Care (AMDTC)** book series seeks to highlight publications on innovative treatment methodologies, diagnosis tools and techniques, and best practices for patient care. Comprised of comprehensive resources aimed to assist professionals in the medical field apply the latest innovations in the identification and management of medical conditions as well as patient care and interaction, the books within the AMDTC series are relevant to the research and practical needs of medical practitioners, researchers, students, and hospital administrators.

Coverage

- Critical Care
- Emergency Medicine
- Patient Interaction
- Diagnostic Medicine
- Medical Procedures
- Disease Prevention
- Patient-Centered Care
- Internal Medicine
- Medical Testing
- Alternative Medicine

IGI Global is currently accepting manuscripts for publication within this series. To submit a proposal for a volume in this series, please contact our Acquisition Editors at Acquisitions@igi-global.com or visit: http://www.igi-global.com/publish/.

The Advances in Medical Diagnosis, Treatment, and Care (AMDTC) Book Series (ISSN 2475-6628) is published by IGI Global, 701 E. Chocolate Avenue, Hershey, PA 17033-1240, USA, www.igi-global.com. This series is composed of titles available for purchase individually; each title is edited to be contextually exclusive from any other title within the series. For pricing and ordering information please visit http://www.igi-global.com/book-series/advances-medical-diagnosis-treatment-care/129618. Postmaster: Send all address changes to above address.

Titles in this Series

For a list of additional titles in this series, please visit: www.igi-global.com/book-series

Global Applications of One Health Practice and Care
Sandul Yasobant (Center for Development Research (ZEF), Germany) and Deepak Saxena (Indian Institute of Public Health Gandhinagar,India)
Medical Information Science Reference • ©2019 • 306pp • H/C (ISBN: 9781522563044) • US $245.00

Pre-Screening Systems for Early Disease Prediction, Detection, and Prevention
Thierry Edoh (Technical University of Munich, Germany) Pravin Pawar (Philips Research, India) and Sagar Mohammad (Philips Research,India)
Medical Information Science Reference • ©2019 • 395pp • H/C (ISBN: 9781522571315) • US $245.00

Advanced Methodologies and Technologies in Medicine and Healthcare
Mehdi Khosrow-Pour, D.B.A. (Information Resources Management Association, USA)
Medical Information Science Reference • ©2019 • 591pp • H/C (ISBN: 9781522574897) • US $325.00

Handbook of Research on Critical Examinations of Neurodegenerative Disorders
Md. Sahab Uddin (Southeast University, Bangladesh) and Md. Shah Amran (University of Dhaka, Bangladesh)
Medical Information Science Reference • ©2019 • 597pp • H/C (ISBN: 9781522552826) • US $345.00

Effective Techniques for Managing Trigeminal Neuralgia
Steven Chang (Stanford University, USA) and Allen Ho (Stanford University, USA)
Medical Information Science Reference • ©2018 • 331pp • H/C (ISBN: 9781522553496) • US $225.00

Handbook of Research on Geriatric Health, Treatment, and Care
Barre Vijaya Prasad (Dharwad Institute of Mental Health and Neurosciences (DIMHANS), India) and Shamsi Akbar (King George's Medical University, India)
Medical Information Science Reference • ©2018 • 604pp • H/C (ISBN: 9781522534808) • US $375.00

Emerging Developments and Practices in Oncology
Issam El Naqa (University of Michigan, USA)
Medical Information Science Reference • ©2018 • 305pp • H/C (ISBN: 9781522530855) • US $245.00

Complementary and Alternative Medicine and Kidney Health
Mayuree Tangkiatkumjai (Srinakharinwirot University, Thailand) Annalisa Casarin (The NIHR Research Design Service East of England, UK) Li-Chia Chen (University of Manchester, UK) and Dawn-Marie Walker (University of Southampton, UK)

IGI Global
DISSEMINATOR OF KNOWLEDGE

701 East Chocolate Avenue, Hershey, PA 17033, USA
Tel: 717-533-8845 x100 • Fax: 717-533-8661
E-Mail: cust@igi-global.com • www.igi-global.com

Editorial Advisory Board

Table of Contents

Detailed Table of Contents

Intellectual disability (ID, also known as mental retardation) is a condition of arrested or incomplete development of the mind. ID is especially characterized by impairment of skills manifested during the developmental period, which contribute to the overall level of intelligence (i.e., cognitive, language, motor, and social abilities). The understanding about intellectual disability, mainly its features, causes and intervention has a long history. Researches on causes of intellectual disability lead to finding of multiple etiological factors which reflected well on its improved management techniques. The changes in terminology used describe intellectual disability also reflected our understanding about it different dimensions including social stigma. This chapter focused to give an overall view about its history, changes in terminology, classification, epidemiology, etiology, comorbidities, and management. Over the years, there are many changes and findings that have happened, yet many questions are unanswered related to this condition.

There is limited evidence base regarding mental health issues in people with intellectual disability (ID), and hence, findings from the general population are often applied to ID groups. Available evidence suggests that individuals with ID experience higher rates of mental health disorders than the general population, although findings are mixed with regard to the determinants of this increased prevalence. Further, the consequences of this comorbidity for individuals, families, and the wider community are often overlooked including the multiple challenges in identifying and managing these concerns. Accurate diagnosis and effective intervention are currently hindered by factors including the applicability of standardized psychiatric classification systems, gaps in service delivery models and access to such services, as well as unmet training needs. It is critical that further research is carried out to examine the specific challenges facing individuals with ID along with facilitating appropriate mental health services to individuals with ID.

School bullying research began in the 1970s through seminal research conducted on these experiences among Norwegian boys. From this initial research, multiple studies have been conducted over the past 40 years, revealing the nature, extent, causes, and consequences of school bullying. More recent investigations have also focused on cyberbullying, bullying using information and communication technologies (e.g., cell phones). Little attention has been given to school bullying involvement among students with disabilities, particularly those with intellectual disabilities. The handful of studies on this topic suggest that these students experience internalizing (e.g., depression, anxiety, loneliness) and externalizing (e.g., aggression, antisocial behaviors) difficulties associated with their involvement in school bullying. The aim of this chapter is to review multidisciplinary research concerning school bullying among students with intellectual disabilities and to make recommendations for public policy and prevention programs as well as future research.

There are many children with intellectual disability (ID) in recent years. The increase in numbers reflects the knowledge regarding the issue, thus creating awareness and increased detection for children for any developmental delay. Consequently, medical services are seeing and treating younger cohorts. Their disability may be mild to moderate, making it difficult even for medical professionals to identify these children. Invariably all parents want to have healthy, intelligent, and capable children who can achieve independence and a successful life. The reality is that parents having children with ID often struggle to understand what is happening with their child, what more how to cope with and help their child. Added to their distress is that even professionals dealing with the children and their family have various ideas and beliefs regarding this issue. Identifying families who are struggling and offering them the appropriate advice is essential as these families need proper guidance and services for their child.

Parents of children with intellectual disability face various stressful situations. However, many of them show resilience even in the midst of challenges and are able to meaningfully contribute to the life of the child. In the present study, the factors of stress that hinder resilience are assessed in a sample of 50 parents of intellectually disabled children. Stress scale for parents of mentally challenged (SPMC) developed by Rejitha, Biji, and Jayan was used to measure the stress of the parents. Resilience was measured using the Bharathiar University resilience scale, developed by Annalakshmi. Results showed extra-familial stress as a significant inverse predictor of resilience. Older parents are relatively more resilient when compared to the younger.

Caregivers are the important and integral part in the lives of people with intellectual disability. As caregiving is extensive and mostly lifelong for this population, the associated burden, stigma, and also wellbeing of the caregivers are also equally important as these are often very directly correlated with the wellbeing of the individuals with intellectual disability. The chapter focused on the issues and impacts of caregiving, mental health problems, wellbeing, and related issues of caregivers. The authors also discuss the various facets of stigma caregivers do face and ways to deal with the stigma.

The need to understand the quality of life of people with intellectual disability is crucial as this mental disability is considered to be a major setback for any individual and his/her family. Current researches focus on creating an equal platform to understand intellectual disability in order to gain more acceptances from the masses, especially for the families who have a member suffering from intellectual disability. The age of the family member and available care taking measures are also of critical value. Models of therapy/interventions drawn from previous evidence-based practices give a bright picture.

Intellectual disability is a neurodevelopment disorder that affects the intellectual and adaptive functioning. The individual fails to meet standards of personal independence and social responsibility in one or more aspects of daily life, including communication, social participation, academic or occupational functioning, and personal independence at home or in community settings. There is an immense need to understand and be aware of the signs and symptoms of the disorder. This chapter focuses on the process of the assessment which is necessary to identify intellectual deficiency and also the issues that should be taken care of during the process. The various principles and tools of assessment, which can be used to measure IQ, are mentioned. It also focuses on the various challenging behaviors and functional analysis. It also focuses on recent and efficient management strategies that can be used to help the affected person cope and acquire new skills.

Intelligence is the general mental capacity that involves reasoning, planning, solving problems, thinking abstractly, comprehending complex ideas, learning efficiently, and learning from experience. Intellectual disability (previously termed "mental retardation") shows significant cognitive deficits (IQ score of below

Preface

I am very happy to come up with the enhanced version of Handbook of Research on Diagnosing, Treating, and Managing Intellectual Disabilities. The success of the Handbook among clinicians, academicians, students and those related to work with intellectual disability reflected the fact that the topic still attracts lots of attention and importance and the condition is a concern for management, rehabilitation and policy making. In the past decades, research in the area of intellectual disability has helped in a phenomenal way to change the attitude toward the condition as well delivery in various multidisciplinary services to affected individuals. New ways for assisting these individuals with focus in understanding and managing significant issues and thereby integrating them into the mainstream society has been the aim every research being conducted.

Previous researches focused on more on the clinical features and its management, and rehabilitation, however later the focus shifted more to the psychosocial issues of the person with intellectual disability and concerns and challenges faced by the family members and care takers. The changes in the terminology, management modalities and policies are reflecting the in depth understanding of the condition of intellectual disability. The awareness and understanding about intellectual disability also highlighted the view point of personal rights and their inclusion in to the society and the new challenges to be faced.

Keeping it in mind this book is designed with the objective of providing students and professionals who work with individuals with intellectual disability a literature which focus on historical development of intellectual disability as a debilitating condition, awareness and attitudes toward intellectual disability, issues pertaining to mental health, schooling, sexuality, parenthood, crime and law, and quality of life of individuals with intellectual disability, issues faced by family members, assessment and management and psychosocial treatment. In the current enhanced version, more emphasis was given to the developmental challenges and various psychosocial issues faced by the individuals with intellectual disability at large.

To be more specific, the book starts with history regarding the understanding about intellectual disability, mainly its features, causes and intervention. Chapter 1 gives an overall view about the history, changes in terminology, classification, epidemiology, etiology, comorbidities and management of intellectual disability. Also, current understanding and latest trends and issues are highlighted.

Chapter 2 deals with developmental vulnerability and mental health issues as individuals with ID experience higher rates of mental health disorders than the general population. It gives an account of the prevalence of psychiatric disorders and its nature in individuals with intellectual disability. It looks into the consequences of this comorbid condition on individuals, families and the wider community, and also the various challenges in identifying and managing these concerns. Issues such as applicability of standardized psychiatric classification systems, gaps in service delivery models and access to such services, as well as unmet training need are also focused in this chapter.

Chapter 3 concentrates on the topic school bullying and students with intellectual disabilities. The history of research in school bullying which has looked into the nature, extent, causes, and consequences of school bullying and recent research on cyber bullying, bullying using information and communication technologies, research on school bullying involvement among students with disabilities, particularly those with intellectual disabilities is provided in this chapter. Along with multidisciplinary research details the chapter also has recommendations for public policy and prevention programs as well as future research.

Chapter 4 discusses the mental health issues among family members of children with mental disability. It looks into the types of problems faced by the children with mental disability, their parents and siblings, including the possible impact on mental health of the family. Parents having children with ID often struggle to understand what is happening with their child, what more how to cope with and help their child. The chapter as well discusses the impact of mental health difficulties in parents and its impact on parenting in detail. It intends to highlight the need to recognize parents who are struggling, what professionals should look for in their assessment of families with children with intellectual disabilities.

Chapter 5 deals with stress and resilience in parents of intellectually disabled children. Parental stress is a major concern as it influences the outcome of management. It presents a study which attempted to find out the factors of stress that could act against the resilience in the parents of intellectually disabled children. The sample consisted of 50 parents of intellectually disabled children from different panchayats in the Calicut, Kannur, Wayanad districts in the state of Kerala, India. Results of the study indicate that extra-familial stress was a negative predictor of resilience in the parents of the intellectually disabled children. Further, the parents who were in a late part of the young adulthood period and old were relatively more resilient than the parents who were in the earlier part of the young adulthood period.

Chapter 6 focuses on the role of family members as caregivers of individuals with intellectual disabilities. Caregivers are the important and integral part in the lives of people with intellectual disability. As caregiving is extensive and mostly lifelong for this population, the associated burden, stigma and also well being of the caregivers are also equally important as these are often very directly correlated with the wellbeing of the individuals with intellectual disability. The chapter focused on the issues and impacts of care giving, mental health problems, wellbeing and related issues of caregiver. It also discusses the various facets of stigma caregivers do face and ways to deal with the stigma.

Chapter 7 explores the quality of life of people with intellectual disability. The need to understand the quality of life of people with intellectual disability is crucial as this mental disability is considered to be a major setback for any individual and his/her family. It is important to improve the quality of life of individuals with ID as it will also reflect in the mental health and overall improvement of the individual. It needs to be highlighted here, that the families of people with intellectual disability also play a crucial role. New research reviews are required to bring policy changes and better tools.

Chapter 8 covers issues and recent trends in the assessment and management of intellectual disability in childhood. It is an attempt to understand disability aspect in general and assessment aspect extensively. Both the classic and latest trends of assessment techniques have been looked into. It includes assessment categories on different dimensions of ability, emotions and behaviours such as intelligence, achievement, adaptive, social behaviour and emotional adjustment, communication/language, sensory status, motor skills, and health status. The issues concerning the assessment of children with intellectual disabilities, including definitional problems, psychometric factors, and practical difficulties is emphasized and measures would be proposed to help students, counselors, teachers and psychologists. The use of current tools and its limitations are important for the clinical practice.

Chapter 9 explores the concerns for individuals with intellectual disability in India. As many parts of world, the stigma on ID exist in India too and the concerns are also high. It focuses on topics like legal services available for persons with intellectual disability, challenges faced by parents, health issues, sexual knowledge, marriage, quality of life, and old age, attitude of society towards the individual with intellectual disability, implications, management and prevention for future improvement for individuals with intellectual disability.

Chapter 10 provides awareness towards intervention for intellectual disability. There are many issues which require attention while dealing with ID like human resources, quality training of clinical psychologists in India, the conflicts among the team approach, acceptance in the family and society and many more. There are 1.5 million people with intellectual disability in India. However, experts working in the field of developmental disabilities feel that prevalence is much higher. The population with ID is increasing but the resources to deal with these issues are few. The mental health profession is a multidisciplinary one. The psychiatrist, the clinical psychologist and the psychiatric social worker all have their significant role in the management of ID. There is a long way to go. Difficulties like lack of human resources, quality training of clinical psychologists in India, scarcity of effective clinical guidelines, conflicts among the team approach, acceptance in the family and society requires attention in current scenario. There are many things that can be offered but what we need is acceptance in our society of such people and awareness towards Intervention. This chapter aims at acknowledging these issues to create awareness amongst the responsible caregivers.

Chapter 11 discusses about attitude towards people with intellectual disabilities (PWID). The attitude makes significant changes in the lives of individuals with disabilities and unfortunately negative attitudes towards them still persist. The chapter delves into the history on PWID to understand the existence of stereotypical attitudes towards PWID. This chapter also presents with the stress, stress related issues faced by families of PWID. It discusses how families often cope with these issues and its effect on providing timely assistance and rehabilitation of PWID. Also, attitude of stakeholders like siblings and relatives, teachers, educationists, health professionals, general public and future recommendations for service and research are also discussed in the light of latest literature.

Chapter 12 aimed to draw attention to the integrated understanding of an individual with intellectual disability. This chapter discusses emotional intelligence in people with intellectual disability and how understanding of this will lead to better management plans for individual with intellectual disability, which will in turn lead to better empowerment. Further this chapter will discuss on the research gaps in this area and future study scope.

Chapter 13 deals with psycho social treatment of intellectual disability and current trends in it. Applied Behaviour Analysis has the most research evidence base for treatment of challenging behaviours and improving the quality of life of these individuals. Applied Behaviour Analysis adopts a systematic approach in assessment and treatment of challenging behaviours. In recent years, 'parenting' has also emerged as a dominant theme among researchers and practitioners. Emerging research evidences are also favouring 'parenting skill based programmes' grounded in behavioural research as intervention strategies to obtain better developmental outcomes for individuals with intellectual disability.

Chapter 14 concentrates on crime and legal issues among intellectually disabled individuals. It presents with research on criminal law and the different forms of aggressive behaviour such as sexual violence, homicide, theft, and arson and alcohol-drug abuse associated with intellectual deficiency. This chapter also provides information on research regarding civil law and the most common problems for individuals with intellectual deficiency, such as financial capacity and capacity for medical consent, issues regarding the trial and conviction for individuals with intellectual deficiency and also recent research on attitudes toward intellectual deficiency and legal issues. Neuropsychological and cross-cultural perspectives of the issues are also presented. The chapter concludes with suggestions for reform of the law relating to ID and the need for further research.

Finally, Chapter 15 deals with sexuality, sexual abuse, marriage, partner violence, parenting skills and associated issues in persons with Intellectual Disability. Sexuality has an active role in the development, evolution, emotional balance and affective stability of the individual. It has a significant role in interpersonal and couple's relationships. As intellectually disabled person approach puberty their control of behaviour and expression of sexuality may manifest in unacceptable ways. Persons with intellectual disabilities are at increased risk for physical, sexual and emotional abuse. This chapter focuses on the issues related to sexual feelings and its expression among intellectually disabled people and the risk for sexual abuse. The necessity of sex education and components of sex education for different group is also explained in detail. The chapter also addresses the parenting skills and problems related with parenthood among individuals with intellectual disability.

This book was aimed to provide the latest empirical research findings in the area of Intellectual disability focusing on epidemiology, assessment, causes, and comorbidities, intellectual disabilities at various stages (childhood, adolescence, and adulthood), educational issues, sexuality, marriage and parenting issues, forensic issues, stigma, and mental health problems among family members. It would also provide a fresh approach and comprehensive knowledge on ID and its various aspects and I think the chapters have done justice to the objective of the book.

I am hopeful that the target audience of this book (composed of professionals and researchers working in the mental health area such as clinicians (especially Psychiatrists, Clinical Psychologists, Pediatricians), academicians, special educators, social workers, Psychiatric nurses, rehabilitation centres, and students in the area of mental health) would be benefited from this handbook. This book is useful for Universities, hospitals, and the public. Moreover, it would provide a deep knowledge on ID and its various issues from a developmental approach and it is valuable as it deals with their sexual issues, marriage, parenting skills and issues faced by the family members. It will further enrich our current knowledge of intellectual disabilities. I hope this book will be another stepping stone to understand intellectual disabilities in a more comprehensive way especially in understanding the various psychosocial issues related to the condition.

The research works cited in this book is referenced according to APA guidelines.

I express my gratitude towards all who have contributed and joined with me in the process of writing this book. I would like to thank my son Harikrishnan for his patience, family members for their encouragements and support. Special thanks to all authors, reviewers and editorial members for their constant support and enthusiasm. My heartfelt thanks to the publisher for their continuous support and suggestions.

Chapter 1
Intellectual Disability (ID): An Overview from History, Terminology, and Classification to Recent Trends

Rejani Thudalikunnil Gopalan
https://orcid.org/0000-0002-5957-8144
Mahatma Gandhi Medical College and Hospital, India

ABSTRACT

Intellectual disability (ID, also known as mental retardation) is a condition of arrested or incomplete development of the mind. ID is especially characterized by impairment of skills manifested during the developmental period, which contribute to the overall level of intelligence (i.e., cognitive, language, motor, and social abilities). The understanding about intellectual disability, mainly its features, causes and intervention has a long history. Researches on causes of intellectual disability lead to finding of multiple etiological factors which reflected well on its improved management techniques. The changes in terminology used describe intellectual disability also reflected our understanding about it different dimensions including social stigma. This chapter focused to give an overall view about its history, changes in terminology, classification, epidemiology, etiology, comorbidities, and management. Over the years, there are many changes and findings that have happened, yet many questions are unanswered related to this condition.

HISTORY OF INTELLECTUAL DISABILITY

Intellectual Disability (ID, also known as mental retardation) is a condition of arrested or incomplete development of the mind. ID is especially characterized by impairment of skills manifested during the developmental period, which contribute to the overall level of intelligence, i.e. cognitive, language, motor, and social abilities (WHO, 1992). It occurs in 2-3% of the general population. Prevalence of mild level of intellectual disability is seven to ten times more than severe level of intellectual disability.

DOI: 10.4018/978-1-7998-1223-4.ch001

The understanding about intellectual disability, mainly its features, causes and intervention has a long history. Both modern and ancient cultures presumed that demon possession caused ID. Similarly, some cultures thought ID was a punishment by God. There were some exceptions. As early as 1500 B.C. some physicians understood IDs as a medical problem. Although translation is imprecise, the therapeutic papyri of Thebes (Luxor), Egypt, 1500 B.C. reference disabilities of the mind due to brain damage. Ancient Greeks and Romans looked upon the condition as a burden on society. Accordingly, persons with ID were treated atrociously. The ancient Greeks and Romans commonly killed infants believed to be defective. Others were sold for entertainment. Since demonic possession or God's wrath was believed the cause, they were treated as less than human. (Reynolds, Zupanick, &Dombeck,2013).

Not much literature is available on mentioning intellectual disability in the past, especially prior to 1700. Jean-Marc Itard (1774-1838) is considered as the pioneer of systematic instruction for intellectually disabled as he tried to educate the boy named Victor with cognitive impairment. The special education for less abled children slowly gained popularity and Edouard Seguin (1812-1880) established an educational program in Paris which emphasized physiological and moral education.One of the major changes occurred in the history of Intellectual disability is the Eugenics movement in the late 19th century. "Eugenics" comes from the Greek words for "good" and "origin," or "good birth" and it is a social philosophy advocating the improvement of human genetic traits through the promotion of higher rates of sexual reproduction for people with desired traits (positive eugenics), or reduced rates of sexual reproduction and sterilization of people with less-desired or undesired traits (negative eugenics), or both (Osborn &Frederick,1937).The term eugenics was first coined by Francis Galton in the late 1800's and he believed that desirable traits could pass through generations based on his studies on intelligence among upper class of Britain. He found that their desired traits such as superior intelligence are hereditary and passes through generations and favored the idea of selective breeding or humanity could be improved by encouraging the fittest members of society to have more children (Norrgard, 2008).The movement became popular in America in the early part of 20th century and it resulted in a negative attitude towards disabled people including mentally ill and intellectually disabled or feeble-minded individuals as they were considered to polluting the gene pool of the country.Such individuals were seen as a threat to society and the probable cause of most of the criminal activity and social problems of the country. In many states, support for the Eugenics movement resulted in legislation requiring mandatory sterilization, incarceration, and in many cases, the castration of persons with disabilities. In each state, hundreds of thousands of people with mental illness or intellectual disabilities were placed in institutions, the largest of which housed as many as 20,000 people(Felty, 2007).

In addition to this, the development of intelligence tests also made remarkable contribution in the history of Intellectual disability. During the early 1900s, Alfred Binet and Theodore Simon developed the first intelligence test as result of the request by the French government to find students with academic difficulties in the school. Terman standardized this test with sample from America and published in 1916, was called the Stanford-Binet Intelligence Scale. Psychological testing, especially intelligence tests used to identify intellectual deficiency and institutionalization was considered as the major remedy for the problem of intellectual disability.On his study on Kallikak family, Goddard (1912) found that feeblemindedness" was inherited which also encouraged institutionalization and sterilization of intellectually disabled people.

Researches on causes of intellectual disability lead to finding of multiple etiological factors which reflected well on its improved management techniques. The changes in terminology used describe intellectual disability also reflected our understanding about it different dimensions including social stigma.

The ideas of normalization evolved in the Scandinavian countries during 1950s-1960s, originated by Niels Eric Bank Mikkelsen. Bank Mikkelsen, who is known as father of Normalization Principle, was the pioneer of the deinstitutionalization movement in the Scandinavian countries. He firstly implemented his ideas of normalization in Denmark, during the 1950s to 1960s. This movement emphasized for providing all the opportunities to all persons with disabilities which are available to a non-disabled person in society, which had a profound positive effect on the lives of the people with disabilities including Intellectually disabled individuals (Kumar, 2013).

The deinstitutionalization movement of the 1970s reflected a concern for the civil rights of mentally retarded.Although deinstitutionalization has been positive for the majority of patients, it also has severe shortcomings. Expectations that community care would lead to fuller social integration have not been achieved; many remain without work, have limited social contacts, and often live in sheltered environments (Fuller, 1997).

Efforts of community integration of disabled individual including intellectually disabled are continuing in different dimensions in terms of education, vocational rehabilitation, social welfare and legal safety. All over the world efforts are taken place in these dimensions and governments, parents organizations, community service centers are working towards this goal though variation can be noticed in developed and developing /under developed countries.

Terminology

Earlier the term simpleton was used to describe people with intellectual disability and it was introduced by S.G.Howe(1846), which was replaced by the term moron invented by Henry Goddard. Changes reflected in the classification of intellectually disabled individuals in to moron (IQ of 51–70), imbecile (26–50), and idiot (0–25) based on IQ tests. For over 50 years, the most frequently used term to refer to individuals with intellectual disabilities was mental retardation. This term reflected widespread and long-term use in the wake of the elimination of the labels of feeblemindedness, moron, imbecile, and idiot (Polloway&Lubin, 2009).Retarded comes from the Latin retardare,which means "to make slow, delay, keep back, or hinder." Mental retardation replaced older terms such as feeblemindedness, idiocy, and mental subnormality that had become pejorative. Now, over 5 decades later, the term 'mental retardation' is being eliminated for similar reasons (Harris, 2013). The consideration of new terminology stressed on a neutral term without stigma and degrading meaning, and value human right aspects. Human rights perspective gained more importance and accordingly the "person first" terminology has been adopted. The more theoretical information leads to the consideration of ID as a neurodevelopmental disorder and the importance of adaptive skills and level of intelligence in the classification also gained importance. In classification, from a neurodevelopmental perspective, a major change has been grouping of ID along with other conditions under the overarching category of neurodevelopmental disorders that have onset in developmental period, affecting the functional abilities of brain, and having a continuous life course presentation. The current classificatory systems have considered various behavioral and clinical indicators of intellectual and adaptive function skills that could be attained across these stages which are line with the lifespan perspective of presentation of ID. The importance on adaptive skills rather relying only on formal IQ scores in diagnosis and classification of ID is a significant trend (Girimai & Pradeep, 2018).

The ICD-10 conceptualization of Mental Retardation is replaced with the concept of intellectual developmental disorders (IDD) in ICD-11. The diagnostic term of mental retardation is replaced by Intellectual Disability in DSM 5. The term "intellectual disability" (ID) has widely replaced MR for policy, administrative and legislative purposes in many countries (Carulla, 2011). There were concerns raised regarding the use of term mental retardation such as it has negative connotations, has become offensive to many people, and often results in misunderstandings about the nature of the disorder and those who have it and thus proposed the term intellectual disability. A federal statute in the United States (Public Law 111-256, Rosa's Law) replaces the term mental retardation with intellectual disability in law and public policy.

It is interesting to note, that in each case, the original term was neutral in meaning. As the term entered public use, it become pejorative. This fact illuminates social cruelty born of ignorance and fear. There are always competing elements of society. Some of people seek respectful, neutral medical terms. Others misuse these same terms as weapons to insult people. For health care professionals, diagnostic labels serve as a form of shorthand communication. Diagnostic labels rapidly communicate a set of symptoms associated with a particular condition. It may simultaneously suggest an appropriate treatment. However, when these conditions carry a social stigma, the diagnostic labels themselves become stigmatizing. The original, medical term loses its intended neutral meaning (Reynolds,. Zupanick, & Dombeck, 2013).

Classification

In ICD-10 criteria, Intellectual disability/mental retardation comes under Mental and Behavioural disorders (F70-F99), specifically from F70 to F79. According to ICD-10 criteria, the coding for degree of mental retardation are: F70 Mild Mental Retardation, F71 Moderate Mental Retardation, F72 Severe Mental Retardation, F73 Profound Mental Retardation, F78 Other Mental Retardation and F79 Unspecified Mental Retardation. In mild mental retardation or intellectual disability, the approximate IQ range from 50 to 69 (in adults, mental age from 9 to under 12 years). This group may have some learning difficulties in school and many adults will be able to work and maintain good social relationships and contribute to society. In moderate level of intellectual disability or Moderate Mental Retardation, the approximate IQ range from 35 to 49 (in adults, mental age from 6 to under 9 years). This category shows marked developmental delays in childhood but most can learn to develop some degree of independence in self-care and acquire adequate communication and academic skills. Adults will need varying degrees of support to live and work in the community. Under severe Mental Retardation or severe level of Intellectual disability, the approximate IQ range from 20 to 34 (in adults, mental age from 3 to under 6 years).This group needs continuous need of support. In Profound Mental Retardation or profound (IQ under 20 (in adults, mental age below 3 years) which results in severe limitation in self-care, continence, communication and mobility(ICD-10,WHO).

In ICD-11 criteria, the term is used asIntellectual Developmental Disorders and the term defines as 'a group of developmental conditions characterized by significant impairment of cognitive functions, which are associated with limitations of learning, adaptive behavior and skills. The levels of severity (mild, moderate, severe, or profound) are proposed to remain unchanged in ICD-11 (Salvador-Carulla, Reed, Vaez-Azizi et al, 2011).

In DSM 5, the diagnostic term of mental retardation is replaced by Intellectual Disability (Intellectual Developmental Disorder) whichis the equivalent term for the ICD-11 diagnosis of Intellectual Developmental Disorders (DSM-5, p. 33). According to DSM 5, Intellectual Disability (Intellectual Developmental Disorder) is a disorder with onset during the developmental period that includes both intellectual and adaptive functioning deficits in conceptual, social, and practical domains.There are three criteria to be considered for making a diagnosis such as deficits in intellectual functions, deficits in adaptive functioning and the onset of intellectual and adaptive deficits during the developmental period. The severity levels for intellectual disability are mild, moderate severe and profound.

There are lot of changes can be noticed in terms of diagnostic criteria in DSM –IV and DSM 5 on Intellectual disability. Apart from change in terms of terminology, reduced importance placed on the intelligence tests or score. According to DSM-IV significantly sub average intellectual functioning; an IQ of approximately 70 or below, is required but DSM 5 emphasis more on adaptive functions. In DSM –IV, onset is considered to be before the age of 18 which is changed as onset of intellectual and adaptive deficits during the developmental period.

Critical components of intelligence proposed in both DSM-5 and the ICD-11 are verbal comprehension, working memory, perceptual reasoning, and cognitive efficacy. The diagnosis in DSM-5 will emphasize both clinical judgment and standardized intelligence testing; however, less emphasis is expected to be placed on the IQ score, but greater emphasis will be placed on the adaptive reasoning in academic, social, and practical settings. The requirement for both intellectual deficits and adaptive deficits that fail to meet the standards for personal independence are proposed to remain in DSM-5, with greater emphasis on linking intellectual deficits to adaptive deficits through adaptive reasoning in the three domains listed (Harris, 2013).

Historically two main approaches have contributed to the development of knowledge-base on ID: a neurodevelopmental-clinical approach and a psychoeducational-social approach. These approaches show a complex interaction throughout the history of IDD and have had a diverse influence on its classification. Although in theory Diagnostic and Statistical Manual (DSM)-5 and ICD adhere to the neurodevelopmental-clinical model, the new definition in the ICD-11 follows a restrictive normality approach to intellectual quotient and to the measurement of adaptive behaviour. On the contrary DSM-5 is closer to the recommendations made by the WHO 'Working Group on Mental Retardation' for ICD-11 for an integrative approach (Salvador-Carulla, Bertelli, Martinez-Leal(2018).

Epidemiology

Epidemiology is essentially the study of a disorder in a given population. Epidemiological research may investigate the causes of a disease, the natural history of a disease, the characteristics of a disease, influenced by such factors as age, sex, social class and ethnic background.Research may be used to test the efficacy and efficiency of healthcare intervention to prevent or treat the disorder. It may also assist in healthcare planning (Prasher& Routhu,2003,2011). Estimation of intellectual disability is important to understand its causes and management.

Prevalence of ID has been reported around 1-3% population in the world (Schalock, Borthwick-Duffy, Bradley, Buntinx, Coulter, Craig, *et al*., 2010). Life span prevalence of ID is found to be 10.37/1000 or 1.04%, ID prevalence of children and adolescents to be 18.3/1000 or 1.83%,and ID prevalence of children/adolescents and adults to range from .05 to 1.55%, and prevalence range for children and adolescents to be from 0.22 to 1.55% . The female-to-male ratio of children and adolescents with ID varied between 0.4 and 1.0 (i.e., four to 10 females with ID for every 10 males with the condition (Maulik, Mascarenhas, Mathers, Dua, & Saxena, 2011; McKenzie, Milton, Smith & Ouellette-Kuntz, 2016). Studies have noticed that highest prevalence is in low income countries (16.41/1000 population), whereas for middle- and high-income countries is around 15.94 and 9.21/1000 population, and the prevalence of ID is more among child/adolescent population (18.30/1000) in comparison with an adult population (4.94/1000) (Harris and Maulik *et al,* 2013).

The prevalence of intellectual disability across Asia appears to be consistent with western estimates at 0.06-1.3% (Jeevanandam, 2009). Prevalence of intellectual disability in India is around 2% for mild level of intellectual disability and 0.5% for severe level of intellectual disability (defined as IQ less than 50) (Srinath&Girimaji, 1999). The causes of severe level of intellectual disability can be determined in 60-70% of cases, as compared to mild level of intellectual disability where 35-55% remain idiopathic (Kabra&Gulati, 2003).A recent study noticed that overall, India has a prevalence of 10.5/1000 in ID. Urban population has slightly higher rate (11/1000) than rural (10.08/1000; $P = 0.044$). Age was found to be highly correlated with prevalence of ID in rural children as well as in children and adults in urban population. The possibility of confounding or the existence of covariates for children in urban settings was noted. Results of this study match findings in other epidemiological studies (Lakhan, Ekúndayò, &Shahbazi, 2015).

Variations in estimation of ID are noticed in many countries.For example, according to census results in 2011, the prevalence of ID is around 13/1000 population in Iran. The prevalence of ID is showed according to age and gender. In general, the prevalence of ID among men (5.3/1000) is more than women (3.5/1000), and it has the highest rate for adolescents and young people.The results in comparison to other studies showed that the prevalence of ID in Iran is lower than global estimates significantly. Because of the different definitions of ID and data collection methods, rates are different in Iran as compared with other countries (Soltani, Khosravi & Salehiniya, 2015).

From an epidemiologic perspective,ID prevalence rates vary according to the definitions and classification system being used. Using IQ<70 as the only criteria, researchers estimated that in the United States the prevalence of ID was around 3%. However, by including other criteria such as deficits in adaptive behavior, or defining less severe ID as learning disabilities, or accounting for variable rates of case identification and mortality across different age-groups, the estimates were reduced to 1% (King et al. 2009). Increasing the IQ cut-off score from 70 to 75 almost doubles the number of PWID because of the general population distribution of intelligence. Even across different states within the U.S., prevalence rates among school children vary, from 3.2/1000 in New Jersey to 25.4/1000 in Kentucky, due to varying case definitions, level of completed education, and income level of the family (Massey and McDermott 1995). Intellectual disability is also conceptualized differently across cultures and countries and this is reflected in the many definitions used across countries (WHO 2007).

In a recent systematic review prevalence of ID, McKenzie, Milton, Smith & Ouellette-Kuntz (2016) noted that over a relatively brief observation period (6 years), a number of studies aimed at determining the prevalence of intellectual disabilities were identified across nine countries; this highlights the global desire for this knowledge. From these studies, it appears that the global prevalence of intellectual disabilities may indeed be lower than 1%. The heterogeneity of studies, however, prohibits definitive conclusions about a potential downward trend. Collaborative national and international efforts to address the issues identified may be needed to ensure increased comparability across studies. Knowing the distribution of intellectual disabilities as a whole in the population (prevalence) informs service planning across multiple sectors from child and youth services, education, health, social services, and aging services. However, to understand variations in the occurrence of intellectual disabilities over time or place requires an appreciation of the shifts and differences in diagnostic practices, population characteristics, and exposure to known risk factors.

Over the past 50 years the prevalence and incidence of mental retardation have been affected by changes in the definition of mental retardation, improvements in medical care and technology, societal attitudes regarding the acceptance and treatment of an individual with mental retardation, and the expansion of educational services to children with disabilities from birth through age 21. The theoretical approach to determining the prevalence of mental retardation uses the normal bell curve to estimate the number of individuals whose IQ falls below the established criterion score. For example, 2.3% of the population of the United States has an IQ score below 70, and 5.5% has an IQ score below 75. However, this estimate does not account for adaptive behaviour skills. Assuming a normal distribution for intelligence with a mean of 100, 2.3% of children would be expected to have an IQ score greater than 2 standard deviations below the mean on an intelligence test, for an estimated prevalence of 23 per 1000. However, prevalence as ascertained from community samples has been shown to be closer to 10 per 1000 (Armatas, 2009 ;Yeargin-Alsoppet al 2008).

Etiology

Though hereditary was considered as the single most reason for ID in earlier days, studies in over many decades found multiple causes and risk factors. These include genetic conditions, metabolic disorders, birth related complications, exposure to toxins, Iodine deficiency (cretinism), and malnutrition. The identification of causes of ID is very important for the management and prevention of the condition.

A recent study reported that genetic factors are responsible for up to 40% developmental disability cases, such as global developmental delay/intellectual disability (GDD/DI). Chromosomal abnormalities and fragile X syndrome are the most frequent causes of developmental disabilities and the techniques employed to detect such genetic disorders should be used as first line investigations of GDD/DI (Miclea, Peca, Cuzmici, Pop, 2015). Previous studies noted that single-gene disorders which are associated with atypical or dysmorphic physical characteristics which include fragile X syndrome, neurofibromatosis, tuberous sclerosis, Noonan's syndrome and Cornelia de Lange's syndromecould lead to intellectual disabilities(Sultana et al., 1995;Jones & Smith, 1997).Because of the high prevalence of developmental disabilities, the high genetic contribution to this type of pathology and insufficient referral for genetic consultation, the American and more recently the European guidelines on this group of diseases state that genetic testing is essential and should become a standardized diagnostic practice. (Miclea, Peca, Cuzmici, Pop, 2015).

Pre- and post-natal exposure to toxins can cause intellectual disabilities, especially lead, mercury or radiations.Diseases like whooping cough, measles, or meningitis can cause mental disability if medical care is delayed or inadequate (Ardinger& Holmes, 2000; Aicardi, 1998).

Birth related complications can cause intellectual disabilities.Several complications and diseases of pregnancy,delivery, and infancy have been found to be more prevalent among the intellectually disabled-than among normal children(Costeff, Cohen, Weller, &Kleckner, 1981). A recent study reported high rate of (74%) pre-natal, peri-natal and post-natal complications among intellectually disabled children (Gopalan, Sharma &Unnikrishnan,2014).Pregnant mothers who use alcohol or drugs during pregnancy or exposure to anticonvulsants,diseases in mother such us heart and kidney disease and diabetes and placental dysfunction, congenital infections such as cytomegalovirus, toxoplasmosis, herpes, syphilis, rubella and human immunodeficiency virus; prolonged maternal fever in the first trimester; untreated maternal phenylketonuria (PKU), low-birth-weight, complications of pregnancy or during deliverycan leads to intellectual deficits (Strømme&Hagberg, 2007; Piecuch et al., 1997; Kolevzon, Gross &Reichenberg, 2007).

Studies also shown that intellectual disability is related with Iodine deficiency, malnutrition, male gender, rural back ground, socioeconomic disadvantage,family history of intellectual disability and mental illness, and increased maternal age(Gopalan, Sharma &Unnikrishnan,2014; Wines, 2006; Emerson& Hatton, 2007;Heikura, Taanila, Hartikainen, Olsen, Linna, Von Wendt, &Järvelin, 2008).

The main risk factors for developmental disorders can be divided into direct factors like male gender, maternal age above 30 years, multiple pregnancies, high birth order, low birth weight, small head circumference, preterm birth, iron and iodine deficiencies, brain injury, and malnutrition, as well as indirect factors, like low parental schooling, maternal depression, low socioeconomic status, and inadequate stimulation (Bergen, 2008). The main causes of ID are genetic abnormalities, prenatal exposure to alcohol or infection, trauma during birth, early childhood infections, exposure to heavy metals, and severe malnutrition. In a study, Karam et al (2016) classified the etiology of ID in to five groups and found environmental factors as 44.4%, genetic factors as 20.5%, idiopathic factor as 12.6%, neonatal sequelae as 13.2%, and other diseases (9.3%). children presented impairment in two or more areas of adaptive behavior. There was no difference in prenatal care attendance or maternal schooling among the groups. For about 40% of children, ID was attributed to nonbiological factors, suggesting that the rate may be reduced with appropriate interventions early in life.

Comorbidities

Intellectual disability is often seen as a predisposing factor for psychiatric disorders and high rates of comorbidity with psychiatric disorders with emotional and behavioural disorders. The risk of psychopathology was found to be significantly increased by moderate intellectual disability, limitations in adaptive behavior, impaired language development, poor socialization, living with one biological parent, and low socio-economic status of the family, child's physical symptoms, family dysfunction, and previous parental mental health (Gopalan, Sharma &Unnikrishnan,2014; Kolaitis, 2008; Koskentausta, Iivanainen & Almqvist, 2007; Wallander, Dekker, &Koot, 2006).

Management

Management of ID requires a detailed case history and assessments. The clinical history must put an emphasis on healthcare during the prenatal, perinatal and postnatal period, genealogical tree for at least three generations and an intentional search for family antecedents of mental delay and psychiatric illnesses and congenital abnormalities. Physical exam should focus on secondary abnormalities and congenital malformations, somatometric measurements and neurological and behavioral phenotype evaluations. The clinical exam should include: head circumference evaluation (microcephaly or macrocephaly may provide useful clues to etiology) and height measurement (short stature could indicate fetal alcohol syndrome or tall stature may suggest fragile X syndrome or Sotos syndrome), neurological consultation (evaluation of muscle tone, coordination, tendon reflexes, abnormal movements, or other modifications), ophthalmologic and otolaryngology evaluation, skin changes (pigmentation abnormalities), facial and extremity dysmorphology or internal malformations assessment (Katz, Lazcano-Ponce, 2008 ;Moeschler&Shevell, 2006).

Intellectual disability is not curable but early identification and managing children with developmental delays may improve the outcomes. The mainstay of ID treatment is the development of a comprehensive management plan for the condition. By considering the comorbidities and multiple disabilities, special inputs would be required from multiple sources such as special educators, language therapists, behavioral therapists, occupational therapists, and community services that provide social support and respite care for families affected by ID. Though no scientifically approved medicines were found to improve the cognitive function of people with ID, they would be benefited from pharmacological treatment for comorbidities such as ADHD, epilepsy, aggressive behaviours.

The current movement of deinstitutionalization (a move from residential to community setting) started affecting the life of individuals with intellectual disability. In a recent review McCarron et al (2019) systematically reviewed thirteen studies to find how deinstitutionalisation affects quality of life (QoL) for adults with intellectual disabilities and found a consistent pattern that moving to the community was associated with improved quality of life compared with the institution.

CONCLUSION

The risk for a psychiatric disorder is greater in persons with ID than in those with intelligence in the normal range. Communication deficits present a challenge to diagnosis, and clinicians must be able to adapt to ensure they ascertain the relevant information that will allow them to make a diagnosis. They should also be alert to the dangers of diagnostic overshadowing. For patients with ID, once a diagnosis of a psychiatric disorder is made, pharmacological treatment does not differ significantly from that in the general population, but care may be required to avoid medication interactions and underdosing or overdosing, as well as the potential to worsen comorbid conditions and individuals with a psychiatric disorder and ID may require additional multidisciplinary support (Kendall & Owen, 2015).

Adults with intellectual disabilities have increased early mortality compared with the general population. However, their extent of multimorbidity (two or more additional conditions) compared with the general population is unknown, particularly with regards to physical ill-health, as are associations between comorbidities, neighbourhood deprivation, and age (Cooper, McLean, Guthrie, McConnachie, Mercer, Sullivan, Morrison & Pract, 2015) and studies are required on this area.

Over these years there are many changes happened to the terminology to define intellectual disability, understanding about different dimensions on classification, co morbidities, etiology and management and prevention, yet, many questions are unanswered related to this condition. Though high prevalent rates are found to be in low income countries, studies are limited from these countries. Awareness about intellectual disability and to deal with stigma related to this conditions are also require great focus and future studies need to address all these issues.

REFERENCES

Aicardi, J. (1998). The etiology of developmental delay. *Seminars in Pediatric Neurology*, *5*(1), 15–20. doi:10.1016/S1071-9091(98)80013-2 PMID:9548636

Armatas, V. (2009). Mental retardation: Definitions, etiology, epidemiology and diagnosis. *Journal of Sport and Health Research*, *1*(2), 112–122.

Bergen, D. C. (2008). Effects of poverty on cognitive function: A hidden neurologic epidemic. *Neurology*, *71*(6), 447–451. doi:10.1212/01.wnl.0000324420.03960.36 PMID:18678828

Carulla, L. S., Reed, G. M., Vaezazizi, L. M., Cooper, S. N., Leal, R. M., Bertelli, M., ... Saxena, S. (2011). Intellectual developmental disorders: Towards a new name, definition and framework for "mental retardation/intellectual disability. *World Psychiatry; Official Journal of the World Psychiatric Association (WPA)*, *10*(3), 175–180. doi:10.1002/j.2051-5545.2011.tb00045.x PMID:21991267

Cooper, S. A., McLean, G., Guthrie, B., McConnachie, A., Mercer, S., Sullivan, F., & Morrison, J. (2015). Multiple physical and mental health comorbidity in adults with intellectual disabilities: Population-based cross-sectional analysis. *BMC Family Practice*, *16*(1), 110. doi:10.118612875-015-0329-3 PMID:26310664

Costeff, H., Cohen, B. E., Weller, L., & Kleckner, H. (1981). Pathogenic factors in idiopathic mental retardation. *Developmental Medicine and Child Neurology*, *23*(5), 484–493. doi:10.1111/j.1469-8749.1981.tb02022.x PMID:7196853

Einfeld, S. L., & Tonge, B. J. (1996). Population prevalence of psychopathology in children and adolescents with intellectual disability: II epidemiological findings. *Journal of Intellectual Disability Research*, *40*(2), 99–109. doi:10.1111/j.1365-2788.1996.tb00611.x PMID:8731467

Emerson, E. (2003). Prevalence of psychiatric disorders in children and adolescents with and without intellectual disability. *Journal of Intellectual Disability Research*, *47*(1), 51–58. doi:10.1046/j.1365-2788.2003.00464.x PMID:12558695

Emerson, E., & Hatton, C. (2008). Poverty, socio-economic position, social capital and the health children with intellectual disability. *Journal of Intellectual Disability Research.*

Fuller, T.E. (1997). Deinstitutionalization: A Psychiatric "Titanic". In *Out of the Shadows: Confronting America's Mental Illness Crisis.* John Wiley & Sons.

Girimaji, S. C., & Pradeep, A. J. (2018). Intellectual disability in international classification of Diseases-11: A developmental perspective. Indian. *Journal of Social Psychiatry*, *34*(Suppl S1), 68–74.

Goddard, H. H. (1912). *The Kallikak family: A study in the heredity of feeble-mindedness*. New York: Macmillan. doi:10.1037/10949-000

Gopalan, R. T., Sharma, R., & Unnikrishnan, M. P. (2014). Socio-Demographic and Clinical Features of Children with Intellectual Disability and Their Parents-an Indian Study. *International Neuropsychiatric Disease Journal*, *2*(6), 289–302. doi:10.9734/INDJ/2014/10610

Harris, J. C. (2006). *Intellectual Disability: Understanding Its Development, Causes, Classification, Evaluation, and Treatment.* New York: Oxford University Press.

Harris, J. C. (2013). New Terminology for Mental Retardation in DSM-5 and ICD-11. *Current Opinion in Psychiatry*, *26*(3), 260–262. doi:10.1097/YCO.0b013e32835fd6fb PMID:23507999

Heikura, U., Taanila, A., Hartikainen, A. L., Olsen, P., Linna, S. L., Von, W. L., & Järvelin, M. R. (2006). Intellectual disability: A prospective longitudinal population-based study. *Intellectual Disability Research*, *50*(4), 259–268. doi:10.1111/j.1365-2788.2005.00792.x PMID:16507030

Jeevanandam, L. (2009). Perspectives of intellectual disability in Asia: Epidemiology, policy, and services for children and adults. *Current Opinion in Psychiatry*, *22*(5), 462–468. doi:10.1097/YCO.0b013e32832ec056 PMID:19625968

Jones, K. L., & Smith, D. W. (1997). *Smith's recognizable patterns of human malformation* (5th ed.). Philadelphia: Saunders.

Kabra, M., & Gulati, S. (2003). Mental retardation. *Indian Journal of Pediatrics, 70*(2), 153–158. doi:10.1007/BF02723745 PMID:12661811

Karam, S. M., Barros, A. J. D., Matijasevich, A., dos Santos, I. S., Anselmi, L., Barros, F., ... Black, M. M. (2016). Intellectual Disability in a Birth Cohort: Prevalence, Etiology, and Determinants at the Age of 4 Years. *Public Health Genomics, 19*(5), 290–297. doi:10.1159/000448912 PMID:27595410

Katz, G., & Lazcano-Ponce, E. (2008). Intellectual disability: Definition, etiological factors, classification, diagnosis, treatment and prognosis. *Salud Pública de México, 50*(2), 132–141. PMID:18470340

Kolevzon, A., Gross, R., & Reichenberg, A. (2007). Prenatal and Perinatal Risk Factors for Autism: A Review and Integration of Findings. *Archives of Pediatrics & Adolescent Medicine, 161*(4), 326–333. doi:10.1001/archpedi.161.4.326 PMID:17404128

Kumar, A. (2013). Normalization: Guiding Principle of Equal Opportunities in Education for Children with Disabilities in India. *American Journal of Epidemiology, 167*, 169–177.

Maulik, P. K., Mascarenhas, M. N., Mathers, C. D., Dua, T., & Saxena, S. (2011). Prevalence of intellectual disability: A meta-analysis of population-based studies. *Research in Developmental Disabilities, 32*(2), 419–436. doi:10.1016/j.ridd.2010.12.018 PMID:21236634

McCarron, M., Lombard-Vance, R., Murphy, E., May, P., Webb, N., Sheaf, G., … O'Donovan, M.A. (2019). Effect of deinstitutionalisation on quality of life for adults with intellectual disabilities: a systematic review. *BMJ Open, 9*(4). doi: . doi:10.1136/bmjopen-2018-025735

McKenzie, K., Milton, M., Smith, G., & Ouellette-Kuntz, H. (2016). Systematic Review of the Prevalence and Incidence of Intellectual Disabilities: Current Trends and Issues. *Current Developmental Disorders Reports, 3*(2), 104–115. doi:10.100740474-016-0085-7

Miclea, D. L., Cuzmici, Z., & Pop, I. V. (2015). Genetic testing in patients with global developmental delay / intellectual disabilities. *A review Med., 88*(3), 288–292. PMID:26609258

Moeschler, J. B., & Shevell, M. (2006). Clinical genetic evaluation of the child with mental retardation or developmental delays. *Pediatrics, 117*(6), 2304–2316. doi:10.1542/peds.2006-1006 PMID:16740881

Norrgard, K. (2008). Human testing, the eugenics movement, and IRBs. *Nature Education, 1*(1), 170.

Osborn, F. (1937). Development of a Eugenic Philosophy. *American Sociological Review, 2*(3), 389–397. doi:10.2307/2084871

Piecuch, R. E., Leonard, C. H., Cooper, B. A., & Sehring, S. A. (1997). Outcome of extremely low birth weight infants (500 to 999 grams) over a 12-year period. *Pediatrics, 100*(4), 633–639. doi:10.1542/peds.100.4.633 PMID:9310517

Polloway, E. A., & Lubin, J. (2009). Feeblemindedness. Encyclopedia of American Disability History of children and adolescents with intellectual disabilities in Britain: A replication. *Journal of Intellectual Disability Research, 51*, 866–874.

Prasher, V. P., & Routhu, S. K. (2003). Epidemiology of learning(intellectual) disability and comorbid conditions. *Psychiatry*, *2*, 8.

Reynolds, T., Zupanick, C. E., & Dombeck, M. (2013). *Historical and Contemporary Perspectives on Intellectual Disabilities*. Intellectual Disabilities.

Salvador-Carulla, L., Reed, G. M., & Vaez-Azizi, L. M. (2011). Intellectual developmental disorders: Towards a new name, definition and framework for 'mental retardation/intellectual disability' in ICD-11. *World Psychiatry; Official Journal of the World Psychiatric Association (WPA)*, *10*(3), 175–180. doi:10.1002/j.2051-5545.2011.tb00045.x PMID:21991267

Sandberg, N. M., & Ahlström, G. (2015). Prevalence of older people with intellectual disability in Sweden: A spatial epidemiological analysis. *Journal of Intellectual Disability Research*, *59*(12), 1155–1167. doi:10.1111/jir.12219 PMID:26306552

Schalock, R. L., Borthwick-Duffy, S. A., Bradley, V. J., Buntinx, W. H., Coulter, D. L., & Craig, E. M. (2010). *Intellectual Disability: Definition, Classification, and Systems of Supports*. Washington, DC: ERIC.

Schalock, R. L., & Ruth, A. (2007). The Renaming of Mental Retardation: Understanding the Change to the Term Intellectual Disability. *Intellectual and Developmental Disabilities*, *45*(2), 116–124. doi:10.1352/1934-9556(2007)45[116:TROMRU]2.0.CO;2 PMID:17428134

Soltani, S., Khosravi, B., & Salehiniya, H. (2015). Prevalence of intellectual disability in Iran: Toward a new conceptual framework in data collection. *Journal of Research in Medical Sciences*, *20*(7), 714–715. doi:10.4103/1735-1995.166234 PMID:26622264

Srinath, S., & Girimaji, S. C. (1999). Epidemiology of child and adolescent mental health problems and mental retardation. *Nimhans Journal*, *17*, 355–366.

Strømme, P., & Hagberg, G. (2007). Aetiology in severe and mild mental retardation: A population-based study of Norwegian children. *Developmental Medicine and Child Neurology*, *42*(2), 76–86. doi:10.1111/j.1469-8749.2000.tb00050.x PMID:10698323

Sultana, S. A. G., Lam-Po-Tang, T. R. L., Wright, F., Linderman, R., & Purvis-Smith, S. (1995). Fragile X mental retardation in an Indonesian family. *Medical Journal of Indonesia*, *4*, 17–17. doi:10.13181/mji.v4i1.885

Tammy Reynolds, T., Zupanick, C. E., & Dombeck, M. (2013). *History Of Stigmatizing Names For Intellectual Disabilities Continued*. Retrieved from https://www.mentalhelp.net/articles/history-of-stigmatizing-names-for-intellectual-disabilities-continued/

Wallander, J.L., Dekker, M.C., & Koot, H.M. (1992). *Variations in prenatal sociodemographic factors associated with intellectual disability*. Academic Press.

Chapter 2
Mental Health Challenges in Children With Intellectual Disabilities

Nisha Elizabeth Mathew
University of New South Wales, Australia

Amelia Walter
University of New South Wales, Australia

Valsamma Eapen
https://orcid.org/0000-0001-6296-8306
University of New South Wales, Australia

ABSTRACT

There is limited evidence base regarding mental health issues in people with intellectual disability (ID), and hence, findings from the general population are often applied to ID groups. Available evidence suggests that individuals with ID experience higher rates of mental health disorders than the general population, although findings are mixed with regard to the determinants of this increased prevalence. Further, the consequences of this comorbidity for individuals, families, and the wider community are often overlooked including the multiple challenges in identifying and managing these concerns. Accurate diagnosis and effective intervention are currently hindered by factors including the applicability of standardized psychiatric classification systems, gaps in service delivery models and access to such services, as well as unmet training needs. It is critical that further research is carried out to examine the specific challenges facing individuals with ID along with facilitating appropriate mental health services to individuals with ID.

DOI: 10.4018/978-1-7998-1223-4.ch002

INTRODUCTION

Despite increased recognition of the prevalence and impact of psychiatric disorders among individuals with Intellectual Disability (ID), the early assessment and treatment of these concurrent comorbidities remains a significant societal challenge and affect the functional skills and intensity of daily support needed for those living with ID. Limitations in current assessment and diagnostic systems prevent the equitable access to services for people with ID in line with Article 25 of the United Nation's Convention on the Rights of Persons with Disabilities which outlines 'the right to the enjoyment of the highest attainable standard of health without discrimination on the basis of disability' (United Nations 2006; Stuart, 2012). Consequently it is critical to further develop and refine standardised diagnostic systems to achieve these aims. Furthermore, in order for intervention to be effective, it must address the multiple risk and resilience factors underlying ID and comorbid mental health problems. Therefore, from a public health perspective, rates of comorbid psychiatric disorders should be taken into account when planning for the equitable provision of services. Similarly, intervention research should consider the role of comorbidity in predicting outcomes and the nature of the barriers that prevent access to services, while basic science research would benefit from increasing understanding of these comorbidities by delineating possible heterogeneous aetiological and neurobiological determinants. This chapter will review and synthesise the literature on the prevalence, impact and determinants of the comorbidity of ID and psychiatric disorders, and discuss important considerations to improve accurate identification and effective management of these concerns.

Background

Intellectual Disability (ID) is characterised by deficits in both intellectual and adaptive functioning beginning during childhood or adolescence (APA, 2013). Adaptive behaviour includes conceptual skills (e.g., language, money and time concepts), social skills (e.g., interpersonal skills and social problem solving), and practical skills (e.g., activities of daily living and occupation) (Maulik, Mascarenhas, Mathers, Dua, & Saxena, 2011).

A comprehensive meta-analysis found that the overall global prevalence of ID was approximately 1%, with higher prevalence rates found in low- and middle-income countries, and among child and adolescent populations (Maulik et al., 2011). Social gradients and ethnic disparities have been reported in previous research on the prevalence of ID. Lower socio-economic status (SES) has been found to be associated with a marked increase in the prevalence of ID, particularly mild ID (Emerson, 2012; Leonard et al., 2005; Leonard & Wen, 2002; Roeleveld & Zielhuis, 1997; Stromme & Magnus, 2000), and higher rates of ID have been found among African-American and Indigenous Australian children (Croen, Grether, & Selvin, 2001; Leonard, Petterson, Bower, & Sanders, 2003; Leonard et al., 2005; Yeargin-Allsopp, Drews, Decouflé, & Murphy, 1995).In a recent epidemiological study it was estimated 5.9% of the Indigenous population lives with ID compared to 2.5% of the non-Indigenous Australian population(Statistics, 2015).

It has been proposed that socioeconomic disadvantage can contribute to both causation and severity of ID. (Durkin & Yeargin-Allsopp, 2018)For instance the etiology of some causes of intellectual disability, such as Down syndrome have been associated with environmental factors and stress that are linked to low SES. Additionally low SES families may not have the resources to provide the early socio-cognitive stimulation that is associated with improved outcomes in ID. Of particular concern is the evidence that an "inverse care law" applies, in that the greater number of risk factors a child may have for ID, the less access they have to preventative and comprehensive health care (Woolfenden et al., 2013). This creates a vicious cycle whereby the risk factors that may predispose a child to ID are also the same risk factors that may mean they are likely to miss out on timely and effective identification and intervention.

CHALLENGES IN THE ASSESSMENT AND MANAGEMENT OF PSYCHIATRIC DISORDERS AMONG INDIVIDUALS WITH INTELLECTUAL DISABILITY

Prevalence of Psychiatric Disorders among Individuals with Intellectual Disability

In a comprehensive systematic review, Einfeld, Ellis, and Emerson (2011) found that between 30 and 50% of children and adolescents with ID had a comorbid mental disorder, and that the relative risk of mental disorder associated with ID, when compared to children and adolescents without ID, ranged from 2.8 to 4.5. Consistent with these findings, a secondary analysis of the 1999 and 2004 Office for National Statistics surveys of the mental health of British children and adolescents estimated that the 3% of British children with ID accounted for 14% of total child and adolescent psychiatric morbidity (Emerson & Hatton, 2007b). Comparing 641 children with ID and 17 774 children without ID, this research found that the prevalence of psychiatric disorders was observed to be 36% among children with ID and 8% among children without (Odds Ratio/OR=6.5). Increased prevalence among children with ID was particularly marked for autism spectrum disorder (OR=33.4), hyperkinesis (OR=8.4) and conduct disorders (OR=5.7). Furthermore, a cumulative effect was observed, with research suggesting that the greater the number of social or environmental risk factors a child with ID is exposed to (e.g., low SES, stressful life events, poor parental mental health), the higher their risk of having mental health problems such as emotional or conduct disorders (Emerson & Hatton, 2007b).

Other studies have also noted an increased relative risk for psychiatric disorders among children and adolescents with ID, and this has been found across a range of diagnoses including anxiety and mood disorders, behaviour disorders and attention deficit hyperactivity disorder (Dekker & Koot, 2003a,b; Emerson, 2003; Emerson & Hatton, 2007b). A secondary analysis of the 1999 Office for National Statistics survey of the mental health of children and adolescents in Great Britain found that the prevalence of any diagnosed ICD-10 disorder, as well as specific disorders such as conduct disorder, anxiety disorder, hyperkinesis and pervasive developmental disorders, was significantly greater among children with ID than among their non-ID peers(Emerson, 2003). A more recent examination of the mental health of adolescents with ID found that they were significantly more likely to report symptoms of anxiety than their peers without ID (King et al., 2019).

Longitudinal studies suggest that comorbid psychiatric disorders among children with ID persist through to adolescence and adulthood (Chadwick, Kusel, Cuddy, & Taylor, 2005; Einfeld et al., 2006; Richardson & Koller, 1996; Tonge & Einfeld, 2000). For example, in a 14-year longitudinal study of children with ID in Australia, high initial levels of behavioural and emotional disturbance decreased only slowly over time, with 31% of participants continuing to meet criteria for a psychiatric disorder in young adulthood (Einfeld et al., 2006). Greater decreases in psychopathology were found among males rather than females, and in participants with mild ID compared to those with severe or profound ID.

Overall findings with regard to rates of mental disorder among adults with ID have been somewhat inconsistent, partially due to differing methods for assessing psychiatric comorbidity. In their meta-analysis, Maulik et al. (2011) found that studies based on diagnosing psychiatric comorbidity using psychological assessments or scales showed higher prevalence compared to those using standard diagnostic systems and disability instruments. When ICD-10 or DSM criteria have been applied, reported rates of psychiatric disorder among adults with ID have been comparable to those found in the general population (Cooper, Smiley, Morrison, Williamson, & Allan, 2007; Deb, Thomas, & Bright, 2001); however, the utility of these criteria among individuals with ID has been questioned (Einfeld & Tonge, 1999; Sturmey, 1995). When psychiatric diagnoses were made by consultant psychiatrists on the basis of clinical interviews, Cooper et al. (2007) found that 41% of adults with ID met diagnostic criteria for at least one mental disorder. This is a significantly higher point prevalence rate than that observed in the general population, where rates have been estimated to be approximately 13.2% (Andrews, Henderson, & Hall, 2001). Indeed, reviews generally indicate a three to four-fold increased prevalence of psychiatric problems among individuals with ID compared to the general population (Harris, 2006; Munir, 2016). As for children and adolescents, a number of psychiatric disorders have been found to be more common among adults with ID than among the general population, including anxiety and affective disorders, psychotic disorders, and behavioural problems(S.-a. Cooper, 1997; Pallab K Maulik & Catherine K Harbour, 2010). Additionally recent cross sectional study of Scottish primary care practices found that people with ID were twice as likely to have one or more concurrent mental health conditions relative to people without ID (Cooper, 1997).

Impact of Psychiatric Disorders among Individuals with Intellectual Disability

Psychopathology associated with ID carries significant consequences for individuals with ID, their families and the wider community. For individuals themselves, for example, the dual disability of ID and psychiatric disorder is a major cause of failure of transition to school programs and community residential placements (Bruininks, Hill, & Morreau, 1988; Einfeld et al., 2006), leads to restricted participation in recreational and educational programs (Parmenter, Einfeld, Tonge, & Dempster, 1998), and is associated with reduced workplace opportunities following school (Anderson, Lakin, Hill, & Chen, 1992). Robust evidence indicates that a lack of early detection and intervention, including interventions directed at improving parental wellbeing, has significant implications for the future academic, behavioural and social functioning of children with ID (Bouras, 2011; Crnic, Neece, McIntyre, Blacher, & Baker, 2017).

Mental health challenges can also be exacerbated by the inaccessibility of services and resources to allow people with disabilities to achieve goals such as independence, to whatever extent possible, from the familial unit. For instance the lack of adequate support during the transition from school to adulthood including a lack of post-school opportunities, such as supported work placements and the inaccessibility of many workplaces for individuals with disabilities has also been identified as contributing to heightened(Young-Southward, Cooper, & Philo, 2017) anxiety and mental health difficulties among youth with ID and their parents. A lack of meaningful daytime activities in addition to negatively affecting mental health is also often associated with a loss of functional skills that had been previously gained and limited formation of socially supportive net words (Gauthier-Boudreault, Gallagher, & Couture, 2017).

Interactions between social environment, family, ID and mental health problems are complex and not unidirectional. It is known that families experiencing additional life stress prior to having children are more likely to have children with ID (Eapen, Al-Gazali, Bin-Othman, & Pramathan, 1998). This is particularly the case with respect to Indigenous families, those from culturally and linguistically diverse backgrounds, and those with a parent who has ID or a mental illness (Leonard et al., 2011; Leonard et al., 2005; To et al., 2004). Hence, a vicious cycle of the development of ID and mental health problems can be seen at an individual level or in population groups experiencing adversity (Whitehouse, Durkin, Jaquet, & Ziatas, 2009; Whitehouse, Watt, Line, & Bishop, 2009). This confluence of factors generates a significant health burden for individuals, families, and communities, as well as inequity in child health resulting in significant health and economic impacts.

The long-term support of individuals with ID places a considerable burden on families and carers (Bourke et al., 2008; Crnic et al., 2017; DeRigne & Porterfield, 2017; Miodrag & Hodapp, 2010), and mothers in particular are at increased risk of mental health problems (Abbeduto et al., 2004; Gilson et al., 2018). Several studies have found that parents of children and adolescents with ID have higher levels of child-related stress and depression than parents of typically developing children (Browne & Bramston, 1998; Dyson, 1997; Olsson & Hwang, 2001; White & Hastings, 2004), and key short- and long-term outcomes for families of individuals with ID may be mediated, at least in part, by mental health difficulties (Eapen, 2014). For example, the mental wellbeing of parents of children and young adults with ID has been shown to be more strongly influenced by the severity of their child's comorbid mental health disorders including emotional and behavioural problems than by the severity of their ID (McIntyre, Blacher, & Baker, 2002; Tonge & Einfeld, 2003). Mental health problems among children and young adults with ID have also been shown to significantly predict parents' feelings of dissatisfaction with the family situation (Maes, Broekman, Došen, & Nauts, 2003), mothers' perceived negative impact of their child on the family, and the family's decision to seek out-of-home placement (Maes et al., 2003; McIntyre et al., 2002). It is interesting to note that stress did not account for significant additional variance in this decision-making (McIntyre et al., 2002), suggesting that mental health problems can significantly impact on the family's ability to care for a young person with ID without requiring out-of-home care arrangements. This adds to the social and financial burden of ID on families and societies, in conjunction with the economic impact of caregiving with mothers of children with ID earning significantly less over the course of their lifetimes than their peers with typically developing children(Parish, Seltzer, Greenberg, & Floyd, 2004). Overall, the inequities relating to the mental health of people with ID and their families relative to the general population has significant implications for service provision and policy development.

A recent meta-analysis based on studies published between 2010 and 2015 (n = 17) found the range of prevalence estimate to be 0.05 to 1.55%.(McKenzie, Milton, Smith, & Ouellette-Kuntz, 2016 ; McKenzie et al 2016). ID is also associated with reduced life expectancy and poorer quality of life (Begg et al., 2007), and high economic costs for governments and families (Doran et al., 2012). It ranks within the top 20 sources of burden of disease (Begg et al., 2007) and is among the 20 most costly disorders (Polder, Meerding, Bonneux, & Van Der Maas, 2002). This burden is compounded when ID is associated with a comorbid mental health disorder, leading to greater economic burden for provision of health care and education, in addition to further reductions in capacity for employment and earning.

Determinants of Mental Health Problems in Intellectual Disability

Given the high prevalence of mental health disorders among individuals with ID, and the impact of this dual diagnosis on individuals, families and the community, there has also been interest in examining specific variables that may influence this comorbidity.

Available evidence from the literature suggests that most variance in developmental vulnerability is associated with the social determinants of health and their interaction with an individual's innate biological susceptibility to adversity (Guralnick, 1997; Zeanah, Boris, & Larrieu, 1997). Cumulative exposure to risk factors over time in the absence of protective factor scan result in changes in neuronal circuitry with long-term consequences (Eapen, 2014).For example, there is evidence of altered brain architecture found in children exposed to abusive environments or who have a history of sensory deprivation, as well as an association between the impact of less extreme adverse environments on brain architecture linked with language and reading skills (Hackman, Farah, & Meaney, 2010; Marmot et al., 2010). Such risk and protective factors have their maximum effect during critical or sensitive periods, especially in the first five years of life (Maggi, Irwin, Siddiqi, & Hertzman, 2010; Siddiqi, Irwin, & Hertzman, 2007). While brain plasticity offers an opportunity for maximum gains with appropriate intervention during the early years, this becomes increasingly difficult the further we move away from childhood.

There is also emerging evidence of a transactional relationship between genes and the environment (A. E. Sameroff, 2009), suggesting that individuals with certain genetic profiles may be more sensitive to favourable and unfavourable environmental influences than those without such genetic makeups (Mitchell et al., 2013). In other instances the behavioural or mental health problem may be part of the behavioural phenotype of the underlying genetic condition as is the case with Lesch-Nyhan syndrome and self-injurious behaviours, Fragile X syndrome and disruptive behaviours, Williams syndrome and exceptional conversational verbal abilities and excessive empathy, Prader-Willi syndrome and temper tantrums and obsessive-compulsive features, and Angelman syndrome and happy affect and hyperactivity (Cassidy & Morris, 2001). Further, when the condition is associated with dysmorphic features or changes in physical appearance, such as short stature or excessive growth, or delayed sexual development or functioning, affected individuals can suffer from low self-esteem and this can, in turn, lead to secondary emotional or behavioural difficulties.

In a recent case-control study using data from the Intellectual Disability and Mental Health Assessing the Genomic Impact on Neurodevelopment (IMAGINE-ID) study, genotype to phenotype associations in children with copy number variants associated with a high risk of neurodevelopmental and psychiatric disorders (referred to as ND-CNVs) was examined. Among individuals with 13 ND-CNVs, a similar range of phenotypic expressions in neurodevelopmental adverse outcomes was observed although there were subtle quantitative and qualitative differences. The findings suggest that the genomic risk for neurodevelopmental and psychiatric disorders has pleiotropic effects involving varying processes and diverse neural circuitry involvement rather than specific or individual phenotypes (Chawner et al., 2019). Due to the transactional and inter-dependent relationship between these factors, developmental vulnerability should be understood, assessed and treated with consideration given to the cumulative impact of multiple factors, both risk and protective, including those related to the individual child, family, psychosocial status, neighbourhood, and service systems and policy (Eapen, 2014).The occurrence and nature of mental health comorbidity in children with ID is therefore influenced by the interaction between biological and environmental risk and protective factors, with the overall risk increasing as the number of risk factors increases (Eapen, 2014).

Exposure to a range of social and environmental risk factors such as poverty, living in a single-parent household, exposure to negative life events, low parental education, and poor maternal mental and physical health, has been found to be associated with increased prevalence of emotional and conduct disorders among children both with and without ID (Emerson & Hatton, 2007b). Importantly, however, exposure to these risk factors was found to be significantly higher among children with ID, with 46% of them having been exposed to three or more potential risk factors compared to 24% of children without ID. While there is limited evidence regarding the specific factors predicting the presence of mental health problems in individuals with ID (Costello & Bouras, 2006), these findings are consistent with the prevailing view that individuals with ID are more vulnerable to psychosocial stress than people without ID, and are therefore more likely to develop psychiatric symptomatology (Deb et al., 2001).

Similar findings were reported by Emerson (2003), who conducted a secondary analysis of data from 10 438 children aged between five and 15 years from the 1999 ONS survey of the Mental Health of Children and Adolescents in Great Britain (Meltzer, Gatward, Goodman, & Ford, 2000). Specific family characteristics were found to be associated with increased rates of particular psychiatric diagnoses, and children living in families belonging to lower social classes, and those from single-parent and lower-income households, were found to be at increased risk for a range of psychiatric disorders, including emotional disorders, anxiety disorders, depression and conduct disorders. A further study specifically examining the contribution of socioeconomic position to the health and mental health status of children and adolescents with ID, using the same sample, found that between-group differences in socioeconomic position and household composition accounted for 24% of the increased risk for poor health, 23% of the increased risk for conduct disorder and 37% of the increased risk for emotional disorder among children and adolescents with ID (Emerson & Hatton, 2007a). The authors concluded that socioeconomic disadvantage may account for a significant proportion of the increased risk for poorer physical and mental health among children and adolescents with ID. Another study, however, failed to find significant differences in the prevalence of psychiatric disorders between children classified as low SES and those classified as medium to high SES (Dekker & Koot, 2003a,b).

Factors related to parents, including parental mental health and parenting practices, have also been found to be an important determinant of mental health problems in children and adolescents with ID (Dekker & Koot, 2003a,b; Emerson, 2003). (Hazarika, Das, & Choudhury, 2017) in a study of parental attitude towards children and adolescents with ID found that while parents exhibited love and acceptance towards their children, there was also evidence of frustration, disappointment, and overprotection. This in turn had a negative impact on the children's adaptive functioning and independent skill development. Further, children whose primary carers reported more frequent use of punitive strategies and who had higher scores on the General Health Questionnaire (a measure assessing risk of developing psychiatric disorders) were more likely to have a range of psychiatric disorders, including an emotional disorder, an anxiety disorder, a conduct disorder and hyperkinesis (Emerson, 2003).

In a systematic review, Einfeld et al. (2011) discuss individual factors that have been associated with mental disorder in children and adolescents with ID. Factors that have been most commonly examined include age, gender and severity of ID, but findings have been largely inconsistent. With regard to age, some studies have found higher rates of psychiatric disorder in younger children when compared to teenagers(Molteno, Molteno, Finchilescu, & Dawes, 2001), but others studies have shown no significant relationships between age and overall rates of mental disorder (Einfeld & Tonge, 1996a, 1996b). Other studies have examined age effects for particular psychiatric disorders. Older children with ID (aged 11 – 16 years) have been found to be more likely to have an emotional disorder, including a depressive disorder, while younger children (aged 5 – 10 years) were more likely to have hyperactivity or a pervasive developmental disorder (Emerson, 2003; Emerson & Hatton, 2007b). Among adults with ID, increasing age has been found to be associated with a higher likelihood of psychiatric illness (S. A. Cooper, 1997; Deb et al., 2001).

Mixed findings have also been noted with regard to the association between gender and risk of mental disorders among children and adolescents with ID. Some studies have found no effect of gender on overall rates of mental disorder (Einfeld & Tonge, 1996a, 1996b; Molteno et al., 2001), but other studies have reported significantly higher overall rates of mental health problems among male children and adolescents with ID (Emerson, 2003; Stromme & Diseth, 2000). Further, some studies of children and adolescents with ID have found that males are significantly more likely to have conduct disorder and hyperactivity than females with ID (Emerson, 2003; Emerson & Hatton, 2007b), while others have shown no gender effects for anxiety, mood or disruptive disorders (Dekker & Koot, 2003a,b). In a study of adults with ID, female gender was associated with increased prevalence of psychiatric disorder (Cooper et al., 2007). In a study of older adults with ID, women with ID were more likely to have been diagnosed with affective disorders or dementia than men with ID and less likely to have been diagnosed with substance use related disorders (Axmon, Sandberg, & Ahlström, 2017). This study also found no gender differences were found for anxiety disorders or psychotic disorders. The research to date has not however been able to elucidate whether these gender differences are due to differences in prevalence, identification or treatment of mental health disorders among adults with ID.

The literature is also unclear about how the severity of ID affects an individual's vulnerability to developing different psychiatric disorders (Costello & Bouras, 2006). Among children and adolescents, several studies have reported no statistically significant association between severity of ID and risk of psychiatric disorder (Einfeld & Tonge, 1996a, 1996b; Stromme & Diseth, 2000), but one study found higher rates of mental disorder in participants with more severe ID (Molteno et al., 2001). Findings are also mixed in adults. Some studies have shown higher rates of psychiatric illness among people with severe ID (Cooper et al., 2007; Gostason, 1985; Lund, 1985), others among individuals with mild ID (Borthwick-Duffy & Eyman, 1990; Iverson & Fox, 1989), and others have found no evidence either way (Corbett, 1979). Intellectual functioning has also been examined, with findings suggesting that depressive feelings, anxiety and antisocial behaviours are more common among those with higher IQs, while psychotic, self-absorbed and autistic behaviours are more likely to be found in children with lower IQs (Dekker & Koot, 2003a,b). The impact of physical disability on psychiatric illness is also unclear. Some studies have found that physical disability is associated with an increased prevalence of mental disorder (Deb et al., 2001), while others report that the absence of severe physical disability and immobility is associated with greater prevalence of psychiatric illness (Cooper et al., 2007).

Challenges in Identification of Psychiatric Disorders among Individuals with Intellectual Disability

There are a number of obstacles to the valid and reliable identification of mental health problems in people with ID (Hatton, 2002). Firstly, standardised psychiatric classification systems are often adopted in studies of mental health problems in people with ID (Costello & Bouras, 2006); however, the applicability of these to this population is questionable. Two factors have been posited to influence the applicability of standardised psychiatric assessment criteria to individuals with ID: linguistic abilities and the presentation of mental health problems (Costello & Bouras, 2006).

Current diagnostic systems such as ICD-10 and DSM-5 rely upon verbal accounts of an individual's symptoms. The utility of these systems is therefore limited by the linguistic skills of the individual being assessed. As Costello and Bouras (2006) note, some features of psychiatric illness are complex, requiring a high level of verbal fluency to describe and differentiate between symptoms. Therefore, the use of these existing diagnostic symptoms may not be appropriate among people with ID, particularly those with severe ID who frequently have limited or no language skills. When examining mental health among individuals with ID, it is therefore necessary to assess the individual's non-verbal behaviour, in addition to gathering historical information and observations from other people such as family members or carers. Importantly, the validity of this information is also dependent on the particular psychiatric condition in question, with informants likely to be more aware of disorders with clear behavioural manifestations rather than subjectively experienced phenomena such as thought disorder or anxiety (Costello & Bouras, 2006).

In addition to concerns with regard to linguistic abilities, the use of standardised classification systems among individuals with ID assumes that mental health problems present in the same way in this population as they do in the general population; however, this may not be the case and may also depend on the severity of ID. For example, in a review of mood disorders among patients with ID, Hurley (2006) reported that individuals with mild ID had a fairly typical presentation and could be assessed using standard practices with minor accommodations. An atypical presentation of mood disorders, however, including increased behavioural problems such as aggression, was more frequent in individuals with moderate to profound ID. Due to limitations in the use of standardised diagnostic symptoms, various instruments (including both self- and informant-report measures) have been either designed specifically or adapted for use with individuals with ID (for a review, see Hatton, 2002).

Differential diagnosis between symptoms that may be an expression of underlying brain damage and those that are related to a psychiatric disorder may also be particularly important when working with individuals with ID (Costello & Bouras, 2006). Disturbances of emotion, attention, activity and thought, and associated behavioural problems, may occur as part of the ID and it is often difficult to ascertain whether these additional difficulties are due to a comorbid psychiatric disorder. For example, it is important to distinguish between ID and the negative symptoms of schizophrenia such as slowness of thought and poverty of speech (Clarke, Littlejohns, Corbett, & Joseph, 1989).

It is likely that many individuals with ID have mental health problems that remain undetected and therefore untreated (Taylor, Hatton, Dixon, & Douglas, 2004). Einfeld et al. (2006), for example, found that only 10% of young adults with ID and definite psychiatric disorder had received specialist mental health intervention. Insufficient numbers of professionals with appropriate training and necessary expertise may impede accurate diagnosis and the adequate provision of mental health services to people with ID (P.K. Maulik & C.K. Harbour, 2010; McCarthy & Boyd, 2002). Diagnostic overshadowing, where a clinician regards the ID as a sufficient explanation for an individual's presenting symptoms rather than attributing them to a psychiatric disorder and making a dual diagnosis, may be partly responsible for the under-recognition of dual disability in clinical settings (Mason & Scior, 2004; Tonge & Einfeld, 2000). Recent linkage of disability services and ambulatory mental health services data in the Australian state of New South Wales further found that people with an ID were more than twice as likely to receive an "unknown" diagnosis as those without ID (Howlett, Florio, Xu, & Trollor, 2015).Recognition of comorbid psychopathology requires detailed interviews using sensitive assessment techniques by specialist staff (P.K. Maulik & C.K. Harbour, 2010). It has been theorized that the rates of mental health disorders in people with ID may be both higher and untreated for longer periods of time than among the general population however no research to date has formally examined this notion(Munir, 2016) .

Furthermore, in the general population, identification of a mental health problem is often prompted by the failure of an individual to maintain social roles such as employment and parenting. In contrast, individuals with ID generally have fewer societal role expectations and the severity of their symptoms therefore does not necessarily relate to the degree of impairment in daily life(Costello & Bouras, 2006).

This reduces the chances that mental health problems will be recognised by carers, and means that conditions such as anxiety and depression may cause significant distress to an individual yet remain undiagnosed(Whittle, Fisher, Reppermund, Lenroot, & Trollor, 2018)

The prevalence, persistence and consequences of comorbid mental health problems in individuals with ID necessitate improvements in the availability of early assessment and diagnostic services for these individuals and their families, for whom there are currently significant gaps in service provision urgently necessitating extensive further research and evaluation (McCarthy & Boyd, 2002; Whittle et al., 2018).

Challenges in Management of Psychiatric Disorders among Individuals with Intellectual Disability

The significant comorbidity between ID and mental health disorders poses considerable challenges to individuals with ID and their families, and for service providers (Eapen & Jairam, 2009), including not only significant barriers in the detection of mental health problems among individuals with ID but also the unique challenges in the management of these concerns. Some of the specific challenges in this regard include the lack of an interdisciplinary service model; lack of dedicated 'space' within mainstream mental health services for individuals with ID; lack of a clear transition model from childhood to adult services; and lack of staff training and expertise. Such deficiencies in service provision, and the associated cognitive, emotional and behavioral problems, combine to increase rates of unemployment, social isolation and depression in individuals with ID and their families, and the consequent healthcare burden for communities and governments.

Additionally as highlighted by a recent systematic review there is a dearth of quality evidence regarding the effectiveness of treatments designed to address the mental health needs of children and adults with severe ID (Vereenooghe et al., 2018). While the scope of this review was broad, only 5 studies were found that examined the mental health related experiences of people with ID and the findings of these studies were largely inconclusive due to small sample sizes, there were a total of 16 participants across the 5 studies examined. Concerningly this review found that the most recent study in the field was published in 1999 with many of the others employing pharmacotherapies that are no longer routinely prescribed. While there is more evidence for treatments that may be promising for adults with mild to moderate ID, the heterogeneity of study designs and the presence of underpowered trials make it difficult for clinicians to make decisions regarding effectiveness of many existing mental health interventions for their patients with ID(Koslowski et al., 2016). Given the limited available evidence, the findings of studies examining the broader population are often applied to manage mental health issues among people with ID. Given that these interventions may not address the specific needs of people with ID, there is an urgent need for further research in the area to facilitate adequate mental health services to children and adults with ID.

Thus, one of the primary targets of intervention when working with children with ID and their families should be to reduce stress and increase wellbeing among parents. This is also important because it is likely that parents of children with ID who report high levels of stress may engage in parenting behaviour that may negatively affect outcomes both in the child with ID and his or her siblings (Hastings & Beck, 2004), thus maintaining a vicious cycle. Indeed, it is likely that complex and multidirectional relationships exist between parents' wellbeing, psychological coping styles, parenting practices, and their child's behavioural problems, and comprehensive and effective intervention should aim to target these various factors.

Several factors have been found to explain stress among parents of children with ID. For example, research has suggested that child characteristics, such as the frequency or severity of behaviour problems, may lead to parental stress (Hassall, Rose, & McDonald, 2005; Hastings, 2002). For example, in a study of Australian children with a disability, the severity of children's behaviour was associated with parents' experience of greater stress in relation to their child, and their own personal wellbeing (Gavidia-Payne, Richdale, Francis, & Cotton, 1997). Thus, interventions that are successful at improving skills or reducing problem behaviours in children with ID also seem to benefit parental wellbeing (Gavidia-Payne & Hudson, 2002; Hastings & Beck, 2004). Other studies, however, have found that different factors are more important in predicting parental stress than child characteristics. For example, the way in which parents define their situation, and the resources available to them, have been found to predict significantly more variance in stress levels in mothers (29% and 42% respectively) and fathers (37% and 33% respectively) than any characteristics of the child, which accounted for only 2% of variance in maternal stress and 8% of variance in paternal stress (Saloviita, Itälinna, & Leinonen, 2003). Similarly, significant variance in mothers' parenting stress has been found to be explained by parental locus of control and parenting satisfaction (Hassall et al., 2005). These findings are encouraging, as changing parents' attitudes and perceptions may be an easier intervention target than ameliorating the child's disability and associated difficulties (Saloviita et al., 2003).

Recent reviews suggest that behavioural family interventions that train parents to respond contingently to child behaviour indicate positive results among both children with ID and their parents (Gavidia-Payne & Hudson, 2002; Hastings & Beck, 2004).For example, Stepping Stones Triple P (Sanders, Mazzecchelli, & Studman, 2003), an adaptation of the Triple P Positive Parenting Program for families of children with developmental disabilities, has been found to lead to fewer maternal-reported child behaviour problems, improved maternal and paternal parenting style, and decreased maternal stress, with gains maintained at the six-month follow-up(Roberts, Mazzucchelli, Studman, & Sanders, 2006). Similarly, parents of children with ID who have been trained in behavioural principles, such as limit setting and use of consequences and rewards, have been found to report increases in their self-efficacy in managing their child's behaviour, as well as lower levels of stress (Feldman & Werner, 2002). While parent training programs have been found to be beneficial, some research has suggested that families with additional psychosocial stressors such as lack of employment and poor marital adjustment may make the least gains (Baker, Landen, & Kashima, 1991). Additionally recent research has identified that parents of children with disabilities facing mental health problems also report greater difficulty in arranging appropriate childcare, financial difficulties and limited service provider availabilities as barriers to accessing treatment for their own psychiatric issues. (Osborn, Roberts, & Kneebone, 2019)

Hastings and Beck (2004) have also reviewed other interventions for stress reduction in parents of children with ID, including parent-to-parent interventions, and group interventions with parents. Although descriptions of various models have been published, strong evaluation data has rarely been reported for parent-to-parent interventions. One exception is a controlled trial of the Parent-to-Parent model (Singer et al., 1999), in which a parent who has experience caring for a child with a disability is paired with and provides emotional support and information to another parent of a child with ID. Although no measure of parental stress was used, the study found that parents' positive perceptions of their child and his or her impact on the family improved significantly in the treatment group, and parents' ratings of progress towards the resolution of their main need showed a clear improvement (Singer et al., 1999). Aside from the value of formal or informal networks of parents, research has also investigated the efficacy of group interventions for decreasing stress among parents of children with ID. Most group interventions have involved elements of cognitive-behavioural therapy (CBT), and suggest a reasonable evidence base for the use of CBT techniques in improving the wellbeing of parents of children with ID (for a review, see Hastings & Beck, 2004). For example, mothers assigned to a Life Skills Training group where sessions focused on CBT techniques including coping and communication skills, problem solving and decision making, and skills to manage and control social networks, had reduced depression and stress and improved social support compared to mothers who were assigned to a non-directive parent support group (Kirkham & Schilling, 1990). Further, mothers in the Life Skills Training group maintained lower depression scores and higher levels of social support at a two-year follow-up (Kirkham, 1993). Furthermore, there is increasing evidence of the buffering role of informal support in the management of young people with ID and mental health problems and their families. For example, parents of adolescents with ID who perceived greater helpfulness from informal supports (e.g., spouse, extended family, friends) reported lower stress, anxiety and depression, even after controlling for child characteristics (White & Hastings, 2004). Typical appropriate supports provided by services for children with ID and their families such as respite services, case management and provision of key workers are also likely to contribute to reductions in parental stress (Hastings & Beck, 2004). Further, the establishment of early family-school partnerships is important in promoting positive outcomes among children with developmental delays and should not be overlooked as children transition to school (McIntyre, Blacher, & Baker, 2006).The importance of school-based intervention programs for mental health difficulties, including among children and adolescents with ID, has been recognised (Christensen et al., 2011). School-based interventions, such as the NSW School-Link initiative in NSW, Australia (NSW Ministry of Health, 2015), and targeted policies, such as the No Child Left Behind Act ("No Child Left Behind Act of 2001," 2002) are vital in ensuring effective intervention is provided to children and adolescents with comorbid mental disorders and ID.

There is also an acute need to be aware of the impact of ID and associated mental health difficulties not only on the individual, but also on the wellbeing of his or her family. Several studies have found that parents of children with ID report higher levels of child-related stress than parents of typically developing children (Browne & Bramston, 1998; Dyson, 1997; Patton, Ware, McPherson, Emerson, & Lennox, 2018), however this heightened stress has not been found to be the case across all causes of intellectual disability (Dabrowska & Pisula, 2010). Parental stress may result from life events that may impact on any family such as marital breakdown, but also from family life-cycle transitions that may be especially relevant to families of children with disabilities, such as the diagnosis of the child's disability, starting school, transition from child to adult services, and increasing age and infirmity of parents (Hastings & Beck, 2004). It has been assumed that the extra stress of caring for a child with disabilities places parents at an increased risk for depression. Indeed, mothers of children with ID have been found to have higher depression scores than mothers of typically developing children. (Olsson & Hwang, 2001). While no differences were reported in the wellbeing of fathers of children with ID in early studies (Olsson & Hwang, 2001), more recent studies have found significantly higher levels of depression and stress than normative data (Giallo et al., 2015).Similarly, having a brother or sister with ID is a risk factor for sibling adjustment problems (Rossiter & Sharpe, 2001). Within their families, siblings may experience extra caregiver burden, differential treatment, and an imbalance of family resources (Lobato & Kao, 2002). Outside their families, siblings may experience limited access to information about the child's condition, negative peer reactions, and disruptions in age-appropriate peer and family activities (Lobato & Kao, 2002). Thus, siblings of children with ID may also require formal support. Studies have investigated the efficacy of combined group interventions for siblings and parents of children with ID that are designed to increase the siblings' understanding of and adjustment to ID. These studies have found significant improvements in siblings' knowledge of the child's disorder, siblings' self-competence, and sibling connectedness, and decreases in parent-reported behavioural problems among siblings (Lobato & Kao, 2002, 2005). Several of these improvements have been shown to be maintained at three-month follow-up (Lobato & Kao, 2002, 2005). Open communication and sharing age-appropriate information with siblings appears to be the best approach, as this reduces uncertainty and confusion, helps the development of family-centred problem solving skills, and allows siblings to support parents in the best way they can. If there are issues of risk to the sibling in terms of violent or aggressive behaviours, appropriate safety steps should also be taken.

Despite this range of interventions, there are significant challenges in providing a comprehensive and integrated service for those with ID and mental health problems. For example, studies from the UK have shown that young people with severe ID and mental health problems fall between a number of healthcare providers, including child and adolescent mental health services, specialist ID services and paediatricians (McCarthy & Boyd, 2002). Working with children with ID and their families likely necessitates a multidisciplinary approach, potentially involving physiotherapy for motor development and coordination, occupational therapy for proprioception and sensory integration, speech therapy for receptive, expressive and pragmatic communication, psychology for assistance with thoughts, feelings and behaviour including social interaction, and medical specialists for assistance with physical health difficulties, just to name a few. In this regard, it is worth noting that severity of ID is associated with an increase in associated medical conditions and complications, with the relationship being complex as they interact with one another and can result in secondary medical and behavioural complications (O'Brien, Barnard, Pearson, & Rippon, 2002). Collaboration and clear communication is also needed between families, health providers, and the various other agencies involved in the patient's care including education, housing and financial support services. Due to the multidisciplinary nature of services required for children with ID and their families, a model where one person works closely with the family and can mediate between the family and various services or professionals may lead to the most positive outcomes for parents (Hastings & Beck, 2004). However, there is often no collaboration or communication to enable a continuum of care. This is further compounded by the fact that different disciplines and agencies use different models of care ranging from patient-centred to those involving the family. Often there is no continuity between various services such as acute inpatient units, emergency departments, outpatient and community services, education services, vocational centres, the juvenile justice system and disability services. Families may be expected to go from one specialist to another, and navigating the complex health system is a significant challenge for both patients and their carers.

Hatton (2002)Reviewed the literature on psychosocial interventions for adults with ID and comorbid mental health problems. Individual and group intervention studies using modified CBT, including one small waiting list controlled trial (Rose, West, & Clifford, 2000), have found reductions in anger and aggressive behaviour among adults with ID. Adaptations of CBT have also shown reasonable outcomes in reducing depression and anxiety among adults with ID, but the reviewed research is limited to case studies and case series (Hatton, 2002). When implementing CBT with adults with ID, Hatton (2002) discusses the importance of assessing the individual's capacity to give informed consent. Wong, Clare, Holland, Watson, and Gunn (2000) found that people with ID and people with dementia were less able to make an informed consent decision than people with a chronic mental health problem or a comparison group. All participants benefited when the informed consent decision-making task was simplified by presenting information as separate elements and reducing the level of expressive verbal ability required to respond (Wong et al., 2000). These considerations may be particularly important when working with adults with comorbid ID and mental health problems. Further, consideration must be given to the person's suitability to engage in CBT, including assessment of communication skills, cognitive aptitude, ability to identify emotions, and capacity to understand the CBT model (Hatton, 2002). Enhancing skills including communication, emotion recognition, problem solving and social skills can lead to increased independence and self-determination, which in turn can improve overall quality of life among individuals with ID (Nota, Ferrari, Soresi, & Wehmeyer, 2007). Assistance with housing, employment, social networks and independent living skills also deserve attention.

As such it is critical to facilitate the development of clinical tools for use by people with ID including those who are non-verbal to allow for better communication with clinicians regarding the nature of concurrent mental health issues in ID. Given the heterogeneous range of functional, behavioral and cognitive features among people with ID, the lack of consensus with regards to the tools to measure functional outcomes presents a significant challenge to health service provision. Once mental health problems have been identified however gaps in the integration and sharing of information between service providers of disability and mental health services, lack of appropriately targeted services and deficits in clinician knowledge act as barriers to access to appropriate health care(Whittle et al., 2018). Risk management is also important when working with individuals with comorbid ID and mental health problems. One particular area that warrants attention is the issue of behavioural change associated with sexual development, which can lead to sexualised behaviours and offending. Social stories appropriate to the mental age of the person with ID and sexual health education are critical in these situations. CBT has also been found to be successful in changing attitudes in sex offenders with ID (Hatton, 2002). Planning for emergencies and crisis situations is an important consideration of treatment, and having a safety plan with contact numbers of case workers or members of the treating team in case a crisis happens can put the mind at ease for both the patient and the family.

While randomised controlled trials concerning the effectiveness of psychotropic medications for people with ID and comorbid mental health problems are virtually absent (Hatton, 2002), psychopharmacology is a treatment option although this is also associated with challenges. It is to be noted that individuals with ID are often more at risk of developing side effects. One example of the potential complexities when treating people with ID who also have mental health problems is evident when these individuals are treated with second generation antipsychotics (SGAs) which considerably decrease the lifespan due to increased risk of weight gain, cardiometabolic changes, metabolic syndrome and related side effects of SGAs. Concerns have also been raised about the inappropriate use of antipsychotics in individuals with ID especially for behavioral problems without a diagnosed mental health condition(O'Dwyer et al., 2019).In this regard, a recent study examining the antipsychotic use in people with ID found that, of the 305 participants, 45.1% received antipsychotics with only 25.9% having evidence of a psychotic disorder with the rest being treated for problem behaviors. This highlights the need for careful consideration of the indication and the justification for the use of antipsychotics in individuals with ID. In either case, attention should also be given to an integrated and comprehensive physical health care plan for people with ID and mental health problems. While such a plan would be a policy direction to aspire to, research is needed in order to understand gaps in attitudes, awareness, and training of staff, resources, and service delivery options.

While various interventions have been found to show efficacy, Dosen (2007) argues that a mono-disciplinary treatment approach to behavioural and psychiatric problems in persons with ID, such as psychotropic medication or behaviour modification alone, has yielded limited success. He argues for an integrative diagnostic and treatment approach consisting of four dimensions – biological, psychological, social and developmental – for people with ID and mental health problems, where the focus should not be primarily directed towards the symptoms of the disorder but towards restoring a person's mental wellbeing. For individuals with an established dual diagnosis of both ID and a psychiatric disorder, treatment goals should include preventing further disability, restoring premorbid functioning, and improving quality of life through restoration of functionality, independent living and rehabilitation.

SOLUTIONS, RECOMMENDATIONS AND FUTURE RESEARCH DIRECTIONS

A developmental-bio-psycho-social-cultural model of service delivery and training and education of professionals involved in the care of people with ID is critical for early identification and appropriate management of comorbid mental health problems. People with ID and mental health problems are some of the most vulnerable people in society and they are often let down by the health care system, funding and service delivery models. Efforts to intervene in a more coordinated and integrated way can significantly improve their outcomes. Further, both the patient and the family or caregiver would need support, advocacy and case management. This would require coordination rather than separate services across types of difficulty, age groups, treatment modalities and disciplines. This should include a focus on the individual in a family context and using skill building models for developmental gains and appropriate management of maladaptive behaviours through an integrated multidisciplinary and multiagency collaborative service.

In order to plan effective and comprehensive prevention and intervention strategies for young people with ID and mental health disorders, it is important that there is a better understanding of the complex interplay of both risk and protective factors at different levels, including individual child factors, family, neighbourhood and society, as well as services, systems and policies. It is also important to consider the perspectives of the family members and support persons and work collaboratively together. Differentiating between behavioural challenges and mental health co-morbidity is also important and in doing so information from multiple sources needs consideration and interpretation (Weise, Fisher, & Trollor, 2018; Weise et al 2018).Given that no factor acts in isolation, and that there is an interaction of these factors at multiple bio-ecological levels, and at multiple time points along the life course, it is essential to have rigorous and relevant epidemiological and statistical techniques that can apply a bio-ecological model using a life course approach(Woolfenden et al., 2014). A cumulative risk index, being the sum of individual risk factors, is one way of conceptualising how risk factors interact over a life course(A. J. Sameroff & Seifer, 1983), but in this model all risk factors are given an equal weight which is a significant disadvantage when compared to a regression model. Structural Equation Modelling and Multilevel Modelling techniques, on the other hand, are based on a proposed hypothesis and, using regression techniques, variables including time are grouped into hierarchical levels(Diez Roux, 2004), and measured to see which model fits best. Future research exploring risk factors should where possible use composite theoretical models, longitudinal study designs and multilevel modelling in order to tease apart risk factors at different levels including individual, family and neighbourhood as well as society, services, systems and policy factors, which might increase vulnerability of people with ID to develop mental health problems. In this context, it is noteworthy that the occurrence of mental health comorbidity in children with ID, and the nature and type of such comorbidity, is shaped by the interplay of biological and environmental risk and resilience factors, mediated by the life course issues as to when these factors are in operation in the child's life.Eapen (2014) has described such a model of a

Developmental Risk Index where appropriate weighted scoring is given to different microsystem (child's most immediate or proximal environment), mesosystem (reciprocal relationships and interconnections), exosystem (distal factors that indirectly impact on the child and their family) and macrosystem (societal, cultural and service or policy) factors. Future studies should also explore biological risk factors including genetic factors, perinatal events, trauma, toxins, infections and immunological factors. Research should also focus on early identification processes that accurately assess the nature and reasons behind behavioural and emotional problems encountered in the context of ID; for example challenging behaviours may be due to the underlying brain pathology, or due to speech and language difficulties resulting in communication problems, or due to lack of stimulation and opportunities resulting in poor quality of life. Such a comprehensive assessment would no doubt facilitate the development of an individualised multidisciplinary treatment model and better outcomes.

Regarding management of co-morbid ID and mental health disorders, a recent study examined a discrete choice experiment (DCE) for assessing care management preferences of parents for their children(N'Dri, Ross, Castillo, Reeves, & Butler, 2019; dos Reis et al 2019). Using mixed methods, this study tested six attributes of care management decisions by parents namely medication use, parental custody, time cost, social interactions, medication effects, and school placement. Among children with ID the common co-morbidities were autism spectrum disorder (55%) and attention-deficit/hyperactivity disorder (76%). The study found that the participants had a preference for using fewer medications and maintaining decision-making authority and that they considered medication effects on the child's mood to be more important than its effects on personality or body weight.

CONCLUSION

There are significant challenges in the detection and characterisation of comorbid mental health problems in the context of ID. For example, for those with limited language and cognitive abilities, can the same diagnostic criteria and measures be used? Identifying the nature and extent of mental health problems is further compounded by the lack of measures specific for ID. There are also difficulties in identifying the nature and extent of ID and the consequent impact on function (measurement of adaptive behavior), as there is considerable variability in the terms and definitions as well as the diagnostic criteria and assessments across settings and across the different parts of the globe. While some of these issues could be addressed through better training of professionals, there are also significant barriers in service delivery models and access to services. In this regard, there are significant gaps in the availability of evidence based intervention programs in general for children with ID and mental health problems. In particular, the needs of those with behavioural or mental health problems and chronic and complex health care problems are not met by mainstream services. There is an urgent need to have a consensus on a statement of minimum standards of care, with clear policy objectives, program outlines and comprehensive training of staff, followed by evaluation of its implementation. Family and support persons perspectives also need due consideration during the management planning and decision making process. Furthermore, improved longitudinal outcomes will only be possible for people with ID and psychiatric disorders if there are opportunities for access to integrated services including better identification and treatment models, and improved knowledge and awareness of health-related conditions for people with ID, enhanced parent or carer support, as well as changes within health and disability service systems to ensure universal coverage of quality services.

ACKNOWLEDGMENT

This research received no specific grant from any funding agency in the public, commercial, or not-for-profit sectors.

REFERENCES

Abbeduto, L., Seltzer, M. M., Shattuck, P., Krauss, M. W., Orsmond, G., & Murphy, M. M. (2004). Psychological well-being and coping in mothers of youths with autism, down syndrome, or fragile x syndrome. *Journal Information, 109*(3).

Anderson, D. J., Lakin, K. C., Hill, B. K., & Chen, T. (1992). Social integration of older persons with mental retardation in residential facilities. *American Journal of Mental Retardation*. PMID:1562307

Andrews, G., Henderson, S., & Hall, W. (2001). *Prevalence, comorbidity, disability and service utilisation* (vol. 178). Academic Press.

APA. (2013). *Diagnostic and statistical manual of mental disorders - fifth edition (dsm-5)*. Washington, DC: American Psychiatric Publishing.

Axmon, A., Sandberg, M., & Ahlström, G. (2017). Gender differences in psychiatric diagnoses in older people with intellectual disability: A register study. *BMC Psychiatry, 17*(1), 192.

Baker, B. L., Landen, S. J., & Kashima, K. J. (1991). Effects of parent training on families of children with mental retardation: Increased burden or generalized benefit? *American Journal of Mental Retardation*. PMID:1930946

Begg, S., Vos, T., Barker, B., Stevenson, C., Stanley, L., & Lopez, A. (2007). *Burden of disease and injury in Australia, 2003*. Australian Institute of Health and Welfare.

Borthwick-Duffy, S. A., & Eyman, R. K. (1990). Who are the dually diagnosed? *American Journal of Mental Retardation*. PMID:2340136

Bouras, N. (2011). Mental health problems and related issues for people with developmental and intellectual disability. *Current Opinion in Psychiatry, 24*(5), 365-366.

Bourke, J., Ricciardo, B., Bebbington, A., Aiberti, K., Jacoby, P., Dyke, P., . . . Leonard, H. (2008). Physical and mental health in mothers of children with down syndrome. *The Journal of Pediatrics, 153*(3), 320-326.

Browne, G., & Bramston, P. (1998). Stress and the quality of life in the parents of young people with intellectual disabilities. *Journal of Psychiatric and Mental Health Nursing, 5*(5), 415-421.

Bruininks, H., Hill, B. K., & Morreau, L. E. (1988). Prevalence and implications of maladaptive behaviors and dual diagnosis in residential and other service programs. In Mental Retardation and Mental Health (pp. 3-29). Springer.

Cassidy, S. B., & Morris, C. A. (2001). Behavioral phenotypes in genetic syndromes: Genetic clues to human behavior. *Advances in Pediatrics, 49*, 59–86. PMID:12214780

Chadwick, O., Kusel, Y., Cuddy, M., & Taylor, E. (2005). Psychiatric diagnoses and behaviour problems from childhood to early adolescence in young people with severe intellectual disabilities. *Psychological Medicine, 35*(5), 751-760.

Chawner, S., Owen, M., Holmans, P., Raymond, L., Skuse, D., Hall, J., . . . Consortium, I.-I. (2019). Genotype-phenotype relationships in children with copy number variants associated with high neuro-psychiatric risk: findings from the intellectual disability & mental health: assessing the genomic impact on neurodevelopment (imagine-id) study. *Biorxiv*, 535708.

Christensen, H., Calear, A., Tait, R., Gosling, J., Griffiths, K., & Murray, K. (2011). *School based intervention programs and shared care collaborative models targeting the prevention of or early intervention in child and adolescent mental health problems: an evidence check rapid review brokered by the sax institute for the nsw ministry of health*. Academic Press.

Clarke, J., Littlejohns, C. S., Corbett, J. A., & Joseph, S. (1989). Pervasive developmental disorders and psychoses in adult life. *The British Journal of Psychiatry, 155*(5), 692–699. doi:10.1192/bjp.155.5.692 PMID:2611600

Cooper. (1997). High prevalence of dementia among people with learning disabilities not attributable to down's syndrome. *Psychological Medicine, 27*(3), 609–616. doi:10.1017/S0033291796004655 PMID:9153681

Cooper, A. (1997). Psychiatry of elderly compared to younger adults with intellectual disabilities. *Journal of Applied Research in Intellectual Disabilities, 10*(4), 303–311. doi:10.1111/j.1468-3148.1997.tb00025.x

Cooper, A., Smiley, E., Morrison, J., Williamson, A., & Allan, L. (2007). Mental ill-health in adults with intellectual disabilities: Prevalence and associated factors. *The British Journal of Psychiatry, 190*(1), 27–35. doi:10.1192/bjp.bp.106.022483 PMID:17197653

Corbett, A. (1979). Psychiatric morbidity and mental retardation. In F. E. James & R. P. Snaith (Eds.), Psychiatric illness and mental handicap (pp. 11-25). London: Royal College of Psychiatry, Gaskell.

Costello, H., & Bouras, N. (2006). Assessment of mental health problems in people with intellectual disabilities. *Israel Journal of Psychiatry and Related Sciences, 43*(4), 241.

Crnic, A., Neece, C. L., McIntyre, L. L., Blacher, J., & Baker, B. L. (2017). Intellectual disability and developmental risk: Promoting intervention to improve child and family well-being. *Child Development, 88*(2), 436–445. doi:10.1111/cdev.12740 PMID:28138976

Croen, A., Grether, J. K., & Selvin, S. (2001). The epidemiology of mental retardation of unknown cause. *Pediatrics, 107*(6), e86–e86. doi:10.1542/peds.107.6.e86 PMID:11389284

Dabrowska, A., & Pisula, E. (2010). Parenting stress and coping styles in mothers and fathers of pre-school children with autism and down syndrome. *Journal of Intellectual Disability Research, 54*(3), 266-280.

Deb, S., Thomas, M., & Bright, C. (2001). Mental disorder in adults with intellectual disability. 1: prevalence of functional psychiatric illness among a community-based population aged between 16 and 64 years. *Journal of Intellectual Disability Research, 45*(6), 495-505.

Dekker, C., & Koot, H. M. (2003a). Dsm-iv disorders in children with borderline to moderate intellectual disability. I: Prevalence and impact. *Journal of the American Academy of Child and Adolescent Psychiatry, 42*(8), 915–922. doi:10.1097/01.CHI.0000046892.27264.1A PMID:12874493

Dekker, C., & Koot, H. M. (2003b). Dsm-iv disorders in children with borderline to moderate intellectual disability. Ii: Child and family predictors. *Journal of the American Academy of Child and Adolescent Psychiatry, 42*(8), 923–931. doi:10.1097/01.CHI.0000046891.27264.C1 PMID:12874494

<unknown>Derigne, L., & Porterfield, S. L. (2017). Employment change among married parents of children with special health care needs. Journal of Family Issues, 38(5), 579-606.</unknown>

Diez Roux, A. V. (2004). The study of group-level factors in epidemiology: rethinking variables, study designs, and analytical approaches. *Epidemiologic Reviews, 26*(1), 104-111. doi:10.1093/epirev/mxh006

Doran, C. M., Einfeld, S. L., Madden, R. H., Otim, M., Horstead, S. K., Ellis, L. A., & Emerson, E. (2012). How much does intellectual disability really cost? First estimates for australia. *Journal of Intellectual and Developmental Disability, 37*(1), 42-49.

Dosen, A. (2007). Integrative treatment in persons with intellectual disability and mental health problems. *Journal of Intellectual Disability Research, 51*(1), 66-74. doi:10.1111/j.1365-2788.2006.00868.x

Durkin, S., & Yeargin-Allsopp, M. (2018). *Socioeconomic status and pediatric neurologic disorders: current evidence.* Paper presented at the seminars in pediatric neurology. 10.1016/j.spen.2018.03.003

Dyson, L. (1997). Fathers and mothers of school-age children with developmental disabilities: Parental stress, family functioning, and social support. *American Journal of Mental Retardation, 102*(3), 267–279. doi:10.1352/0895-8017(1997)102<0267:FAMOSC>2.0.CO;2 PMID:9394135

Eapen, V., & Jairam, R. (2009). Integration of child mental health services to primary care: challenges and opportunities. *Mental Health in Family Medicine, 6*(1), 43.

Eapen, V. (2014). Developmental and mental health disorders: two sides of the same coin. *Asian Journal of Psychiatry, 8*, 7-11.

Eapen, V., Al-Gazali, L. I., Bin-Othman, S., & Pramathan, T. (1998). Learning disorders in school-going children–detection and diagnosis. *Journal of Tropical Pediatrics, 44*(4), 192-193.

Einfeld, L., Piccinin, A. M., Mackinnon, A., Hofer, S. M., Taffe, J., Gray, K. M., ... Tonge, B. J. (2006). Psychopathology in young people with intellectual disability. *Journal of the American Medical Association, 296*(16), 1981–1989. doi:10.1001/jama.296.16.1981 PMID:17062861

Einfeld, L., & Tonge, B. J. (1996a). Population prevalence of psychopathology in children and adolescents with intellectual disability: I rationale and methods. *Journal of Intellectual Disability Research, 40*(2), 91–98. doi:10.1111/j.1365-2788.1996.tb00610.x PMID:8731466

Einfeld, L., & Tonge, B. J. (1996b). Population prevalence of psychopathology in children and adolescents with intellectual disability: Ii epidemiological findings. *Journal of Intellectual Disability Research, 40*(2), 99–109. doi:10.1111/j.1365-2788.1996.tb00611.x PMID:8731467

Einfeld, L., & Tonge, B. J. (1999). Observations on the use of the icd-10 guide for mental retardation. *Journal of Intellectual Disability Research, 43*(5), 408–412. doi:10.1046/j.1365-2788.1999.043005408.x PMID:10546965

Einfeld, S. L., Ellis, L. A., & Emerson, E. (2011). Comorbidity of intellectual disability and mental disorder in children and adolescents: a systematic review. *Journal of Intellectual and Developmental Disability, 36*(2), 137-143.

Emerson, E., & Hatton, C. (2007a). Contribution of socioeconomic position to health inequalities of british children and adolescents with intellectual disabilities. *Journal Information, 112*(2).

Emerson, E., & Hatton, C. (2007b). Mental health of children and adolescents with intellectual disabilities in Britain. *The British Journal of Psychiatry, 191*(6), 493-499.

Emerson, E. (2003). Prevalence of psychiatric disorders in children and adolescents with and without intellectual disability. *Journal of Intellectual Disability Research, 47*(1), 51-58.

Emerson, E. (2012). Deprivation, ethnicity and the prevalence of intellectual and developmental disabilities. *Journal of Epidemiology and Community Health, 66*(3), 218-224.

Feldman, A., & Werner, S. E. (2002). Collateral effects of behavioral parent training on families of children with developmental disabilities and behavior disorders. *Behavioral Interventions, 17*(2), 75–83. doi:10.1002/bin.111

Gauthier-Boudreault, C., Gallagher, F., & Couture, M. (2017). Specific needs of families of young adults with profound intellectual disability during and after transition to adulthood: What are we missing? *Research in Developmental Disabilities, 66*, 16–26. doi:10.1016/j.ridd.2017.05.001 PMID:28577424

Gavidia-Payne, S., Richdale, A., Francis, A., & Cotton, S. (1997). *The parenting hassles scale: measuring stress in parents of children with disabilities.* Paper presented at the 121st annual meeting of the american association on mental retardation, New York, NY.

Gavidia-Payne, S., & Hudson, A. (2002). Behavioural supports for parents of children with an intellectual disability and problem behaviours: An overview of the literature. *Journal of Intellectual & Developmental Disability, 27*(1), 31–55. doi:10.1080/13668250120119626

Giallo, R., Seymour, M., Matthews, J., Gavidia-Payne, S., Hudson, A., & Cameron, C. (2015). Risk factors associated with the mental health of fathers of children with an intellectual disability in Australia. *Journal of Intellectual Disability Research, 59*(3), 193-207.

Gilson, M., Davis, E., Johnson, S., Gains, J., Reddihough, D., & Williams, K. (2018). Mental health care needs and preferences for mothers of children with a disability. *Child: Care, Health and Development, 44*(3), 384–391. doi:10.1111/cch.12556 PMID:29430692

Gostason, R. (1985). Psychiatric illness among the mentally retarded. *Acta Psychiat. Scand, 318*(suppl 71), 1-117.

Guralnick, J. (1997). Effectiveness of early intervention for vulnerable children: A developmental perspective. *American Journal of Mental Retardation, 102*(4), 319–345. doi:10.1352/0895-8017(1998)102<0319:EOEIFV>2.0.CO;2 PMID:9475942

Hackman, A., Farah, M. J., & Meaney, M. J. (2010). Socioeconomic status and the brain: Mechanistic insights from human and animal research. *Nature Reviews. Neuroscience, 11*(9), 651–659. doi:10.1038/nrn2897 PMID:20725096

Harris, J. C. (2006). *Intellectual disability: Understanding its development, causes, classification, evaluation, and treatment*. Oxford University Press.

Hassall, R., Rose, J., & McDonald, J. (2005). Parenting stress in mothers of children with an intellectual disability: the effects of parental cognitions in relation to child characteristics and family support. *Journal of Intellectual Disability Research, 49*(6), 405-418.

Hastings, P. (2002). Parental stress and behaviour problems of children with developmental disability. *Journal of Intellectual & Developmental Disability, 27*(3), 149–160. doi:10.1080/1366825021000008657

Hastings, P., & Beck, A. (2004). Practitioner review: Stress intervention for parents of children with intellectual disabilities. *Journal of Child Psychology and Psychiatry, and Allied Disciplines, 45*(8), 1338–1349. doi:10.1111/j.1469-7610.2004.00357.x PMID:15482495

Hatton, C. (2002). Psychosocial interventions for adults with intellectual disabilities and mental health problems: a review. *Journal of Mental Health, 11*(4), 357-374.

Hazarika, M., Das, S., & Choudhury, S. (2017). Parents' attitude towards children and adolescents with intellectual developmental disorder. *International Journal of Child Development and Mental Health, 5*(1), 11.

Howlett, S., Florio, T., Xu, H., & Trollor, J. (2015). Ambulatory mental health data demonstrates the high needs of people with an intellectual disability: results from the new south wales intellectual disability and mental health data linkage project. *Australian & New Zealand Journal of Psychiatry, 49*(2), 137-144.

Hurley, D. (2006). Mood disorders in intellectual disability. *Current Opinion in Psychiatry, 19*(5), 465–469. doi:10.1097/01.yco.0000238471.84206.0a PMID:16874117

Iverson, C., & Fox, R. A. (1989). Prevalence of psychopathology among mentally retarded adults. *Research in Developmental Disabilities, 10*(1), 77–83. doi:10.1016/0891-4222(89)90030-9 PMID:2928581

King, T. L., Milner, A., Aitken, Z., Karahalios, A., Emerson, E., & Kavanagh, A. M. (2019). Mental health of adolescents: Variations by borderline intellectual functioning and disability. *European Child & Adolescent Psychiatry*, 1–10. PMID:30759281

Kirkham, A. (1993). Two-year follow-up of skills training with mothers of children with disabilities. *American Journal of Mental Retardation*. PMID:7681675

Kirkham, A., & Schilling, R. F. II. (1990). Life skills training with mothers of handicapped children. *Journal of Social Service Research, 13*(2), 67–87. doi:10.1300/J079v13n02_05

Koslowski, N., Klein, K., Arnold, K., Koesters, M., Schuctzwohl, M., Salize, H. J., & Puschner, B. (2016). Effectiveness of interventions for adults with mild to moderate intellectual disabilities and mental health problems: systematic review and meta-analysis. *The British Journal of Psychiatry, 209*(6), 469-474.

Leonard, H., & Wen, X. (2002). The epidemiology of mental retardation: challenges and opportunities in the new millennium. *Mental Retardation and Developmental Disabilities Research Reviews, 8*(3), 117-134.

Leonard, H., Glasson, E., Nassar, N., Whitehouse, A., Bebbington, A., Bourke, J., . . . Bower, C. (2011). Autism and intellectual disability are differentially related to sociodemographic background at birth. *PloS One, 6*(3), e17875.

<unknown>Leonard, H., Petterson, B., Bower, C., & Sanders, R. (2003). Prevalence of intellectual disability in western australia. Paediatric and Perinatal Epidemiology, 17(1), 58-67.</unknown>

Leonard, H., Petterson, B., De Klerk, N., Zubrick, S. R., Glasson, E., Sanders, R., & Bower, C. (2005). Association of sociodemographic characteristics of children with intellectual disability in Western Australia. *Social Science & Medicine, 60*(7), 1499-1513.

Lobato, J. (2002). Integrated sibling-parent group intervention to improve sibling knowledge and adjustment to chronic illness and disability. *Journal of Pediatric Psychology*, *27*(8), 711–716. doi:10.1093/jpepsy/27.8.711 PMID:12403861

Lobato, J., & Kao, B. T. (2005). Brief report: Family-based group intervention for young siblings of children with chronic illness and developmental disability. *Journal of Pediatric Psychology*, *30*(8), 678–682. doi:10.1093/jpepsy/jsi054 PMID:16260437

Lund, J. (1985). The prevalence of psychiatric morbidity in mentally retarded adults. *Acta Psychiatrica Scandinavica, 72*(6), 563-570.

Maes, B., Broekman, T. G., Došen, A., & Nauts, J. (2003). Caregiving burden of families looking after persons with intellectual disability and behavioural or psychiatric problems. *Journal of Intellectual Disability Research, 47*(6), 447-455. doi:10.1046/j.1365-2788.2003.00513.x

Maggi, S., Irwin, L. J., Siddiqi, A., & Hertzman, C. (2010). The social determinants of early child development: an overview. *Journal of Paediatrics and Child Health, 46*(11), 627-635.

Marmot, M. G., Allen, J., Goldblatt, P., Boyce, T., McNeish, D., Grady, M., & Geddes, I. (2010). *Fair society, healthy lives: strategic review of health inequalities in England post-2010*. Academic Press.

Mason, J., & Scior, K. (2004). 'Diagnostic overshadowing' amongst clinicians working with people with intellectual disabilities in the UK. *Journal of Applied Research in Intellectual Disabilities, 17*(2), 85-90.

Maulik, K., Mascarenhas, M. N., Mathers, C. D., Dua, T., & Saxena, S. (2011). Prevalence of intellectual disability: A meta-analysis of population-based studies. *Research in Developmental Disabilities*, *32*(2), 419–436. doi:10.1016/j.ridd.2010.12.018 PMID:21236634

Maulik, P. K., & Harbour, C. K. (2010). Epidemiology of intellectual disability. *International Encyclopaedia of Rehabilitation.*

Maulik, P. K., & Harbour, C. K. (2010). Epidemiology of intellectual disability. *International Encyclopedia of Rehabilitation, 2*.

McCarthy, J., & Boyd, J. (2002). Mental health services and young people with intellectual disability: is it time to do better? *Journal of Intellectual Disability Research, 46*(3), 250-256.

Mcintyre, L., Blacher, J., & Baker, B. L. (2002). Behaviour/mental health problems in young adults with intellectual disability: The impact on families. *Journal of Intellectual Disability Research, 46*(3), 239–249. doi:10.1046/j.1365-2788.2002.00371.x PMID:11896809

Mcintyre, L. L., Blacher, J., & Baker, B. L. (2006). The transition to school: Adaptation in young children with and without developmental delays. *Journal of Intellectual Disability Research, 50*(5), 349–361. doi:10.1111/j.1365-2788.2006.00783.x PMID:16629928

McKenzie, K., Milton, M., Smith, G., & Ouellette-Kuntz, H. (2016). Systematic review of the prevalence and incidence of intellectual disabilities: current trends and issues. *Current Developmental Disorders Reports, 3*(2), 104-115.

Meltzer, H., Gatward, R., Goodman, R., & Ford, T. (2000). *Mental health of children and adolescents in Great Britain*. London: The Stationery Office.

Miodrag, N., & Hodapp, R. M. (2010). Chronic stress and health among parents of children with intellectual and developmental disabilities. *Current Opinion in Psychiatry, 23*(5), 407-411.

Mitchell, C., McLanahan, S., Brooks-Gunn, J., Garfinkel, I., Hobcraft, J., & Notterman, D. (2013). Genetic differential sensitivity to social environments: implications for research. *American Journal of Public Health, 103*(s1), s102-s110.

Molteno, G., Molteno, C. D., Finchilescu, G., & Dawes, A. R. L. (2001). Behavioural and emotional problems in children with intellectual disability attending special schools in Cape Town, South Africa. *Journal of Intellectual Disability Research, 45*(6), 515-520.

Munir, M. (2016). The co-occurrence of mental disorders in children and adolescents with intellectual disability/intellectual developmental disorder. *Current Opinion in Psychiatry, 29*(2), 95–102. doi:10.1097/YCO.0000000000000236 PMID:26779862

N'dri, L., Ross, M., Castillo, W. C., Reeves, G., & Butler, b. (2019). Care management for youth with co-morbid developmental and mental health conditions: A discrete choice experiment pilot study. *Academic Pediatrics*. PMID:31128382

<unknown>No child left behind act of 2001, 20 u.s.c., pub. L. No. 107-110 (2002).</unknown>

<unknown>Nota, L., Ferrari, L., Soresi, S., & Wehmeyer, M. (2007). Self-determination, social abilities and the quality of life of people with intellectual disability. Journal of Intellectual Disability Research, 51(11), 850-865.</unknown>

NSW Ministry of Health. (2015). *NSW school-link strategy and action plan 2014-2017*. Sydney, Australia: NSW Ministry of Health.

O'Brien, G., Barnard, L., Pearson, J., & Rippon, L. (2002). Physical health and clinical phenotypes. *Physical Health of Adults With Intellectual Disabilities*, 35-62.

O'Dwyer, C., McCallion, P., Henman, M., McCarron, M., O'Leary, E., Burke, E., . . . O'Dwyer, M. (2019). Prevalence and patterns of antipsychotic use and their associations with mental health and problem behaviours among older adults with intellectual disabilities. *Journal of Applied Research in Intellectual Disabilities*. PMID:31038275

Olsson, B., & Hwang, C. P. (2001). Depression in mothers and fathers of children with intellectual disability. *Journal of Intellectual Disability Research*, *45*(6), 535–543. doi:10.1046/j.1365-2788.2001.00372.x PMID:11737541

Osborn, R., Roberts, L., & Kneebone, I. (2019). Barriers to accessing mental health treatment for parents of children with intellectual disabilities: A preliminary study. *Disability and Rehabilitation*, 1-7.

Parish, L., Seltzer, M. M., Greenberg, J. S., & Floyd, F. (2004). Economic implications of caregiving at midlife: Comparing parents with and without children who have developmental disabilities. *Mental Retardation*, *42*(6), 413–426. doi:10.1352/0047-6765(2004)42<413:EIOCAM>2.0.CO;2 PMID:15516174

Parmenter, R., Einfeld, S. L., Tonge, B. J., & Dempster, J. A. (1998). Behavioural and emotional problems in the classroom of children and adolescents with intellectual disability. *Journal of Intellectual & Developmental Disability*, *23*(1), 71–77. doi:10.1080/13668259800033591

Patton, A., Ware, R., McPherson, L., Emerson, E., & Lennox, N. (2018). Parent-related stress of male and female carers of adolescents with intellectual disabilities and carers of children within the general population: A cross-sectional comparison. *Journal of Applied Research in Intellectual Disabilities*, *31*(1), 51–61. doi:10.1111/jar.12292 PMID:27704663

Polder, J. J., Meerding, W. J., Bonneux, L., & van der Maas, P. J. (2002). Healthcare costs of intellectual disability in the netherlands: a cost-of-illness perspective. *Journal of Intellectual Disability Research, 46*(2), 168-178.

<unknown>Richardson, S. A., & Koller, H. (1996). Twenty-two years: Causes and consequences of mental retardation. Harvard University Press.</unknown>

Roberts, C., Mazzucchelli, T., Studman, L. J., & Sanders, M. R. (2006). Behavioral family intervention for children with developmental disabilities and behavioral problems. *Journal of Clinical Child and Adolescent Psychology, 35*(2), 180-193.

<unknown>Roeleveld, N., & Zielhuis, G. A. (1997). The prevalence of mental retardation: a critical review of recent literature. Developmental Medicine & Child Neurology, 39(2), 125-132.</unknown>

Rose, J., West, C., & Clifford, D. (2000). Group interventions for anger in people with intellectual disabilities. *Research in Developmental Disabilities, 21*(3), 171-181. doi:10.10160891-4222(00)00032-9

Rossiter, L., & Sharpe, D. (2001). The siblings of individuals with mental retardation: a quantitative integration of the literature. *Journal of Child and Family Studies, 10*(1), 65-84.

Saloviita, T., Itälinna, M., & Leinonen, E. (2003). Explaining the parental stress of fathers and mothers caring for a child with intellectual disability: A double abcx model. *Journal of Intellectual Disability Research, 47*(4-5), 300-312.

Sameroff, A. E. (2009). *The transactional model of development: how children and contexts shape each other*. American Psychological Association.

Sameroff, J., & Seifer, R. (1983). Familial risk and child competence. *Child Development, 54*(5), 1254–1268. doi:10.2307/1129680 PMID:6354632

Sanders, M. R., Mazzecchelli, T. G., & Studman, L. J. (2003). *Practitioner's manual for standard stepping stones triple p: for families with a child who has a disability*. Brisbane, Australia: Triple P International.

Siddiqi, A., Irwin, L. G., & Hertzman, C. (2007). *The total environment assessment model of early child development*. Evidence report for the world health organization's commission on the social determinants of health, oms.

Singer, G. H. S., Marquis, J., Powers, L. K., Blanchard, L., Divenere, N., Santelli, B., . . . Sharp, M. (1999). A multi-site evaluation of parent to parent programs for parents of children with disabilities. *Journal of Early Intervention, 22*(3), 217–229. doi:10.1177/105381519902200305

Statistics, A. B. (2015). Disability, ageing and carers, Australia: Summary of findings. *Retrieved Januari, 18*, 2018.

Stromme, P., & Diseth, T. H. (2000). Prevalence of psychiatric diagnoses in children with mental retardation: data from a population-based study. *Developmental Medicine & Child Neurology, 42*(04), 266-270.

Stromme, P., & Magnus, P. (2000). Correlations between socioeconomic status, iq and aetiology in mental retardation: a population-based study of Norwegian children. *Social Psychiatry and Psychiatric Epidemiology, 1*(35).

Stuart, H. (2012). United nations convention on the rights of persons with disabilities: a roadmap for change. *Current Opinion in Psychiatry, 25*(5), 365-369.

Sturmey, P. (1995). Dsm-iii-r and persons with dual diagnoses: conceptual issues and strategies for future research. *Journal of Intellectual Disability Research, 39*(5), 357-364.

Taylor, L., Hatton, C., Dixon, L., & Douglas, C. (2004). Screening for psychiatric symptoms: Pas-add checklist norms for adults with intellectual disabilities. *Journal of Intellectual Disability Research, 48*(1), 37–41. doi:10.1111/j.1365-2788.2004.00585.x PMID:14675229

To, T., Guttmann, A., Dick, P. T., Rosenfield, J. D., Parkin, P. C., Tassoudji, M., . . . Harris, J. K. (2004). Risk markers for poor developmental attainment in young children: results from a longitudinal national survey. *Archives of Pediatrics & Adolescent Medicine, 158*(7), 643-649.

Tonge, B., & Einfeld, S. (2000). The trajectory of psychiatric disorders in young people with intellectual disabilities. *Australian and New Zealand Journal of Psychiatry, 34*(1), 80-84.

Tonge, B., & Einfeld, S. L. (2003). Psychopathology and intellectual disability: the australian child to adult longitudinal study. *International Review of Research in Mental Retardation, 26*, 61-91.

Vereenooghe, L., Flynn, S., Hastings, R. P., Adams, D., Chauhan, U., Cooper, S.-A., . . . Jahoda, A. (2018). Interventions for mental health problems in children and adults with severe intellectual disabilities: a systematic review. *BMJ Open, 8*(6), e021911.

Weise, J., Fisher, K. R., & Trollor, J. N. (2018). What makes generalist mental health professionals effective when working with people with an intellectual disability? A family member and support person perspective. *Journal of Applied Research in Intellectual Disabilities, 31*(3), 413-422.

White, N., & Hastings, R. P. (2004). Social and professional support for parents of adolescents with severe intellectual disabilities. *Journal of Applied Research in Intellectual Disabilities, 17*(3), 181-190.

Whitehouse, J. O., Durkin, K., Jaquet, E., & Ziatas, K. (2009). Friendship, loneliness and depression in adolescents with asperger's syndrome. *Journal of Adolescence*, *32*(2), 309–322. doi:10.1016/j.adolescence.2008.03.004 PMID:18692233

Whitehouse, J. O., Watt, H. J., Line, E. A., & Bishop, D. V. M. (2009). Adult psychosocial outcomes of children with specific language impairment, pragmatic language impairment and autism. *International Journal of Language & Communication Disorders*, *44*(4), 511–528. doi:10.1080/13682820802708098 PMID:19340628

Whittle, L., Fisher, K. R., Reppermund, S., Lenroot, R., & Trollor, J. (2018). Barriers and enablers to accessing mental health services for people with intellectual disability: A scoping review. *Journal of Mental Health Research in Intellectual Disabilities*, *11*(1), 69–102. doi:10.1080/19315864.2017.1408724

Wong, J. G., Clare, I. C. H., Holland, A. J., Watson, P. C., & Gunn, M. (2000). The capacity of people with a 'mental disability' to make a health care decision. *Psychological Medicine, 30*(2), 295-306.

Woolfenden, S., Goldfeld, S., Raman, S., Eapen, V., Kemp, L., & Williams, K. (2013). Inequity in child health: the importance of early childhood development. *Journal of Paediatrics and Child Health, 49*(9), e365-e369.

Woolfenden, S., Williams, K., Eapen, V., Mensah, F., Hayen, A., Siddiqi, A., & Kemp, L. (2014). Developmental vulnerability–don't investigate without a model in mind. *Child: Care, Health and Development.*

Yeargin-Allsopp, M., Drews, C. D., Decouflé, P., & Murphy, C. C. (1995). Mild mental retardation in black and white children in metropolitan Atlanta: A case-control study. *American Journal of Public Health*, *85*(3), 324–328. doi:10.2105/AJPH.85.3.324 PMID:7892913

Young-Southward, G., Cooper, S.-A., & Philo, C. (2017). Health and wellbeing during transition to adulthood for young people with intellectual disabilities: A qualitative study. *Research in Developmental Disabilities*, *70*, 94–103. doi:10.1016/j.ridd.2017.09.003 PMID:28918309

Zeanah, H., Boris, N. W., & Larrieu, J. A. (1997). Infant development and developmental risk: A review of the past 10 years. *Journal of the American Academy of Child and Adolescent Psychiatry*, *36*(2), 165–178. doi:10.1097/00004583-199702000-00007 PMID:9031569

KEY TERMS AND DEFINITIONS

Cognitive-Behavioral Therapy: A type of psychotherapy that helps individuals to identify and teaches skills to modify unhelpful thinking patterns, feelings, and behaviors.

Indigenous Australians: The original inhabitants of the Australian continent and nearby islands, including Aboriginal people and Torres Strait Islanders.

Intellectual Disability: A disability characterized by significantly impaired intellectual and adaptive functioning, formerly known as mental retardation.

Multidisciplinary: Drawing on expertise from multiple disciplines to accurately define and manage complex situations including health concerns.

Chapter 3
School Bullying Among Students With Intellectual Disabilities:
Predictors, Outcomes, and Recommendations

Michelle F. Wright
Pennsylvania State University, USA

ABSTRACT

School bullying research began in the 1970s through seminal research conducted on these experiences among Norwegian boys. From this initial research, multiple studies have been conducted over the past 40 years, revealing the nature, extent, causes, and consequences of school bullying. More recent investigations have also focused on cyberbullying, bullying using information and communication technologies (e.g., cell phones). Little attention has been given to school bullying involvement among students with disabilities, particularly those with intellectual disabilities. The handful of studies on this topic suggest that these students experience internalizing (e.g., depression, anxiety, loneliness) and externalizing (e.g., aggression, antisocial behaviors) difficulties associated with their involvement in school bullying. The aim of this chapter is to review multidisciplinary research concerning school bullying among students with intellectual disabilities and to make recommendations for public policy and prevention programs as well as future research.

INTRODUCTION

Students with disabilities benefit from inclusion in the same schools as their nondisabled peers. Research findings also suggest that nondisabled peers benefit from this inclusion as well (Buckley, Bird, Sacks, & Archer, 2002; Lindsay & McPherson, 2012; Richardson, 1996; Sailor, Wolf, Choi, & Roger, 2009; Tomasik, 2007). Therefore, disabled and nondisabled students benefit from having an inclusive school environment where there is potential for social interactions among a variety of students with different

DOI: 10.4018/978-1-7998-1223-4.ch003

backgrounds. There is also evidence that such inclusion does not reduce test scores, grades, or instructional time, further suggesting the necessity of inclusion for students with disabilities (Sirlopu et al., 2008; Stahmer, Carter, Baker, & Miwa, 2003; Salend & Duhaney, 1999; York, Vandercook, MacDonald, Heise-Neff, & Caughey, 1992).

The total number of students with disabilities in inclusion education varies based on students' location within the United States. In particular, students from the Eastern United States are more frequently assigned to segregated classrooms (Kurth, 2014). In addition, some states (e.g., Iowa, Minnesota, West Virginia) favor inclusion, while other states (e.g., Florida, New Jersey, South Carolina) prefer the restrictive setting for students with disabilities. Overall, 50% of disabled students from the ages of 6 to 11 are

in regular classrooms around 80% of the day, while 30% of disabled students from the ages of 12 and higher are in such classrooms (Maryland Coalition for Inclusive Education, 2011). Regardless of the differences in these rates, it is clear that a variety of students with disabilities spend some time learning in the regular classroom.

Although there are benefits to the inclusion of students with disabilities in the school environment, additional attention is needed to promote a more welcoming environment as these students are often victims of school bullying (Mishna, 2003). Welcoming school environments are not always something students with disabilities experience as bullying is frequently a direct result of their disability, especially if the students' disability is more visible in inclusion environments (Verdugo, Bernejo, & Fuertes, 1995; Waldman, Swerdloff, & Perlman, 1999; Whitney, Smith & Thompson, 1994). In addition, students with disabilities are also rejected by their peers, a risk factor associated with victimization and bullying perpetration (Fox, 1989; Kistner & Gatlin, 1989; Martlew & Hodson, 1991; Morrison, Furlong, & Smith, 1994). Being rejected by one's peers can lead to isolation and other consequences, such as depression, loneliness, and anxiety. Furthermore, peer rejection can affect academic engagement and achievement, which are vital to the long-term functioning of these students.

Some students with disabilities are also vulnerable to school bullying involvement because they have inadequate protection in the inclusion environment and their tendency to react aggressively (Lagerheim, 1986; Nabuzoka & Smith, 1993; Sprafkin & Gadow, 1987). This inadequate protection stems from these students being socially rejected by their peers, which diminishes their odds of having good quality friendships, a protective factor associated with reduced bullying incidences. Reacting aggressively to benign situations or in situations when it is not warranted increases children's and adolescents' risk of being rejected by their peers. This increased risk also makes them vulnerable to victimization. Students with intellectual disabilities are also at risk for victimization because they have fewer resources to cope with this experience (Cunningham, Clark, Heaven, Durrant, & Cunningham, 1989; Lagerheim, 1986; Nabuzoka & Smith, 1993; Zeitlin & Williamson, 1990).

The purpose of this chapter is to examine school bullying perpetration and victimization among students with intellectual disabilities in elementary, middle, and high schools. The chapter utilizes multidisciplinary qualitative, quantitative, and mixed-design research methodologies drawn from psychology, special education, sociology, social work, and criminology to review research on students with intellectual disabilities' involvement in school bullying, incorporating both cross-sectional and longitudinal research designs.

This chapter has six main purposes, including describing:

- The Nature of School Bullying: Discussion of the definition, forms and types, prevalence rates, and associated psychosocial adjustment difficulties;

- The prevalence and consequences of school bullying among students with disabilities;
- The predictors of school bullying among students with intellectual disabilities;
- Solutions and Recommendations: Description of public policy and school bullying prevention programs concerning students with intellectual disabilities;
- Future Research Directions: The focus is on longitudinal research designs as well as recommending more research dedicated to understanding risk factors and protective factors associated with school bullying involvement among students with intellectual disabilities;
- Conclusion: Final remarks concerning the state of the literature on school bullying among students with intellectual disabilities.

The Nature of School Bullying

School bullying is a common experience for many students in the United States and throughout the world. It is defined as the intentional use of physical force or power against another person or group (Espelage & Swearer, 2003; Hemphill, Tollit, Kotevski, & Florent, 2015; Hong et al., 2014). It includes behaviors which cause physical and/or psychological harm and are perceived as unwanted by the target of these behaviors. Over the last forty years, research on school bullying has been evolving, providing an important foundation for understanding the nature, extent, causes, consequences, intervention strategies, and the prevention of these behaviors (Hymel & Swearer, 2015).

The recent attention given to school bullying by the public is the result of many high profile cases and news reports regarding school shootings and victims committing suicide. Although some of the research awareness and concern over school bullying is the result of the 1999 Columbine school shooting, the study of school bullying began in Norway during the 1970s. This systematic study of school bullying began with Olweus's 1973 book, *Aggression in the Schools: Bullies and Whipping Boys.* In his book, Olweus described boys' experiences with school bullying in Scandinavian countries. Most of the earliest research spurred by Olweus's book occurred across Europe as a result of the 1978 translation of his book into English. The book generated further interest and 10 years later the first European conference was held on school bullying. At this time, Olweus developed an intervention campaign designed to prevent school bullying among Norwegian students. Other European countries, like England, Wales, and Scotland, launched similarly designed intervention programs. A couple of years later, research and awareness began in Canada, the United States, Australia, and New Zealand. Most current research has focused attention on school bullying in Asia, Africa, and South America. The typically used definition of school bullying comes from Olweus's (1993) work. Like the definition provided in the previous paragraph, Olweus's definition emphasizes three essential elements of school bullying, including:

- The behavior is aggressive and negative (i.e., it is unwanted and causes emotional distress to the victim),
- The behavior is carried out repeatedly (i.e., it occurs often and over time), and
- The behavior occurs in a relationship where there is an imbalance of power between the individuals involved.

School bullying behaviors are further delineated into two modes, direct and indirect. Direct forms of school bullying include physical aggression in which the victim is openly attacked, while indirect forms include social exclusion or social rejection. Indirect forms of bullying are often employed by girls while direct forms are more often used by boys (Banks, 1997; Brighi, Guarini, Melotti, Galli, & Genta, 2012; Carbone-Lopez, Esbensen, & Brick, 2010; Carney & Merrell, 2001; Crick & Grotpeter, 1995; Ericson, 2001). Socialization processes throughout childhood and adolescence are thought to account for gender differences in the use of direct and indirect forms of bullying.

As a result of gender differences in bullying involvement, researchers argue that it is important to distinguish between indirect and direct forms of school bullying. Other researchers, like Underwood and colleagues (2001), suggest that referring to some school bullying behaviors as indirect implies that the behavior does not involve direct or overt interaction with the victim, which might diminish beliefs about the severity of this type of bullying. By diminishing the belief that indirect forms of bullying are severe, schools, parents, and students might not take these behaviors seriously and consider them harmful to victims' well-being. Instead of using the terminology of indirect bullying, some researchers utilize social aggression to categorize the indirect forms of school bullying that Olweus (1993) described.

As a result of the different forms of school bullying, researchers have categorized these behaviors into four types, including physical (e.g., pushing, hitting), verbal (e.g., name-calling), relational (e.g., exclusion, spreading rumors), and damage to property (Olthof & Goossens, 2008; Wang, Iannotti, Luk, & Nansel, 2010). Bullying can also include bullying in other contexts, such as those behaviors which occur electronically. Electronic forms of bullying are referred to as cyberbullying, and typically these behaviors are perpetrated or experienced through social networking websites, email, chatrooms, or chat programs (Lapidot & Dolev-Cohen, 2015; Waasdorp & Bradshaw, 2015). Sexual bullying is another type of bullying which can occur in the school setting. It occurs when a person is bullied based on his or her sex or sexual activity, and it can include physical, verbal, or emotional forms (Duncan, 1999).

Another important element of the school bullying definition is that the behaviors occur among school-aged students, 5 to 18 years of age, and it doesn't include aggression or bullying perpetrated by siblings. The definition also does not include bullying that might occur within romantic relationships. Furthermore, the definition excludes any bullying and abuse which might be perpetrated by adults or behaviors directed to adults. Children and adolescents can hold a variety of different roles in the bullying situation. They can be victims, bullies, bully-victims (both victim and perpetrator), bystanders (i.e., witnesses to the bullying situation), and uninvolved (Noorden, Haselager, Cillessen, & Bukowski, 2015; Psalti, 2012). Students experience a variety of academic and psychosocial adjustment consequences associated with the specific role they have in school bullying. In particular, bully-victims usually have the worst psychological, social, behavioral, and academic outcomes when compared to victims, bullies, bystanders, and uninvolved children and adolescents, with victims having worse outcomes than the other roles.

Prevalence rates of school bullying vary, depending on the definitions employed, samples used, the measurement of school bullying, and the age of the participants. Variations found in the general population range from 13% to 75% based on a variety of factors that impact students' reporting of school bullying (Swearer, Siebecker, Johnsen-Frerichs, & Wang, 2010). Usually, researchers report prevalence rates between 30% and 32%, with 10.6% of students categorized as victims, 13.0% as bullies, and 6.3% as bully-victims (Dinkes, Kemp, Baum, & Snyder, 2009; Nansel et al., 2001). Research has also revealed that boys were more likely to report victimizing others when compared to girls while girls were more likely to report being victimized (Charach, Pepler, & Ziegler, 1995; Craig & Pepler, 1995). However, when researchers specified different forms of bullying, girls were more often involved in relational forms, while boys were more often engaged in physical forms (Banks, 1997; Brighi et al., 2012; Carbone-Lopez et al., 2010; Carney & Merrell, 2001; Crick & Grotpeter,1995; Ericson, 2001). Furthermore, relational forms of school bullying increase in adolescence, while physical forms tend to decrease from childhood into adolescence (Boyes, Bowes, Cluver, Ward, & Badcock, 2014; Bradshaw, Waasdrop, & Johnson, 2015; Ryoo, Wang, & Swearer, 2015). Findings from these studies underscore the importance of considering both gender and age when examining school bullying involvement.

Researchers, parents, and educators are particularly concerned with school bullying because of its linkages to academic (e.g., poor academic achievement, lower academic engagement), behavioral (e.g., delinquency), and psychosocial (e.g., depression, anxiety, loneliness) adjustment difficulties. School bullying victimization is a strong predictor of interpersonal problems and internalizing emotional problems, such as anxiety, depression, and loneliness (Graham, Bellmore, & Mize, 2006; Hawker & Boulton, 2000; Kelly et al., 2015; Nishina, Juvonen, & Witkow, 2005; Perren, Dooley, Shaw, & Cross, 2010; Thomas et al., 2015). Such psychosocial problems contribute to victimized students' poor academic performance, often as a result of frequent absences from school and impaired concentration (Card & Hodges, 2008; Espelage, Low, & Jimerson, 2014; Hong et al., 2014; Nishina et al., 2005). Victims might not attend school because they fear further victimization. In addition, their concentration is impaired because they might repeatedly ruminate over their experience and be concerned about the chances of experiencing other attacks. Victimized students are also at risk for psychiatric problems and suicidal ideation (Dickerson Mayesa et al., 2014; Kumpulainen, Rasanen, & Puura, 2001; Rigby & Slee, 1991; Skapinakis et al., 2011). It is unclear whether victimization is a cause of psychiatric problems and suicidal ideation or whether psychiatric problems and suicidal ideation reduce children's and adolescents' coping abilities, leading them to be vulnerable to victimization. Many victimized children believe that they deserve to be bullied, which further contributes to the helplessness they feel, creating a vicious cycle of peer victimization. This cycle might make it difficult for them to believe that they can ever escape victimization.

Students who bully others also experience depression and suicidal ideation, and they are also at risk for antisocial behavioral tendencies, such as abusing drugs, drinking alcohol, and property theft (Hertz, Donato, & Wright, 2013; Kaltiala-Heino, Rimpela, Marttunen, Rimpela, & Rantanen, 1999; Cummings, Pepler, Mishna, & Craig, 2006). They also engage in academic misconduct, such as cheating and skipping school, and have lower academic achievement (Atik & Guneri, 2013; Berthold & Hoover, 2000; Carlson & Cornell, 2008; Rigby & Cox, 1996). Later in life, bullies are likely to be diagnosed with a psychiatric problem and to engage in substance abuse and criminal misconduct (Baldry & Farrington, 2000; Kumpulainen et al., 2001; Luukkonen, Riala, Hakko, & Rasanen, 2010; Nansel et al., 2001; Radliff, Wheaton, Robinson, & Morris, 2012; Rigby & Cox, 1996). Although there are overlaps in negative adjustment consequences between bullies and victims, there are differences in the type of consequences experienced. For instance, bullies typically experience more externalizing problems, while victims usually experience more internalizing problems.

Bully-victims experience the highest levels of these externalizing (e.g., antisocial behavior, rage, anger) and internalizing (e.g., depression, anxiety, loneliness) behaviors when compared to students who are either bullies or victims only (Kelly et al., 2015; Marini et al., 2009; Ozdemir & Stattin, 2011; Sansone & Sansone, 2008). Given that bully-victims experience elevated levels of internalizing and externalizing problems when compared to bullies and victims, it is imperative that researchers consider the multiple roles that students can have in school bullying.

Nowadays, the education of students with disabilities occurs in schools with their peers without disabilities. Because peer victimization is a concern in the school environment, researchers began to focus their attention on investigating the school bullying experiences of disabled students.

Prevalence and Consequences of School Bullying

Although many studies have been conducted on school bullying involvement among the general population of students, less attention has been given to examining students with disabilities' involvement in these behaviors, especially those with intellectual disabilities. The lack of attention to these students might be the result of the mistaken belief that such students cannot adequately express their opinions about their experiences with peers. As a result, some researchers might not include students with disabilities in their samples. Furthermore, ethical considerations might require special provisions for including students with disabilities in research, and many researchers might not have the resources necessary to ensure that they have the tools to aid in data collection that would allow these students' participation.

Most of the research on school bullying among students with disabilities utilizes school-aged samples of children and adolescents with disabilities between the ages of 5 and 18. Such research is important as there are consistent findings concerning students with disabilities being at an increased risk for school bullying when compared to their peers without disabilities (Rose, Espelage, & Monda-Amaya, 2009; Rose, Monda-Amaya, & Espelage, 2011; Sheard, Clegg, Standen, & Cromby, 2001). In particular, some research indicates that these students are more vulnerable to school bullying in comparison to nondisabled peers, while other research suggests that there are no differences in their risk for experiencing school bullying. The researchers that conclude that students with disabilities are more prone to school bullying propose that these students are at an increased risk for peer victimization because they have fewer resources to cope with this experience. Having better coping strategies makes it easier for students with disabilities to handle the challenges that they encounter and to "bounce back" from such challenges. When compared to the general population of students, students with disabilities are 5 times more likely to report victimization by school bullying (Rose et al., 2009; Rose et al., 2011). In addition, research indicates that students with disabilities were more likely to experience peer victimization when placed in remedial classes and regular education classes when compared to students without disabilities. To explain these results, Rose and colleagues (2009, 2011) proposed that these students' physical or mental disability makes them particularly salient in the classroom, increasing the likelihood that they will be noticed and that others will be aware that they are different in some way. Being different from the average, might heightened the chance that students with disabilities will be victimized.

In one of the few longitudinal studies to examine school bullying among students with disabilities, students between the ages of 3 and 6 were followed for three years (Son, Parish, & Peterson, 2012). Employing parent reports, Son and colleagues found that 19% of 3 and 4 years old experienced one or more types of peer victimization, and that 25% of 5 years old experienced one or more types of peer victimization. The experience of peer victimization increased to 30% at the age of 6. The developmental trajectory of peer victimization reveals increases in these experiences from elementary to middle school, with declines beginning in early high school. Similar to their peers without disabilities' experiences with school bullying, peer victimization peaks in middle school. The patterns concerning the increase in peer victimization experiences from ages 3 to 6 is not unique among students with disabilities, but the odds of exposure are a bit higher than among students without disabilities. In particular, 34.1% of students with disabilities in one sample reported peer victimization compared with 24.5% in elementary school and 26.6% in high school (Blake et al., 2012). Other research revealed that rates of victimization among children with disabilities peaked in 3rd grade and declined afterward, somewhat in contrast to findings from the previous research (Bear, Mantz, Glutting, Yang, & Boyer, 2015).

So far, only one study has examined the prevalence rates of cyberbullying involvement among students with intellectual disabilities. In their study, Didden et al. (2009) found that between 4% and 9% of students with intellectual disabilities were involved in cyberbullying as either the perpetrator or the victim. Students with disabilities are also at an elevated risk of school bullying perpetration (Carter & Spencer, 2006; Doren, Bullis, & Benz, 1996; Estell et al., 2009; Rose et al., 2009; Whitney et al., 1994). Students with disabilities also report more incidences of physical bullying, sexual abuse, and emotional abuse (Cappadocia, Weiss, & Pepler, 2012; Mishna, 2003; Reiter, Bryen, & Shachar, 2007). For example, Whitney and colleagues (1994) found that one-third of students with disabilities in their sample engaged in school bullying perpetration when compared to one-sixth of students without disabilities. In another study comparing prevalence rates between students with disabilities and students without, Dickson and colleagues (2005) found that 28% of students with disabilities in their sample reported being victims of school bullying when compared to 9.8% of students without. Given that students with disabilities are more likely to be exposed to school bullying, they might experience extreme distress from such exposure. This distress might reduce their ability to deal with peer victimization, making them utilize ineffective coping strategies. One such way they might cope with peer victimization is by aggressing against others, maybe even those responsible for their victimization.

Thus far, much of the research reviewed on school bullying perpetration among students with disabilities did not specify whether school bullying was a function of revenge, specifically that the bully was retaliating against someone who had previously bullied him or her first. This provoked type of school bullying is more common among students with disabilities, and they are more often classified as bully-victims (Carter & Spencer, 2006; Reiter & Lapidot-Lefler, 2007; Roberts & Smith, 1999; Whitney et al., 1994; Van Cleave & Davis, 2006). Considering that students with disabilities are at risk for being bully-victims, it is important for research to focus more attention on these students' experiences with school bullying as bully-victims experience the worse psychological, social, behavioral, and academic consequences when compared to victims and bullies only. Thus, students with disabilities who are bully-victims might be at an elevated risk for these consequences.

The statistics discussed in the previous paragraphs involve studies in which researchers combined samples of students with physical disabilities as well as intellectual and social disabilities without delineating different types of disability (Dawkins, 1996; Llewellyn, 2000). Such a consideration is important as risk factors associated with disability, like aggressiveness, anger, hostility, low impulsive control, hyperactivity, poor social information processing, poor social skills, low self-esteem, and social rejection, are what contribute to school bullying involvement, and these factors vary depending on the specific type of disability (Kavale & Forness, 1995; Kavale & Forness, 1996; Lewandowski & Barlow, 2000; McNamara, Willoughby, Chalmers, & YLC-CURA, 2005; Nabuzoka, 2003; Rose & Espelage, 2012).

Therefore, it is important to take into consideration the type of disability that students might have when examining their experience of school bullying. Students with intellectual disabilities typically have more problems with anger, aggression, information processing, and self-control than students with other types of disabilities (Jahoda, Pert, & Trower, 2006a; Jahoda, Pert, & Trower, 2006b; Novaco & Taylor, 2004). Among students with mild developmental and intellectual disabilities, Reiter and Lapidot-Lefler (2007) found that half of the 12 through 18 year old students in their sample were involved in school bullying as perpetrators. About 83% of students in their sample were victims of physical, social, and verbal forms of school bullying. Similar patterns were found in later studies, citing prevalence rates between 50% and 80% among students with mild developmental and intellectual disabilities (Emerson, 2010; Glumbic & Zunic-Pavlovic, 2010). It is often difficult to compare school bullying experiences for students with different disabilities, due to the challenging with sampling and having access to students with these disabilities.

Variations in prevalence rates might be the result of measurement and definitional differences among the studies. Despite such variations, it is clear that researchers need to delineate the type of disability when examining school bullying. Such a consideration is also important for research comparing students with disabilities to students without disabilities. The research is mixed as to whether students with intellectual disabilities are more at risk for peer victimization in special education placement settings or inclusive placement settings. In particular, research indicates that rates of peer victimization are much higher in more restrictive special education placements (Norwich & Kelly, 2004; Rose et al., 2009), while other studies reveal that inclusive placement relates to greater school bullying involvement (Sterzing, Shattuck, Narendorf, Wagner, & Cooper, 2012; Whitney, Nabuzoka, & Smith, 1992; Zablotsky, Bradshaw, Anderson, & Law, 2013). Furthermore, research on cyberbullying suggested that placement in special education settings increased the risk of cyberbullying involvement among students with intellectual disabilities (Didden et al., 2009). Additional research attention should be given to understanding their experience of cyberbullying as children and adolescents, even students with intellectual disabilities, are spending more time utilizing information and communication technologies, a known risk factor associated with cyberbullying involvement (Flander, Stimac, Bagaric, & Vinscak, 2014; Kopecky, 2014; Lindfors, Kaltiala-Heino, & Rimpela, 2012; Mishna, Khoury-Kassabri, Gadalla, & Daciuk, 2012; Sourander et al., 2010). Biased-based cyberbullying involving hate-filled speech and/or teasing regarding disabilities is something that students with intellectual disabilities might experience. Studies on cyberbullying among these students often assess their experiences more generally. It might be a fruitful direction in this research to also examine the specific types of cyberbullying they experience as cyberbullying based on disability can be experienced by these students.

Students with disabilities are at risk for a variety of adjustment difficulties resulting from their involvement in school bullying. In this literature, students with disabilities experience depression, anger, hostility, and lower self-esteem as a result of their bullying involvement, no matter their role as victims or perpetrators (Bauminger, Solomon, & Rogers, 2010; Larkin, Jahoda, MacMahon, & Pert, 2012; Rose, Forber-Pratt, Espelage, & Aragon, 2013). Similar patterns were found for victims and perpetrators of cyberbullying (Didden et al., 2009). They also experience increased levels of loneliness, delinquency, greater difficulties in their social interactions with their peers, and higher levels of social exclusion and peer rejection (Andreou, Didaskalou, & Vlachou, 2013; Jahoda et al., 2012; Nadeau & Tessier, 2006; Pearl & Bay, 1999). In addition, Davis and Nixon (2010) found that students with disabilities were more likely to experience severe trauma as a result of peer victimization when compared to students without disabilities. The associations between adjustment difficulties and school bullying are much stronger when students with disabilities are identified as bully-victims. In particular, Farmer and colleagues (2012) found that students with disabilities who were classified as bully-victims were at an increased risk for experiencing emotional (e.g., depression) and behavioral (e.g., antisocial behavior) problems when compared to students who were identified as either victims or bullies. Taken together, this research indicates that more consideration should be given to predictors of students with disabilities' involvement in school bullying as understanding such predictors can help identify students who are at an increased risk for experiencing these behaviors. Identification of these students is important as specific intervention strategies can be implemented to mitigate their involvement in school bullying. In addition, identifying such students could help with including them in school bullying prevention programs.

Predictors of School Bullying

Little attention has been given to the risk factors related to students with intellectual disabilities' involvement in school bullying. In the literature, behavioral problems (e.g., uncontrolled anger) are risk factors associated with school bullying perpetration among students with disabilities (Reiter & Lapidot-Lefler, 2007). In particular, temper tantrums, unruly and quarrelsome behavior, and a tendency to lie and steal increase these students' school bullying involvement as bullies and as bully-victims. Other findings revealed that emotional and interpersonal problems (e.g., poor social skills) increase these students' vulnerability to peer victimization. Their higher levels of depression, anxiety, and loneliness, and frequent conflicts within their friendships are significant predictors of peer victimization as well (Matheson, Olsen, & Weisner, 2007; Zeedyk, Rodriguez, Tipton, Baker, & Blacher, 2014). Students with intellectual disabilities also have lower adaptive behaviors and poorer social skills (i.e., social problems, social withdrawal), which increase their risk for peer victimization (Neece & Baker, 2008). Because they have lower adaptive behavioral skills, students with disabilities might not be able to effectively deal with changes in their routine, which could reduce their ability to cope with changes. Their reduced capacity to cope might increase their susceptibility to peer victimization. Furthermore, having poorer social skills might also increase students with intellectual disabilities' saliency in the peer group as well. Individuals from the peer group might notice the lack of social skills among students with intellectual disabilities, subsequently perceiving these students as targets, especially easy targets, for school bullying. Prevention and intervention programs should be designed to help students with intellectual disabilities develop adaptive coping strategies to deal with school bullying. It might be even more helpful for these programs to be part of the classroom curriculum.

Another study found that poor social skills increased students with intellectual disabilities' susceptibility to peer victimization from middle childhood through early adolescence (Christensen, Fraynt, Neece, & Baker, 2012). Given that bullying increases in early adolescence, it might be likely that having poor social skills increases these students' vulnerability to peer victimization. Findings from Christensen et al. (2012) demonstrate the need for social skills training programs for these students as a lack of such skills perpetuates the cycle of peer victimization. A fruitful direction in this area of study is for researchers to consider implementing social skills training for all students, especially those with intellectual disabilities. Many times, prevention and intervention programs do not include students with intellectual disabilities. This is a limitation as they might benefit from such programs to reduce their risk of experiencing school bullying. Therefore, it is important for schools, parents, researchers, and the government to join together to help mitigate students with disabilities' involvement in school bullying.

SOLUTIONS AND RECOMMENDATIONS

To better understand and prevent school bullying among students with intellectual disabilities, federal programs should be developed to help fund research and bullying prevention incentives (Flynt & Morton, 2007). Access to funding can make conducting research on bullying among students with intellectual disabilities more feasible for researchers who might not have the funds necessary to revise data collection tools to fit this population. Furthermore, increased funding can also help researchers design more large-scale projects devoted to understanding more about school bullying among students with intellectual disabilities. Funding might also make it possible for researchers to purchase reusable means of data collection methods. For example, funds for school bullying research could be used to purchase devices (e.g., iPads) that can be used and reused for data collection purposes. The purchasing of such devices might also be attractive for funders because it might provide an alternative and much cheaper option for data collection from students with intellectual disabilities. With grant funding, researchers are also able to collect better data with more representative samples of students with intellectual disabilities, which strengths the results of such research.

Research plays a major role in the development of bullying prevention programs and additional funds should be allocated to better serve students with intellectual disabilities in anti-bullying efforts. Individualized Education Programs could also be a source of bullying prevention. Expanding technical assistance within these programs can help to protect students with intellectual disabilities from school bullying involvement as well as provide effective ways for addressing specific bullying behaviors relatedto students' disabilities. Furthermore, school-wide bullying prevention programs should be modified to accommodate students with intellectual disabilities in an effort to guarantee that these students benefit from such programs. Most bullying prevention and intervention strategies have not been empirically evaluated for application to students with intellectual disabilities. However, the available programs do have some evidence that they decrease anger as well as school bullying victimization and perpetration among students with intellectual disabilities (Rose, West, & Clifford, 2000; Whitney et al., 1994). Many programs are designed and implemented for use with students without disabilities. Therefore, the application and effectiveness of such programs for students with intellectual disabilities is untestable, making the implementation of these programs particularly problematic, especially if the cost of implementation is high. With funding, it might be possible to conduct more elaborative studies to evaluate and determine the effectiveness of school bullying programs for students with intellectual disabilities. This could involve being able to conduct more detailed randomized controlled trials of these school bullying programs. Such a "gold standard" of assessment might increase the likelihood that such programs are evaluated properly. Funding can also help with the dissemination of these programs as researchers might be able to include more schools and students to have a more representative sample of students with intellectual disabilities and other disabilities.

Social policy should also mandate the development of a system used to notify parents of incidences involving school bullying. The aims of such a system would be to notify parents of their children's involvement in bullying, as either victims or perpetrators, as well as when other children are involved in these incidences. This notification system might be especially important for students with intellectual disabilities who might have communication issues which could prevent their reporting of school bullying incidences to their parents. For instance, an incident might have occurred at school, but parents could only have an awareness of the event, not really knowing what really happened. It might be difficult for a student with intellectual disabilities to explain the event to their parents, which might make parents panic. Receiving information from the notification system might reduce parents' worries and their complaints to schools. The system could also allow parents to report incidences of school bullying that their child might experience. It might be easier for them to utilize a website to "log" their complaint, even with identifying information, than to come to the school campus to discuss with school staff. Parents are busy and so are school staff, and having such a system might streamline the process, making it easier for parents to report incidences at all times and for school staff to review these incidences at any time as well.

FUTURE RESEARCH DIRECTIONS

Based on the literature reviewed in this chapter, there are some clear gaps concerning students with intellectual disabilities' involvement in school bullying that should be addressed in future research. First, much of the literature involves cross-sectional designs, making it difficult to draw conclusions concerning the long-term extent, causes, and consequences of school bullying among students with intellectual disabilities. Such research can determine the risk factors associated with school bullying involvement and the long-term outcomes of students with intellectual disabilities' involvement as bullies and victims. Furthermore, this longitudinal research will shed light on whether students with intellectual disabilities experience more severe consequences associated with their involvement in school bullying when compared to their peers without intellectual disabilities. Longitudinal designs will also be helpful for testing prevention and intervention programs that are specifically designed for students with intellectual disabilities. With the advances in information and communication technologies, it is possible to better control attrition rates associated with longitudinal designs and to more cheaply facilitate longitudinal data collection with students who have intellectual disabilities.

Much of the research does not compare school bullying involvement among students with different intellectual disabilities, which is important as some individuals might be more susceptible to these behaviors when compared to other individuals with intellectual disabilities. That is, students with physical disabilities might experience school bullying at different rates when compared to students with intellectual disabilities. This knowledge might also be important for the development of more sensitive prevention and intervention programs. In addition, some disabilities might differentially relate to different risks for school bullying involvement from childhood to adolescence, as well as increase the severity of adjustment difficulties related to school bullying. For example, students with physical disabilities might experience different levels of psychological, social, behavioral, and academic difficulties after experiencing school bullying in comparison to students with intellectual disabilities. It might be difficult to have the sample size necessary to compare students with different types of disabilities but with the increasing availability of online data collection methods it might be possible to "cast a wider net" for having a representative sample. Furthermore, the advances in information and communication technologies also make it possible to accommodate students with different disabilities. More about the role of information and communication technologies in data collection with students who have disabilities is discussed at the end of this section.

Even students with intellectual disabilities are online and utilize other information and communication technologies. Such use increases their risk of negative experiences online, such as cyberbullying. Furthermore, oftentimes experiences online overlap into experiences offline; that is, victims of school bullying are often victims of cyberbullying, and typically cyberbullying incidences involve peers from the same school. Few studies have focused on cyberbullying among students with intellectual disabilities, or even other disabilities. Longitudinal studies on this topic are also limited as well. Therefore, researchers should focus on the predictors and long-term outcomes of cyberbullying among students with intellectual disabilities. Objective assessments of technology use might be a fruitful direction in this future research because it allows a more accurate assessment. It might also be appropriate to include other informants when assessing risk factors and long-term outcomes of cyberbullying for students with intellectual disabilities. Such informants might include teachers, peers, and parents. This research might also aim to determine if there are unique or different risk factors and outcomes of cyberbullying for students with disabilities versus general education students.

Another topic worth investigating is the role of protective factors. It is currently unknown whether there are protective factors associated with school bullying among students with intellectual disabilities. Understanding these protective factors might benefit the development of prevention programs and intervention strategies as they can be promoted to reduce these students' involvement in school bullying. Raising awareness of protective factors that can reduce involvement with school bullying and the negative psychological consequences of school bullying is important as schools and parents can implement new strategies to address this problem. This research will also address a gap in the literature on protective factors associated with school bullying among students with intellectual disabilities, as much of the existing literature focuses on risk factors.

Another important future direction for this research is to consider the intersection of different experiences with studying school bullying among students who have intellectual disabilities. The intellectual disability might not be the only experience that could alter this students' experience with school bullying. For example, consider Mary who has Downs Syndrome. However, Mary is also African American whose family is of the Muslim faith. Being an African American student and of the Muslim religion might also represent other characteristics of Mary that could increase her risk for school bullying. Therefore, with increasing ability to assess students with intellectual disabilities, researchers might want to consider assessing other characteristics of these students to further understand their experiences of school bullying.

Methodology it can be challenging to include students with intellectual disabilities or other disabilities in research. Failing to include these students in studies on school bullying does not allow for students with intellectual disabilities experiences and unique voices to be heard. With the explosion of information and communication technologies, it might be possible for researchers to overcome the challenges associated with conducting research with these students. Technology could be used as a data collection method and it could be used to facilitate data collection. For example, using an iPad with an online survey that can be read to the students can overcome issues associated with reading comprehension. It also might be easier to use these devices to make data collection easier for use with students who have some sort of physical issue, along with their intellectual disability. Devices could be used to increase font size of text as well for students with visual disabilities. Another benefit of information and communication technologies is that such devices can be utilized multiple times with different samples of students with intellectual disabilities. It can be expensive to incorporate technology in data collection, but with increasing focus on funding for researchers interested in providing comprehensive assessments of school bullying, it might be more feasible to purchase such devices.

CONCLUSION

In summary, the literature reveals that students with intellectual disabilities are involved in school bullying as victims, perpetrators, and bully-victims. Furthermore, the research also suggests that they experience victimization by school bullying more often than their peers without intellectual disabilities. They also have similar risk factors and adjustment difficulties related to their experience of school bullying as their nondisabled peers. More research needs to be conducted to provide a better understanding of students with disabilities' involvement in school bullying and the associated risk factors and psychosocial adjustment difficulties. Such research is important as it serves as a foundation for the much needed policies and prevention and intervention programs aimed at reducing school bullying involvement among students with intellectual disabilities.

REFERENCES

Andreou, E., Didaskalou, E., & Vlachou, A. (2013). Bully/victim problems among Greek pupils with special educational needs: Associations with loneliness and self-efficacy for peer interactions. *Journal of Research in Special Educational Needs.*

Atik, G., & Guneri, O. Y. (2013). Bullying and victimization: Predictive role of individual, parental, and academic factors. *School Psychology International*, *34*(6), 658–673. doi:10.1177/0143034313479699

Baldry, A. C., & Farrington, D. (2000). Bullies and delinquents: Personal characteristics and parental styles. *Journal of Community & Applied Social Psychology*, *10*(1), 17–31. doi:10.1002/(SICI)1099-1298(200001/02)10:1<17::AID-CASP526>3.0.CO;2-M

Banks, R. (1997). *Bullying in Schools.* Washington, DC: U.S. Government Printing Office.

Bauminger, N., Solomon, M., & Rogers, S. J. (2010). Externalizing and internalizing behaviors in ASD. *Autism Research*, *3*(3), 101–112. doi:10.1002/aur.131 PMID:20575109

Bear, G. G., Mantz, L. S., Glutting, J. J., Yang, C., & Boyer, D. E. (2015). Differences in bullying victimization between students with and without disabilities. *School Psychology Review*, *44*(1), 98–116. doi:10.17105/SPR44-1.98-116

Berthold, K., & Hoover, J. (2000). Correlates of bullying and victimization among intermediate students in Midwestern USA. *School Psychology International*, *21*(1), 65–79. doi:10.1177/0143034300211005

Blake, J. J., Lund, E. M., Zhou, Q., Kwok, O., & Benz, M. (2012). National prevalence rates of bully victimization among students with disabilities in the United States. *School Psychology Quarterly*, *27*(4), 2100–2222. doi:10.1037pq0000008 PMID:23294235

Boyes, M. E., Bowes, L., Cluver, L. C., Ward, C. L., & Badcock, N. A. (2014). Bullying victimization, internalizing symptoms, and conduct problems in South African children and adolescents: A longitudinal investigation. *Journal of Abnormal Child Psychology*, *42*(8), 1313–1324. doi:10.100710802-014-9888-3 PMID:24882504

Bradshaw, C. P., Waasdorp, T. E., & Johnson, S. L. (2015). Overlapping verbal, relational, physical, and electronic forms of bullying in adolescence: Influence of school context. *Journal of Clinical Child and Adolescent Psychology*, *44*(3), 494–508. doi:10.1080/15374416.2014.893516 PMID:24738548

Brighi, A., Guarini, A., Melotti, G., Galli, S., & Genta, M. L. (2012). Predictors of victimization across direct bullying, indirect bullying and cyberbullying. *Emotional & Behavioural Difficulties*, *17*(3-4), 375–388. doi:10.1080/13632752.2012.704684

Buckley, S., Bird, G., Sacks, B., & Archer, T. (2002). A comparison of mainstream and special school education for teenagers with Down syndrome: Effects of social and academic development. *Down's Syndrome: Research and Practice*, *2*(2), 46–54.

Cappadocia, M. C., Weiss, J. A., & Pepler, D. (2012). Bullying experiences among children and youth with autism spectrum disorders. *Journal of Autism and Developmental Disorders*, *42*(2), 266–277. doi:10.100710803-011-1241-x PMID:21499672

Carbone-Lopez, K., Esbensen, F. A., & Brick, B. T. (2010). Correlates and consequences of peer victimization: Gender differences in direct and indirect forms of bullying. *Youth Violence and Juvenile Justice*, *8*(4), 332–350. doi:10.1177/1541204010362954

Card, N. A., & Hodges, E. V. E. (2008). Peer victimization among schoolchildren: Correlations, causes, consequences, and considerations in assessment and intervention. *School Psychology Quarterly*, *23*(4), 451–461. doi:10.1037/a0012769

Carlson, I. W., & Cornell, D. W. (2008). Differences between persistent and desistent middle school bullies. *School Psychology International*, *29*(4), 442–451. doi:10.1177/0143034308096433

Carney, A., & Merrell, K. (2001). Bullying in schools: Perspectives on understanding and preventing an international problem. *School Psychology International*, *21*(3), 364–382. doi:10.1177/0143034301223011

Carter, B. B., & Spencer, V. G. (2006). The Fear Factor: Bullying and Students with Disabilities. *International Journal of Special Education*, *21*(1). Retrieved from http://www.forockids.org/PDF Docs/Bullying.pdf

Charach, A., Pepler, D., & Ziegler, S. (1995). Bullying at school. *Education Canada*, *37*, 12–18.

Christensen, L., Fraynt, B., Neece, C. L., & Baker, B. L. (2012). Bullying adolescents with intellectual disability. *Journal of Mental Health Research in Intellectual Disabilities*, *5*(1), 49–65. doi:10.1080/19315864.2011.637660

Craig, W. M., & Pepler, D. J. (1995). Peer processes in bullying and victimization: An observational study. *Exceptionality Education Canada*, *5*, 81–95.

Crick, N. R., & Grotpeter, J. K. (1995). Relational aggression, gender, and social-psychological adjustment. *Child Development*, *66*(3), 710–722. doi:10.2307/1131945 PMID:7789197

Cummings, J., Pepler, D. J., Mishna, F., & Craig, W. M. (2006). Bullying and victimization among children with exceptionalities. *Exceptionality Education Canada*, *16*, 193–222.

Cunningham, C. E., Clark, M. L., Heaven, R. K., Durrant, J., & Cunningham, L. H. (1989). The effects of coping-modelling problem solving and contingency management procedures on the positive and negative interactions of learning disabled and attention deficit disordered children with an autistic peer. *Child & Family Behavior Therapy*, *11*(3-4), 89–106. doi:10.1300/J019v11n03_06

Davis, S., & Nixon, C. (2010). *The youth voice research project: Victimization and strategies*. Retrieved from: http://njbullying.org/documents/YVPMarch2010.pdf

Dawkins, J. L. (1996). Bullying, physical disability and the pediatric patient. *Developmental Medicine and Child Neurology*, *38*(7), 603–612. doi:10.1111/j.1469-8749.1996.tb12125.x PMID:8674911

Dickerson Mayes, S., Baweja, R., Calhoun, S. L., Syed, E., Mahr, F., & Siddiqui, F. (2014). Suicide ideation and attempts and bullying in children and adolescents: Psychiatric and general population samples. *Crisis*, *35*(5), 301–309. doi:10.1027/0227-5910/a000264 PMID:25115491

Dickson, K., Emerson, E., & Hatton, C. (2005). Self-reported anti-social behaviour: Prevalence and risk factors amongst adolescents with and without intellectual disability. *Journal of Intellectual Disability Research*, *49*(11), 820–826. doi:10.1111/j.1365-2788.2005.00727.x PMID:16207279

Didden, R., Scholte, R. H. J., Korzilius, H., De Moor, J. M. H., Vermeulen, A., O'Reilly, M., & Lancioni, G. E. (2009). Cyberbullying among students with intellectual and developmental disability in special education settings. *Developmental Neurorehabilitation*, *12*(3), 146–151. doi:10.1080/17518420902971356 PMID:19466622

Dinkes, R., Kemp, J., Baum, K., & Snyder, T. (2009). *Indicators of school crime and safety: 2009 (NCES 2010–012/NCJ 228478)*. Washington, DC: National Center for Education Statistics, Institute of Education Sciences, U.S. Department of Education, and Bureau of Justice Statistics, Office of Justice Programs, U.S. Department of Justice.

Doren, B., Bullis, M., & Benz, M. R. (1996). Predictors of victimization: Experiences of adolescents with disabilities in transition. *Exceptional Children*, *63*(1), 7–18. doi:10.1177/001440299606300101

Duncan, N. (1999). *Sexual bullying: Gender conflict and pupil culture in secondary schools*. New York, NY: Routledge.

Emerson, E. (2010). Self-reported exposure to disablism is associated with poorer self-reported health and well-being among adults with intellectual disabilities in England: A cross-sectional survey. *Public Health*, *124*(12), 682–689. doi:10.1016/j.puhe.2010.08.020 PMID:21035153

Ericson, N. (2001). *Addressing the problem of juvenile bullying*. Washington, DC: U.S. Government Printing Office; doi:10.1037/e317892004-001

Espelage, D. L., Low, S. K., & Jimerson, S. R. (2014). Understanding school climate, aggression, peer victimization, and bully perpetration: Contemporary science, practice, and policy. *School Psychology Quarterly*, *29*(3), 233–237. doi:10.1037pq0000090 PMID:25198615

Espelage, D. L., & Swearer, S. M. (2003). Research on school bullying and victimization: What have we learned and where do we go from here? *School Psychology Review*, *32*, 365–383.

Estell, D. B., Farmer, T. W., Irvin, M. J., Crowther, A., Akos, P., & Boudah, D. J. (2009). Students with exceptionalities and the peer group context of bullying and victimization in late elementary school. *Journal of Child and Family Studies*, *18*(2), 136–150. doi:10.100710826-008-9214-1

Farmer, T. W., Irvin, M. J., Motoca, L. M., Leung, M., Hutchins, B. C., Brooks, D. S., & Hall, C. M. (2015). Externalizing and internalizing behavior problems, peer affiliations, and bullying involvement across the transition to middle school. *Journal of Emotional and Behavioral Disorders*, *23*(1), 3–16. doi:10.1177/1063426613491286

Farmer, T. W., Petrin, R., Brooks, D. S., Hamm, J. V., Lambert, K., & Gravelle, M. (2012). Bullying involvement and the school adjustment of rural students with and without disabilities. *Journal of Emotional and Behavioral Disorders*, *20*(1), 19–37. doi:10.1177/1063426610392039

Flander, G. B., Stimac, D., Bagaric, E. S., & Vinscak, M. (2014). Patterns of and copying with cyberbullying in Croatia. *International Journal of Person Centered Medicine*.

Flynt, S. W., & Morton, R. C. (2007). Bullying prevention and students with disabilities. *National Forum of Special Education Journal, 19*(1), 1-6.

Fox, C. L. (1989). Peer acceptance of learning disabled children in the regular classroom. *Exceptional Children, 56*(1), 50–59. doi:10.1177/001440298905600108

Glumbic, N., & Zunic-Pavlovic, V. (2010). Bullying behavior in children with intellectual disability. *Procedia: Social and Behavioral Sciences, 2*(2), 2784–2788. doi:10.1016/j.sbspro.2010.03.415

Graham, S., Bellmore, A. D., & Mize, J. (2006). Peer victimization, aggression, and their co-occurrence in middle school: Pathways to adjustment problems. *Journal of Abnormal Child Psychology, 34*(3), 363–378. doi:10.100710802-006-9030-2 PMID:16648999

Hawker, D. S., & Boulton, M. J. (2000). Twenty years' research on peer victimization and psychosocial maladjustment: A meta-analytic review of cross sectional studies. *Journal of Child Psychology and Psychiatry, and Allied Disciplines, 41*(4), 441–455. doi:10.1111/1469-7610.00629 PMID:10836674

Hemphill, S. A., Tollit, M., Kotevski, A., & Florent, A. (2015). Bullying in schools: Rates, correlates and impact on mental health. In J. Lindert & I. Itzhak (Eds.), *Violence and mental health: Its manifold faces* (pp. 185–205). Springer.

Hertz, M. F., Donato, I., & Wright, J. (2013). Bullying and suicide: A public health approach. *The Journal of Adolescent Health, 53*(1), S1–S3. doi:10.1016/j.jadohealth.2013.05.002 PMID:23790194

Hong, J. S., Davis, J. P., Sterzing, P. R., Yoon, J., Choi, S., & Smith, D. C. (2014). A conceptual framework for understanding the association between school bullying victimization and substance misuse. *The American Journal of Orthopsychiatry, 84*(6), 696–710. doi:10.1037/ort0000036 PMID:25545436

Hong, J. S., Peguero, A. A., Choi, S., Lanesskog, D., Espelage, D. L., & Lee, N. Y. (2014). Social ecology of bullying and peer victimization of Latino and Asian youth in the United States: A review of the literature. *Journal of School Violence, 13*(3), 315–338. doi:10.1080/15388220.2013.856013

Hymel, S., & Swearer, S. M. (2015). Four decades of research on school bullying. *The American Psychologist, 70*(4), 293–299. doi:10.1037/a0038928 PMID:25961310

Jahoda, A., Pert, C., & Trower, P. (2006a). Socioemotional understanding and frequent aggression in people with mild to moderate intellectual disabilities: Recognition of facial affect and role-taking abilities. *American Journal of Mental Retardation, 111*(2), 77–89. doi:10.1352/0895-8017(2006)111[77:SUAFAI]2.0.CO;2 PMID:16466287

Jahoda, A., Pert, C., & Trower, P. (2006b). Frequent aggression and attribution of hostile intent in people with mild to moderate intellectual disabilities: An empirical investigation. *American Journal of Mental Retardation, 111*(2), 90–99. doi:10.1352/0895-8017(2006)111[90:FAAAOH]2.0.CO;2 PMID:16466288

Kaltiala-Heino, R., Rimpela, M., Marttunen, M., Rimpela, A., & Rantanen, P. (1999). Bullying, depression, and suicidal ideation in Finnish adolescents: School survey. *British Medical Journal, 319*(7206), 438–451. doi:10.1136/bmj.319.7206.348 PMID:10435954

Kavale, K. A., & Forness, S. R. (1995). Social skill deficits and training: A meta-analysis of the research in learning disabilities. *Advances in Learning and Behavioral Disabilities, 9*, 119–160.

Kavalc, K. A., & Forness, S. R. (1996). Social skill deficits and learning disabilities: A meta-analysis. *Journal of Learning Disabilities*, *29*(3), 226–237. doi:10.1177/002221949602900301 PMID:8732884

Kelly, E. V., Newton, N. C., Stapinski, L. A., Slade, T., Barrett, E. L., Conrod, P. J., & Teesson, M. (2015). Suicidality, internalizing problems and externalizing problems among adolescent bullies, victims and bully-victims. *Preventive Medicine*, *73*, 100–105. doi:10.1016/j.ypmed.2015.01.020 PMID:25657168

Kistner, J. A., & Gatlin, D. F. (1989). Sociometric differences between learning-disabled and non-handicapped students: Effects of sex and race. *Journal of Educational Psychology*, *81*(1), 118–120. doi:10.1037/0022-0663.81.1.118

Kopecky, K. (2014). Cyberbullying and other risks of internet communication focused on university students. *Procedia: Social and Behavioral Sciences*, *112*, 260–269. doi:10.1016/j.sbspro.2014.01.1163

Kumpulainen, K., Rasanen, E., & Puura, K. (2001). Psychiatric disorders and the use of mental health services among children involved in bullying. *Aggressive Behavior*, *27*(2), 102–110. doi:10.1002/ab.3

Kurth, J. A. (2014). Educational placement of students with autism: The impact of state of residence. *Focus on Autism and Other Developmental Disabilities*.

Lagerheim, B. (1986). Preparing disabled children for coping with adolescent stress. *International Journal of Adolescent Medicine and Health*, *2*(4), 309–316.

Lapidot-Lefler, N., & Dolev-Cohen, M. (2015). Comparing cyberbullying and school bullying among school students: Prevalence, gender, and grade level differences. *Social Psychology of Education*, *18*(1), 1–16. doi:10.100711218-014-9280-8

Larkin, P., Jahoda, A., MacMahon, K., & Pert, C. (2012). Interpersonal sources of conflict in young people with and without mild to moderate intellectual disabilities at transition from adolescent to adulthood. *Journal of Applied Research in Intellectual Disabilities*, *25*(1), 29–38. doi:10.1111/j.1468-3148.2011.00652.x PMID:22473946

Lewandowski, L. J., & Barlow, J. R. (2000). Social cognition and verbal learning disabilities. *Journal of Psychotherapy in Independent Practice*, *4*(4), 35–47. doi:10.1300/J288v01n04_04

Lindfors, P. J., Kaltiala-Heino, R., & Rimpela, A. H. (2012). Cyberbullying among Finnish adolescents – a population-based study. *BMC Public Health*, *12*(1), 1027. doi:10.1186/1471-2458-12-1027 PMID:23176715

Lindsay, S., & McPherson, A. C. (2012). Strategies for improving disability awareness and social inclusion of children and young people with cerebral palsy. *Child: Care, Health and Development*, *38*(6), 809–816. doi:10.1111/j.1365-2214.2011.01308.x PMID:21880056

Llewellyn, A. (2000). Perceptions of mainstreaming: A systems approach. *Developmental Medicine and Child Neurology*, *42*(2), 106–115. doi:10.1017/S0012162200000219 PMID:10698328

Luukkonen, A. H., Riala, K., Hakko, H., & Rasanen, P. (2010). Bullying behavior and substance abuse among underage psychiatric inpatient adolescents. *European Psychiatry*, *25*(7), 382–389. doi:10.1016/j.eurpsy.2009.12.002 PMID:20435448

Marini, Z. A., Dane, A. V., Bosacki, S. L., & Cura, Y. (2006). Direct and indirect bully-victims: Differential psychosocial risk factors associated with adolescents involvement in bullying and victimization. *Aggressive Behavior, 32*(6), 551–569. doi:10.1002/ab.20155

Martlew, M., & Hodson, J. (1991). Children with mild learning difficulties in an integrated and in a special school: Comparisons of behavior, teasing and teachers' attitudes. *The British Journal of Educational Psychology, 61*(3), 355–372. doi:10.1111/j.2044-8279.1991.tb00992.x PMID:1786214

Maryland Coalition for Inclusive Education. (2011). *Quality indicators for inclusive building based practices*. Retrieved from: http://www.mcie.org/usermedia/application/8/quality-indicators---building-based-practices-(2011).pdf

Matheson, C., Olsen, R. J., & Weisner, T. (2007). A good friend is hard to find: Friendship among adolescents with disabilities. *American Journal of Mental Retardation, 112*(5), 319–329. doi:10.1352/0895-8017(2007)112[0319:AGFIHT]2.0.CO;2 PMID:17676957

McNamara, J. K., Willoughby, T., & Chalmers, H. (2005). Psychosocial status of adolescents with learning disabilities with and without comorbid attention deficit hyperactivity disorder. *Learning Disabilities Research & Practice, 20*(4), 234–244. doi:10.1111/j.1540-5826.2005.00139.x

Mishna, F. (2003). Learning disabilities and bullying: Double jeopardy. *Journal of Learning Disabilities, 36*(4), 336–347. doi:10.1177/00222194030360040501 PMID:15490906

Mishna, F., Khoury-Kassabri, M., Gadalla, T., & Daciuk, J. (2012). Risk factors for involvement in cyber bullying: Victims, bullies, and bully-victims. *Children and Youth Services Review, 32*(1), 63–70. doi:10.1016/j.childyouth.2011.08.032

Morrison, G. M., Furlong, M. J., & Smith, G. (1994). Factors associated with the experience of school violence among general education, leadership class, opportunity class, and special day class pupils. *Journal of Education and Treatment of Children, 17*, 356–369.

Nabuzoka, D. (2003). Teacher ratings and peer nominations of bullying and other behavior of children with and without learning difficulties. *Educational Psychology, 23*(3), 307–321. doi:10.1080/0144341032000060147

Nabuzoka, D., & Smith, P. K. (1993). Sociometric status and social behaviour of children with and without learning difficulties. *Journal of Child Psychology and Psychiatry, and Allied Disciplines, 34*(8), 1435–1448. doi:10.1111/j.1469-7610.1993.tb02101.x PMID:8294529

Nadeau, L., & Tessier, R. (2006). Social adjustment of children with cerebral palsy in mainstream classes: Peer perception. *Developmental Medicine and Child Neurology, 48*(05), 331–336. doi:10.1017/S0012162206000739 PMID:16608539

Nansel, T. R., Overpeck, M., Pilla, R. S., Ruan, W. J., Simons-Morton, B., & Scheidt, P. (2001). Bullying behaviors among US youth: Prevalence and association with psychosocial adjustment. *Journal of the American Medical Association, 285*(16), 2094–2100. doi:10.1001/jama.285.16.2094 PMID:11311098

Neece, C., & Baker, B. L. (2008). Predicting maternal parenting stress in middle childhood: The roles of child intellectual status, behavior problems and social skills. *Journal of Intellectual Disability Research, 52*(12), 1114–1128. doi:10.1111/j.1365-2788.2008.01071.x PMID:18513339

Nishina, A., Juvonen, J., & Witkow, M. (2005). Sticks and stones may break my bones, but names will make me sick: The consequences of peer harassment. *Journal of Clinical Child and Adolescent Psychology*, *34*, 37–48. doi:10.120715374424jccp3401_4 PMID:15677279

Noorden, T. H. J., Haselager, G. J. T., Cillessen, A. H. N., & Bukowski, W. M. (2015). Empathy and involvement in bullying in children and adolescents: A systematic review. *Journal of Youth and Adolescence*, *44*(3), 637–657. doi:10.100710964-014-0135-6 PMID:24894581

Norwich, B., & Kelly, N. (2004). Pupils' views on inclusion: Moderate learning difficulties and bullying in mainstream and special schools. *British Educational Research Journal*, *30*(1), 43–65. doi:10.1080/0141192031000l629965

Novaco, R. W., & Taylor, J. L. (2004). Assessment of anger and aggression among male offenders with developmental disabilities. *Psychological Assessment*, *16*(1), 42–50. doi:10.1037/1040-3590.16.1.42 PMID:15023091

O'Brennan, L. M., Bradshaw, C. P., & Sawyer, A. L. (2009). Examining development differences in the social-emotional problems among frequent bullies, victims, and bully/victims. *Psychology in the Schools*, *46*(2), 100–115. doi:10.1002/pits.20357

Olthof, T., & Goossens, F. A. (2008). Bullying and the need to belong: Early adolescents' bullying-related behavior and the acceptance they desire and receive from particular classmates. *Social Development*, *17*(1), 24–46.

Olweus, D. (1978). *Aggression in the schools: Bullies and whipping boys*. Washington, DC: Hemisphere Press.

Olweus, D. (1993). *Bullying at school: What we know and what we can do*. Blackwell Publishing.

Ozdemir, M., & Stattin, H. (2011). Bullies, victims, and bully-victims: A longitudinal examination of the effects of bullying-victimization experiences on youth well-being. *Journal of Aggression, Conflict and Peace Research*, *3*(2), 97–102. doi:10.1108/17596591111132918

Pearl, R., & Bay, M. (1999). Psychosocial correlates of learning disabilities. In V. L. Schwean & D. H. Saklofske (Eds.), *Handbook of psychosocial characteristics of exceptional children* (pp. 443–470). New York, NY: Kluwer Academic / Plenum Publishers. doi:10.1007/978-1-4757-5375-2_17

Perren, S., Dooley, J., Shaw, T., & Cross, T. (2010). Bullying in school and cyberspace: Associations with depressive symptoms in Swiss and Australian adolescents. *Child and Adolescent Psychiatry and Mental Health*, *23*(4), 28. doi:10.1186/1753-2000-4-28 PMID:21092266

Psalti, A. (2012). Bullies, victims, and bully-victims in Greek schools: Research data and implications of practice. *Hellenic Journal of Psychology*, *9*(2), 132–157.

Radliff, K. M., Wheaton, J. E., Robinson, K., & Morris, J. (2012). Illuminating the relationship between bullying and substance use among middle and high school youths. *Addictive Behaviors*, *37*(4), 569–572. doi:10.1016/j.addbeh.2012.01.001 PMID:22277772

Reiter, S., Bryen, D., & Shachar, I. (2007). Adolescents with intellectual disabilities as victims of abuse. *Journal of Intellectual Disabilities*, *11*(4), 371–387. doi:10.1177/1744629507084602 PMID:18029413

Reiter, S., & Lapidot-Leflet, N. (2007). Bullying among special education students with intellectual disabilities: Differences in social adjustment and social skills. *Journal of Intellectual & Developmental Disability*, *45*(3), 174–181. doi:10.1352/1934-9556(2007)45[174:BASESW]2.0.CO;2 PMID:17472426

Richardson, S. O. (1996). Coping with dyslexia in the regular classroom: Inclusion or exclusion. *Annals of Dyslexia*, *46*(1), 37–48. doi:10.1007/BF02648170 PMID:24234266

Rigby, K., & Cox, I. K. (1996). The contributions of bullying and low self-esteem to acts of delinquency among Australian teenagers. *Personality and Individual Differences*, *21*(4), 609–612. doi:10.1016/0191-8869(96)00105-5

Rigby, K., & Slee, P. T. (1991). Bullying among Australian school children: Reported behaviour and attitudes to victims. *The Journal of Social Psychology*, *131*(5), 615–622. doi:10.1080/00224545.1991.9924646 PMID:1798296

Roberts, C. M., & Smith, P. R. (1999). Attitudes and behavior of children towards peers with disabilities. *International Journal of Disability Development and Education*, *46*(1), 35–50. doi:10.1080/103491299100713

Rose, C. A., & Espelage, D. L. (2012). Risk and protective factors associated with the bullying involvement of students with emotional and behavioral disorders. *Behavioral Disorders*, *37*(3), 133–148. doi:10.1177/019874291203700302

Rose, C. A., Espelage, D. L., & Monda-Amaya, L. E. (2009). Bullying and victimization rates among students in general and special education: A comparative analysis. *Educational Psychology*, *29*(7), 761–776. doi:10.1080/01443410903254864

Rose, C. A., Forber-Pratt, A. J., Espelage, D. L., & Aragon, S. R. (2013). The influence of psychosocial factors on bullying involvement of students with disabilities. *Theory into Practice*, *52*(4), 272–279. doi:10.1080/00405841.2013.829730

Rose, C. A., Monda-Amaya, L. E., & Espelage, D. L. (2011). Bullying perpetration and victimization in special education: A review of the literature. *Remedial and Special Education*, *32*(2), 114–130. doi:10.1177/0741932510361247

Rose, J., West, C., & Clifford, D. (2000). Group intervention for anger in people with intellectual disabilities. *Research in Developmental Disabilities*, *21*(3), 171–181. doi:10.1016/S0891-4222(00)00032-9 PMID:10939316

Ryoo, J. H., Wang, C., & Swearer, S. M. (2015). Examination of the change in latent statuses in bullying behaviors across time. *School Psychology Quarterly*, *30*(1), 105–122. doi:10.1037pq0000082 PMID:25111466

Sailor, W., Wolf, N., Choi, H., & Roger, B. (2009). Sustaining positive behavior support in a context of comprehensive school reform. In W. Sailor, G. Dunlop, G. Sugai, & R. Horner (Eds.), *Handbook of positive behavior support* (pp. 633–669). New York: Springer Publishing. doi:10.1007/978-0-387-09632-2_26

Salend, S. J., & Duhaney, L. M. G. (1999). The impact of inclusion on students with and without disabilities and their educators. *Remedial and Special Education*, *20*(2), 114–126. doi:10.1177/074193259902000209

Sansone, R. A., & Sansone, L. A. (2008). Bully victims: Psychological and somatic aftermaths. *Psychiatry, 5*(6), 62–64. PMID:19727287

Sheard, C., Clegg, J., Standen, P., & Cromby, J. (2001). Bullying and people with severe intellectual disability. *Journal of Intellectual Disability Research, 45*(5), 407–415. doi:10.1046/j.1365-2788.2001.00349.x PMID:11679046

SirlopuD.GonzalezR.BohnerG.SieblerF.OrdonnezG.MillarA., & De

Skapinakis, P., Bellos, S., Gkatsa, T., Magklara, K., Lewish, G., Araya, R., & .... (2011). The association between bullying and early stages of suicidal ideation in late adolescents in Greece. *BMC Psychiatry, 11*(1), 1–9. doi:10.1186/1471-244X-11-22 PMID:21303551

Son, E., Parish, S. L., & Peterson, N. A. (2012). National prevalence of peer victimization among young children with disabilities in the United States. *Children and Youth Services Review, 34*(8), 1540–1545. doi:10.1016/j.childyouth.2012.04.014

Sourander, A., Klomek, A. B., Ikonen, M., Lindroos, J., Luntamo, T., Koskelainen, M., & .... (2010). Psychosocial risk factors associated with cyberbullying among adolescents: A population based study. *Archives of General Psychiatry, 67*(7), 720–728. doi:10.1001/archgenpsychiatry.2010.79 PMID:20603453

Sprafkin, J., & Gadow, K. (1987). An observational study of emotionally disturbed and learning-disabled children in school settings. *Journal of Abnormal Child Psychology, 15*(3), 393–408. doi:10.1007/BF00916457 PMID:3668086

Sterzing, P. R., Shattuck, P. T., Narendrof, S. C., Wagner, M., & Cooper, B. P. (2012). Bullying involvement and autism spectrum disorders: Prevalence and correlates of bullying involvement among adolescents with an autism spectrum disorder. *Archives of Pediatrics & Adolescent Medicine, 166*(11), 1058–1064. doi:10.1001/archpediatrics.2012.790 PMID:22945284

Swearer, S. M., Siebecker, A. B., Johnsen-Frerichs, L., & Wang, C. (2010). Assessment of bullying/victimization: The problem of comparability across studies and across methodologies. In S. R. Jimerson, S. M. Swearer, & D. L. Espelage (Eds.), *Handbook of bullying in schools: An international perspective* (pp. 305–327). New York, NY: Routledge.

Tezanos-Pinto, P., & .... (2008). Promoting positive attitudes toward people with Down syndrome: The benefit of school inclusion programs. *Journal of Applied Social Psychology, 38*(11), 2710–2736. doi:10.1111/j.1559-1816.2008.00411.x

Tomasik, M. (2007). Effective inclusion activities for high school students with multiple disabilities. *Journal of Visual Impairment & Blindness, 101*(10), 657–659. doi:10.1177/0145482X0710101012

Underwood, M. K., Galen, B. R., & Paquette, J. A. (2001). Top ten challenges for understanding gender and aggression in children: Why can't we all just get along? *Social Development, 10*(2), 248–266. doi:10.1111/1467-9507.00162

Van Cleave, J., & Davis, M. M. (2006). Bullying and peer victimization among children with special health care needs. *Pediatrics, 118*(4), 1212–1219. doi:10.1542/peds.2005-3034 PMID:17015509

Verdugo, M. A., Bermejo, B. G., & Fuertes, J. (1995). The maltreatment of intellectually handicapped children and adolescents. *Child Abuse & Neglect, 19*(2), 205–215. doi:10.1016/0145-2134(94)00117-D PMID:7780782

Waasdorp, T. E., & Bradshaw, C. P. (2015). The overlap between cyberbullying and traditional bullying. *The Journal of Adolescent Health, 56*(5), 483–488. doi:10.1016/j.jadohealth.2014.12.002 PMID:25631040

Waldman, H. B., Swerdloff, M., & Perlman, S. P. (1999). A "dirty secret": The abuse of children with disabilities. *ASDC Journal of Dentistry for Children, 66*(3), 197–202. PMID:10476359

Wang, J., Iannotti, R. J., Luk, J. W., & Nansel, T. R. (2010). Co-occurrence of victimization from five subtypes of bullying: Physical, verbal, social exclusion, spreading rumors, and cyber. *Journal of Pediatric Psychology, 35*(10), 1103–1112. doi:10.1093/jpepsy/jsq048 PMID:20488883

Whitney, I., Nabuzoka, D., & Smith, P. K. (1992). Bullying in schools: Mainstream and special needs. *Support for Learning, 7*(1), 3–7. doi:10.1111/j.1467-9604.1992.tb00445.x

Whitney, I., Smith, P. K., & Thompson, D. (1994). Bullying and children with special educational needs. In P. K. Smith & S. Sharp (Eds.), *School bullying: Insights and perspectives* (pp. 213–240). London: Routledge.

York, J., Vandercook, T., MacDonald, C., Heise-Neff, C., & Caughey, E. (1992). Feedback about integrating middle school students with severe disabilities in general education classes. *Exceptional Children, 58*(3), 244–257. doi:10.1177/001440299105800307 PMID:1839896

Zablotsky, B., Bradshaw, C. P., Anderson, C., & Law, P. A. (2013). The association between bullying and the psychological functioning of children with autism spectrum disorders. *Journal of Developmental and Behavioral Pediatrics, 34*(1), 1–8. doi:10.1097/DBP.0b013e31827a7c3a PMID:23275052

Zeedyk, S. M., Rodrigeuz, G., Tipton, L. A., Baker, B. L., & Blacher, J. (2014). Bullying of youth with autism spectrum disorder, intellectual disability, or typical development: Victim and parent perspectives. *Research in Autism Spectrum Disorders, 8*(9), 1173–1183. doi:10.1016/j.rasd.2014.06.001 PMID:25285154

Zeitlin, S., & Williamson, G. (1990). Coping characteristics of disabled and nondisabled young children. *The American Journal of Orthopsychiatry, 60*(3), 404–411. doi:10.1037/h0079183 PMID:2143354

ADDITIONAL READING

Basquill, M., Nezu, C. M., Nezu, A. M., & Klein, T. L. (2004). Aggression-related hostility bias and social problem-solving deficits in adult males with mental retardation. *American Journal of Mental Retardation, 109*(3), 255–263. doi:10.1352/0895-8017(2004)109<255:AHBASP>2.0.CO;2 PMID:15072517

Ebeling, H., & Nurkkala, H. (2002). Children and adolescents with developmental disorders and violence. *International Journal of Circumpolar Health, 61*(0), 51–60. doi:10.3402/ijch.v61i0.17502 PMID:12585820

Fenning, R. M., Baker, J. K., Baker, B. L., & Crnic, K. A. (2007). Parenting children with borderline intellectual functioning: A unique risk population. *American Journal of Mental Retardation, 112*(2), 107–121. doi:10.1352/0895-8017(2007)112[107:PCWBIF]2.0.CO;2 PMID:17295551

Horner-Johnson, W., & Drum, C. E. (2006). Prevalence of maltreatment of people with intellectual disabilities: A review of recently published research. *Mental Retardation and Developmental Disabilities Research Reviews*, *12*(1), 57–69. doi:10.1002/mrdd.20097 PMID:16435331

Loveland, K. A., & Kelley, M. L. (1988). Development of adaptive behavior in adolescents and young adults with autism and Down syndrome. *American Journal of Mental Retardation*, *93*, 84–92. PMID:2970861

Luckasson, R., Borthwick-Duffy, S., Buntinx, W. H. E., Coulter, D. L., Craig, E. M., Reeve, A., & … . (2002). *Mental retardation: Definition, classification, and systems of supports*. Washington, DC: American Association on Mental Retardation.

Mitchell, L. M., & Buchele-Ash, A. (2000). Abuse and neglect of individuals with disabilities: Building protective supports through public policy. *Journal of Disability Policy Studies*, *10*(2), 225–243. doi:10.1177/104420730001000206

Murphy, N. (2011). Maltreatment of children with disabilities: The breaking point. *Journal of Child Neurology*, *26*(8), 1054–1056. doi:10.1177/0883073811413278 PMID:21775619

Nettelbeck, T., & Wilson, C. (2002). Personal vulnerability to victimization of people with mental retardation. *Trauma, Violence & Abuse*, *3*(4), 289–306. doi:10.1177/1524838002237331

Olweus, D. (1991). Bully/victim problems among school children: Some basic facts and effects of a school-based intervention program. In D. Pepler & K. Rubin (Eds.), *The development and treatment of childhood aggression* (pp. 411–448). Hillsdale, NJ: Erlbaum.

Chapter 4
Struggles of a Child with ID and Their Family Members:
The Child's and Their Family's Difficulties and Factors Affecting Their Well-Being

Aili Hanim Hashim
University Malaya, Malaysia

Manveen Kaur Sachdev
University Malaya, Malaysia

Norharlina Bahar
Selayang Hospital, Malaysia

Wan Salwina Wan Ismail
Universiti Kebangsaan Malaysia, Malaysia

ABSTRACT

There are many children with intellectual disability (ID) in recent years. The increase in numbers reflects the knowledge regarding the issue, thus creating awareness and increased detection for children for any developmental delay. Consequently, medical services are seeing and treating younger cohorts. Their disability may be mild to moderate, making it difficult even for medical professionals to identify these children. Invariably all parents want to have healthy, intelligent, and capable children who can achieve independence and a successful life. The reality is that parents having children with ID often struggle to understand what is happening with their child, what more how to cope with and help their child. Added to their distress is that even professionals dealing with the children and their family have various ideas and beliefs regarding this issue. Identifying families who are struggling and offering them the appropriate advice is essential as these families need proper guidance and services for their child.

DOI: 10.4018/978-1-7998-1223-4.ch004

INTRODUCTION

Though it is difficult to precisely state the prevalence of children with intellectual disabilities (ID) in any country, in reality, there are many more children with ID in recent years. Consequently, the medical services are seeing and treating younger children as the focus is early diagnosis and prompt intervention. However, in many of the children with ID, their disability may be mild to moderate. Thus, making it difficult even for medical professionals to identify these children.

In many societies, intelligence and success are still highly valued, and these two factors are of utmost importance for any individual to gain social standings and respect. Consequently, parenting a child with intellectual disabilities is challenging. Many people misunderstand these children and often blame the parents for not trying hard enough. The truth is that parents of children with ID are themselves unable to understand what is going on with their child, why is their child different and struggling, and what can they do to help their child. The fact is that for many parents, they continue to look for answers.

The child's disabilities pose many challenges for the child, their parents, and siblings. As the disability affects the child's development globally, understandably the child struggles to preform according to their biological age and as well as their healthy functioning peers.

The reality is that parents of these disabled children are themselves unable to grasp what is happening with their child, what more to cope with the child. In truth, many parents struggle firstly to understand what is going on with their child. Then, the parents have many thoughts regarding what to do with the child so that they can perform as the rest of the healthier children, and most importantly be independent.

Then, there are many children with mild ID and are not identified. These children with mild ID are struggling to function well in society, particularly in schools. This group of children is at risk as many of them look normal, and people misunderstand them as not trying hard enough. Additionally, it frustrates their parents as the adults are not aware of the real difficulties, and many adults continue to push the children to excel academically. It is tough for the children to excel or to catch up as ID is about deficits in the child's intellectual functioning and affecting their adaptive functioning and performance.

The chapter discusses problems faced by the children with Intellectual disability, their parents and siblings, including the possible impact on mental health of the family. The chapter will as well discuss the impact of the mental health difficulties in parents and its consequences on their parenting, and vice versa. The chapter highlights the need to recognize parents who are struggling, and what should professionals looked for in their assessment of families with children with intellectual disabilities. Identifying families who are struggling is important as the family environment has an impact on every family members' functioning and, consequently, their mental health.

Professionals working with children with ID and their families must be aware of these issues and additionally, consider their experience, values and attitudes to ensure that they respond appropriately to the children with ID and their families.

UNDERSTANDING CHILDREN WITH INTELLECTUAL DISABILITY

Intelligence or the individual's mental capacity is essential to all humans. Human intelligence is vital for one's mental functioning. We need our intelligence to acquire and apply the knowledge, ideas and consequently develop further and appropriate thoughts, opinions and acquire skills to help us think, ascertain and deal with things around us effectively.

Struggles of a Child with ID and Their Family Members

Many more children with intellectual disability (ID)[1] are surviving now than they did a century ago (DeWeaver and Kropf, 1992). Intellectual disability is a state whereby the individuals have a varying degree of impairments in their mental abilities with consequence on their learning, performance and adaptive functioning (American Psychiatric Association, 2013; American Association on Intellectual & Developmental Disabilities, 2012). Humans need an adequate level of intelligence to be able to function independently. They need an adequate level of intelligence to regulate themselves accordingly and to manage their various tasks and challenges effectively.

A child's intellectual functioning is vital. In several cultures, children are predominantly judged based on their intellectual abilities especially their academic performance. Children are expected to do well in their school performance, and those not doing as well are often side-lined or thought of as not putting in much effort. While some parents are more mindful that children develop differently, others expect their child to pick up and eventually learn enough to be independent and consequently successful. Likewise, it is stressful for families with children who are slow to learn and not performing as well as their peers.

What is the significance of an individual with reduced cognitive ability or mental functioning? Children with ID have reduced cognitive development affecting their ability to acquire knowledge and manage themselves adequately. The reduced cognitive ability has consequences on the children's capacity to learn, understand and develop ideas and concepts. The disability as well affects the person's ability to remember and utilize the knowledge taught to them. Thus, the affected children are unable to learn and perform as well or as much as the other children of similar age group.

It is easier to pick up the impairment if the child has any physical signs or illness, or if the impairment is severe. For those who are less impaired and with no physical signs are often not recognized until much later. The situations where the child has less impairment and look physically well, are often stressful for the child and their parents. The children may pick up speaking, reading and writing albeit slower or inadequately than the rest. However, our experiences have discovered that because they have no evidence of any disorders, it is hard for people to believe the children may have ID. Besides, the children themselves have less understanding regarding their situation, and may not be able to verbalize their difficulties and struggle well enough for the adults to understand what is going on.

Furthermore, a common scenario often made is that many adults do not pick up or dismissed the child's difficulties in understanding what they read, write or have learned. Many adults often dismissed the matter with the notion that the child 'will eventually pick up and manage.' The adults are not able to see the significance of the child's simple thinking and are developing way below their biological age. The child is not behaving as such on purpose. It is a reflection of their cognition ability, i.e., mental functioning. Our experiences found that children in such situations are pushed to do 'better,' and often labeled as not trying hard enough.

The child's simple thinking reflects the child's reduced ability to acquire and apply the knowledge taught to them (World Health Organization, 1992; American Association on Intellectual & Developmental Disabilities, 2012). Consequently, the reduced ability to acquire and to apply the knowledge affects all areas of their daily living (World Health Organization, 1992; American Association on Intellectual & Developmental Disabilities, 2012) and is seen in their inadequacy to adapt and to the handle themselves with the daily demands of their social environment.

The children often struggle even with simple things in their daily routine (Table 1). Parents helping their child get ready for school in the pre-school age will experience the child continues to need their help as they enter the primary school going age. They may need help waking up, getting ready adequately, and on time and need assistance to organize things for school.

The difficulties with their mental abilities become more significant as the child starts schooling (Table 1). The child will struggle in areas such as reading and writing, remembering things taught and doing the tasks expected of them. The child will battle in areas needing them to reason things out, to plan and think about things or issues. As the child enters the higher levels of schooling time, i.e., mid-primary school stage, their struggles become more noticeable. Their thinking and problem-solving process do not come naturally or quickly for the affected children. The children are slow to make sense of and remember instructions and to go about with their daily activities.

Furthermore, their defective problem-solving abilities results in them not completing or understanding their tasks or school work. They will struggle with handling the work given by their teachers, and often need continued aid from adults or their peers to do or complete the tasks. Again, left on their own the child will not be able to do or to complete their tasks adequately. Due to their limited understanding of the situation, many children with mild to borderline ID cannot fully comprehend the matter. They may not understand why they have to complete the work, or why the adults reprimand them for not completing or adequately doing their work.

In other instances, the child would often prefer to play or be on their own and while some join in peer groups and seem less mature than their peers. The quiet child is afraid and is often unable to understand and manage relationships with their peers. In the latter scenario, the child is particularly playful and unable to understand the norms of social relationships. They are unable to understand there are some rules regarding relationships, for example, give and take and taking turns. While some are followers, others want to lead, and they get upset if the rest of their friends do not follow or do as they suggest.

Then, they are less interested in things related to school. Even if they are interested in some books, they are often looking at the pictures rather than reading or trying to understand the content of the page.

The child's impairment continues to affect their functioning and seen across the other activities of their daily living, e.g., in their personal care, keeping their schedules or routines, and their safety (Table 1). As their level of thinking is way below their biological age the affected children often do things similar to children below their age. The children frequently need assistance from people around them with their daily routines. Going about carrying out their day-to-day tasks is a struggle as they are unable to comprehend and remember there is a routine to follow, and how to go about it. It is hard for them to understand how things work, how to go about doing things 'routinely.' They will struggle to remember these personal tasks and to decide on simple issues. The adults often need to repeatedly tell the child what to do, how to behave, how to do things or tasks, etc. The child with ID would follow as shown or told, while some unfazed and do as they seemed suitable, the tasks left undone or hurriedly done.

Furthermore, another complication of their defective state is that they do not understand the consequences of their behavior and act without thinking of the consequences of their actions. Many of the children with ID act and behave in ways which are detrimental to their well-being. Some children have taken money from their parents and spend the amount on their friends or simple stuff such as food or toys. Some leave the class, or their home and returned when they felt they should go home. They are not aware of the concept of money, time added to their inability to think about the consequences of their actions. In this matter, we have come across children with ID following and doing things their friends said to them to do. They follow their friends' instructions to take money from their parents, to buy things for their friends and even to follow their friends' home or to go hang out at the malls. In such instances, children with ID have gotten into serious trouble as they pick up smoking, and follow their peers commit crimes.

Thus, daily the children and their family struggles. Parents worry or become anxious when their child lacks behind their siblings and peers, or why the child is unable to consider things appropriate for their age. Some parents become frustrated and, in many instances, the child is unable to realize what the fuss is all about. In many situations, most people view the children as being "childish" and not of their biological age. It is frustrating for people around them as the child is unable to cope well without help or their supervision.

As stated above the deficits in the child's global functioning impact their quality of life and everyday functioning (American Psychiatric Association, 1994; Einfeld et al., 2006; American Association on Intellectual & Developmental Disabilities, 2012). Comparisons are often made as the child does not live up to the expectations of their parents, and teachers. Aggravating the situation is that despite the aid given, they continue to lack behind their peers. Their differences are often highlighted, with many pushed and punished to do better. For some, the adults in their environment or others often labeled the child as defiant, stubborn, lazy, etc. The adults do not equate or understand the child's struggles are due to the deficits in the child's global functioning.

Possible presentations children may have reduced reduce intellectual ability (Table 1).

Table 1.

Developmental Stage	Possible Scenarios
Pre-school	• may still need aid with their self-care and handling their personal needs, • slow to adapt going to school; • playful and not attentive in class; • quiet and shy; • unable or slow to understand, and remember instructions or lessons; • needs constant help with reading and writing and doing the work expected of them,
Schooling age	During this stage children should progressively be able to learn and remember the information taught to them and consequently develop more ideas, insight and skills. Thus, possible signs of a child with ID: • may still need aid with their self-care and handling their personal needs; • needing constant reminders handling self-care and personal needs; • personal care not up to par with the child's age; • still struggling with reading, writing and simple calculations despite considerable time in preschool and help given to the child; • needs constant help with understanding and doing the work expected of them; • playful at home and in school; • avoiding or unable to do the school work without aid; • prefer playing and fitting in better with younger children; • unable to understand and follow social rules or behaviour of same age peers. They may be seen as too playful and rough in their manner of play and not able to behave as expected by the peer group or family; • able to provide simple answers or ideas while struggling with more complex tasks and responsibilities.
Adolescents	During the adolescent stage children should be thinking in ways that are more advanced, and complex. They can use their thinking to generate ideas and attempt to deal with more complex situations. Thus, possible signs of a child with ID: • performing way below par in terms of their academic performance; • still struggling with reading, writing and understanding concepts; • struggling to handle money and poor concept of time and organizing one-self; • playful at home and avoiding or unable to do the school work without aid; • prefer playing with younger children; • needing constant reminders handling self-care and personal needs; • simple ideas and thinking and below biological age. Often gives short and simple answers, and adults often have to ask many times to get much information from the adolescent; • self-care, self-regulation and motivation below biological age; • follow more delinquent peers and may start smoking, using illicit drugs and progressively gravitate to delinquent activities, i.e., stealing, leaving home without informing their parents.

The presentation of the difficulties varies according to the severity of the child's deficiency, which corresponds approximately to the level of IQ scores (American Psychiatric Association, 2013; American Association on Intellectual & Developmental Disabilities, 2012). The levels are categorized as mild, moderate, severe and profound difficulties, and are discussed elsewhere in the book.

Consequences of Having Deficits in Intellectual Disability

Children with ID experience more physical, emotional and behavioral problems and manifest more social issues when compared to typically developing children (Dekker et al., 2002; E. and Hatton, 2007; Witwera and Lecavaliera, 2008; Mazzucchelli and Sanders, 2011; Vrijmoeth et al., 2011; Gray et al., 2011).

Parents with children with mental disabilities will have to deal with:

1. Behavioural and emotional problems (Parmenter et al., 1998; Crnic et al., 2004; Witwera and Lecavaliera, 2008; Emerson et al., 2014).

As discussed in the section above, parents and teachers often report their child's behaviours as being problematic at home and in social settings, describing their children as:

- Being uncooperative as the child does not listen well to them. Thus, many adults label the children as being 'stubborn;'
- The child is unable to keep on with simple and repeated requests or tasks;
- Not being able to verbalise their daily experience and needs adequately;
- Continually relying on them or others even to do 'simple' things;
- Fussy with their food intake;
- Uninterested and lack behind in their school performance and tasks;
- They seemed to play most times, and unable to cope well when left on their own.

As demonstrated above a central theme of the child's problems and it emerges as the child struggles to keep up with the many age-appropriate expectations. Frequently the behavior problems are as a result of the child trying to cope with the demands and expectations placed on them. Several researchers believe the behavioral problems often emerge as a sign of the children communicating their distress (Bakken et al., 2010; Caplan et al., 2015). Many are unable to make sense of what the expectations are, why and how they will cope. Moreover, they are unable to communicate their stress and distress.

Their inability to organize their behavior coherently and consistently, and to address the tasks expected of them becomes frustrating for many adults (Fenning et al., 2014; Schuiringa et al., 2015) and the child. The problematic behaviors are more visible over time as the child ages. The child is seen becoming more dependent on others and unable to cope when left on their own. While some parents worry, many others become frustrated.

Further problematic behavior includes the children are more likely to be destructive, over-activity, self-injurious behavior, sleeping difficulties, physical aggression, attention-seeking behavior and temper tantrums (Crnic et al., 2004). Other challenging behaviours faced by parents are some of the children are 'self-absorbed' as they often prefer to be by themselves (Molteno et al., 2001; Einfeld et al., 2006; Alimovic, 2013; Emerson et al., 2014). Then there are others who are more disruptive and aggressive in their interaction (Molteno et al., 2001; Einfeld et al., 2006; Alimovic, 2013; Emerson et al., 2014).

In these instances, the children often intimidate others using inappropriate words, or inappropriate behaviors in public.

Additional common and distressing behaviours seen among children with ID are self-injurious behaviors, and they can be extreme or erratic in their moods (Einfeld et al., 2006; Allen, 2008). In many instances, the emergence of behavioral problems is indicative of the presence of psychiatric disorders (Bakken et al., 2010; Caplan et al., 2015). The presence of these behaviors causes added distress to their parents who often worry about possible harm to the child and others. In these situations, their peers often isolate or exclude the child from their friendship groups.

In situations when their peers isolate or exclude the child from their friendship groups may as well have negative consequences on the child as discussed below. The strained and fewer friendship opportunities may lead the child to have feelings of sadness and commonly loneliness which is an inescapable state in children with ID (Gilmore and Cuskelly, 2014). Consequently, such uncooperative and challenging behaviors upset the family environment as well.

Behavior problems are harder to manage in older children. With increasing age, there is a lack of school and post-schooling options. Likewise, in events of much self-injurious behavior and aggression, the capacity of families to continue to provide care is more challenging (Orsmond et al., 2003). Then, with the worsening of behavioral problems concerns may arise with regards to living arrangements.

2. Social difficulties (Cermak and Aberson, 1998; Kemp and Carter, 2002; Fenning et al., 2014):

People learn social skills as they progress in age. These skills or socially acceptable behaviours are necessary for humans to fit into their environment and for others to accept them (Elliott and Gresham, 1993; Cermak and Aberson, 1998). These behaviours include behaving appropriately with others, having respectable and adequate emotional control, being cooperative and responsible, helpful and many more (Elliott and Gresham, 1993; Cermak and Aberson, 1998).

Due to their limited cognitive abilities, children with ID have difficulties learning, understanding and remembering social norms. In social settings, children with ID have more problems fitting in and settling in their environment (Howell et al., 2007). They seemed awkward and unable to handle themselves adequately in many social settings (Guralnick et al., 2006; Howell et al., 2007).

Their 'child-like' or 'immature' behaviours make others view them as a problematic child, and their parents often worry about their child as not being able to manage oneself independently. They are unable to understand and follow social rules or behaviours of the same age peers. The child may not be able to control their impulse and continue to be in a playful mode while others have stopped playing and are serious with their work. In these situations, the children are at risk of others isolating them as they may not be able to be patient and learn to take their turn, or they may always want to be the person to win or for people to listen to them. In other instances, the child will follow what their peers do or say. In such situations, the child might get into trouble repeatedly as they cannot consider the consequences of their mates' actions or instructions.

Howell et al. (2007) found that children with ID as more hyperactivity and impulsivity than children with healthy functioning children. Thus, the child's inability to comprehend their behaviour and actions aggravates their disruptive situation.

They may think their friends are people to play with, and they have difficulties managing the social norms of making and maintaining relationships. In other instances, the child with ID may not recognize their peers take advantage or bully them. In some others, they are quiet in the peer group and follow what their friends do, while some prefer to be alone and possibly have one close friend.

These are examples of the deficits in their cognition, i.e., understanding social norms and the inability to understand and regulate their behaviour (Guralnick, 1977; Howell et al., 2007). Moreover, making and choosing friends is worrying in the child with ID as they may not understand the meaning of friendships and the consequences of theirs's and peers' behaviors and actions fully.

3. Difficulties in areas of scholastic attainment (Parmenter et al., 1998; E. and Hatton, 2007; Fenning et al., 2014).

The difficulties are evident as the child enters preschool, but many adults are less worried as pre-school is still time for play. However, by the time, they reach primary school, many continue to struggle even with basic reading, writing, and calculations. While in some children with ID they may eventually learn to read or recognize words, they are not as fluent or as quick as their normally functioning peers. Still, the most critical issue is that the child would not be able to comprehend, i.e., understand what they read or write, and what they have to do. Their thinking and skills are simplistic. Thus, they frequently need constant help to understand concepts, and to carry out and complete their tasks. Alternatively, the child's level of understanding regarding the tasks or situations is simple and not to the expected level of understanding as for their biological age. The difficulties are a consequence of the mental functioning difficulties associated with their intellectual disability and again not easily recognized and understood by the adults.

If the parents were less concerned about their child's performance at the pre-school level by the time the child is in primary school and struggling to keep up, many parents would start to worry. Being in school is stressful in some children with mild intellectual disability. Parents, teachers and even peers see them behaving and performing way below their biological age. Invariably, countless parents organize more classes to provide opportunities for their child to try to catch up to their peers. However, due to the child's intellectual deficiencies they often are unable to catch up, and many continue to perform below average. The parents' worries increase over time as they begin to recognize that despite more time and aid provided for the child, the latter continues to struggle. Again, due to the child's limited understanding abilities, some children continue to go to school as they see the situation as an opportunity for them to play. In others, the child starts to worry or seemed unperturbed as they are not able to comprehend fully what the fuss is all about. Correspondingly, the child is unable to verbalize their concerns fully.

Many adults, parents, including teachers, believe all children have the same thinking and performing ability. Adults feel knowledge and success will be gained with child learning and working hard. Adults may not realize the child is having a disability and what the disability entails. Commonly, the expectation placed on the child is similar to that of a normally functioning child.

At some stage, some parents begin to recognize, and worry will their child ever be able to cope with the academic journey? The parents recognize the child's struggle and are more appropriate in dealing with the difficulties. They realize their child actually cannot cope with the mainstream school program. In others, they continue to push their child to deliver. They are made to attend more tuition classes hoping the child would eventually catch up.

It does not help the child or their parents as in many instances the school or others continue to put expectations on the child to perform. Many parents experience countless negative contacts with educators or other family members, and this worsens the situation. In our experience, we encounter many people are not receptive about the possibility of the disability and dismiss the situation as the child not putting in enough effort or having no interest. The adults are not aware of the actual matter of the disorder and believe more academic training and more effort will help the child improve. The situation is more often seen in children with mild disability.

Similarly, in our experience, many people continue to consider the situation as the child is not trying hard enough. They believe that the child can still manage and go through the mainstream school lessons and program despite the below average performance. Only in some instances that the adults realize their child actually cannot cope with the regular school program. In time, they are more open to understanding what is happening with their child and looking at other options.

As the child ages, many parents rightly worry about what employment prospects would be suitable for their child. The reality is that many will be at the risk of not finding suitable employment. They will continue to rely on their families in their adulthood as most cannot establish enough finances on their own, or have anyone else to help look after them (Wells et al., 2003; Wolfe et al., 2014).

IMPACT OF CO-MORBIDITY

Additionally, children with ID are prone to develop psychiatric disorders (Deb et al., 2001; Einfeld et al., 2006; Witwera and Lecavaliera, 2008; Bakken et al., 2010; Tremblay et al., 2010; Reardon et al., 2015). The presence of a psychiatric diagnosis signifies more challenging behaviours (Moss et al., 2000; Myrbakk and von Tetzchner, 2008; Bakken et al., 2010; Baker et al., 2010; Caplan et al., 2015); in addition to the increasing impairment in their functioning (Dekker and Koot, 2003; Einfeld et al., 2011).

The presence of these co-morbidities is discussed in the other chapters of the book

IMPACT OF HAVING A CHILD WITH ID

Most couples are ecstatic with the arrival of a new child in their family. Parents are often bursting with optimistic expectations and plans for the new-born child. Every parent hopes for a healthy child thus when told their child is having difficulties, and the difficulties may be life long, the feelings of joy and hopes inevitably fades (Feniger-Schaal and Oppenheim, 2013; Barak-Levy and Atzaba-Poria, 2013).

It is often an unexpected situation and at times traumatic for any parent learning that one's child has a disability (Kazak and Marvin, 1984; Pianta and Marvin, 1996; Sheeran et al., 1997; Schuengel et al., 2009). The news of having a child with a disability often place them into a quandary and at times crisis (Sheeran et al., 1997; Nimbalkar et al., 2014). Many are left feeling confused, helpless and at times angry. Having a child with ID requires many life adjustments for the parents and family (Gupta and Harpreet, 2010).

Many parents go through an initial period of a mixture of reactions from shock, anger, denial, guilt and even rejection of the possible truth (Kazak and Marvin, 1984; Trute, 1990; Pianta and Marvin, 1996; Schuengel et al., 2009). Blacher (1984) reports that some parents go through a period of mourning, i.e., grieving and sadness for the loss of a healthy child while some parents reported feeling stress and anxiety (Schuengel et al., 2009).

Invariably, most parents try to comprehend what they are facing i.e., the reality of their child's disability and their faded wish and desire to have a healthy child (Trute, 1990; Pianta and Marvin, 1996; Marvin and Pianta, 1996; Sheeran et al., 1997; Jessop et al., 1998). While others may feel they are punished for sins in their past, while others blame their spouses or partners, while some reach a stage of despair.

The process of grief continues with differences in parental expectations regarding the disability and the needs of the child (Wikler, 1981; Eakes, 1995). Bruce et al. (1994) describe parents going through a continuing sense of loss with the presence of the disability being an ongoing source of stress, with mothers more affected than fathers. Eakes (1995) and other researchers (Trute, 1990; Bruce et al., 1994; Eakes et al., 1998) speak of parents going through chronic sorrow. They not only have they to come to terms with the loss of a healthy functioning child, they invariably have to go through the tedious process of many medical examinations and procedures, and at the same time continuing to manage their child. Many parents know that having children with chronic difficulties place additional challenges for them.

Then, there are situations where many parents have difficulties receiving or accepting their child's diagnosis. Many children with borderline to mild ID look very ordinary. Many of these children too can speak and continue attending school. However, their performance is below par. Their developmental delay may be very subtle and not as visible as a child with more severe ID. When told their child may have intellectual disability many parents may initially dismiss the news or disagrees with the results of the assessment. As time passes, the child's difficulties are seen across the many areas of their development (Table 1). A particularly common situation would be that the child does not attain a satisfactory academic performance or is continually performing below average.

The presence of prolonged and complicated emotional reactions of anxiety, distress, and even sadness may interfere with the parents' availability as caregivers for their child (Schuengel et al., 2009). The sense of loss continues throughout the time the parents have to handle their child and may resurface with other significant life events (Trute, 1990; Bruce et al., 1994) such as the delivery of a healthy child, weddings and for some, family gatherings maybe stressful occasions. Family gatherings are stressful particularly in families with children with mild ID as it tough for many people to understand why and how the deficiencies affect the child and their family. In many instances, there are often difficulties in the family members themselves during their childhood days, e.g., delay in talking, not interested in academics yet they could survive their childhood. These scenarios make it harder for parents and families to comprehend and accept the difficulties in the child. Often in such situations, people may think the child has to try harder or that the adults are not trying hard enough to help the child.

Various demands persist throughout their childhood and possibly into their adult years. Often there is a broad range of difficulties impacts the child and on the lives of their family (Baker et al., 2003; Baker et al., 2005; McConkey et al., 2008; Woodman et al., 2011; Fenning et al., 2014; Reardon et al., 2015). However, the child may not be the only factor that affects his family's life and dynamics. Researchers have shown the parents' behavior, parenting styles, and mental health positively or negatively affects the child's development.

1. Parenting, family functioning and relationship:

It is challenging to deal with a less independent child. Handling the child is time-consuming and requires much patience to handle their daily needs. Added to the situation, the presence of for some children with ID self-injurious, aggressive and destructive behaviours increase the family distress (MacLean Jr. et al., 2010; Petty et al., 2014).

Invariably, every child needs a healthy family environment for them to develop optimally. A 'normal and healthy' family has parents who are supportive and able to provide a nurturing environment for their children. The unique caretaking demands in parents with children ID places many limitations on the family, and the presence of other family stressors such as financial constraint increases the emotional distress for all family members. Almost all parents feel the stress, and distress handling a child with ID and the situation would complicate the parent-child relationship (Baker et al., 2002).

The parenting behaviors and styles play a pivotal in the life of a child with ID. An ideal situation is the existence of a nurturing environment. A nurturing environment is where the children can feel safe and connected to their parents (Maccoby and Martin, 1983; Reder and Lucey, 1995). In these nurturing and supportive environments, the adults recognize the children have varying needs and wants at different times.

The parenting the children receives is associated with many aspects of the child development, including cognitive, social, and behavioral outcomes (Maccoby and Martin, 1983; Ainsworth, 1985; Ainsworth and Bowlby, 1991; Reder and Lucey, 1995). Even with children with ID, the parenting quality mutually affects the child's maladaptive behaviors and developmental outcomes (Fenning et al., 2014; Brown et al., 2011).

Consequently, researchers have found that children with ID are exposed to additional environmental adversity compared to healthier children (Emerson et al., 2014; Fenning et al., 2014). No doubt the child's behaviors including maladaptive behaviors (e.g., disruptive or aggressive behaviors, stereotyped or abusive behaviors) impact the family environment. It is common to see in children with mild ID, parents are often perplexed why the adults have to remind their child to do things continuously, or why they have to explain things many times, and over and over again. It is distressing for any person to keep reminding or explaining the same things to the same individual. Similarly, the siblings may be upset with the behavior of their sibling(s) with ID. Hauser-Cram et al. (1999) strongly showed these early-related aspects of the family environment are predictive of the child's communication, social and daily living skills.

Invariably, the child's with ID behaviors and emotions are influenced directly by the parenting, parental behaviors and external environment (Floyd and Zmich, 1991; Arim et al., 2012). Inevitably, the parenting stress is evident even in early childhood and across disabilities. However, when there is a lack of parental responsiveness such as intrusiveness, demanding or critical parenting, and using harsh discipline, the situation is associated with an increase in the children's disruptive behavior (Fenning et al., 2014; Norlin et al., 2014; Arim et al., 2012). Brown et al. (2011) disclosed that having a child with developmental delay was the most significant predictor of subsequent negative parenting. Likewise, Norlin et al. (2014) established more fathers of children with disabilities (than in fathers with healthy children) admitted using aggression at least once.

The presence of a responsive mother-child behavior certainly helps the child, mainly when the child is unable to understand what the environment expects from them. Hauser-Cram et al. (1999) indicated that more proper performance of the child's social behavior might be seen if the child is in a calm environment. The pattern of interaction in the presence of a caring and supportive mum provides a calm environment that helps soothe the child down and encourages their development and helps promote more socially acceptable behaviours (Hauser-Cram et al., 1999; Guralnick, 1999). In a calm and supportive environment, the appropriate reactions and actions of the parent influence the child's modelling prosocial behavior and possibly their motivation to improve their skills even with their limitations.

Fenning et al. (2014) found among parents of children with borderline ID they were often negative while dealing with their child's problematic behaviors. They are often impatient, distress or frustrated. Many parents view the child as demanding more of their time and attention. This is particularly true in the situation when the parents do not understand or are unaware of their child's difficulties and limitations. In these situations, many parents too understandably generally view their child's behaviour as undesired, stubborn or oppositional. Invariably, the parents' views and their interactions turn negative particularly when they perceive their child is frequently bidding for their attention and it is getting too much, too frequently or is inappropriate (Brown et al., 2011). It frustrates many parents to know their child is incapable of handling themselves despite their growing age.

Additionally, Emerson et al. (2014) found the presence of inconsistent parenting among parents of children with borderline ID. It is understandable as the parents may not know about the child's condition unless they have had the child's assessed by professionals. In situations when the parents know about their child's condition, they forget or are unsure what ID means while some may not comprehend the impact of ID on the child adequately. We frequently find parents still consider their child as having normal intellectual functioning and expect the child to have some understandings of their expectations including handling themselves adequately. The parents' understanding of their child's situation is that the child is slow to do things. Many people do not and cannot fully understand the 'child's slowness' is related to the child's mental and adaptive functioning which has a major impact on the child's learning and doing things, understanding, figuring and reasoning things out and thus significantly impact on their thinking and functioning. The situation adds to the stressful state as managing the child means having to oversee their self-care and daily activities continually.

Likewise, some parents with children with ID are overprotective and over-intrusive (Arim et al., 2012; Fenning et al., 2007; Brown et al., 2011). Greene et al. (1983) found an association between birth complications with intrusive parenting and its negative impact. No doubt many parents having a child with a disability are often worried about their child's functioning. However, the parents' intrusiveness may affect the child wanting to learn to handle some social skills and personal care on their own. Egeland et al. (1993) and Stevenson and Crnic (2013) found that even in healthy functioning children parents' intrusive behavior significantly impacted the child's academic, social, emotional, and behavioral development. Encouraging the child and using positive reinforcements often motivate the child to keep trying to the best of their ability particularly in children with mild impairment. A child with mild impairment may learn to reach an acceptable level of self-care, communication skills, and school readiness skills, though they often still need help with independent living and learning.

In children with ID, parental intrusiveness and overprotectiveness impair the child's social developmental competency, and it may create a situation whereby especially in children with mild ID, they become dependent or even controlling their parents. In these situations, the parent may display more negative affect and are impatient, often doing or completing the child's tasks. Thus, the child experiences and learns their parents' step-in and complete their tasks. Consequently, the child loses the motivation to master any tasks as they experience and understand to some extent their parents will do the tasks despite expecting the child to do as told.

Kennedy (1994) and Granic and Patterson (2006) are among researchers who found a significant link between negative-parenting corresponded with an exacerbation of the child's behavioral difficulties. In reality, many parents do struggle handling the child with ID. In our experience many parents view their child as demanding their attention and time, and some resort to using physical punishments or using more intrusive parenting style. The parents hope that such decision would lead to an improvement in the child's behavior. Even though in the short term the use of physical punishment or constantly telling off or criticizing the child often leads to increase in desirable behaviours, in the long-term it is associated with increased oppositional and uncooperative behaviours, and aggressiveness (Straus and Stewart, 1999;

Straus and Donnelly, 2001). The use of physical punishment, or constantly telling off or criticizing the child is often equates with heightened levels of negative affect.

The family and the home environment is essential for every child's development and well-being (Bowlby, 1988a; Bowlby, 1988b). Bradley et al. (2001) found that learning occurs and is affected by the presence of the different types of stimulation, maternal responsiveness and perception, and the use of punishment. Ainsworth et al. (1978) and Ainsworth (1985) speaks about how the environment stimulates and encourages certain behaviors with

Thus as discussed above, the parent-child relationship plays a crucial role in the mental health development of every child (Bowlby, 1989; Bowlby, 1988a) even in children with ID. A critical component of any parent-child relationship is the emotional element of parents' expression (Ainsworth, 1985). In typically healthy children the parents' expressions of positive emotions contribute to better social development while negative and controlling parenting behaviours are linked with externalizing behaviours problems and poorer adjustment (Ainsworth, 1985).

Fittingly Nihira et al. (1985) observed that parenting quality and maladaptive child behaviors mutually influence each other. The relations between parents' psychological distress and child behaviours is bidirectional, with each individual influencing the other over time (Brown et al., 2011; Baker et al., 2003). Thus, as discussed the presence of family connectedness and being responsive helps with the development of the child's social and communicative skills (Hauser-Cram et al., 1999). Indeed, the adult's ability to preserve a positive interactional style and to maintain patience improves resilience in this population. A positive interactional style which provides a supportive and comforting environment predicted significant developmental gains, including adaptive cognitive, language, social-emotional, and behavioral outcomes in these children with developmental problems (Fenning et al., 2014; Warren and Brady, 2007; Landry et al., 2008). Bandura (1991) hypothesizing children learn behaviours from the environment by watching, observing and imitating actions of others. Chiefly, in children with ID, an encouraging environment can provide the children with learning more adaptive and functioning behavior.

The matter is further backed up with research consistently demonstrating the association between maternal distress and increasing challenging behavior in children (Nihira et al., 1985; Orsmond et al., 2003). The finding is not surprising as maternal distress is not associated with a calm state. Distress mothers are often impatient, and they tend to use more punitive methods to handle the child's daily hassles. Understandably, trying to understand the child is a complicated process and is difficult to achieve for many parents. These negative expressed emotions have significant consequences on the child's learning (Hastings et al., 2006; Hastings and Lloyd, 2007) as the child has limited mental capacity and tries to make sense of what is going on and what he or she has to do. Sensing the parents' adverse reaction is often scary or worrying to the child.

In other circumstances, Emerson et al. (2014) found that children with intellectual disability were significantly more likely to be exposed to household poverty, and low maternal education. Conversely, poverty is often associated with lower levels of affective parental expression, sensitivity, and with more frequent use of power-assertive control techniques (McLoyd and Wilson, 1990; McLoyd, 1990).

2. The couple's relationship:

Consequently, Emerson and Hatton (2007) state that the strength of the relationship between the parents supporting a child with disability lessens the very high rates of disadvantage faced by a lone parent.

The daily handling of the child added with the presence of the child's challenging behaviors invariably affects the parents' emotional well-being as well their marital relationship (Baker et al., 2005; Robinson and Neece, 2015). A pertinent issue in this matter is related to the quality of the couple's marriage and relationship and if there are any presence of conflicts, particularly chronic conflicts (Kersh et al., 2006; Robinson and Neece, 2015).

Mothers are often the primary carer for the child as often the father works to bring in the income to support the family. MacDonald and Hastings (2010), Dyer et al. (2009) and Quesenberry et al. (2007) are among many researchers who spoke about the importance of the father's presence and role in families with children with ID. Earlier research suggested fathers were more in the peripheral and the invisible parent. The findings postulated that the fathers withdrew with having a child with ID (Fenning et al., 2014). However, recent findings reported that fathers were motivated to have increased involvement in the family and to help raise their children (Dyer et al., 2009). MacDonald and Hastings (2010) postulated the emergence of the attachment theory and family systems theory, changing trends with more women going out to work, and fewer extended family support may have contributed to more fathers becoming more involved in their child's care.

Moreover, many studies on father's involvement in their child's development and in particular low-income groups supports the father's involvement contributed significantly to the child's social and language development (Cabrera et al., 2007; Shannon et al., 2002; Pancsofar et al., 2010). Thus, it is not surprising that research among children with ID found evidence that the father's presence plays a vital role in their child's development (De Falco et al., 2008; Flippin and Crais, 2011; Hodapp, 2002). De Falco et al. (2008) found in a study among children with Down's syndrome, the father's involvement contributed significantly to an increased in the child's exploratory and symbolic play. Shannon et al. (2002) and (de Falco et al., 2009) supported the findings that father's emotional involvement did lead to enhanced cognitive functioning in children with ID and suggested more fathers be involved in caring for their child with special needs. Additionally, Shannon et al. (2002) found that fathers can be as responsive and less intrusive which would encourage the child to respond correspondingly. Besides, there are many tasks involving the child which are much easier for the fathers to do than for the mothers. Fathers are often stronger to carry or lift the child, and the children often perceive their fathers as the stricter parent.

Without a doubt, having a special needs child is challenging. Having a special need child often result in the couple being distant to each other, or it may bring the couple closer (Baker et al., 2005; McCarthy et al., 2006). Bringing the couple together strengthens their marriage. The latter is not surprising as the presence of both parents working together helps relieve the stress of just one parent handling the child. A couple working together as well improves their communication and understanding each other. Likewise, a healthier marital relationship undoubtedly helps reduce the stress as parents share responsibility and support each other.

3. The stress level of the family:

Having a child with ID is stressful for many families (Lopez et al., 2008; Al-Krenawi et al., 2011; Ritzema and Sladeczek, 2011; Robinson and Neece, 2015). Parents having children with ID reported having higher levels of child-related tension than parents of typically developing children (Gallagher et al., 2008; Azar and Badr, 2010; Cramm and Nieboer, 2011; Gray et al., 2011; Lin et al., 2014; Gallagher and Hannigan, 2014). Hence, it is not surprising that parents of children with ID have more reduced levels of both good mental and physical health (Bourke-Taylor et al., 2012; Bazzano et al., 2015).

Struggles of a Child with ID and Their Family Members

The ID is a permanent condition. Therefore, it creates an additional burden for both the individual and the family across the child's life span. Thus, their stress often persists throughout childhood and into the child's adult years. Invariably stress occurs with the continuous and significant challenge with looking after the child (Dabrowska and Pisula, 2010; Pisula, 2011).

For the parents, the stress is related to a combination of issues, i.e., the child's diagnosis, their condition added with the increase in the care-giving necessity that is often required daily. The presence of the behaviors already discussed above frequently tests the parents' capacity to manage the child adequately.

The adults or siblings often forget about the affected child's limitation. In many households, the interactions with the child is often similar to the other healthier children. Often tasks need to be done repetitively and broken down into more uncomplicated steps for the child to be able to follow. Likewise, their communication is different compared to parents communicating with their healthier children. Frequently parents forget to be mindful of their child's limitations and expect the child to manage their challenges effectively.

Recurrently there will be a crisis to attend to, and often this requires an instant and quick response by the parents to manage the crises. Similarly to typically developing children, the presence of negative-parenting behavior is associated with an exacerbation of the child's behavioral difficulties in children with ID (Granic and Patterson, 2006; Mullineaux et al., 2009; Fenning et al., 2014).

Very often the experience of the child-related stress begins in the preschool period with parents having to face and handle the hassles daily (Azad et al., 2013), e.g., getting the child up, bath and dressed. Due to the deficiencies in their mental functioning, the child will need help as he or she has trouble seeing how things or how events are, and how they relate to each other. This is due to the limitation in their understanding, reasoning, remembering and problem-solving abilities. They often require reminders or cues to help them manage even 'normally simple' and repetitive tasks. The children often need more structure and support for them to carry out necessary skills and tasks, such as dressing, getting ready for school, playing or interacting with others and for some even feeding themselves.

In our experience, many parents are often left wondering how else to handle the child, as, despite their many reminders or teaching, the child still poorly understands and forgets instructions. The prolonged period and energy invested in dealing with the child invariably result in the parents' questioning their parenting ability and self-worth. It is not surprising that many parents report handling one's child is challenging as well as tiring. Invariably it often evokes a mixture of emotions in the parents. Thus, it is not surprising that many parents report feeling they have failed. Consequently, the adults see that they are not able to change the situation added to them feeling helpless as the parents do not know whereas can they get the help that they need.

The stress level remains relatively stable and then increases over time. The increase in the stress level is mainly related to the emergence of behavior issues (Baker et al., 2002; Azad et al., 2013). Children with ID have heightened levels of problematic or challenging behaviors (Emerson et al., 2014), and a correlation is seen between the child's cognitive ability and severity of behavior problems (Baker et al., 2002; Crnic et al., 2004). Consequently, the occurrence of high levels of behavior problems and with their low levels of understanding put mothers of children with ID at the most risk for heightened stress levels (Neece and Baker, 2008). It is not surprising as the presence of more challenging behavior stresses the parents (Baker et al., 2005) as invariably, the children require closer supervision.

For sure, these behaviors are exhausting, distressing, and time-consuming for the family. The child customarily needs constant care to ensure their safety. Studies support parents' psychological health, and well-being tends to decrease as children's behavior problems increase (Hastings, 2003; Baker et al.,

2005; McCarthy et al., 2006; Robinson and Neece, 2015). Correspondingly, research supports many more mothers experience higher levels of stress than fathers (McCarthy et al., 2006; Bourke-Taylor et al., 2010; Lee, 2013; Fairthorne et al., 2015) and they report higher depressive scores (Olsson and Hwang, 2001; Lee, 2013).

The parents' concerns are legitimate. Moreover, the reality of parental concerns and the stress for their child increases as the child grows older (Hallum, 1995). There are continuous learning problems and delays in development, and the deficiency limits the child's prospects of being independent and self-directed in their functioning. Parents have anxiety concerning the child's sexualized behavior, menstruation, and many more (Hallum, 1995). The parents' worry about their child's future is legitimate, and this is the most significant concern for many parents (Hallum, 1995). Doctors are asked again and again by the same parents what will happen to their child? Can they look after themselves? Who will take care of them?

Understandably, there is a significant reduction in the parents' personal and social satisfactoriness as their routines often include being mindful of their child who struggles with their day-to-day tasks (Plant and Sanders, 2007; Ritzema and Sladeczek, 2011). Handling the child's daily needs invariably adds further strain and stress for the parent. The physically demanding and repetitive tasks are time-consuming and often disrupt the family routines and activities as well. The child often takes a longer time to get ready and having to supervise and wait for the child always is frequently for the others tiring and frustrating. Adjustments are required to accommodate the needs of the child, and it not only affects the parents but the whole family. Thus, it is not surprising that high portion parents of children with ID are anxious and depressed (Azeem et al., 2013).

Undoubtedly, stress and worries are an important determinant of family functioning, interactions and relationships and consequently the individual's wellbeing (Deater-Deckard, 2005; Gerstein et al., 2009; Baker et al., 2010). Any parent feeling overwhelmed by the continuous strain of handling the daily hassles and challenges of their child will invariably have greater problems managing and interacting with their children. Also, stressful parents have negative implications for the family. When stress, their parenting is often characterized by more impatience, harsh and critical attitudes when handling their child. Added to this is the presence of inconsistent discipline (Deater-Deckard, 2005). It would be difficult for parents to react more positively and calmly when upset or stressed.

The presence of other vulnerabilities in the family e.g., ongoing conflicts or the presence of mental health problems places the family at increased risk of having more difficulties in coping and making the adjustments needed.

As discussed above the parental stress, ill-health or continuing conflicts within the family even interferes with getting adequate help or intervention programs for the child. When one or both parents disagree about their child's difficulties, along with the stigma of receiving help from mental health facilities and special education, many families do not seek or refuse help.

Interestingly, studies found as the child settles, e.g., being in a more structured school environment or receiving a school-based intervention or the child spends more time in school, the parenting stress reduces (Blacher et al., 2009). However if the child is unable to cope with the requirements of the school as the school may place many new demands on their academic performance, social, and self-regulatory skills, then the parents' stress level perpetually increases (Eisenhower et al., 2007; Azad et al., 2013) again.

However, when parents can cope well with the unique childcare demands, they can enhance the social and emotional adjustment of their child. When this occurs, it as well avoids much distress and disruption for the other family members (Bourke-Taylor et al., 2012).

Among factors, which may affect the stress, level, and functioning of the family are:

1. The more challenging the child's behavior is, the higher is the stress level (Bourke-Taylor et al., 2010). As many of these behavioral problems persist into adolescence and adulthood, it aggravates the family's stress level (Einfeld et al., 2006; Gray et al., 2011).

The thoughts often wondered by parents are: "What will my child's life be as an adult? Will college or employment be possible?" "Who will look after my child when I am no longer around?"

Longitudinal studies show increasing behavior, and mental health problems in an adult with ID are associated with maternal depression and pessimism (Orsmond et al., 2003; Gray et al., 2011). Parents experience increase stress as their child ages. Gray et al. (2011) found mothers of older children (above 12 years old) report feeling more distress compared to mothers with younger children with mild disability.

Likewise, the presence of family cohesiveness and harmony helps with more positive social-emotional functioning (Hauser-Cram et al., 1999; Floyd and Zmich, 1991).

Other factors, which affect the stress level and functioning of the family, are:

2. The level of disability (Mitchell and Hauser-Cram, 2008; DeLambo et al., 2011; Esbensen, 2011; Baker et al., 2010). The child's features and level of disabilities often predict their cognitive, social and daily living difficulties and needs.

Interestingly the onset of psychopathology and its chronicity has been shown in several studies to be predicted by family dysfunction, parental mental health state, and the child's physical symptoms (Wallander et al., 2006; Koskentausta et al., 2007).

Schuiringa et al. (2015) state that the frequency and severity of the child's difficulties are strongly associated with the parent-child relationship. The elevated level and frequency of behavioral problems and severity of disability add considerable challenge to the extent that mothers of an adult with ID report more caregiving burden and are more pessimistic about the future caring for their adult son or daughter (Orsmond et al., 2003). The presence of maternal pessimism invariably affects their quality in the parent-adult child relationship and additionally mothers were found to have higher levels of anxiety and depression.

3. The age of the parents.
4. The mother's appraisal of the difficulties including the mothers' sense of empowerment (Bourke-Taylor et al., 2010; Bourke-Taylor et al., 2012). The mother's perception includes that of her managing the child's disability and needs, along with other family matters.

Mothers are often the primary carers of children in families. Thus, it is not surprising that there is a important link between the functional status of the child and the mental health status of the mother. Mothers of children with ID experience poorer psychological well-being compared to mothers with normal healthy functioning children (Hauser-Cram et al., 2001; Baker et al., 2002; Mitchell and Hauser-Cram, 2008; Eisenhower et al., 2013; Fairthorne et al., 2015). Additional to this, mothers experience more restriction in their freedom and development (Holroyd, 1974; Holroyd and McArthur, 1976) as often they are the primary caregivers. Invariably the child's behavior problems are a chronic stressor for the mother. If the mothers' appraisal of the events is positive and she copes appropriately using positive and supportive parenting, it will help in the child's social-emotional adjustment.

Over the last decade, despite more employment opportunity for women to enter the workforce, many mothers leave their job or are unemployed when having a special child (Shearn and Todd, 2000; Gray et al., 2011). Having a special need child significantly affects many mothers' decision to seek employment. Shearn and Todd (2000) found that work restrictions were due to the timing and nature of work, lack of adequate and affordable childcare and even finding suitable employment. Unmet parental expectations in work and minimal to none child-care opportunities are factors of distress for mothers when thinking about working (Gray et al., 2011).

Over the years with more fathers taking extra responsibility and interest in child-care matters a change is seen in parenting practices. It has been helpful for many mothers in such practicing household. The fathers are around to share mothers' stress of handling the child's behaviors (McCarthy et al., 2006) and most importantly provide some respite for the other parent.

Furthermore, the level of parents' functioning is much affected by the parents' reaction to the diagnosis and the difficulties and invariably their level of acceptance (Sheeran et al., 1997). Pianta and Marvin (1996) suggest a link between resolutions of receiving the child's diagnosis with the subsequent managing of the difficulties.

5. Single-parent and two-parent families (Olsson and Hwang, 2001). Being in a single-family home, invariably the single parent has many tasks to shoulder, from finances to being solely responsible for their child/ children. Single mothers and having children with ID were more vulnerable to severe depression than in mothers living with partners.
6. Family functioning particularly parenting behaviors and coping styles (Irazábal et al., 2011; Dabrowska and Pisula, 2010; Schuiringa et al., 2015).
7. Participation in health promoting activities (Mitchell and Hauser-Cram, 2008; Bourke-Taylor et al., 2012).
8. Availability of support (Bernard, 2009; Dabrowska and Pisula, 2010; Bourke-Taylor et al., 2012).
9. Social exclusion: research suggests for children with ID, the risk of social exclusion is higher (Emerson, 2015).
10. Being able to work or be financially stable (Brehaut et al., 2004; Bourke-Taylor et al., 2010; Dyson, 2010; Irazábal et al., 2011; Bourke-Taylor et al., 2012).

Thus, as discussed above, the parents and the child's difficulties affect each other. The presence of difficulties and challenges, impact the interaction of the parents with their child with ID with parents expressing less positive interaction and engagement with the child compared to a child with healthy development (Fenning et al., 2014). Consequently, the magnitude of stress and worries about their child and their future, impact the parents' appraisal and subsequent handling of their child. As the child develops and times moves on, the family must begin coping with long-term uncertainty regarding the child's present and future functioning (Kazak and Marvin, 1984). With the raised levels of parental stress invariably the environment is often associated with the presence of inappropriately, or negative feelings. The heightened level of parental stress invariably creates an environment associated with possibly increased expression of negative emotions. The presence of more negative emotional expression will significantly impact the interactions of the parents' and siblings' relationship with the child.

Fortunately, most families attempt to make things as practical and manageable as possible, and they do better with the support and understanding from others.

4. The families' finances:

In many cases, having a child with ID incurs added costs (Emerson and Hatton, 2007). The increase in expenses is likely to cause financial stress to the couple (Ouyang et al., 2014; Goudie et al., 2014; Ou et al., 2015; Emerson and Hatton, 2007). The family's economic status is often associated with caring for children, and the more severe the disability, the higher the likelihood of finance-related problems is (Emerson and Hatton, 2007; Goudie et al., 2014).

The financial difficulties are much related to:

1. Higher expenditure related to the direct cost of handling and raising the child from their daily needs, medical, and at times educational expenses;
2. Cutting back on work or working hours;
3. Having someone to look after the child;
4. Single parent or as a couple; and
5. Health and insurance coverage.

Health and insurance coverage help cover medical costs and alleviates the family's finances. However, not all children with a disability receive health and insurance coverage.

The Impact on Siblings

It is not easy having a brother or sister with disability (Scelles, 1997; Dyson, 1999; Meyer et al., 2011; Petalas et al., 2012; De Caroli and Sagone, 2013). Siblings of children ID faced numerous challenges, at times similar to their parents. They often experience a range of emotions (Dyson, 1999; Hosseinkhanzadeh and Yeganeh, 2013).

The situation of siblings with their brothers or sisters with ID and the function of the type of disability of the child is not a simple relationship (De Caroli and Sagone, 2013). Over time, the siblings become aware that something is not right with their sibling. Siblings become subtly aware they have a brother or sister who needs a significant portion of the family time and attention. They become conscious that their parents are not physically or mentally available to them even to participate in their daily activities.

Many parents spoke of numerous periods when their other and well children struggled as the parents handle their child with ID. For example, their other children are often left unattended as the parents have to make numerous hospital visits. The parents recognize their other off-springs face additional demands due to the parents' unavailability (Dyson, 1999; Hosseinkhanzadeh and Yeganeh, 2013). A period when the parents' attention is turned more on their child with the disability is when the child experiences significant physical and psychological changes while their non-effected siblings are similarly having their challenges in their development from childhood to adolescent (Dyson, 1999).

Children who have a sibling(s) with disabilities often take on added or unique roles. Often the unaffected siblings are often involved in caregiving responsibilities (Longo and Bond, 1984; Sherman and Cocozza, 1984; Dyson, 1999; Wolfe et al., 2014). Many are required to take the role as a caretaker, leader or helper for the affected child. Many children speak about having to look after their affected siblings at home or when the family goes out. Additionally, many children have to be mindful of their siblings with ID when they are in school. The parents would expect their unaffected child to look after their siblings with ID and to help them to do things when the siblings are attending the same school. While some children may not mind, there are others who report feeling overwhelmed, unattended or neglected while some reported feeling angry or upset with the added responsibility. For many children taking on the role added may restrict them (Dyson, 1999) primarily when the situation occurs repeatedly.

The non-affected siblings may develop behaviour problems as a result of:

1. Role strains (Farber, 1959). Often their parents want their healthy child to understand and help look after their child with ID;
2. High parental expectations (Gath and Gumley, 1987) and pressure to make up for the deficiency of the siblings with disabilities (Farber, 1959; Cleveland and Miller, 1977; Gath and Gumley, 1987); or
3. Reduced parental attention and family resources (Sieman, 1984).

Studies show mixed results with regards to impact on non-affected siblings, with studies showing the unaffected siblings may be at risk of developing:

1. Lesser social competency due to stress related to caring for a brother or sister with disabilities (Cleveland and Miller, 1977; McHale and Gamble, 1989; Wolfe et al., 2014);
2. Lower self-esteem; and
3. Higher social withdrawal.

Breslau and Prabucki (1987) found the siblings manifested an excess in depressive affect and social isolation compared to controls. The findings are not surprising as there is definitely reduce family recreational time as the parents devote more time to child-care and possibly a lack of respite care which will definitely make the siblings feel short-changed (Benderix and Sivberg, 2007). While other siblings have reported feelings of bitterness and resentment because of the extra and much needed attention given to the child with disability (Benderix and Sivberg, 2007; Van Riper, 2000), while some report feeling guilty because of their good health (Benderix and Sivberg, 2007).

Another issue, which may affect the siblings, is the stigma associated with having a sibling with ID (Hughes et al., 2005; Ali et al., 2012; Jones et al., 2012). People with disabilities are at increased risk of societal stigma, and discrimination just because of their needs for personal assistance with daily living. Many siblings find it difficult to manage the public perceptions of the sibling and family. The unaffected siblings may themselves be teased or isolated by their peers, neighbors, etc. The teasing and stigma may impact their relationship with their sibling, giving rise to feelings of fear and resentment towards their sibling.

Studies are reporting positive outcomes occurring in the siblings. Mandleco et al. (2003) reported that the siblings had increased self-control. The siblings develop more self-control as they try to understand and adapt to their affected sibling's problematic behaviours. Thus, they develop more tolerance and improvement in their social skills.

Dyson (2010) showed in the instances described in the above paragraph the unaffected siblings might have an accelerated growth as they take on responsibilities earlier in their childhood. The findings were significant among female siblings who were noted to be more protective, caring and understanding of others.

The family functioning mainly the parental well-being particularly maternal state, presence of marital conflict, stress level, and family resources predicted the siblings' well-being (Van Riper, 2000; Mandleco et al., 2003).

A family which continues to emphasize personal growth, and family cohesion, with the adults offering as much support as possible to their children improves the family outcome. McCubbin (1993) reported that the family having a repertoire of problem-solving and coping strategies helps with the family adaptation and increases the resilience of the affected families. Having a repertoire of problem-solving and coping strategies comes handy when the family is faced with unexpected and numerous challenges which often disrupt their routine and functioning.

Family Outcome

Parents eventually become aware of the impact of their inability to support, be available or to give the attention needed by the non-disabled siblings. These factors including pessimism about the future will affect the parent-child relationship including the siblings of children with ID and their psychosocial functioning (Abbott and Meredith, 1986; Scelles, 1997; Orsmond et al., 2003).

The disability and difficulties can severely disrupt family functioning leading to some families breaking down and in some instances, the child possibly needing institutionalization (Blacher and Bromley, 1990; Chan and Sigafoos, 2001). It is never comfortable thinking of placing any child in an out of the home facility, and it stresses the family (Cramm and Nieboer, 2011). Moreover, it does not help with society continuing to believe the parents are the best people to care for the child. However, with worsening of their psychological well-being or the child's condition, some parents are unable to meet the long-term needs of their child.

Although many families do not cope well with the challenges of caring for a child with disability, there are families who have made positive adjustments and report positive experiences (Holroyd, 1974; Kazak and Marvin, 1984; Abbott and Meredith, 1986; Kishore, 2011; De Caroli and Sagone, 2013; Mandleco et al., 2003). In these instances, the family is brought together and their bonds closer. The presence of a more positive environment is where parents are understanding, patient, tolerant and supportive, paves the way for the off-springs to learn and model positive coping skills and express emotions. The positive adaptation is associated with better family functioning, as parents' optimism, positive affect, a better internal locus of control, and the use of meaning-focused and problem-focused coping strategies (Bourke-Taylor et al., 2012; McConnell et al., 2014) are present and utilized. The positive environment results in the siblings benefiting from the association and dealing with the affected child in a more helpful and supportive caregiving role.

The collaborative relationship between parents and their children's doctors is significant in helping parents cope (Galil et al., 2006; Horrell et al., 2006; Mitchell and Hauser-Cram, 2008; Bourke-Taylor et al., 2012; Fairthorne et al., 2015). The majority of these children with ID live at home with their family. In some children, the problem of co-morbid psychopathology is indeed substantial and persistent which suggests the need for medical intervention (Einfeld et al., 2006; Gray et al., 2011). Mitchell and Hauser-Cram (2008) found a significant association with utilization and satisfaction with children's health services helps parents cope not just with their child's difficulties as well as a reduction in the parents' stress level.

The Role of Professionals

In recent years, advocates for support of families with children with ID, have risen. A significant number of these children and their families need professional help (Dekker and Koot, 2003; Jansen et al., 2013). Many children with ID eventually age and live with, or are under the supervision of their family, and for the majority of their lives (Abbott and Meredith, 1986; Orsmond et al., 2003). Invariably, parents and siblings are the mainstays of their emotional and physical support (Abbott and Meredith, 1986; Orsmond et al., 2003; Dyson, 2010). Therefore, unsurprisingly, managing children with ID involves ensuring that their families are emotionally well, because of high levels of distress and burden among caregivers.

Thus, support for families having children with ID is crucial. The developmental course, chronicity, and comorbidities of the disorder highlight to medical and mental health practitioners, the impact of the disability on the child and his/her family. Numerous reports suggest the need to understand bio-psychosocial factors, that contribute to improvements and decline, in the functioning of families of children with ID. Day to day challenges such as changes in the daily routine, or changes in the child's environment such as for example, the loss of a sibling, where the sibling might have moved out of home, or the child facing difficulties in managing relationships with peers in school, can present as behavioral or emotional outbursts. Therefore, health care professionals need to explore triggering factors within the child's environment, in order to better understand the inner world of the child and support them effectively.

Families themselves are often able to cope better, with the presence of child-care facilities that cater to the child's needs, including both therapeutic and educational opportunities, that assist the children's skills development and inclusion. Even to this time, having a child with ID is sadly perceived as a source of shame and guilt by some. Many still hold prejudice that parents are to blame, or one or both parents are deficient. This lack of understanding of the child's condition and the probable causes of precipitates social ostracism and deprives the family's ability, to obtain the help and support they so require.

Very relevant is the need to intervene early and swiftly, especially when there are symptoms suggestive of psychopathology (Floyd and Gallagher, 1997). Improved detection and intervention of associated difficulties, potentially reduce both the human suffering and economic burden to the family. Pianta and Marvin (1996) found in parents with unresolved parental reaction to the crisis, where the parents have difficulties accepting the child's diagnosis and condition, leads to increased stressful handling of their child. Understandably so, the ability for acceptance has a link with the quality of attachment to their child. Hence, parental perception and assessment of their child affect the quality of the relationship between parent and child. Therefore, a family's resilience is greatly influenced by their perception of their child, their ability to set realistic expectations, and establishing the role the child plays in the context of the family system.

Besides, despite the advancement in the medical field and improved knowledge dissemination, many parents who turn to professionals for help are frequently met with disappointment, frustration, and further confusion. Many professionals have little or no knowledge of the condition; while some minimize or dismiss the situation, telling parents, "their child will outgrow the difficulties."

Roos (1977) speaks of unhelpful professional attitudes as:

1. Lack of expertise and ignorant of technology advancement;
2. Sense of hopelessness and "incurable" disease;
3. Lack of acceptance of such a diagnosis/ disorder; and
4. Reluctance to share proper information with the clients.

The presence of such unhelpful attitudes may result in many parents switching therapist or doctor shopping, in the hope of finding more satisfactory answers. Worse still, they would not seek any help or intervention.

The holistic assessment and management of these children and their families require a multidisciplinary team, involving a range of experienced professionals. The multidisciplinary teams consist of primary care doctors, speech therapists, physical and occupational therapists, social workers, educational staff, neurologists/developmental pediatricians, psychologists, child psychiatrists, and others. The ultimate aim of treatment is to enable the child to achieve their full potential and to maintain emotional wellbeing. Given the complexity of their needs, the treatment has to be multi-modal. The roles of clinicians involve ensuring the child's wellbeing, such as detecting symptoms of depression or mood changes, identifying psychotic symptoms, assessing for difficulties in social skills, behavioral problems, learning difficulties and comorbid medical problems as well. These roles are diverse due to the large comorbidities often associated with the ID.

Once an adequate assessment and diagnosis of the child and the family are determined, an individualized program is constructed. An integral component of the treatment naturally involves the family. Parents themselves need support to enable them to assist their child effectively. The child also requires therapeutic and educational opportunities, which hopefully can assist skill development and inclusion into schools.

Bernard (2009) proposed that the assessment should consider:

1. A functional analysis of the behavioral disturbance, i.e., what factors could precipitate, aggravate or predispose to the challenging behaviors;
2. The overall cognitive level of the child and specific areas of deficit and needs of the child, including academic needs;
3. Psychiatric assessment entails looking at any underlying psychopathology including emotional, behavioral, mood disorders and the presence of psychosis;
4. An organic workout, e.g. hematological, biochemical, etc.;
5. Family functioning and assessment of risk. A critical evaluation covers factors affecting the family from within and factors outside, i.e., the environment. The intervention has to be tailored for the affected child.

Clark and Ladd (2000) and Fenning et al. (2014) believed in the huge impact that parents and caregivers have on their children's emotional and social development. The influence of caregivers were mainly linked to the parents' role in their child's developmental deficits, vulnerabilities, and outcomes. Likewise, there is a strong relationship between the functional status of the child and the mental health status of the mother, particularly in families with a child with chronic illness or difficulties (Jessop et al., 1998).

The central role played by the child within the family unit, the nature of his/her relationships and interactions with siblings and other family members, along with the parental perceptions and expectations of their child, have to be explored. Identifying pathological relationships, unhealthy perceptions, and treating mental health difficulties of the child's caregivers, are essential.

Therefore, the treating team cannot ignore the emotional needs of parents or caregivers, and siblings. There is a need to examine the impact of the child's behavior on the entire family unit. The role of caregiving can impact the psychological wellbeing of the family. Supportive psychotherapy, family therapy, working with parents and parenting skills therapy to the caregivers/parents, are modalities of treatment that health professionals can offer to families. Often, as parents grieve upon the realization of a loss of a healthy child, the therapist needs to support them by acknowledging and effectively assisting them, to ensure smooth transitions to support their child better. The mainstay of treatment involves working with families to facilitate the process of working through, facilitating acceptance and improving quality of life, for both the child and his/her family.

Pianta and Marvin (1996) added that the resolution of matters impacts the parents' mental representation of strategies in managing their difficulties. When parents reconcile and are able to adjust what they want for their children, themselves and their family, they can meet their challenges better.

Pianta and Marvin (1996) found a significant link between the presence of a support system including marital and partner relationship, with eventual acceptance and working towards resolution of the crisis. This finding makes sense as the existence of other crisis, and for example, marital conflict serves to distract the family, towards finding a possible intervention for their child's difficulties. The presence of support provides the comfort and security needs for the adult in times of their crisis. Consequently, management strategies need to be aimed at parents' belief systems, to increase parental optimism towards their child. (Baker et al., 2005).

Clinicians and mental health professionals working with children and their families need to be aware of the impact of family functioning, on the child and their family. Ignoring and not being aware of family dysfunctions and not utilizing family intervention strategies, may lead to the family decompensating (Di Nuovo and Buono, 2007). In the work done by Pianta and Marvin (1996), the manner by which parents learned the diagnosis of their child's chronic difficulties, have significant implication for practitioners and the bearer of news. Parents report feeling angry and resentful when hearing or knowing the news:

1. From letters between practitioners not intended for parents;
2. Knowing from someone else other than their health care providers;
3. The use of highly technical information and not well understood by them;
4. Secrets or truth kept away from them; and
5. Being made to wait months to know the diagnosis.

Health care providers need to aware of factors within the child's environment that could precipitate and perpetuate challenging behaviors. The presence of the child's behavioral difficulties, communication and sensory difficulties, co-morbid medical disorders, restricted range of coping strategies, and effects of medications, have an astounding impact on the child's behavior. As discussed, these children often have high rates of mental health difficulties, which often lead to them presenting at child psychiatric services (Edelstein and Glenwick, 1977). These conditions are often unrecognized and undiagnosed.

Equally important to keep in mind is that behavioral problems among children, in turn, predict parental stress and exacerbates dysfunction within families. Clinicians need to be on the alert that some behaviors may be more distressing to some families than others (Nimbalkar et al., 2014). If parental stress is not recognized and treated, this can, in turn, lead to worsening of behavioral difficulties in the child (Baker et al., 2003; Eisenhower et al., 2013).

Treatment of children and adolescents with such difficulties, needs a diverse approach. Supportive therapy for parents/caregivers and working with families are modalities of treatment that mental health professionals need to offer. Assisting with issues that can be easily tackled, parenting skills, balancing the needs of siblings, understanding the interplay of relationships within the family, and understanding patterns of behavior of the child are all part of the management. Other areas of emphasis are limit setting, the need for consistency of implemented measures, the capability to advocate for services, and the participation in support activities such as parents' organizations. Parents receiving help have favorable developmental and behavioral outcomes (Jansen et al., 2013; McConnell et al., 2014; Cantwell et al., 2014).

Group therapy has been helpful especially in emotional regulation, improving communication skills, effective problem solving and social skills training. It is essential that any information presented to the child has to be comprehensible to the child. Indications for therapy include conflicts in relationships, and distress over one's impairments in social skills. In addition, parent support groups are beneficial for parents to facilitate understanding and acceptance, to enable them to cope better.

Other modalities of treatment are Applied Behavioral Analysis. This technique is a natural science-based approach that aims to change socially significant behavior, based on the fundamental principles of learning, i.e. respondent and operant conditioning. This technique is the first-line psychosocial treatment for behavioral and psychiatric disorders in people with ID (Rush and Frances, 2000; Mafifei-Almodovar and Sturmey, 2012). Cognitive Behavior Therapy (CBT) consists of behavioral interventions, including skills training, self-instruction, relaxation training, and cognitive interventions, such as reframing maladaptive patterns of thinking. CBT has become increasingly popular as a treatment for anger and depression.

Clinicians offer pharmacological treatment to treat difficult behaviors. Medications employed range from the use of mood stabilizers, antidepressants and antipsychotic medications that are used to treat self-injurious behaviors, psychotic symptoms, agitation or severe mood disorders. Clinicians are still faced with limited choices, as there is still a dearth of research in this area.

In conclusion, treating young people with ID is indeed complex. The diversity of needs of the child requires a multifaceted treatment, with collaboration of health professionals from various specialties. Healthcare professionals need to tailor their treatment according to the family's values and needs and ensure compatibility with their aims too. The role of mental health professionals is essential, in understanding the psychological and emotional needs of the child, understanding his or her role in the family, and playing a role in supporting the family as a whole. The task that clinicians undertake is indeed challenging, and yet rewarding, when young people with ID can resume living enriching and fulfilling lives.

CONCLUSION

There is still a lot more we can do to help children with ID and their family. Factors that would bring significant help in caring for these affected children is early diagnosis and providing the necessary intervention, improving parenting behavior while involving fathers in caring for the children and increasing support from the necessary professionals and services in the community. Work is as well needed in lessening the social stigma.

REFERENCES

Abbott, D. A., & Meredith, W. H. (1986). Strengths of parents with retarded children. *Family Relations*, *35*(3), 371–375. doi:10.2307/584363

Ainsworth, M. D. (1985). Attachments across the life span. *Bulletin of the New York Academy of Medicine*, *61*, 792–812. PMID:3864511

Ainsworth, M. S., Blehar, M. C., & Everett Waters, E. (1978). *Patterns of attachment: A psychological study of the strange situation*. New York: Lawrence Erlbaum.

Ainsworth, M. S., & Bowlby, J. (1991). An ethological approach to personality development. *The American Psychologist*, *46*(4), 333–341. doi:10.1037/0003-066X.46.4.333

Al-Krenawi, A., Graham, J. R., & Al Gharaibeh, F. (2011). The impact of intellectual disability, caregiver burden, family functioning, marital quality, and sense of coherence. *Disability & Society*, *26*(2), 139–150. doi:10.1080/09687599.2011.543861

Ali, A., Hassiotis, A., Strydom, A., & King, M. (2012). Self stigma in people with intellectual disabilities and courtesy stigma in family carers: A systematic review. *Research in Developmental Disabilities*, *33*(6), 2122–2140. doi:10.1016/j.ridd.2012.06.013 PMID:22784823

Alimovic, S. (2013). Emotional and behavioural problems in children with visual impairment, intellectual and multiple disabilities. *Journal of Intellectual Disability Research*, *57*(2), 153–160. doi:10.1111/j.1365-2788.2012.01562.x PMID:22563696

Allen, D. (2008). The relationship between challenging behaviour and mental ill-health in people with intellectual disabilities: A review of current theories and evidence. *Journal of Intellectual Disabilities*, *12*(4), 267–294. doi:10.1177/1744629508100494 PMID:19074934

American Association on Intellectual & Developmental Disabilities. (2012) *Definition of Intellectual Disability*. Author.

American Psychiatric Association. (1994). *Diagnostic and Statistical Manual of mental disorders: DSM-IV*. Washington, DC: Author.

American Psychiatric Association. (2013). *Diagnostic and Statistical Manual of Mental Disorders* (5th ed.). American Psychiatric Publishing, Incorporated.

Arim, R. G., Garner, R. E., Brehaut, J. C., Lach, L. M., MacKenzie, M. J., Rosenbaum, P. L., & Kohen, D. E. (2012). Contextual influences of parenting behaviors for children with neurodevelopmental disorders: Results from a Canadian national survey. *Disability and Rehabilitation*, *34*(26), 2222–2233. doi:10.3109/09638288.2012.680650 PMID:22663074

Azad, G., Blacher, J., & Marcoulides, G. A. (2013). Mothers of children with developmental disabilities: Stress in early and middle childhood. *Research in Developmental Disabilities*, *34*(10), 3449–3459. doi:10.1016/j.ridd.2013.07.009 PMID:23920028

Azar, M., & Badr, L. K. (2010). Predictors of coping in parents of children with an intellectual disability: Comparison between Lebanese mothers and fathers. *Journal of Pediatric Nursing*, *25*(1), 46–56. doi:10.1016/j.pedn.2008.11.001 PMID:20117676

Azeem, M.W., Dogar, I.A., & Shah, S. (2013). Anxiety and Depression among Parents of Children with Intellectual Disability in Pakistan. *Journal of the Canadian Academy of Child and Adolescent Psychiatry*, *22*(4), 290-296.

Baker, B. L., Blacher, J., Crnic, K. A., & Edelbrock, C. (2002). Behavior problems and parenting stress in families of three-year-old children with and without developmental delays. *American Journal of Mental Retardation, 107*(6), 433–444. doi:10.1352/0895-8017(2002)107<0433:BPAPSI>2.0.CO;2 PMID:12323068

Baker, B. L., Blacher, J., & Olsson, M. B. (2005). Preschool children with and without developmental delay: Behaviour problems, parents' optimism and well-being. *Journal of Intellectual Disability Research, 49*(8), 575–590. doi:10.1111/j.1365-2788.2005.00691.x PMID:16011551

Baker, B. L., McIntyre, L. L., Blacher, J., Crnic, K., Edelbrock, C., & Low, C. (2003). Pre-school children with and without developmental delay: Behaviour problems and parenting stress over time. *Journal of Intellectual Disability Research, 47*(4-5), 217–230. doi:10.1046/j.1365-2788.2003.00484.x PMID:12787154

Baker, B. L., Neece, C. L., Fenning, R. M., Crnic, K. A., & Blacher, J. (2010). Mental disorders in five-year-old children with or without developmental delay: Focus on ADHD. *Journal of Clinical Child and Adolescent Psychology, 39*(4), 492–505. doi:10.1080/15374416.2010.486321 PMID:20589561

Bakken, T. L., Helverschou, S. B., Eilertsen, D. E., Heggelund, T., Myrbakk, E., & Martinsen, H. (2010). Psychiatric disorders in adolescents and adults with autism and intellectual disability: A representative study in one county in Norway. *Research in Developmental Disabilities, 31*(6), 1669–1677. doi:10.1016/j.ridd.2010.04.009 PMID:20493660

Bandura, A. (1991). Social cognitive theory of self-regulation. *Theories of Cognitive Self-Regulation, 50*, 248–287.

Barak-Levy, Y., & Atzaba-Poria, N. (2013). Paternal versus maternal coping styles with child diagnosis of developmental delay. *Research in Developmental Disabilities, 34*(6), 2040–2046. doi:10.1016/j.ridd.2013.02.026 PMID:23584184

Bazzano, A., Wolfe, C., Zylowska, L., Wang, S., Schuster, E., Barrett, C., & Lehrer, D. (2015). Mindfulness Based Stress Reduction (MBSR) for parents and caregivers of individuals with developmental disabilities: A community-based approach. *Journal of Child and Family Studies, 24*(2), 298–308. doi:10.100710826-013-9836-9

Benderix, Y., & Sivberg, B. (2007). Siblings' experiences of having a brother or sister with autism and mental retardation: A case study of 14 siblings from five families. *Journal of Pediatric Nursing, 22*(5), 410–418. doi:10.1016/j.pedn.2007.08.013 PMID:17889735

Bernard, S. H. (2009). Mental health and behavioural problems in children and adolescents with learning disabilities. *Psychiatry, 8*(10), 387–390. doi:10.1016/j.mppsy.2009.06.017

Blacher, J. (1984). Sequential stages of parental adjustment to the birth of a child with handicaps: Fact or artifact? *Mental Retardation, 22*, 55–68. PMID:6234448

Blacher, J., Baker, B. L., & Eisenhower, A. S. (2009). Student–teacher relationship stability across early school years for children with intellectual disability or typical development. *American Journal on Intellectual and Developmental Disabilities, 114*(5), 322–339. doi:10.1352/1944-7558-114.5.322 PMID:19928015

Blacher, J., & Bromley, B. E. (1990). Correlates of out-of-home placement of handicapped children: Who places and why? *Journal of Children in Contemporary Society*, *21*, 3–41. doi:10.1300/J274v21n03_02

Bourke-Taylor, H., Law, M., Howie, L., & Pallant, J. F. (2010). Development of the Child's Challenging Behaviour Scale (CCBS) for mothers of school-aged children with disabilities. *Child: Care, Health and Development*, *36*(4), 491–498. doi:10.1111/j.1365-2214.2009.01055.x PMID:20047597

Bourke-Taylor, H., Pallant, J. F., Law, M., & Howie, L. (2012). Predicting mental health among mothers of school-aged children with developmental disabilities: The relative contribution of child, maternal and environmental factors. *Research in Developmental Disabilities*, *32*(6), 1732–1740. doi:10.1016/j.ridd.2012.04.011 PMID:22699247

Bowlby, J. (1988a). *A secure base: clinical applications of attachment theory*. Hove, NY: Brunner-Routledge, Taylor & Francis Group.

Bowlby, J. (1988b). *A secure base: Parent-child attachment and healthy human development*. New York: Basic Books.

Bowlby, J. (1989). *The Making and Breaking of Affectional Bonds*. New York: Routledge, Taylor and Francis Group.

Bradley, R. H., Corwyn, R. F., Burchinal, M., McAdoo, H. P., & Garcia Coll, C. (2001). The home environments of children in the United States Part II: Relations with behavioral development through age thirteen. *Child Development*, *72*(6), 1868–1886. doi:10.1111/1467-8624.t01-1-00383 PMID:11768150

Brehaut, J. C., Kohen, D. E., Raina, P., Walter, S. D., Russell, D. J., Swinton, M., ... Rosenbaum, P. (2004). The health of primary caregivers of children with cerebral palsy: How does it compare with that of other Canadian caregivers? *Pediatrics*, *4*(2), e182–e191. doi:10.1542/peds.114.2.e182 PMID:15286255

Breslau, N., & Prabucki, K. (1987). Siblings of disabled children: Effects of chronic stress in the family. *Archives of General Psychiatry*, *44*(12), 1040–1046. doi:10.1001/archpsyc.1987.01800240014003 PMID:2961319

Brown, M. A., McIntyre, L. L., Crnic, K. A., Baker, B. L., & Blacher, J. (2011). Preschool children with and without developmental delay: Risk, parenting, and child demandingness. *Journal of Mental Health Research in Intellectual Disabilities*, *4*(3), 206–226. doi:10.1080/19315864.2011.596990 PMID:22778798

Bruce, E. J., Schultz, C. L., Smyrnios, K. X., & Schultz, N. C. (1994). Grieving related to development: A preliminary comparison of three age cohorts of parents of children with intellectual disability. *The British Journal of Medical Psychology*, *67*(1), 37–52. doi:10.1111/j.2044-8341.1994.tb01769.x PMID:7515655

Cabrera, N. J., Shannon, J. D., & Tamis-LeMonda, C. (2007). Fathers' influence on their children's cognitive and emotional development: From toddlers to pre-K. *Applied Developmental Science*, *11*(4), 208–213. doi:10.1080/10888690701762100

Cantwell, J., Muldoon, O. T., & Gallagher, S. (2014). Social support and mastery influence the association between stress and poor physical health in parents caring for children with developmental disabilities. *Research in Developmental Disabilities*, *35*(9), 2215–2223. doi:10.1016/j.ridd.2014.05.012 PMID:24927515

Caplan, B., Neece, C. L., & Baker, B. L. (2015). Developmental level and psychopathology: Comparing children with developmental delays to chronological and mental age matched controls. *Research in Developmental Disabilities*, *37*, 143–151. doi:10.1016/j.ridd.2014.10.045 PMID:25498740

Cermak, S. A., & Aberson, J. R. (1998). Social skills in children with learning disabilities. *Occupational Therapy in Mental Health*, *13*(4), 1–24. doi:10.1300/J004v13n04_01

Chan, J. B., & Sigafoos, J. (2001). Does respite care reduce parental stress in families with developmentally disabled children? *Child and Youth Care Forum*, *30*(5), 253–263. doi:10.1023/A:1014467226528

Clark, K. E., & Ladd, G. W. (2000). Connectedness and autonomy support in parent–child relationships: Links to children's socioemotional orientation and peer relationships. *Developmental Psychology*, *36*(4), 485–498. doi:10.1037/0012-1649.36.4.485 PMID:10902700

Cleveland, D. S., & Miller, N. B. (1977). Attitudes and life commitments of older siblings of mentally retarded adults: An exploratory study. *Mental Retardation*, *15*, 38–41. PMID:875727

Cramm, J. M., & Nieboer, A. P. (2011). Psychological well-being of caregivers of children with intellectual disabilities: Using parental stress as a mediating factor. *Journal of Intellectual Disabilities*, *15*(2), 101–113. doi:10.1177/1744629511410922 PMID:21750213

Crnic, K., Hoffman, C., Gaze, C., & Edelbrock, C. (2004). Understanding the emergence of behavior problems in young children with developmental delays. *Infants and Young Children*, *17*(3), 223–235. doi:10.1097/00001163-200407000-00004

Dabrowska, A., & Pisula, E. (2010). Parenting stress and coping styles in mothers and fathers of preschool children with autism and Down syndrome. *Journal of Intellectual Disability Research*, *54*(3), 266–280. doi:10.1111/j.1365-2788.2010.01258.x PMID:20146741

De Caroli, M. E., & Sagone, E. (2013). Siblings and disability: A study on social attitudes toward disabled brothers and sisters. *Procedia: Social and Behavioral Sciences*, *93*, 1217–1223. doi:10.1016/j.sbspro.2013.10.018

De Falco, S., Esposito, G., Venuti, P., & Bornstein, M. H. (2008). Fathers' play with their Down syndrome children. *Journal of Intellectual Disability Research*, *52*(6), 490–502. doi:10.1111/j.1365-2788.2008.01052.x PMID:18373561

de Falco, S., Venuti, P., Esposito, G., & Bornstein, M. H. (2009). Mother–child and father–child emotional availability in families of children with Down syndrome. *Parenting, Science and Practice*, *9*(3-4), 198–215. doi:10.1080/15295190902844381

Deater-Deckard, K. (2005). Parenting stress and children's development: Introduction to the special issue. *Infant and Child Development*, *13*(2), 111–115. doi:10.1002/icd.383

Deb, S., Thomas, M., & Bright, C. (2001). Mental disorder in adults with intellectual disability: Prevalence of functional psychiatric illness among a community-based population aged between 16 and 64 years. *Journal of Intellectual Disability Research*, *46*(6), 495–505. doi:10.1046/j.1365-2788.2001.00374.x PMID:11737536

Dekker, M. C., & Koot, H. M. (2003). DSM-IV Disorders in Children With Borderline to Moderate Intellectual Disability. I: Prevalence and Impact. *Journal of the American Academy of Child and Adolescent Psychiatry*, *42*(8), 915–922. doi:10.1097/01.CHI.0000046892.27264.1A PMID:12874493

Dekker, M. C., Koot, H. M., van der Ende, J., & … . (2002). Emotional and behavioral problems in children and adolescents with and without intellectual disability. *Journal of Child Psychology and Psychiatry, and Allied Disciplines*, *43*(8), 1087–1098. doi:10.1111/1469-7610.00235 PMID:12455929

DeLambo, D., Chung, W., & Huang, W. (2011). Stress and age: A comparison of Asian American and Non-Asian American parents of children with developmental disabilities. *Journal of Developmental and Physical Disabilities*, *23*(2), 129–141. doi:10.100710882-010-9211-3

DeWeaver, K. L., & Kropf, N. P. (1992). Persons with mental retardation: A forgotten minority in education. *Journal of Social Work Education*, *28*(1), 36–46. doi:10.1080/10437797.1992.10778756

Di Nuovo, S. F., & Buono, S. (2007). Psychiatric syndromes comorbid with mental retardation: Differences in cognitive and adaptive skills. *Journal of Psychiatric Research*, *41*(9), 795–800. doi:10.1016/j.jpsychires.2006.02.011 PMID:16697412

Dyer, W. J., McBride, B. A., & Jeans, L. M. (2009). A longitudinal examination of father involvement with children with developmental delays: Does timing of diagnosis matter? *Journal of Early Intervention*, *31*(3), 265–281. doi:10.1177/0192513X09340386

Dyson, L. (2010). Unanticipated effects of children with learning disabilities on their families. *Learning Disability Quarterly*, *33*(1), 43–55. doi:10.1177/073194871003300104

Dyson, L. L. (1999). The psychosocial functioning of school-age children who have siblings with developmental disabilities: Change and stability over time. *Journal of Applied Developmental Psychology*, *20*(2), 253–271. doi:10.1016/S0193-3973(99)00016-7

Eakes, G. G. (1995). Chronic sorrow: The lived experience of parents of chronically mentally ill individuals. *Archives of Psychiatric Nursing*, *9*(2), 77–84. doi:10.1016/S0883-9417(95)80004-2 PMID:7755411

Eakes, G. G., Burke, M. L., & Hainsworth, M. A. (1998). Middle range theory of chronic sorrow. *Journal of Nursing Scholarship*, *30*(2), 179–184. doi:10.1111/j.1547-5069.1998.tb01276.x PMID:9775562

Edelstein, T. M., & Glenwick, D. S. (1977). Referral reasons for psychological services for adults with mental retardation. *Research in Developmental Disabilities*, *18*(1), 45–59. doi:10.1016/S0891-4222(96)00037-6 PMID:9085429

Egeland, B., Pianta, R., & O'brien, M. A. (1993). Maternal intrusiveness in infancy and child maladaptation in early school years. *Development and Psychopathology*, *5*(3), 359–370. doi:10.1017/S0954579400004466

Einfeld, S. L., Ellis, L. A., & Emerson, E. (2011). Comorbidity of intellectual disability and mental disorder in children and adolescents: A systematic review. *Journal of Intellectual & Developmental Disability*, *36*(2), 137–143. doi:10.1080/13668250.2011.572548 PMID:21609299

Einfeld, S. L., Piccinin, A. M., Mackinnon, A., Hofer, S. M., Taffe, J., Gray, K. M., ... Tonge, B. J. (2006). Psychopathology in young people with intellectual disability. *Journal of the American Medical Association, 296*(16), 1981–1989. doi:10.1001/jama.296.16.1981 PMID:17062861

Eisenhower, A., Blacher, J., & Baker, B. L. (2013). Mothers' perceived physical health during early and middle childhood: Relations with child developmental delay and behavior problems. *Research in Developmental Disabilities, 34*(3), 1059–1068. doi:10.1016/j.ridd.2012.12.002 PMID:23306002

Eisenhower, A. S., Baker, B. L., & Blacher, J. (2007). Early student–teacher relationships of children with and without intellectual disability: Contributions of behavioral, social, and self-regulatory competence. *Journal of School Psychology, 45*(4), 363–383. doi:10.1016/j.jsp.2006.10.002 PMID:21490876

Elliott, S. N., & Gresham, F. M. (1993). Social skills interventions for children. *Behavior Modification, 17*(3), 287–313. doi:10.1177/01454455930173004 PMID:8343100

Emerson, E., Blacher, J., Einfeld, S., Hatton, C., Robertson, J., & Stancliffe, R. J. (2014). Environmental risk factors associated with the persistence of conduct difficulties in children with intellectual disabilities and autistic spectrum disorders. *Research in Developmental Disabilities, 35*(12), 3508–3517. doi:10.1016/j.ridd.2014.08.039 PMID:25238636

Emerson, E., & Hatton, C. (2007). The socio-economic circumstances of children at risk of disability in Britain. *Disability & Society, 22*(6), 563–580. doi:10.1080/09687590701560154

Emerson, E., & Hatton, C. (2007). Mental health of children and adolescents with intellectual disabilities in Britain. *The British Journal of Psychiatry, 191*(6), 493–499. doi:10.1192/bjp.bp.107.038729 PMID:18055952

Esbensen, A. J. (2011). Families of individuals with intellectual disability and comorbid mental health problems. *Journal of Mental Health Research in Intellectual Disabilities, 4*(3), 140–157. doi:10.1080/19315864.2011.597018

Fairthorne, J., Jacoby, P., Bourke, J., de Klerk, N., & Leonard, H. (2015). Onset of maternal psychiatric disorders after the birth of a child with intellectual disability: A retrospective cohort study. *Journal of Psychiatric Research, 61*, 223–230. doi:10.1016/j.jpsychires.2014.11.011 PMID:25499469

Farber, B., & Kirk, S. A. (1959). Effects of a severely retarded child on family integration. *Monographs of the Society for Research in Child Development, 24*(2), 1–112. doi:10.2307/1165597

Feniger-Schaal, R., & Oppenheim, D. (2013). Resolution of the diagnosis and maternal sensitivity among mothers of children with Intellectual Disability. *Research in Developmental Disabilities, 34*(1), 306–313. doi:10.1016/j.ridd.2012.08.007 PMID:22983017

Fenning, R. M., Baker, J. K., Baker, B. L., & Crnic, K. A. (2007). Parenting children with borderline intellectual functioning: A unique risk population. *American Journal of Mental Retardation, 112*(2), 107–121. doi:10.1352/0895-8017(2007)112[107:PCWBIF]2.0.CO;2 PMID:17295551

Fenning, R. M. B., Baker, J. K., & Crnic, B. L. (2014). Parent-child interaction over time in families of young children with borderline intellectual functioning. *Journal of Family Psychology, 28*(3), 326–335. doi:10.1037/a0036537 PMID:24707801

Flippin, M., & Crais, E. R. (2011). The need for more effective father involvement in early autism intervention: A systematic review and recommendations. *Journal of Early Intervention*, *33*(1), 24–50. doi:10.1177/1053815111400415

Floyd, F. J., & Gallagher, E. M. (1997). Parental stress, care demands, and use of support services for school-age children with disabilities and behavior problems. *Family Relations*, *46*(4), 359–371. doi:10.2307/585096

Floyd, F. J., & Zmich, D. E. (1991). Marriage and the parenting partnership: Perceptions and interactions of parents with mentally retarded and typically developing children. *Child Development*, *62*(6), 1434–1448. doi:10.2307/1130817 PMID:1786726

Galil, A., Bachner, Y. G., Merrick, J., Flusser, H., Lubetzky, H., Heiman, N., & Carmel, S. (2006). Physician-parent communication as predictor of parent satisfaction with child development services. *Research in Developmental Disabilities*, *27*(3), 233–242. doi:10.1016/j.ridd.2005.03.004 PMID:15998579

Gallagher, S., & Hannigan, A. (2014). Depression and chronic health conditions in parents of children with and without developmental disabilities: The growing up in Ireland cohort study. *Research in Developmental Disabilities*, *35*(2), 448–454. doi:10.1016/j.ridd.2013.11.029 PMID:24361813

Gallagher, S., Phillips, A. C., Oliver, C., & Carroll, D. (2008). Predictors of psychological morbidity in parents of children with intellectual disabilities. *Journal of Pediatric Psychology*, *33*(10), 1129–1136. doi:10.1093/jpepsy/jsn040 PMID:18430761

Gath, A., & Gumley, D. (1987). Retarded children and their siblings. *Journal of Child Psychology and Psychiatry, and Allied Disciplines*, *28*(5), 715–730. doi:10.1111/j.1469-7610.1987.tb01554.x PMID:2959672

Gerstein, E. D., Crnic, K. A., Blacher, J., & Baker, B. L. (2009). Resilience and the course of daily parenting stress in families of young children with intellectual disabilities. *Journal of Intellectual Disability Research*, *53*(12), 981–997. doi:10.1111/j.1365-2788.2009.01220.x PMID:19874449

Gilmore, L., & Cuskelly, M. (2014). Vulnerability to loneliness in people with intellectual disability: An explanatory model. *Journal of Policy and Practice in Intellectual Disabilities*, *11*(3), 192–199. doi:10.1111/jppi.12089

Goudie, A., Narcisse, M. R., Hall, D. E., & Kuo, D. Z. (2014). Financial and psychological stressors associated with caring for children with disability. *Families, Systems & Health*, *32*(3), 280–290. doi:10.1037/fsh0000027 PMID:24707826

Granic, I., & Patterson, G. R. (2006). Toward a comprehensive model of antisocial development: A dynamic systems approach. *Psychological Review*, *113*(1), 101–131. doi:10.1037/0033-295X.113.1.101 PMID:16478303

Gray, K. M., Piccinin, A. M., Hofer, S. M., Mackinnon, A., Bontempo, D. E., Einfeld, S. L., ... Tonge, B. J. (2011). The longitudinal relationship between behavior and emotional disturbance in young people with intellectual disability and maternal mental health. *Research in Developmental Disabilities*, *32*(3), 1194–1204. doi:10.1016/j.ridd.2010.12.044 PMID:21295442

Greene, J. G., Fox, N. A., & Lewis, M. (1983). The relationship between neonatal characteristics and three-month mother-infant interaction in high-risk infants. *Child Development, 54*(5), 1286–1296. doi:10.2307/1129682 PMID:6354634

Gupta, R. K., & Harpreet, K. (2010). Stress among parents of children with intellectual disability. *Asia Pacific Disability Rehabilitation Journal*, 21.

Guralnick, M. J. (1977). Peer social networks of young boys with developmental delays. *American Journal of Mental Retardation, 101*, 595–612. PMID:9152475

Guralnick, M. J. (1999). Family and child influences on the peer-related social competence of young children with developmental delays. *Mental Retardation and Developmental Disabilities Research Reviews, 5*(1), 21–29. doi:10.1002/(SICI)1098-2779(1999)5:1<21::AID-MRDD3>3.0.CO;2-O

Guralnick, M. J., Hammond, M. A., Connor, R. T., & Neville, B. (2006). Stability, change, and correlates of the peer relationships of young children with mild developmental delays. *Child Development, 77*(2), 312–324. doi:10.1111/j.1467-8624.2006.00872.x PMID:16611174

Hallum, A. (1995). Disability and the transition to adulthood:Issues for the disabled child, the family, and the pediatrician. *Current Problems in Pediatrics, 25*(1), 12–50. doi:10.1016/S0045-9380(06)80013-7 PMID:7720408

Hastings, R. P. (2003). Child behaviour problems and partner mental health as correlates of stress in mothers and fathers of children with autism. *Journal of Intellectual Disability Research, 47*(4-5), 231–237. doi:10.1046/j.1365-2788.2003.00485.x PMID:12787155

Hastings, R. P., Daley, D., Burns, C., & Beck, A. (2006). Maternal distress and expressed emotion: Cross-sectional and longitudinal relationships with behavior problems of children with intellectual disabilities. *American Journal of Mental Retardation, 111*(1), 48–61. doi:10.1352/0895-8017(2006)111[48:MDAEEC]2.0.CO;2 PMID:16332156

Hastings, R. P., & Lloyd, T. (2007). Expressed emotion in families of children and adults with intellectual disabilities. *Mental Retardation and Developmental Disabilities Research Reviews, 13*(4), 339–345. doi:10.1002/mrdd.20173 PMID:17979206

Hauser-Cram, P., Warfield, M. E., & Shonkoff, J. P. (2001). Children with disabilities: A longitudinal study of child development and parent wellbeing. *Monographs of the Society for Research in Child Development, 66*, 1–131. PMID:11677873

Hauser-Cram, P., Warfield, M. E., Shonkoff, J. P., Krauss, M. W., Upshur, C. C., & Sayer, A. (1999). Family influences on adaptive development in young children with Down syndrome. *Child Development, 70*(4), 979–989. doi:10.1111/1467-8624.00071 PMID:10446730

Hodapp, R. M. (2002). Parenting children with mental retardation. In M. H. Bornstein (Ed.), Handbook of Parenting (pp. 355–381). London: Lawrence Erlbaum Associates.

Holroyd, J. (1974). The Questionnaire on Resources and Stress: An instrument to measure family response to a handicapped family member. *Journal of Community Psychology, 2*(1), 92–94. doi:10.1002/1520-6629(197401)2:1<92::AID-JCOP2290020133>3.0.CO;2-A

Holroyd, J., & McArthur, D. (1976). Mental retardation and stress on the parents: A contrast between Down's syndrome and childhood autism. *American Journal of Mental Deficiency*, *80*, 431–436. PMID:129006

Horrell, S.C.V., MacLean, W.E., & Conley, V.M. (2006) Patient and parent/guardian perspectives on the health care of adults with mental retardation. *Mental Retardation, 44*(4), 239-248.

Hosseinkhanzadeh, A. A., & Yeganeh, T. (2013). A study of the siblings relationships in families with mentally disable children. *Procedia: Social and Behavioral Sciences*, *84*, 864–868. doi:10.1016/j.sbspro.2013.06.663

Howell, A., Hauser-Cram, P., & Kersh, J. E. (2007). Setting the stage: Early child and family characteristics as predictors of later loneliness in children with developmental disabilities. *American Journal of Mental Retardation*, *112*(1), 18–30. doi:10.1352/0895-8017(2007)112[18:STSECA]2.0.CO;2 PMID:17181387

Hughes, K., Bellis, M. A., Jones, L., Wood, S., Bates, G., Eckley, L., ... Officer, A. (2005). Prevalence and risk of violence against adults with disabilities: A systematic review and meta-analysis of observational studies. *Lancet*, *379*(9826), 1621–1629. doi:10.1016/S0140-6736(11)61851-5 PMID:22377290

Irazábal, M., Marsà, F., & García, M. (2011). Family burden related to clinical and functional variables of people with intellectual disability with and without a mental disorder. *Research in Developmental Disabilities*, *32*, 796–803. PMID:22245729

Jansen, S. L., van der Putten, A. A., & Vlaskamp, C. (2013). What parents find important in the support of a child with profound intellectual and multiple disabilities. *Child: Care, Health and Development*, *39*(3), 432–441. doi:10.1111/j.1365-2214.2012.01381.x PMID:22515566

Jessop, D. J., Riessman, C. K., & Stein, R. E. (1998). Chronic childhood illness and maternal mental health. *Journal of Developmental and Behavioral Pediatrics*, *9*, 147–156. PMID:3403730

Jones, L., Bellis, M. A., Wood, S., Hughes, K., McCoy, E., Eckley, L., ... Officer, A. (2012). Prevalence and risk of violence against children with disabilities: A systematic review and meta-analysis of observational studies. *Lancet*, *380*(9845), 899–907. doi:10.1016/S0140-6736(12)60692-8 PMID:22795511

Kazak, A. E., & Marvin, R. S. (1984). Differences, difficulties and adaptation: Stress and social networks in families with a handicapped child. *Family Relations*, *33*(1), 67–77. doi:10.2307/584591

Kemp, C., & Carter, M. (2002). The social skills and social status of mainstreamed students with intellectual disabilities. *Educational Psychology*, *22*(4), 391–411. doi:10.1080/0144341022000003097

Kennedy, C. H. (1994). Manipulating antecedent conditions to alter the stimulus control of problem behavior. *Journal of Applied Behavior Analysis*, *27*(1), 161–170. doi:10.1901/jaba.1994.27-161 PMID:8188556

Kersh, J., Hedvat, T. T., Hauser-Cram, P., & Warfield, M. E. (2006). The contribution of marital quality to the well-being of parents of children with developmental disabilities. *Journal of Intellectual Disability Research*, *50*(12), 883–893. doi:10.1111/j.1365-2788.2006.00906.x PMID:17100949

Kishore, M. T. (2011). Disability impact and coping in mothers of children with intellectual disabilities and multiple disabilities. *Journal of Intellectual Disabilities*, *15*(4), 241–251. doi:10.1177/1744629511431659 PMID:22158461

Koskentausta, T., Iivanainen, M., & Almqvist, F. (2007). Risk factors for psychiatric disturbance in children with intellectual disability. *Journal of Intellectual Disability Research, 51*(1), 43–53. doi:10.1111/j.1365-2788.2006.00871.x PMID:17181602

Landry, S. H., Smith, K. E., Swank, P. R., & Guttentag, C. (2008). A responsive parenting intervention: The optimal timing across early childhood for impacting maternal behaviors and child outcomes. *Developmental Psychology, 44*(5), 1335–1353. doi:10.1037/a0013030 PMID:18793067

Lee, J. (2013). Maternal stress, well-being, and impaired sleep in mothers of children with developmental disabilities: A literature review. *Research in Developmental Disabilities, 34*(11), 4255–4273. doi:10.1016/j.ridd.2013.09.008 PMID:24080069

Lin, L.-P., Hsu, S.-W., Kuo, M.-T., Wu, J.-L., Chu, C., & Lin, J.-D. (2014). Onset aging conditions of adults with an intellectual disability associated with primary caregiver depression. *Research in Developmental Disabilities, 35*(3), 632–638. doi:10.1016/j.ridd.2013.12.013 PMID:24467811

Longo, D. C., & Bond, B. (1984). Families of the handicapped child: Research and practice. *Family Relations, 33*(1), 57–65. doi:10.2307/584590

Lopez, V., Clifford, T., & Minnes, P. (2008). Parental stress and coping in families of children with and without developmental delays. *Journal on Developmental Disabilities, 14*, 99–103.

Maccoby, E. E., & Martin, J. A. (1983). *Socialization in the context of the family: Parent-child interaction*. New York: Wiley.

MacDonald, E. E., & Hastings, R. P. (2010). *Fathers of children with developmental disabilities*. John Wiley & Sons.

MacLean, W. E. Jr, Tervo, R. C., Hoch, J., Tervo, M., & Symons, F. J. (2010). Self-Injury among a community cohort of young children at risk for intellectual and developmental disabilities. *The Journal of Pediatrics, 157*(6), 979–983. doi:10.1016/j.jpeds.2010.05.052 PMID:20630541

Mafifei-Almodovar, L., & Sturmey, P. (2012). Evidence-based practice and crisis intervention. In D. D. Reed, R. F. D. DiGennaro, & J. K. Luiselli (Eds.), *Handbook of crisis intervention for individuals with developmental disabilities*. New York: Springer.

Mandleco, B., Olsen, S. F., Dyches, T., & Marshall, E. (2003). The relationship between family and sibling functioning in families raising a child with a disability. *Journal of Family Nursing, 9*(4), 365–396. doi:10.1177/1074840703258329

Marvin, R.S., & Pianta, R.C. (1996). Mothers' reactions to their child's diagnosis: Relations with security of attachment. *Journal of Clinical Child Psychology, 25*(4), 436-445.

Mazzucchelli, T. G., & Sanders, M. R. (2011). Preventing behavioural and emotional problems in children who have a developmental disability: A public health approach. *Research in Developmental Disabilities, 32*(6), 2148–2156. doi:10.1016/j.ridd.2011.07.022 PMID:21831592

McCarthy, A., Cuskelly, M., van Kraayenoord, C. E., & Cohen, J. (2006). Predictors of stress in mothers and fathers of children with fragile X syndrome. *Research in Developmental Disabilities, 27*(6), 688–704. doi:10.1016/j.ridd.2005.10.002 PMID:16361079

McConkey, R., Truesdale-Kennedy, M., Chang, M.-Y., Jarrah, S., & Shukri, R. (2008). The impact on mothers of bringing up a child with intellectual disabilities: A cross-cultural study. *International Journal of Nursing Studies*, *45*(1), 65–74. doi:10.1016/j.ijnurstu.2006.08.007 PMID:17022985

McConnell, D., Savage, A., & Breitkreuz, R. (2014). Resilience in families raising children with disabilities and behavior problems. *Research in Developmental Disabilities*, *35*(4), 833–848. doi:10.1016/j.ridd.2014.01.015 PMID:24491480

McCubbin, H. I. (1993). Families coping with illness: The resiliency model of family stress, adjustment, and adaptation. In Families, Health & Illness: Perspectives on coping and intervention. Winstead & Fry.

McHale, S. M., & Gamble, W. C. (1989). Sibling relationships of children with disabled and nondisabled brothers and sisters. *Developmental Psychology*, *25*(3), 421–429. doi:10.1037/0012-1649.25.3.421

McLoyd, V. C. (1990). The impact of economic hardship on Black families and children: Psychological distress, parenting, and socioemotional development. *Child Development*, *61*(2), 311–346. doi:10.2307/1131096 PMID:2188806

McLoyd, V. C., & Wilson, L. (1990). Maternal behavior, social support, and economic conditions as predictors of distress in children. *New Directions for Child and Adolescent Development*, *1990*(46), 49–69. doi:10.1002/cd.23219904605 PMID:2348935

Meyer, K. A., Ingersoll, B., & Hambrick, D. Z. (2011). Factors influencing adjustment in siblings of children with autism spectrum disorders. *Research in Autism Spectrum Disorders*, *5*(4), 1413–1420. doi:10.1016/j.rasd.2011.01.027

Mitchell, D. B., & Hauser-Cram, P. (2008). The well-being of mothers of adolescents with developmental disabilities in relation to medical care utilization and satisfaction with health care. *Research in Developmental Disabilities*, *29*(2), 97–112. doi:10.1016/j.ridd.2006.12.002 PMID:17267176

Molteno, G., Molteno, C. D., Finchilescu, G., & Dawes, A. R. L. (2001). Behavioural and emotional problems in children with intellectual disability attending special schools in Cape Town, South Africa. *Journal of Intellectual Disability Research*, *45*(6), 515–520. doi:10.1046/j.1365-2788.2001.00368.x PMID:11737538

Moss, S., Emerson, E., Kiernan, C., Turner, S., Hatton, C., & Alborz, A. (2000). Psychiatric symptoms in adults with learning disability and challenging behaviour. *The British Journal of Psychiatry*, *177*(5), 452–456. doi:10.1192/bjp.177.5.452 PMID:11060000

Mullineaux, P. Y., Deater-Deckard, K., Petrill, S. A., & Thompson, L. A. (2009). Parenting and child behaviour problems: A longitudinal analysis of non-shared environment. *Infant and Child Development: An International Journal of Research and Practice*, *18*(2), 133–148. doi:10.1002/icd.593 PMID:19436771

Myrbakk, E., & von Tetzchner, S. (2008). Psychiatric disorders and behaviour problems in people with intellectual disability. *Research in Developmental Disabilities*, *29*(4), 316–332. doi:10.1016/j.ridd.2007.06.002 PMID:17616450

Neece, C., & Baker, B. (2008). Predicting maternal parenting stress in middle childhood: The roles of child intellectual status, behaviour problems and social skills. *Journal of Intellectual Disability Research*, *52*(12), 1114–1128. doi:10.1111/j.1365-2788.2008.01071.x PMID:18513339

Nihira, K., Mink, I. T., & Meyers, C. E. (1985). Home environment and development of slow-learning adolescents: Reciprocal relations. *Developmental Psychology*, *21*(5), 784–794. doi:10.1037/0012-1649.21.5.784

Nimbalkar, S., Raithatha, S., & Shah, R. (2014). *A qualitative study of psychosocial problems among parents of children with cerebral palsy attending two tertiary care hospitals in Western India*. ISRN Family Medicine. doi:10.1155/2014/769619

Norlin, D., Axberg, U., & Broberg, M. (2014). Predictors of harsh parenting practices in parents of children with disabilities. *Early Child Development and Care*, *184*(9-10), 1472–1484. doi:10.1080/03004430.2013.845562

Olsson, M. B., & Hwang, C. P. (2001). Depression in mothers and fathers of children with intellectual disability. *Journal of Intellectual Disability Research*, *45*(6), 535–543. doi:10.1046/j.1365-2788.2001.00372.x PMID:11737541

Orsmond, G. I., Seltzer, M. M., Krauss, M. W., & Hong, J. (2003). Behavior problems in adults with mental retardation and maternal well-being: Examination of the direction of effects. *American Journal of Mental Retardation*, *108*(4), 257–271. doi:10.1352/0895-8017(2003)108<257:BPIAWM>2.0.CO;2 PMID:12780337

Ou, J.-J., Shi, L.-J., Xun, G.-L., Chen, C., Wu, R.-R., Luo, X.-R., ... Zhao, J.-P. (2015). Employment and financial burden of families with preschool children diagnosed with autism spectrum disorders in urban China: Results from a descriptive study. *BMC Psychiatry*, *15*(1), 42–57. doi:10.118612888-015-0382-4 PMID:25608486

Ouyang, L., Grosse, S. D., Riley, C., Bolen, J., Bishop, E., Raspa, M., & Bailey, D. B. Jr. (2014). A comparison of family financial and employment impacts of fragile X syndrome, autism spectrum disorders, and intellectual disability. *Research in Developmental Disabilities*, *35*(7), 1518–1527. doi:10.1016/j.ridd.2014.04.009 PMID:24755230

Pancsofar, N., & Vernon-Feagans, L. (2010). Fathers' early contributions to children's language development in families from low-income rural communities. *Early Childhood Research Quarterly*, *25*(4), 50–463. doi:10.1016/j.ecresq.2010.02.001 PMID:21057648

Parmenter, T. R., Einfeld, S. L., Tonge, B. J., & Dempster, J. A. (1998). Behavioural and emotional problems in the classroom of children and adolescents with intellectual disability. *Journal of Intellectual & Developmental Disability*, *23*(1), 71–77. doi:10.1080/13668259800033591

Petalas, M. A., Hastings, R. P., Nash, S., Hall, L. M., Joannidi, H., & Dowey, A. (2012). Psychological adjustment and sibling relationships in siblings of children with Autism Spectrum Disorders: Environmental stressors and the Broad Autism Phenotype. *Research in Autism Spectrum Disorders*, *6*(1), 546–555. doi:10.1016/j.rasd.2011.07.015

Petty, J. L., Bacarese-Hamilton, M., Davies, L. E., & Oliver, C. (2014). Correlates of self-injurious, aggressive and destructive behaviour in children under five who are at risk of developmental delay. *Research in Developmental Disabilities, 35*(1), 36–45. doi:10.1016/j.ridd.2013.10.019 PMID:24216345

Pianta, R. C., Marvin, R. S., Britner, P. A., & Borowitz, K. C. (1996). Mothers' resolution of their children's diagnosis: Organized patterns of caregiving representations. *Infant Mental Health Journal, 17*(3), 239–256. doi:10.1002/(SICI)1097-0355(199623)17:3<239::AID-IMHJ4>3.0.CO;2-J

Pisula, E. (2011). Parenting stress in mothers and fathers of children with autism spectrum disorders In A Comprehensive Book on Autism Spectrum Disorders. InTech. doi:10.5772/18507

Plant, K. M., & Sanders, M. R. (2007). Predictors of care-giver stress in families of preschool-aged children with developmental disabilities. *Journal of Intellectual Disability Research, 51*(2), 109–124. doi:10.1111/j.1365-2788.2006.00829.x PMID:17217475

Quesenberry, A., Ostrosky, M. M., & Corso, R. (2007). Skilled and knowledgeable caregivers: The role of fathers in supporting young children's development. *Young Exceptional Children, 10*(4), 11–19. doi:10.1177/109625060701000402

Reardon, T. C., Gray, K. M., & Melvin, G. A. (2015). Anxiety disorders in children and adolescents with intellectual disability: Prevalence and assessment. *Research in Developmental Disabilities, 36*, 175–190. doi:10.1016/j.ridd.2014.10.007 PMID:25462478

Reder, P., & Lucey, C. (1995). *Assessment of parenting: Psychiatric and psychological contributions.* Hove, NY: Brunner-Routledge, Taylor and Francis Group.

Ritzema, A.M., & Sladeczek, I.E. (2011). Stress in parents of children with developmental disabilities over time. *Journal of Developmental Disabilities, 17*, 21-34.

Robinson, M., & Neece, C. L. (2015). Marital satisfaction, parental stress, and child behavior problems among parents of young children with developmental delays. *Journal of Mental Health Research in Intellectual Disabilities, 8*(1), 23–46. doi:10.1080/19315864.2014.994247

Roos, P. (1977). Parents of mentally retarded people. *International Journal of Mental Health, 6*(1), 96–119. doi:10.1080/00207411.1977.11448758

Rush, A. J., & Frances, A. T. (2000). The expert consensus guidelines: Treatment of psychiatric and behavioral problems in mental retardation. *American Journal of Mental Retardation, 105*, 159–1228.

Scelles, R. (1997). The impact of a person's disability on his or her sibling. *International Journal of Rehabilitation Research. Internationale Zeitschrift fur Rehabilitationsforschung. Revue Internationale de Recherches de Readaptation, 20*(2), 129–137. doi:10.1097/00004356-199706000-00002 PMID:9226496

Schuengel, C., Rentinck, I. C. M., Stolk, J., Voorman, J. M., Loots, G. M. P., Ketelaar, M., ... Becher, J. G. (2009). Parents' reactions to the diagnosis of cerebral palsy: Associations between resolution, age and severity of disability. *Child: Care, Health and Development, 35*(5), 673–680. doi:10.1111/j.1365-2214.2009.00951.x PMID:19320906

Schuiringa, H., van Nieuwenhuijzen, M., & de Castro, B. O. (2015). Parenting and the parent–child relationship in families of children with mild to borderline intellectual disabilities and externalizing behavior. *Research in Developmental Disabilities*, *32*, 1–12. doi:10.1016/j.ridd.2014.08.018 PMID:25262097

Shannon, J. D., Tamis-LeMonda, C. S., London, K., & Cabrera, N. (2002). Beyond rough and tumble: Low-income fathers' interactions and children's cognitive development at 24 months. *Parenting, Science and Practice*, *2*(2), 77–104. doi:10.1207/S15327922PAR0202_01

Shearn, J., & Todd, S. (2000). Maternal employment and family responsibilities: The perspectives of mothers of children with intellectual disabilities. *Journal of Applied Research in Intellectual Disabilities*, *13*(3), 109–131. doi:10.1046/j.1468-3148.2000.00021.x

Sheeran, T., Marvin, R. S., & Pianta, R. C. (1997). Mothers' resolution of their child's diagnosis and self-reported measures of parenting stress, marital relations, and social support. *Journal of Pediatric Psychology*, *22*(2), 197–212. doi:10.1093/jpepsy/22.2.197 PMID:9114643

Sherman, B. R., & Cocozza, J. J. (1984). Stress in families of the developmentally disabled: A literature review of factors affecting the decision to seek out-of-home placements. *Family Relations*, *33*(1), 95–103. doi:10.2307/584594

Sieman, M. (1984). Siblings of the chronically ill or disabled child. *The Nursing Clinics of North America*, *19*, 295–307. PMID:6233538

Stevenson, M., & Crnic, K. (2013). Intrusive fathering, children's self-regulation and social skills: A mediation analysis. *Journal of Intellectual Disability Research*, *57*(6), 500–512. doi:10.1111/j.1365-2788.2012.01549.x PMID:22458354

Straus, M. A., & Stewart, J. H. (1999). Corporal punishment by American parents: National data on prevalence, chronicity, severity, and duration, in relation to child and family characteristics. *Clinical Child and Family Psychology Review*, *2*(2), 55–70. doi:10.1023/A:1021891529770 PMID:11225932

Straus, M. S., & Donnelly, D. A. (2001). *Beating the devil out of them. Corporal punishment in American families and its effects on children*. New Brunswick, NJ: Transaction Publishers.

Tremblay, K. N., Richer, L., Lachance, L., & Côté, A. (2010). Psychopathological manifestations of children with intellectual disabilities according to their cognitive and adaptive behavior profile. *Research in Developmental Disabilities*, *31*(1), 57–69. doi:10.1016/j.ridd.2009.07.016 PMID:19700260

Trute, B. (1990). Child and parent predictors of family adjustment in households containing young developmentally disabled children. *Family Relations*, *39*(3), 292–297. doi:10.2307/584874

Van Riper, M. (2000). Family variables associated with well-being in siblings of children with down syndrome. *Journal of Family Nursing*, *6*(3), 267–286. doi:10.1177/107484070000600305

Vrijmoeth, C., Monbaliu, E., & Lagast, E. (2011). Behavioral problems in children with motor and intellectual disabilities: Prevalence and associations with maladaptive personality and marital relationship. *Research in Developmental Disabilities*, *32*, 1027–1038. PMID:22502827

Wallander, J. L., Dekker, M. C., & Koot, H. M. (2006). Risk factors for psychopathology in children with intellectual disability: A prospective longitudinal population-based study. *Journal of Intellectual Disability Research, 50*(4), 259–268. doi:10.1111/j.1365-2788.2005.00792.x PMID:16507030

Warren, S. F., & Brady, N. C. (2007). The role of maternal responsivity in the development of children with intellectual disabilities. *Mental Retardation and Developmental Disabilities Research Reviews, 13*(4), 330–338. doi:10.1002/mrdd.20177 PMID:17979201

Wells, T., Sandefur, D., & Hogan, D. P. (2003). What happens after the high school years among young persons with disabilities? *Social Forces, 82*(2), 803–832. doi:10.1353of.2004.0029

Wikler, L. (1981). Chronic stresses of families of mentally retarded children. *Family Relations, 30*(2), 281–288. doi:10.2307/584142

Witwera, A. N., & Lecavaliera, L. (2008). Psychopathology in children with intellectual disability: Risk markers and correlates. *Journal of Mental Health Research in Intellectual Disabilities, 1*(2), 75–96. doi:10.1080/19315860801988327

Wolfe, B., Song, J., Greenberg, J. S., & Mailick, M. R. (2014). Ripple effects of developmental disabilities and mental illness on nondisabled adult siblings. *Social Science & Medicine, 108*, 1–9. doi:10.1016/j.socscimed.2014.01.021 PMID:24607704

Woodman, A. C., Mawdsley, H. P., & Hauser-Cram, P. (2011). Parenting stress and child behavior problems within families of children with developmental disabilities: Transactional relations across 15 years. *Research in Developmental Disabilities, 32*, 264–276. PMID:25462487

World Health Organization. (1992) The ICD-10 classification of mental and behavioral disorders: Clinical descriptions and diagnostic guidelines. Geneva, Switzerland: WHO.

ENDNOTE

1 Intellectual Disability

Chapter 5
Role of Stress and Age in Resilience Among Parents of the Children with Intellectual Disability

Santhosh Kareepadath Rajan
https://orcid.org/0000-0003-1423-5428
Christ University (Deemed), India

ABSTRACT

Parents of children with intellectual disability face various stressful situations. However, many of them show resilience even in the midst of challenges and are able to meaningfully contribute to the life of the child. In the present study, the factors of stress that hinder resilience are assessed in a sample of 50 parents of intellectually disabled children. Stress scale for parents of mentally challenged (SPMC) developed by Rejitha, Biji, and Jayan was used to measure the stress of the parents. Resilience was measured using the Bharathiar University resilience scale, developed by Annalakshmi. Results showed extra-familial stress as a significant inverse predictor of resilience. Older parents are relatively more resilient when compared to the younger.

INTRODUCTION

Raising a child with an intellectual disability is a stressful experience for the parents (McConnel & Savage, 2015; Khadi & Hidangmayum, 2012). The birth of the child would be like an accident happened in the family (Walsbren, 1980). Initially, parents would have difficulty to accept reality. Later, when they were ready to accept, close and distant relatives would formulate intricate speculations regarding the associated reflections and stigmatizations in the society. Interpersonal and intrapersonal responses of the parents to the accepted reality depends on how much they identify these speculations as true or false. Along with the speculations, various other stressors related to the parent-child relationship will together interplay in bringing down the hope and expectations and ultimately, the self-esteem of the

DOI: 10.4018/978-1-7998-1223-4.ch005

parents. Distress in parents, as a whole, is multidimensional and more than the sum of its parts (Gohel, Mukherjee, & Choudhary, 2011).

Stressors faced by the parents include comments by others on the errors committed by them to have such a child, remarks by the observers on the deficits in the child and flaws in parenting, stigmatization while attending the public functions, dilemma in facing the mental health professionals, financial difficulties due to the investment in the treatment, behaviour of the child and so on (Minnes, 1988; Dervishaliaj, 2013). All these factors are potential inverse contributors to the low quality of life of the parents. The most predominant among these is the problem behavior of the child (Mulder, Tudor, & Walsh, 2013), which acts as a moderator in the relationship between pain experienced by the parents and their stress. To prevent this stressor, parents may show a tendency to separate the child from the family. Some parents had reported high suicidal ideation due to this stressor.

Another most recurrently observed stressor is financial difficultie (Serrata, 2012). The treatment, as there are no medicines but only behavioral interventions that demand longitudinal care, which costs more than half of the income of a middle-class family in a country like India. Moreover, a significant chunk of the population and the policymakers are not yet aware of and convinced with the role of psychology and allied science professionals in modifying the behavior of the child with different abilities. Financial support from the part of the government seems to be more towards the special-education sector, which is also important but can only be effective when accompanied by the support of psychotherapy, occupational therapy, speech therapy. Hence, parents are compelled to spend a considerable part of their income on providing the therapies that help their child to achieve acceptability in the mainstream. Those who are from the moderate and low-socioeconomic background the expenses are unaffordable.

Some parents are stressed while taking the child to a mental health professional (Singer and Todis, 1991). They fear stigmatization by the public. By the time, they might have already reformulated and readopted their roles and identities as the parents of children with intellectual disability (Walsbren, 1980). Observation of the public on the challenging behavior and self-mutilation of the child resulting in the comments and comparisons with mainstream lead the parents to experience the stigma, rather than the child (Dervishaliaj, 2013). While explaining the issues related to the behavior of the child to the professional, they re-experience this stigma and hence get stressed.

Some of them fear the change in the behavior of the child due to the exposure to the other disabled children in the mental health center. They were also anxious about the care, given by the professionals to their child, as there are more such children in the center. As the children demanded constant care (Minnes, 1988), they tend to continue committing most of their time and energy in caretaking. While leaving the child in the mental health center makes them feel insecure, as the child is not with them for some time. This feeling of insecurity will persist until they develop a convincing and good relationship with the mental health professional.

There are situations when parents change the therapists recurrently due to this feeling of insecurity. They will be doubtful regarding the perception of the professional on the child's disability. While interacting, they will constantly be looking at the signs and reflections, which they can relate themselves with the professional. Whenever there is a gap in this relatedness, a lack of trust emerges. The recurrent feeling of the breach in the trust would lead to show the tendency to quit and approach a new professional.

Constant care for a period of time, and the dependency of the child may lead to an unhealthy attachment style between the parent and the child (Mulder, Tudor, & Walsh, 2013). Parents might have started considering their child as a part of themselves. They fear to expose the child to an inclusive classroom, as they are anxious about the stigma that will be experienced by their child from their classmates as well as the educators. Educational institutions are also not happy in entertaining inclusive education, even if the government encourages it. At least some educational institutions consider reduced academic performance as a sin. They fear the loss of reputation and the later consequences of the reduction among the stakeholders of their services.

Stress differs concerning disability and its intensity (Minnes, 1988). For instance, according to Abbeduto, et al. (2004), mothers of fragile X syndrome children have reduced levels of well-being when compared to those of down-syndrome children, but increased levels than those of autistic children. Here the source of stress is the deficits in the characteristics of the child, including the lack of communication skills, or difficulty in performing a behavior. As there is a need for special health care, parents have to accompany their child continuously. Such constant supervision limits the possibilities of the parents to take rest, have fun, and dedicate some time to themselves (Herring, et al., 2006).

Studies indicate that responses of the parents to these stressors differ a lot; many are showing the capacity to bounce back from the despair and report resilience and growth, accepting the reality, but some doomed to frustration and dissatisfaction (Heiman, 2002). A significant part of the literature discusses the negative influence of the disability on the quality of life of the parents. As per the observation of Gavidia-Payne and Stoneman (2006), couples with intellectually disabled children tend to consider their marriages deleterious. Their relationship satisfaction is also low. Reduced, as well as unproductive interaction and little marital satisfaction, lead to counter-productive responses to the child (Ahmedani & Hock, 2012). Floyd and Zmich (1991) indicated the reluctance of these couples, to open their issues even to close friends or to seek help from a mental health professional, which had made situations worse.

Moreover, the parents are deficient in maintaining social capital, including their relationship with the neighbors (Ahmedani & Hock, 2012). Their social participation is meager and employment status, lower even if they are similar in education, physical health, and marital status while comparing to the parents of the healthy children (Floyd, Greenberg, Hong, Pettee, & Seltzer, 2001). Lack of protective factors associated with social support results in the vulnerability to psychosocial issues (Serrata, 2012). The resilient parents, on the other hand, realize the availability of the resources and shows readiness to maintain them (Heiman, 2002).

The gender of the parents is also a deciding factor in their response to the stress. Krauss (1993) identified that stress in father is more associated with the temperament and interpersonal relationship behaviors of the child. Mother's stress is linked with the personal consequences of general parenting. Mothers suffer significantly more daily hassles than fathers (Gavidia-Payne & Stoneman, 2006). They involve more in self-criticism, emotional stress, and are not able to withstand without social support factors. In the observation of Rogner and Wessels (1994), they are subjected to undergo a complex process of adaptation.

Specific studies on mothers with intellectually disabled children, differentiating with others, showed that they have high levels of stress and unfortunate mental health (Bradshaw, Stuart, & Zablotsky, 2013). Mothers with more than one intellectually disabled children, compared to those with only one child, showed severe symptoms of depression and anxiety, and lower family adaptability and cohesion (Lin, Orsmond, & Seltzer, 2007).

Some of the parents, while trying to bring positive changes in their social life adopts methods that are counterproductive (Blumberg, et al., 2004). Blumberg et al. (2004), for instance, notes the tendency of certain parents to practice a coercive family process. Two types of coercive methods routinely used by parents are attention driven and escape driven. In the attention driven coercive processes, parents will be occupied in non-child centered task. The child engages in problem behavior until s/he gets parental attention, which reinforces the child to perform in the same way when the parents are non-attentive. As the child stops problem behavior, the parents also get reinforced to attend the child, while showing problem behavior. In escape driven coercive processes, the parent makes a demand on the child. The child responds by engaging in problem behavior until the parent terminates the demand. The child gets reinforced and will perform problem behavior whenever the demand arises. Termination of the problem behavior reinforces the parent to withdraw the demand in a subsequent similar situation. Even if the coercive processes are not healthy and unsuccessful in the children with intellectual disability (Lucyshyn, et al., 2004), these are indications of the tendency shown by the parents to achieve resiliency.

Higher education in the parents seems to be one of the mediating or moderating factors that could influence certain regional or cultural inputs to resilience. For instance, in the study by Upadhyaya and Havalappanavar (2008), conducted in a sample from India, extrinsic protective factors of the parents included higher education level. Other identified protective factors were non-agricultural occupation, higher income, and urban status of the family. However, higher educational level need not always help (Ravindranadan & Raju, 2007; Floyd, Greenberg, Hong, Pettee, & Seltzer, 2001). Cohesion among the family members and flexibility in them are influenced by the education level, which in turn, contributing to resilience (Jones & Passey, 2005; McGrail & Rieger, 2013). Other most significant factors that contribute to resilience include family belief systems, positive outlook of the parents, family hardiness, resourcefulness, flexible and committed family environment, predictable and open communication patterns, social support and higher economic factors (Greef & Van der Walt, 2010; Bauman, 2004). Empowerment oriented practices by professionals are identified to have a mediating effect in controlling family stress (Bauman, 2004).

Participation in the programs, along with other similar parents, alike in the profession, helps them feel accepted and respected, contributing to resilience (Crowe, Cunningham-Sabo, Helitzer, & Vanleit, 2002). Coping skills are enhanced among the parents who attend activities and programs on how to bring up the children in an improved way. The new coping skills thus learned enabled them to be relieved from over-expectations and enhanced their capacity to practice self-care (Crowe, Cunningham-Sabo, Helitzer, & Vanleit, 2002).

Parents differ with respect to gender in identifying and using resources and coping strategies to achieve resiliency (Gavidia-Payne & Stoneman, 2006; Upadhyaya & Havalappanavar, 2008). Fathers showed the tendency to adopt more problem-focused coping strategies than emotion-focused, except if they were irritated by the daily hassles (Upadhyaya & Havalappanavar, 2008). They are higher in problem-solving, positive distraction, negative distraction, acceptance-redefinition, and social support. The study conducted by Rodrigue, Morgan, and Geffken (1992), showed that fathers of intellectually disabled children could be equally resilient like those of the children with mainstream abilities, with a similarity in perceived parenting competence, marital satisfaction, and social support. Such successful parents were skilled in keeping contact with other families in the same situation and had a positive appraisal of life circumstances (Singer & Todis, 1991).

Mothers focus on making their support network splendid (Krauss, 1993). Resources in the form of emotional and social support from the neighborhood enable them to overcome high-stress levels and the risk of poor mental health (Bradshaw, Stuart, & Zablotsky, 2013). They also tend to seek shelter in religion and faith. However, such mothers show the habit of denial and blaming (Upadhyaya & Havalappanavar, 2008). Mothers who had their first child intellectually disabled showed mastery over those who had a disabled second child (Rogner & Wessels, 1994). However, mothers with the first child with intellectual disability showed a negation or delay in the subsequent childbearing. They recognized the extensive needs of the first child and wanted to maximize their potential to provide that (Macinnes, 2008). Moreover, they feared the possibility of the next child having a disability (Kimura & Yamazaki, 2017). A study based on the lived experiences of the 11 mothers of children with intellectual disability conducted at Ghana by Oti-Boadi (2017), revealed that spiritual beliefs, hope, and support as the major coping strategies they used.

Literature is splendid with the findings on stress, as well as resilience, of the parents of intellectually disabled children. Stigmatization, financial difficulties, the intensity of the disability, and constant care that has to be provided are some of the factors that contribute to the stress. Cultural values of social support, rewards of caregiving, and spirituality protect the parents from stress, enhancing resilience. However, there is a lack of information regarding the relationship between stress and resilience. The present study attempts to find out the dimensions of stress that challenge the resilience of the parents of the intellectually disabled children. The study also assesses if the age of the parents has a significant influence on their resilience.

HYPOTHESES

1. There is no significant relationship between stress and resilience in the parents of intellectually disabled children
2. Factors of stress do not include the factors that predict resilience in the parents of intellectually disabled children
3. Parents who are in early adulthood do not differ from the parents who are in late adulthood and old age in their resilience

METHOD

Sample

Fifty parents of the intellectually disabled children were selected purposively from different child mental health clinics at Kozhikode, Kannur and Wayanad district in the state of Kerala, India. Only the parents who have their children living along with them in the same house were considered in the sample. Parents who were diagnosed to have a psychiatric disorder and who had regular usage of substances were excluded from the study.

Measures

1. BU Resilience Scale (Form A), developed by Annalakshmi (2009) consists of 30 Likert-type items. The scale purports to measure resilience with reference to seven domains including duration for getting back to normalcy, reaction to negative events, response to risk factors (specifically, disadvantaged environment) in life, perception of effect of past negative events, defining problems, hope/confidence in coping with future and openness to experience and flexibility. The scale has adequate reliability (reliability coefficient of Spearman-Brown, 0.84; Guttman, 0.84; and Cronbach alpha, 0.86) as found on a sample of 577 post-graduate students. The scale was validated against

Friborg's Resilience Scale for Adults (r = 0.401) and Bell's Adjustment Inventory (r = -0.392). Higher scores indicate higher resiliency, and lower scores indicate lower resiliency.

2. Stress Scale for Parents of mentally challenged (SPMC); developed by Rejitha, Biji & Jayan (2005) consist of 20 items. The scale purports to measure stress concerning four domains such as financial, intra-familial, extra-familial, and emotional factors. As per the authors, the tool has adequate reliability and validity

RESULTS

To find out if there is a significant relationship between stress and resilience in the parents of intellectually disabled children, correlation analysis was administered. Results are given in table 1

Correlation analysis showed that resilience among the parents of intellectually disabled children has a significant moderate negative correlation ($r = -0.47$, $p < 0.01$) with their extra-familial stress. Also, resilience showed a significant moderate negative correlation ($r = 0.4$, $p < 0.01$) with an overall stress score of the parents of intellectually disabled children.

To find out if extra-familial stress can predict resilience in the parents of intellectually disabled children, one variable regression analysis was done. Table 2 summarizes the results

Results indicated that extra-familial stress could predict ($\beta = -0.473$, $t = 3.72$, $p < 0.01$) resilience in the parents of intellectually disabled children. Extra-familial stress showed a negative relationship with resilience. Hence, when extra-familial stress increases, resilience decreases.

To find out if parents who are in early adulthood differ from the parents who are in late adulthood in their resilience, the t-test is used. Table 3 summarizes the results of the t-test.

Table 1. Correlation analysis – the relationship between the resilience and various factors of stress in parents of intellectually disabled children

Variables	Stress				Overall Stress
	Financial	Intra-familial	Extra-familial	Emotional	
Intra-familial	0.34*				
Extra-familial	0.21	0.58**			
Emotional	-0.08	0.09	-0.15		
Overall stress	0.48**	0.80**	0.78**	0.34**	
Resilience	0.06	-0.20	-0.47**	-0.163	-0.40**

**P < 0.01, *P < 0.05

Table 2. Regression model-Extra-familial stress predicting regression

DV	Predictor	β	t	F	R^2
Resilience	Extra-familial stress	-0.473	3.724**	13.87**	0.224

**P < 0.01

Table 3. Summary of the group statistics which differentiate parents in early adulthood from the parents in late adulthood and old age in their resilience

DV	Age	N	Mean	S.D	"t"
Resilience	Late adulthood	23	98.69	10.64	3.07**
	Early adulthood	27	89.48	10.35	

**P < 0.01

As per the findings, parents in the late adulthood differ ($t = 3.07$, $p < 0.01$) from the parents in the early adulthood in their resilience. Parents in the late adulthood ($M = 98.69$, S.D. = 10.64) is higher in resilience when compared to the parents in the early adulthood ($M = 89.48$, S.D. = 10.35).

DISCUSSION

In collectivistic countries like India, people are more concerned with the opinions and affiliations received from extra-familial situations (Hui & Triandis, 1986). Lack of affiliation and contradictory opinions may lead individuals to stress (Popa, Guillet, & Mullet, 2014). Parents of the children with intellectual disabilities would be experiencing isolation and negative recognition from the society, and hence might not be satisfied in the affiliation from the community. Comments from the mainstream society regarding the deficits in the child, flaws in parents, stigmatization, demotivating comments by the professionals and financial difficulties, along with the feeling of lack of affiliation (Minnes, 1988; Dervishaliaj, 2013) might be the components of the extra-familial stress. Consequently, they lack the courage to take the child out, even if it is to meet a mental health professional or an educational institution (Singer and Todis, 1991).

As per the findings of Chandravanshi, et al. (2017), factors related to extra-familial stress also have an association with psychological issues, including depression. The study indicated an increase in the prevalence of depression of the mothers of the children with intellectual disability to those reported by the previous research. Oti-Boadi (2017) supports this by showing possibilities of contracting with other disorders such as anxiety and psychosomatic related. Along adapting with the new role of meeting the unique needs of the child, the parents have to deal with the financial challenges and social demands.

Parents might be feeling difficulty in presenting the child to the professionals. Interactions with the professionals, however, would enhance their insight about the reality of the disability of the child. At the same time, some parents fear such insights that may take away hope and expectations. They understand the limitation of their child to behave as mainstream children. Consequently, pessimism, hostility, and shame will rule their thoughts. Initial responses may be denial, projection of blame, grief, withdrawal, rejection. Parents are reported to feel helpless, inadequate, anger, shock, and guilt. Acceptance of the situation will only happen after periods of disbelief, depression, and self-blame, which may vary from person to person.

Parents who are in the later part of adulthood were indicated as more capable of accepting the disability of the child. Similar results were found out by Gandotra (1985) when the parents aged less than 35years were compared with parents above 35 years. Results of the study indicated that lower be the age of parents, higher was the stress (Gandotra, 1985). Older parents might be better in maintaining social capital than the younger. Due to significant social interaction, older parents will be skilled in finding out the resources.

Moreover, while becoming old, their network with other parents with a similar situation would have increased (Rodrigue, Morgan, & Geffken, 1992). Also, accepting the child with intellectual disability as a part of the family would be contributing to the cohesion and flexibility among the family members (Jones & Passey, 2005). Altogether, they would be relieved from the extra-familial stress, which in turn would increase resilience.

CONCLUSION AND RECOMMENDATION

The study shows that extra-familial stress is a significant inverse predictor of resilience in the parents of the intellectually disabled children. This relationship may be an indication that the mainstream public continues to observe individuals with intellectual disabilities and their families differently. Or it may be in the other way; the parents of the intellectually disabled children perceive that their family was observed differently by the public. The negative feelings in the parents would have an association with discrimination, stigmatization, and isolation, which they perceive to be experienced by their children with intellectual disability.

The study also reveals that parents who are in the younger stages of young adulthood are more vulnerable to stress. However, the findings cannot be generalized, as the sample is selected from a limited part of the population. At the same time, the study brings out a specific factor that may be active in most of the similar population. Further inquiries comparing the same factors of stress and resilience have to be done in different cohorts. In the case of repeated results, intervention strategies that could help the parents overcome extra-familial stress shall be designed and tested. More researches to find out the factors which could help enhance the resilience of the parents of intellectually disabled people are recommended.

REFERENCES

Abbeduto, L., Krauss, M. W., Murphy, M. M., Orsmond, G., Seltzer, M. M., & Shattuck, P. (2004). Psychological well-being and coping in mothers of youths with autism, down syndrome, or fragile x syndrome. *American Journal of Mental Retardation, 109*(3), 237–254. doi:10.1352/0895-8017(2004)109<237:PWACIM>2.0.CO;2 PMID:15072518

Ahmedani, B. K., & Hock, R. (2012). Parent perceptions of autism severity: Exploring social-ecological context. *Disability and Health Journal, 5*(4), 298–304. doi:10.1016/j.dhjo.2012.06.002 PMID:23021742

Annalakshmi, N. (2009). Bharathiar University Resilience Scale. In Research Methodology Tools and Techniques, (pp. 105-121). Retrieved from Google Scholar.

Bauman, S. (2004). *Parents of children with mental retardation, coping mechanisms and support needs.* College Park: Dissertation, Faculty of the Graduate School of University of Maryland.

Blumberg, E. R., Horner, R. H., Irvin, L. K., Laverty, R., Lucyshyn, J. M., & Sprague, J. R. (2004). Validating the construct of coercion in family routines: Expanding the unit of analysis in behavioral assessment with families of children with developmental disabilities. *Research and Practice for Persons with Severe Disabilities, 29*(2), 104–121. doi:10.2511/rpsd.29.2.104 PMID:26321883

Bradshaw, C. P., Stuart, E. A., & Zablotsky, B. (2013). The association between mental health, stress, and coping supports in mothers of children with autism spectrum disorders. *Journal of Autism and Developmental Disorders*, *43*(6), 1380–1393. doi:10.100710803-012-1693-7 PMID:23100053

Chandravanshi, G., Sharma, K. K., Jilowa, C. S., Meena, P. S., Jain, M., & Prakash, O. (2017). Prevalence of depression in mothers of intellectually disabled children: A cross-sectional study. *Medical Journal of Dr. D.Y. Patil Vidyapeeth*, *10*(2), 156–161.

Crowe, T. K., Cunningham-Sabo, L. D., Helitzer, D. L., & Vanleit, B. (2002). Perceived changes in self-image and coping strategies of mothers of children with disabilities. *The Occupational Therapy Journal of Research*, *22*(1), 25–33.

Dervishaliaj, E. (2013). Parental stress in families with disabilities: A literature review. *Journal of Educational and Social Research*, *3*(7), 579–584.

Floyd, F. J., Greenberg, J. S., Hong, J., Pettee, Y., & Seltzer, M. M. (2001). Life course impacts of parenting a child with a disability. *American Journal of Mental Retardation*, *106*(3), 265–286. doi:10.1352/0895-8017(2001)106<0265:LCIOPA>2.0.CO;2 PMID:11389667

Floyd, F. J., & Zmich, D. E. (1991). Marriage and the parenting partnership: Perceptions and interactions of parents with mentally retarded and typically developing children. *Child Development*, *62*(6), 1434–1448. doi:10.2307/1130817 PMID:1786726

Gavidia-Payne, S., & Stoneman, Z. (2006). Marital adjustment in families of young children with disabilities: Associations with daily hassles and problem-focused coping. *American Journal of Mental Retardation*, *111*(1), 1–14. doi:10.1352/0895-8017(2006)111[1:MAIFOY]2.0.CO;2 PMID:16332152

Gohel, M., Mukherjee, S., & Choudhary, S. K. (2011). Psychosocial impact on the parents of mentally retarded children in Anand District. *Healthline (Bhavnagar)*, *2*(2), 62–66.

Greef, A. P., & van der Walt, K. J. (2010). Resilience in families with an autistic child. *Education and Training in Autism and Developmental Disabilities*, *45*(3), 347–355.

Heiman, T. (2002). Parents of Children with Disabilities: Resilience, Coping, and Future Expectations. *Journal of Developmental and Physical Disabilities*, *14*(2), 159–171. doi:10.1023/A:1015219514621

Herring, S., Gray, K., Taffe, J., Tonge, B., Sweeney, D., & Einfeld, S. (2006). Behaviour and emotional problems in toddlers with pervasive developmental disorders and developmental delay: Associations with parental mental health and family functioning. *Journal of Intellectual Disability Research*, *50*(Pt 12), 874–882. doi:10.1111/j.1365-2788.2006.00904.x PMID:17100948

Hui, C. H., & Triandis, H. C. (1986). Individualism-Collectivism: A study of cross-cultural researchers. *Journal of Cross-Cultural Psychology*, *17*(2), 225–248. doi:10.1177/0022002186017002006

Jones, J., & Passey, J. (2005). Family adaptation, coping, and resources: Parents of children with developmental disabilities and behaviour problems. *Journal on Developmental Disabilities*, *11*(1), 31–46.

Khadi, P. B., & Hidangmayum, N. (2012). Parenting stress of normal and mentally challenged children. *Karnataka Journal of Agricultural Sciences*, *25*(2), 256–259.

Kimura, M., & Yamazaki, Y. (2017). Having another child without intellectual disabilities: Comparing mothers of a single child with disability and mothers of multiple children with and without disability. *Journal of Intellectual Disabilities*, *23*(2), 216–232. doi:10.1177/1744629517749129 PMID:29284333

Krauss, M. W. (1993). Child related and parenting stress: Similarities and differences between mothers and fathers of children with disabilities. *American Journal of Mental Retardation*, *97*(4), 393–404. PMID:8427694

Lin, L. Y., Orsmond, G. I., & Seltzer, M. M. (2007). Mothers of adolescents and adults with autism: Parenting multiple children with disabilities. *Intellectual and Developmental Disabilities*, *45*(4), 257–270. doi:10.1352/1934-9556(2007)45[257:MOAAAW]2.0.CO;2 PMID:17627373

Lucyshyn, J., Irvin, L. K., Blumberg, E. R., Laverty, R., Horner, R. H., & Sprague, J. R. (2004). Validating the construct of coersionin family routines: Expanding the unit of analysis in behavioural assessment in families of children with developmental disabilities. *Research and Practice for Persons with Severe Disabilities*, *29*(2), 104–121. doi:10.2511/rpsd.29.2.104 PMID:26321883

Macinnes, M. D. (2008). One's enough of now: Children, disability, and subsequent childbearing of mothers. *Journal of Marriage and the Family*, *70*(3), 758–771. doi:10.1111/j.1741-3737.2008.00519.x PMID:23946550

McConnel, D., & Savage, A. (2015). Stress and resilience among families caring for children with disability: Expanding the research agenda. *Current Developmental Disorders Reports*, *2*(2), 100–109. doi:10.100740474-015-0040-z

McGrail, J. P., & Rieger, A. (2013). Coping humor and family functioning in parents of children with disabilities. *Rehabilitation Psychology*, *58*(1), 89–97. doi:10.1037/a0031556 PMID:23438005

Minnes, P. M. (1988). Family stress associated with a developmentally handicapped child: A multidimensional perspective. In N. W. Bray (Ed.), *International Review of Research in Mental Retardation* (pp. 195–226). Birmingham, AL: University of Alabama.

Mulder, E., Tudor, M. E., & Walsh, C. E. (2013). Predictors of parent stress in a sample of children with ASD: Pain, problem behaviour, and parental coping. *Research in Autism Spectrum Disorders*, *7*(2), 256–264. doi:10.1016/j.rasd.2012.08.010

Oti-Boadi, M. (2017). Exploring the Lived Experiences of Mothers of Children With Intellectual Disability in Ghana. *SAGE Open*, *7*(4), 1–12. doi:10.1177/2158244017745578

Popa, B., Guillet, L., & Mullet, E. (2014). Cultural differences in the appraisal of stress. *Psicológica (Valencia)*, *35*, 745–760.

Ravindranadan, V., & Raju, S. (2007). Adjustment and attitude of parents of children with mental retardation. *Journal of the Indian Academy of Applied Psychology*, *33*(1), 137–141.

Rodrigue, J. R., Morgan, S. B., & Geffken, G. R. (1992). Psychosocial adaptation of fathers of children with autism, Down syndrome, and normal development. *Journal of Autism and Developmental Disorders*, *22*(2), 249–263. doi:10.1007/BF01058154 PMID:1385591

Serrata, C. A. (2012). Psychosocial aspects of parenting a child with autism. *Journal of Applied Rehabilitation Counseling*, *43*(4), 29–35. doi:10.1891/0047-2220.43.4.29

Singer, G., & Todis, B. (1991). Stress and stress management in families with adopted children who have severe disabilities. *The Journal of the Association for Persons with Severe Handicaps*, *16*(1), 3–13. doi:10.1177/154079699101600102

Upadhyaya, G. R., & Havalappanavar, N. B. (2008). Coping in parents of the mentally challenged. *Journal of the Indian Academy of Applied Psychology*, *34*(2), 221–225.

Walsbren, S. E. (1980). Parents' reactions after the birth of a developmentally disabled child. *American Journal of Mental Deficiency*, *84*(4), 345–351. PMID:6444494

Chapter 6
Mental Health Issues, Wellbeing, and Related Issues Among Caregivers of Individuals With Intellectual Disability

Tanay Maiti
AIIMS Bhubaneswar, India

ABSTRACT

Caregivers are the important and integral part in the lives of people with intellectual disability. As caregiving is extensive and mostly lifelong for this population, the associated burden, stigma, and also wellbeing of the caregivers are also equally important as these are often very directly correlated with the wellbeing of the individuals with intellectual disability. The chapter focused on the issues and impacts of caregiving, mental health problems, wellbeing, and related issues of caregivers. The authors also discuss the various facets of stigma caregivers do face and ways to deal with the stigma.

INTRODUCTION

Care giving to individuals with disability is laborious and associated with many mental health issues and related problems. In a longitudinal study on the well-being of parents of individuals included in the Australian Rett Syndrome Database over the period from 2002 to 2011, Mori, Downs, Wong, & Leonard (2019) reported that poorer parental physical well-being was related with residential remoteness, the child being a teenager at baseline, having frequent sleep disturbances or behavioural problems, and being a single parent or on a low income was associated with later poorer physical well-being, while the child having enteral feeding was associated with later poorer emotional well-being. Laurvick, Msall, Silburn, Bower, de Klerk, & Leonard (2006) reported in a study on mothers (n = 135, age ranged from 21 to 60 years) of children with Rett syndrome (age between 3 and 27 years) that the most important predictors of maternal physical and emotional health are child behavior, caregiver demands, and family function. The scenario is not much different with caregivers of individual with intellectual disability.

DOI: 10.4018/978-1-7998-1223-4.ch006

Many researches focused on the management of individuals with intellectual disability, the mental health issues, stress and burden of the care givers of intellectually disabled individuals are equally important as indicated by the recent researches. In some cases, family members neglect the disabled individuals. Enoch, Mprah, Isaac & Joseph (2018) have reported in a study from Ghana that most parents refuse to visit their children with intellectual disability in school. However, due to deinstitutionalization and perspective of inclusion in to society, most of the intellectually disabled children, adults and older adults are taken care at home and at least one of the family members to be the primary care taker. Such scenario gives importance for the needs and difficulties for the caregiver. The chapter focused on the issues and impacts of care giving, mental health problems, wellbeing and related issues of caregiver.

Care giving and Mental Health Issues

The negative impact of caregiving on the mental health of caregivers is well documented in the literature. In a population based study, Schofield et al., (1998) found less life satisfaction, less positive affect, and more negative affect among caregivers compared with non caregivers regardless of age or marital status. Caregivers experienced depression, anxiety and stress symptoms and these symptoms were found to be significantly higher among caregivers of individuals with intellectual disability than those with Psychiatric illness (Panicker & Ramesh, 2019). Similar findings were reported in other studies too. For example, in a study on family burden in people with intellectual disability with or without mental disorders, higher levels of family burden were related to higher functional disability in all the areas, lower intelligence quotient, diagnosis of ID with mental disorders and presence of organic, affective, psychotic and behavioral disorders. Stepwise multiple regression showed that behavioral problems, affective and psychotic disorder, disability in participation in society, disability in personal care and presence of ID-MD explained more than 61% of the variance in family burden (Irazábal, Marsà, García, Gutiérrez-Recacha, Martorell, Salvador-Carulla, & Ochoa, 2012). In another study, higher family impact was found between caregivers to people with mental health disorders - intellectual disability. The interaction of both conditions (ID and mental health problems) results in a higher degree of burden on families (Martorell, Gutiérrez-Recacha, Irazábal, Marsà, & García, 2011).

Maternal depression in families having a child with a disability has been the subject of considerable research over four decades. Bailey, Golden, Roberts, Ford (2007) reviewed 42 articles on maternal depression and found that only eight were clinically diagnosed depression; most of them used a scale rating depressive symptoms. Across the studies, mothers of children with disabilities generally exhibited a higher than average rate of depressive symptoms and are more at risk for clinical depression, but the incidence may be lower than reported in previous literature. Child behavior problems, maternal stress, coping style, and support were consistently associated with depressive symptoms. The distinction between clinical depression and depressive symptoms may be important in conceptualizing how a child with a disability can influence family members and the nature of support that may need to be provided.

Many studies on mental health issues of caregivers of intellectually disabled individuals in different cultural settings consistently reported increased maternal distress and burden. Australian Bureau of Statistics (ABS) (1998) reported that, approximately 30% of caregivers reported that their well-being had been affected by caregiving, and that they were often worried or depressed. McConkey, Truesdale-Kennedy, Chang, & Jarrah, Shukri (2008) have studied 206 mothers with intellectually disabled children in three different countries and reported that mothers experienced poor mental health, increased levels of child-related stress and poorer family functioning. Their child's behaviour problems were a major factor in this. The impacts on mothers' well-being were not alleviated by access to professional supports or use of coping strategies. John (2012) assessed stress among mothers of young children with intellectual disabilities in urban India and examined the extent to which child functioning and maternal coping predict maternal stress. Three-fourths of the sample obtained a clinically significant stress score, and maternal coping emerged as a robust predictor of stress for mothers of boys with intellectual disabilities. Qualitative analyses indicated positive and negative maternal experiences related to self, child, family and community. In a study involved secondary analysis of data from the 2011 Survey on the Actual Conditions of Individuals with Developmental Disabilities, conducted by the Ministry of Health and Welfare of Korea reported that all components of caregiving burden and depression (effects of caregivers' characteristics, caregiving time and cost, and perceptions of time and cost, on depression) were significantly higher in the 1st grade, designating the most severe disabilities. Overall, caregiving burden tended to be higher in female caregivers, the unemployed, parents, co-residents, and people with health problems. Caregivers' characteristics such as spouse relationship, having health problems, and perception of caregiving time and cost were associated with depression (Nam & Park, 2017). Studies across the world confirming the fact that caregivers experience stress, burden and various mental health issues.

Gardiner, Miller & Lach (2018) have tried to identify functional predictors of perceived impact of childhood disability among families of children with neurodevelopmental disorders and disabilities. They examined the relationship between sub-domains of adaptive and problematic behaviour and perceived family impact, and whether the same sub-domains would emerge as significant after controlling for the impact of child diagnosis, including autism spectrum disorder, cerebral palsy and intellectual disability. Caregivers of 216 children and adolescents with neurodevelopmental disorder and disability completed measures of children's practical, conceptual and social skills (i.e. adaptive behaviour), behaviour problems and positive and negative family impact. Indices of child adaptive and problematic behaviour were only significantly associated with perceived negative family impact. Children's practical and social skills, as well as emotional symptoms, emerged as significant predictors of perceived negative family impact, with emotional symptoms accounting for greatest variance. The study findings suggest that it is not children's most impaired domains of functioning that are perceived as significantly impactful by the family. The findings highlight the importance of devoting consideration to the ways in which the functional limitations experienced by children with chronic developmental health conditions similarly impact family life and well-being, regardless of disorder designation. Future studies are required on this direction.

Care Giving and Wellbeing

The impact associated with long term care giving has been indicated that care givers are burned out with poor subjective well being, life satisfaction and social support. Gebeyehu, Sahile, & Ayalew (2019) reported in a study on level of burden, social support, and life satisfaction of seventy four caregivers (parents, grandparents, and siblings of the child) of children with intellectual disability that caregivers are experiencing much level of burden with inadequate social support and have pitiable satisfaction in their life. Burden is negatively correlated with social support and life satisfaction, but social support is positively correlated with satisfaction in life. The authors emphasized the need of result social support for caregivers in order to reduce the level of burden and enhance their satisfaction in life.

The impact of care giving and compound caregiving (i.e. multiple caregiving roles) on caregivers are different in many ways. Compared with the non-compound caregivers, the compound caregivers of adult children with intellectual disabilities had increased desire to place their care recipient into residential care. They also spent an average of 12 additional hours per week undertaking the compound caregiving role. Overall findings indicated that caregivers reported giving more tangible and emotional support than they vii received, but considerable variability was evident. Relative disadvantage in tangible reciprocity was associated with increased depressive symptomatology, poorer mental health, and reduced desire for residential placement of the care recipient, but not with physical health or life satisfaction (Perkins, 2009).

In order to compensate for the disadvantages of caring, researches tried to identify factors associated to caregivers' subjective well-being (SWB). Hope is found to have significant impact on social self-care, mental health and conscientiousness of staff working with people with intellectual disabilities (Oliver, Revuelto, Fernández, Simó-Algado, & Galiana,2019).

Caregiver Impact on Management

Attitude and perception of the caregiver influence the service selection and outcome of management. The responsibility of choosing the kind of services to be provided to the disabled individuals is also related to the knowledge and attitude of the caregiver. Werner, Stern, Roth, & Tenenbaum (2019) have examined the roles of stigma and of enabling factors in help-seeking by parental caregivers of individuals with intellectual disabilities and dual diagnosis. Questionnaires were completed by 195 family caregivers. Lower family stigma was related to higher personal enabling factors (e.g. knowledge about services and previous experience in seeking help), which in turn was related to higher help-seeking behaviors. Higher professional enabling factors (e.g. attitude of the professional, services in the vicinity) were related to higher intentions to seek help, which were related to higher help-seeking behaviors. Professionals can help families achieve a greater sense of self-efficacy in their own help-seeking process by providing them with knowledge about services and facilitating a more positive experience in the process.

The involvement of caregiver in the intervention programs for intellectually disabled individuals could predict the success of the intervention. For example, many weight reduction programs fail to show positive and sustainable impacts due to not involving parents, who are usually unavailable to attend school-based health programs. The mHealth interactive interventions were carried out in September 2015-August 2016 by Lee, Brown, Leung, Chen, Louie, Chen, & Lee (2019), engaging carers to monitor and sustain their children's healthy lifestyle behaviours at home. Twenty family carers were recruited and four themes emerged such as improving family carer-child interactions and communications, gaining useful and practical health information from experts, supporting each other via an mHealth platform and appreciating the collaborative effort between school personnel and family carers. Family carers stressed the usefulness of the mHealth interactive interventions in monitoring and sustaining the children's healthy lifestyle behaviours at home. The mHealth interactive interventions for increasing family carers' involvement and monitoring were well received. The findings provide new insights into using mHealth interventions in future weight management programmes involving parental participation in the home environment.

Carer mental health literacy and help seeking are areas that are not well researched in the intellectual disability field. Man & Kangas (2019) aimed to explore the above including service utilization experiences of Australian parents with an offspring with an intellectual disabilityand a comorbid psychiatric disorder. Forty-one parents took part in an online survey assessing satisfaction and helpfulness ratings of received services. Twenty-six parents also completed items to assess mental health literacy and attitudinal barriers to help seeking. Parents showed good mental health literacy with depression and with challenging behaviour associated with autism and poorer literacy with mixed presentations. Parents reported varied helpfulness and satisfaction ratings with disability and mental health services and they are capable of recognizing the need to seek professional help for their offspring.

The relationship between ethnicity, service use and perceptions of service effectiveness is inconclusive. The study examined differences in service use and perceptions of service effectiveness between Israeli Jewish (Jewish) and Israeli Arab (Arab) parental caregivers of individuals with intellectual disabilities and dual diagnosis of psychopathology. Arab parental caregivers perceived health services to be more accessible than did Jewish caregivers, but there was no difference between the two groups in the use of the services. Overall, greater enabling factors and accessibility were associated with higher use of education and social services. No differences were found between the groups in their perceptions of service effectiveness.Arab family caregivers use education and social services less than do their Jewish peers, possibly because they have fewer enabling resources. The finding that both groups reported similar use of health services may be explained by a shared perception that informal help may not be suitable for dealing with situations of psychopathology. The similar perceptions of service effectiveness may be explained by extensive services available in Israel, to the satisfaction of both groups, or by the fact that participants perceived these services as their only alternative, and therefore fear losing them (Werner, 2019).

Stigma and Caregivers

Stigma, can be understood as mark of social disgrace, where discrimination happens based on variable factors like disability, mental health problems, ethnicity etc. Both the individuals with intellectual disability and their respective caregivers do face significant amount of stigma and prejudices, resulting in added disability and obstacles restricting their human rights. Stigma can be conceptualized as an attitude or belief which lead people to reject or avoid others who are 'percieved' to be different. The word is greek in origin which initially meant a cut or burn mark in skin used as identification mark for slaves or criminals.

Among the various type of stigmas described; family, courtesy or associative stigma has been described for the people or caregivers associated with targeted individuals, who are subjected to stigmatization by common people. Both associative and affiliate stigma has been researched in details and Mak et al (Mak WWS et. J Appl Res Intellect Disabil 2008) has mentioned about three components of family stigma; i.e. affect, cognitions and behavioral responses whereas Mak & Cheung's Affiliate Stigma Scale(MakWWS et al 2008)measures the extent of self stigmatization with good predictive value on subjective burden, even after controlling the factors like extent of caregiving involvement and caregiving stress.

Researches from India has shown direct correlation of lower parental education belongingness to low socio economic strata and low paying high labouring job of the parents with the prevalence of intellectual disability, all of which definitely increases the burden of caregiving leading to a further vicious circle. (Naskar S, et al . Int J Med Sci Public Health 2016. In a country like india, with 21 million people living with disability(as per census 2011), of which nearly 75% staying in rural background, without basic resources and minimum facilities, the burden of caregiving is immense. Stigma certainly make things even worse. The legislation related to intellectual disability(PWD Act 1995, National Trust Act 1999, UNCRPD 2007), simplified procedure of issuing disability certificates, multiple educational facilities(acceptance of 'Child with Special Needs', CWSN into regular school, The Right of Children to Free and Compulsory Education (RTE) Act, 2009, under Article 21-A) along with employment benefits might have changed the Indian scenario partially, but the social stigma alone hindering access to maximum benefit to this population.

Other than legislation and policy making at the government level, village gatherings and support from community or religious leaders can turn very useful to deal these stigmas of caregivers in a developing country like India (McConkey et al 2016) McConkey proposed four key strategies to challenege the negative perception about intellectual disability, which include nurturing the child's development, inclusion in the society and also in the peer group, information about myths, superstitions and advocacy about their needs and rights. (McConkey, R., Kahonde, C., & McKenzie, J. 2016). Cross et al mentions about matrix of intervention plans which could be explained at various levels, like intrapersonal, interpersonal, organisational or at community level. For the first three level the labelling, stereotyping, status loss and discrimination out of it need to be dealt specifically however government lead policy and favourable legislation can change the scenario over time.

Stigma by now, is more than a belief. It's a social, cultural and moral process, whose complex interaction within the socio cultural environment affects not only the stigmatised individuals but also their caregivers, in multiple domains. The anthropological researches on stigma has emphasised about the moral standing of an individual determined by their local social world, and local social obligations and norms further maintains one's morality.

CONCLUSION

Understanding the disability impact on parenting and caregiving is important for intervention. Despite variations in coping pattern, both positive and negative coping strategies were observed in caregivers and positive coping does not rule out negative coping strategies (Kishore, 2011). Use of appropriate coping styles can reduce the negative impact of care giving. The factors positively associated with better maternal physical health were the mother working full-time or part-time outside the home, having some high school education, having private health insurance, the child not having breathing problems in the last 2 years, the child not having home-based structured therapy, and high scores on the Family Resource Scale (indicating adequacy of time resources for basic and family needs). The factors positively associated with better maternal mental health: were the mother working full-time or part-time outside the home, the child not having a fracture in the last 2 years, lesser reporting of facial stereotypes and involuntary facial movements, being in a well-adjusted marriage, and having low stress scores (Panicker & Ramesh(2019); Laurvick, Msall, Silburn, Bower, de Klerk &, Leonard (2006). The amount and quality of social support available to caregivers is an important factor in moderating the impact of caregiving and social support can be provided both informally, by family, friends, neighbours, social groups and so on, and formally, by professionals and agencies (Dunst, Trivette & Deal, 1988).

Factors such as the type of disability of the care recipient and where the caregiver is in the caregiving process will affect the impact caring has on the caregiver's mental health, and thus the type of supports most appropriate for the caregiver. The important role of moderators of the impact of caring, such as the caregiver's financial situation and coping strategies used, should also be considered by service providers when planning how to assist caregivers. Greater consideration of some of these factors may assist in more efficient use of the resources available to support caregivers. Attention should be paid to the individual situation of each caregiver. Careful assessment of caregivers' needs should consider the factors associated with a negative impact of caregiving and of the various mediators of this impact.

It is also important to acknowledge the positive aspects of the caring role to ensure that these are not obstructed by interventions to assist caregivers. Global responses to the needs of all caregivers will not provide the most benefit to individuals (Sally Savage & Susan Bailey (2004).

It is important to give attention to various issues of caretaking and negative impact of care giving and to implement appropriate intervention strategies and policies to deal with such issues.

REFERENCES

Bailey, D. B. Jr, Golden, R. N., Roberts, J., & Ford, A. (2007). Maternal depression and developmental disability: Research critique. *Mental Retardation and Developmental Disabilities Research Reviews, 13*(4), 321–329. doi:10.1002/mrdd.20172 PMID:17979207

Enoch, A., Mprah, W.K., Isaac, O., & Joseph, B. (2018). Role of Caregivers of Children with Intellectual Disabilities and Support Systems Available to them in Ghana. *Disability, CBR & Inclusive Development, 28*(4), 80-95. doi:. doi:10.5463/dcid.v28i4.645

Gardiner, E., Miller, A. R., & Lach, L. M. (2018). Family impact of childhood neurodevelopmental disability: Considering adaptive and maladaptive behaviour. *Journal of Intellectual Disability Research, 62*(10), 888–899. doi:10.1111/jir.12547 PMID:30230656

Gebeyehu, F., Sahile, A., & Ayalew, M. (2019). Burden, Social Support, and Life Satisfaction Among Caregivers of Children With Intellectual Disability: The Case of Felege Abay and Shembt Primary Schools, Bahir Dar, Ethiopia. *International Quarterly of Community Health Education, 39*(3), 147–153. doi:10.1177/0272684X18819974 PMID:30602336

Groce, N., & McGeown, J. (2013). *Witchcraft, Wealth and Disability: Reinterpretation of a folk belief in contemporary urban Africa* (Working Paper Series: No. 30). Leonard Cheshire Disability and Inclusive Development Centre, UCL.

Irazábal, M., Marsà, F., García, M., Gutiérrez-Recacha, P., Martorell, A., Salvador-Carulla, L., & Ochoa, S. (2012). Family burden related to clinical and functional variables of people with intellectual disability with and without a mental disorder. *Research In Developmental Disabilities, 33*(3), 796-803. doi:10.1016/j.ridd.2011.12.002

John, A. (2012). Stress among mothers of children with intellectual disabilities in urban India: Role of gender and maternal coping. *Journal of Applied Research in Intellectual Disabilities, 25*(4), 372–382. doi:10.1111/j.1468-3148.2011.00672.x PMID:22711485

Jokinen, N., Gomiero, T., Watchman, K., Janicki, M. P., Hogan, M., Larsen, F., ... Crowe, J. (2018). Perspectives on family caregiving of people aging with intellectual disability affected by dementia: Commentary from the International Summit on Intellectual Disability and Dementia. Journal. *Journal of Gerontological Social Work, 61*(4), 411–431. doi:10.1080/01634372.2018.1454563 PMID:29583104

Kishore, M. T. (2011). Disability impact and coping in mothers of children with intellectual disabilities and multiple disabilities. *Journal of Intellectual & Developmental Disability, 15*(4), 241–251. doi:10.1177/1744629511431659 PMID:22158461

Laurvick, C. L., Msall, M. E., Silburn, S., Bower, C., Klerk, N., & Leonard, H. (2006). Physical and mental health of mothers caring for a child with Rett syndrome. *Pediatrics, 118*(4), e1152–e1164. doi:10.1542/peds.2006-0439 PMID:16966392

Lee, R. L. T., Brown, M., Leung, C., Chen, H., Louie, L., Chen, J. L., & Lee, P. H. (2019). Family carers' experiences of participating in a weight management programme for overweight children and adolescents with intellectual disabilities: An exploratory study. *Journal of Advanced Nursing, 75*(2), 388–399. Epub2018Oct8. doi:10.1111/jan.13845 PMID:30187576

Low, L.P., Chien, W.T, Lam, L.W., & Wong, K.K. (2017). A qualitative study protocol of ageing carers' caregiving experiences and their planning for continuation of care for their immediate family members with intellectual disability. *BMC Geriatrics, 17*(1), 81. doi:10.118612877-017-0473-9

Man, J., & Kangas, M. (2019). Service satisfaction and helpfulness ratings, mental health literacy and help seeking barriers of carers of individuals with dual disabilities. *Journal of Applied Research in Intellectual Disabilities, 32*(1), 184-193. doi:10.1111/jar.12520

Martorell, A., Gutiérrez-Recacha, P., Irazábal, M., Marsà, F., & García, M. (2011). Family impact in intellectual disability, severe mental health disorders and mental healthdisorders in ID. A comparison. *Research in Developmental Disabilities, 32*(6), 2847–2852. doi:10.1016/j.ridd.2011.05.021 PMID:21641769

McConkey, R., Kahonde, C., & McKenzie, J. (2016). Tackling Stigma in Developing Countries: The Key Role of Families. In K. Scior & S. Werner (Eds.), *Intellectual Disability and Stigma: Stepping Out from the Margins*. Palgrave Macmillan. doi:10.1057/978-1-137-52499-7_12

McConkey, R., Truesdale-Kennedy, M., Chang, M. Y., Jarrah, S., & Shukri, R. (2008). The impact on mothers of bringing up a child with intellectual disabilities: A cross-cultural study. *International Journal of Nursing Studies, 45*(1), 65–74. doi:10.1016/j.ijnurstu.2006.08.007 PMID:17022985

Mori, Y., Downs, J., Wong, K., & Leonard, H. (2019). Longitudinal effects of caregiving on parental well-being: the example of Rett syndrome, a severe neurological disorder. *European Child and Adolescent Psychiatry, 28*(4), 505-520. doi:10.100700787-018-1214-0

Nam, S. J., & Park, E. Y. (2017). Relationship between caregiving burden and depression in caregivers of individuals with intellectual disabilities in Korea. *Journal of Mental Health (Abingdon, England), 26*(1), 50–56. doi:10.1080/09638237.2016.1276538 PMID:28084102

Naskar, S., & Nath, K. (2016). A clinical study on intellectual disability in northeastern India: Insight into the sociodemographic risk factors of a developing country. *International Journal of Medical Science and Public Health, 5*(9), 1789–1797. doi:10.5455/ijmsph.2016.23122015323

Oliver, A., Revuelto, L., Fernández, I., Simó-Algado, S., & Galiana, L. (2019). An integrative model of the subjective well-being of staff working in intellectual disabilityservices. *Research in Developmental Disabilities, 87*, 1–8. doi:10.1016/j.ridd.2019.01.007 PMID:30685682

Perkins, E. A. (2009). Caregivers of adults with intellectual disabilities: The relationship of compound caregiving and reciprocity to quality of life. *Graduate Theses and Dissertations*. Retrieved from https://scholarcommons.usf.edu/etd/2140

Savage, S., & Bailey, S. (2004). The impact of caring on caregivers' mental health: A review of the literature. *Australian Health Review*, *27*(1), 103–109. doi:10.1071/AH042710111 PMID:15362303

Werner, S. (2019). Service use and perceptions of service effectiveness by parents of individuals with intellectualdisabilities: Comparing Jewish and Arab Israeli parental caregivers. *Journal of Intellectual Disability Research*, *18*. doi:10.1111/jir.12611 PMID:30775831

Werner, S., Stern, I., Roth, D., & Tenenbaum, A. (2019). Help-Seeking by Parental Caregivers of Individuals with Intellectual Disabilities and Dual Diagnosis. *Administration and Policy in Mental Health*, *46*(3), 321–333. doi:10.100710488-018-00915-w PMID:30604003

Chapter 7
Living With Intellectual Disability:
Quality of Life

Mansi Jadeja
The Maharaja Sayajirao University of Baroda, India

Jamila Firdaus
Navrachana Higher Secondary School, Baroda

ABSTRACT

The need to understand the quality of life of people with intellectual disability is crucial as this mental disability is considered to be a major setback for any individual and his/her family. Current researches focus on creating an equal platform to understand intellectual disability in order to gain more acceptances from the masses, especially for the families who have a member suffering from intellectual disability. The age of the family member and available care taking measures are also of critical value. Models of therapy/interventions drawn from previous evidence-based practices give a bright picture.

INTELLECTUAL DISABILITY

Intellectual disability, formerly labelled "mental retardation," is defined by the Individuals with Disabilities Education Act (IDEA) as "significantly sub-average general intellectual functioning, existing concurrently [at the same time] with deficits in adaptive behavior and manifested during the developmental period, that adversely affects a child's educational performance." There are two key components within this definition: a student's IQ and his or her capability to function independently usually referred to as adaptive behavior. The deficits in "adaptive behavior" cited by IDEA prove trickier to evaluate. Factors considered include the ability to comprehend and participate in a conversation, to understand and follow social norms and to perform activities such as getting dressed and using the restroom. NICHCY explains that the causes of intellectual disabilities vary from pregnancy issues and complications at birth to genetic conditions (such as Down syndrome and fragile X syndrome) and health problems early in life, including diseases like measles and contact with poisonous substances such as lead and mercury.

DOI: 10.4018/978-1-7998-1223-4.ch007

A number of traits can point to an intellectual disability. The National Institute of Child Health and Human Development (NICHD, 2016) lists the following among early indicators:

- Delay in reaching developmental milestones such as sitting up and talking
- Difficulty remembering things
- Trouble comprehending accepted social behaviors and/or understanding the consequences to actions
- Poor problem-solving skills

The term Intellectual Disability has its roots in the term 'mental retardation' and 'developmental disability' (Health Commission, 1981; Thompson & O'Quinn, 1979; Wolfe, 1992) and its epidemiology is usually developmental or subsequent to traumatic brain injury. Individuals may have mild, moderate or severe intellectual disabilities depending on the assessments of their cognitive abilities (Arthur, 1998; Hogg & Sebba, 1987).Intellectual disability could be defined as an inability to carry out everyday adaptive functions which make living simple. These deficits could result in difficulties in communication, social participation and independent living across multiple environments such as home, school, workplace and community. On more complex level, intellectual functions of reasoning, problem solving, planning, abstract thinking, judgment, academic learning and learning from experiences could also be hindered.

According to the DSM-V, intellectual disability is defined as a ''disorder with onset during the developmental period that includes both intellectual and adaptive functioning deficits in conceptual, social and practical domains."(DSM-V, 2013).The World Health Organization's definitions of impairment, disability and handicap are generally regarded as authoritative, although multiple interpretations militate against a consensus (Bowe, 1978; Fulcher, 1989; Smyer, McHale, Birkel, & Madle, 1988). A very basic disagreement is whether the disability is a personal tragedy for the individual or is it more of a social problem arising because of disabling barriers within the environment (Abberley, 1987; Bickenbach, 1993; Gleeson, 1995).

Many terms, definitions and various descriptions of people with an intellectual disability see them in a 'deficit perspective'. Such a perspective does not give much importance to the social place, humanity and abilities of people with intellectual disabilities (Bickenbach, 1993; Schalock, 2004). On the other hand, the 'similarity perspective' focuses on capabilities. It supports the argument that all persons can learn, irrespective of the degree or complexity of their disabilities (Oliver, 1996).

General definitions of quality of life prevail in the literature reviews. Schalock (1997) referred to perceived quality of life as satisfaction with the main areas of one's own life. Brown (1994) stated that enhancement of quality of life was related to reduction in the discrepancy between an individual's achieved and unmet needs. Brown (1998) also mentioned that quality of life is the extent to which individuals have increasing control of their environments. Heal (1994) described it in terms of global satisfaction with one's lifestyle and control over resources that produced satisfaction.

A strong literature review supports the idea that conceptualization and assessment of quality of life of people with intellectual disability should be done in a manner similar to those which are done for people without such a disability. Schalock's (1999) core dimensions of quality of life of people with intellectual disability included emotional well-being, personal development, physical well being, self-determination, social inclusion and rights. Emphasis was also put upon individual improvement rather than population improvement (Brown, 1998; Cummins, 1996; Zapf, 1987). It was also argued that people with intellectual disabilities should be more involved in decision-making about policies and programs aimed at improving their quality of life (Brown, 1995; Brown, McLinden, & Porter, 1998, Goode and Hogg (1994), Nankervis (1997), Schalock (2002), and Schalock and Verdugo (2002).

Fabian (1991) identified three approaches of quality of life. The first two approaches view quality of life as an objective social indicator for specific groups and viewing it as a broad subjective measure of life satisfaction. The third approach is a measure of adaptive functioning which was identified as an alternative for individuals who were unable to self report or whose life experiences were inequitably limited.

Relationship Between Intellectual Disability and Quality of Life

The Convention on the Rights of Persons with Disabilities (United Nations 2006) acknowledges that people with disabilities continue to face rights violations and barriers to equal participation in society. There is growing recognition of the need to ensure that all people who have disabilities enjoy human rights on an equal basis with others. These rights pertain to a range of life domains. While there is no international consensus on what constitutes a human rights approach to social policy and services (Gruskin & Loff 2002), human rights treaties and documents explicitly or implicitly include the right of people with a disability to expect and receive effective evidence-based services and care.

Regardless of a country's human rights perspective or economic status, the lives of adults with ID, especially those who have severe and profound ID, mental illness and those who exhibit challenging behaviors, differ significantly from others in the community (Cummins 2005; United Nations 2006). Historically, service systems have failed to adequately meet the needs of people with ID and have not met the obligations articulated within the Convention on the Rights of Persons with Disabilities. Services have been crisis-driven, ad hoc, have denied human dignity and have failed to facilitate or encourage meaningful community engagement. Service responses have included restrictive practices including: physical/mechanical and chemical restraint, and systematic neglect resulting in adverse physical and psychological effects for consumers and carers (Bernal & Hollins 1995; Deveau & McGill 2009; Sanders 2009).

Within a human rights framework people with intellectual disability (ID) have the right to accessible, appropriate, evidence-based services that enable them to achieve personal goals and to enjoy a quality of life (QOL) equal to that of people who do not have a disability.There is a pressing need within the ID service system for more consistent and responsive services which facilitate positive outcomes. Quality-based reform movements within health, mental health, education and disability fields increasingly emphasise the importance of accountability and the establishment of quality frameworks that include reporting mechanisms to monitor service and resource effectiveness and congruence with consumer needs (Pirkis et al. 2005; Brown et al. 2009).

Quality monitoring systems are required in ID services as for any other disability group. Routine outcome measurement systems constitute an important part of a quality system and can promote effective evidence-based policy and service development, planning and delivery. Comprehensive outcome data include individual and population outcomes, service level outcomes including levels of service utilisation, efficiency, effectiveness, accessibility, equity and appropriateness (Bickman et al. 1998; Hensel 2001), and economic data including resource use and costs at the level of individual users, their families and the community. A comprehensive outcome measurement system includes measures that assess individual consumer outcomes or changes in an individual, which are wholly attributable to the ID service or intervention. Human rights frameworks recognise the right of people with a disability to have full and effective participation equal to other members of society generally and particularly in relation to matters directly concerning them. Consumer outcome measurement must therefore include the perspective of the individual service user as well as family members and the service provider. Consumer outcome measurement should be 'embedded' in routine service delivery and data should be collected on entry to a service and at regular intervals while the individual is using the service. Consumer outcomes should be directly relevant to the goals articulated in individual service users' plans including person-centred plans or positive behaviour support plans. A key individual outcome domain is QOL.The concept of QOL has evolved within ID since the 1980s (Verdugo et al. 2005; Zuna et al. 2009). Areas of focus have shifted from the effects of institutionalisation and untenable environments to 'higher order' aspects of QOL (Cummins & Lau 2003). QOL is associated with human values including happiness, satisfaction, general feelings of well-being and opportunities to achieve personal potential (Cummins 1991; Schalock 2000; Brown & Brown 2009). Quality of life is a multidimensional phenomenon composed of core domains and elements that are influenced by personal characteristics and environmental and contextual variables (Verdugo et al. 2005). Domains and specific indicators of QOL have been identified and critically assessed (Brown & Brown 2009). QOL domains include those that are common to all humans and additional domains that may be unique to the individual (Lyons 2005; Verdugo et al. 2005). There is international consensus about the dimensions of QOL (Schalock et al. 2002; Brown & Brown 2009). Eight core QOL domains have been identified and validated in a series of cross-cultural studies: emotional wellbeing, interpersonal relationships, material wellbeing, personal development, physical well-being, self-determination, social inclusion and rights (Schalock 2000; Beadle-Brown et al. 2009; Wang et al. 2010).When aggregated, these domains represent the total QOL construct. QOL outcomes may be impacted upon by variables within several domains, for example, the nature of service delivery, the consumer's life experience, their physical environment, and the number and nature of people with whom the consumer lives and with whom they interact. Individual QOL varies over time and is substantially influenced by cultural environments, individual interests and circumstances. As a measurement, QOL should be considered holistically and family QOL should also be considered (Schalock et al. 2009).

Some aspects of QOL can be objectively measured through direct observation and assessed and verified against commonly held standards, for example, medical health and wealth (McGillivray et al. 2009). Other aspects of QOL can only be assessed from the subjectively perceived experience of the individual through self-report. QOL domains should therefore include separately measured subjective and objective indicators (Verdugo et al. 2005; Beadle-Brown et al. 2009). It is important to note that subjective and objective indicators are typically not highly correlated (Schalock et al. 2002, 2008; Cummins 2005b). As a consumer outcome measure, QOL enables impact studies, cross-cultural and country comparisons, and provides a framework for service principles and service design, delivery and evaluation that is congruent with human rights frameworks (Schalock 2004; Schalock et al. 2008; Brown et al. 2009). QOL outcome data can inform a range of stakeholders as to whether and to what extent service users experience changes in their QOL as a result of service interventions and whether personal outcomes are being achieved (Bonham et al. 2004; Brown & Brown 2005; Schalock et al. 2008). It can guide quality improvement strategies at individual, service and community levels (Schalock et al. 2002, 2008; Hoffman et al. 2006; D'Eath et al. 2009; Kober & Eggleton 2009) and influence political development and reform (Cummins & Lau 2003). Quality of life is developing from a concept to a measurable and socially valid construct (Claes et al. 2009).There is growing acceptance of the need for QOL to be measured, over time and in relation to services received (Brown et al. 2009; Claes et al. 2009; Griffith & Owen2009; Isaacs et al.

2009; Murphy 2009). Hughes et al.(1995; cited in Claes et al. 2009) found over 1243 measures of QOL reported in the ID literature by the mid-1990s; however, there are no systematic reviews or comparative analyses of QOL measures for people with ID against key criteria.

People may have difficulty in "knowing" a person with an intellectual disability. It is usually difficult to understand what their feelings, interests, wants, preferences and inner life is like. Several authors have attempted to have a look at these aspects and have described that "knowing" a person with intellectual disability would emerge when a person spends more time with the disabled person. This 'knowing" would become a central part of the quality of relationship and create a better understanding (Gustiatas & Young, 1986; Goode, 1984; Keenan, 1992; & Sacks, 1995).

There is growing concern for a need to ensure that all individuals with an intellectual disability enjoy life as beautifully as others and share equal rights. Such rights cover many aspects of life out of which quality of living or quality of life is a part. One may wonder as to how a person with an intellectual disability would communicate and express his/her feelings regarding various aspects of quality of life? One would at least require basic level of intelligence in order to carry this out.

Quality of Life

The earliest known reference to Quality of Life is made by Aristotle who used the term 'eudemonia' or 'the good life'. However, this notion did not enter into social sciences, particularly sociology and psychology, as a defining concept until the beginning of the 20th century and only began being researched in the field of disability in the 1980's and 1990's. Since this time there has been a large growth in the use of the concept and its application within the field of intellectual and allied disabilities (Brown et al. 1989; Schalock 1990; Goode 1994; Felce & Perry 1996; Cummins 1996).

Quality of Life is an integrating concept, which takes into account a number of previous approaches and concepts such as normalization, inclusion, and empowerment, though the development of Quality of Life is resulting in some modification to those practices. For example, the application of personal choice within a developmental framework may set limits for some individuals on the degree to which they wish or feel comfortable with inclusion. Thus it is important to recognize individual and family variability. there are further principles integrated within this holistic concept including, for example, self-image, lifespan, perception, inter and intra personal variability (Schalock & Verdugo 2002; Brown & Brown 2003; Turnbull et al. 2004). Domains cover all areas of individual and family living. Examples are health, finance, community, family, employment, education (see Felce & Perry 1996; Brown et al. 2003, 2006). It is recognized that all of the domains are linked and are activated through such principles as choice. For example, recreation and leisure may for some people the best way to improve physical health and employment. It is this notion of holism that makes Quality of Life an interesting prism through which to examine policies and practices for individuals with disabilities, their families and social network (Brown & Brown 2003).

Much used in international public policy are the domains used by the World Health Organization: physical health, psychological well-being, social relations and environment (Murphy et al. 2000). Brown & Brown (2003) consolidated these ideas for practice in disability services into three core domains and nine sub-domains: Being (namely physical, psychological and spiritual well-being), Belonging (namely physical, social and community belonging) and Becoming (namely practical, leisure and growth becoming). Another widely used set of domains is described by Schalock & Verdugo (2002), namely: emotional well-being, interpersonal relations, material well-being, personal development, physical well-being, self-determination, social inclusion, and rights. The various domains discussed by different researchers have a wide degree of commonality though different labels are sometimes employed. All the recent domain structures cover similar ground and reflect the particular context involved.

Many authors have regarded quality of life as a multidimensional concept that covers life satisfaction and other aspects like psychological and subjective well being (Abbey & Andrews, 1986; Headey & Wearing, 1992; Pavot & Diener, 1993). Quality of life seems to be more than the subjective experience of life satisfaction. Schalock (1996) explained three definitions of quality of life which were most representative:

1. Quality of life is experienced when a person's basic needs are met and he has opportunities to pursue and achieve goals.
2. Quality of life is a multidimensional concept involving a number of core dimensions relating to well being.
3. Quality of life reflects a person's desired conditions of living and health and wellness.

The terms subjective well being and subjective quality of life refer to the perceptions of the individual. Life satisfaction means the degree to which the individual's life is perceived to match some implicit or explicit internal standard or referent (Evans, 1994). Subjective quality of life is a personal phenomenon more closely related to the broader concept of quality of life.

Researches in the 1980s focused on individuals with intellectual disability affected by deinstitutionalization (Hughes, 1995; Parmenter, Cummins, Shaddock & Stancliffe, 1994; Richmond, 1983; Schalock, 1994). Clear links between quality of life and normalization, deinstitutionalization, integration, choice and empowerment were established (Brown, 1994; Edgerton, 1996; Goode & Hogg, 1994; Goode, 1992; Parmenter, 1995; Romney, 1994; Schalock, 1994).

The broad emphasis in quality of life research during 1990s was to improve population quality of life. The World Health Organization placed the study and improvement of population quality of life as a primary goal (Evans, 1994). Researchers sought to inform decision-making for public programs and services that purported to improve quality of life (Cheng, 1988; Evans, 1994; Faden & Laplege, 1992; Goodinson & Singleton, 1989; Halpern, 1993; Hatton, 1998; Hughes & Hwang, 1996; Social Policy Directorate, 1994).

COMMUNICATION

Individuals with intellectual disability are most varied, particularly in terms of their abilities to communicate with others around them (Cirrin & Rowland, 1985).Thus, it becomes important to understand the different communication challenges faced by these people in order to understand them and their quality of life. Communicative competence is crucial (Butterfield, Arthur, & Linfoot, 1992) and so establishing meaningful communication is a major challenge for their families, caregivers and service providers (Feil, 1993).

Researchers have developed specific strategies to minimize these communication deficits. The life sharing approach described by Goode and Hogg (1994) is a method in which adult clients and caregivers share and record life histories and biographies to enhance communication and understanding. Systematic gathering of information from communication partners was utilized by Shaddock, Dowse, Richards and Spinks (1998) to represent the views of adults with intellectual disability at formal tribunal hearings.

Literature demonstrates consensus that communicative behaviors of people with intellectual disability are diverse and frequently difficult to interpret (Arthur, 1998; Goode, 1997). Contemporary research about communication training recognized the potential of communicative intent of subtle, idiosyncratic and non-symbolic behaviors. Some learners communicate effectively without the need for conventional symbols (Carter & Hook, 1998). The most ethical approach seems to be of that in which communication with these individuals is taken seriously and they are considered as an authentic communicator (Tetzchner and Jensen, 1999).

In 1988 the NINDS (NIH) estimated that 90% of children with severe ID manifested some type of language disorder (McLean et al., 1999); likewise adults with mild to moderate ID often exhibit difficulties with speech and language (Cheslock et al., 2008). Research has shown that adults with ID exhibit deficits in multiple aspects of communication, including written, expressive, and receptive modes (Berry, 1972; Merrill & Mar, 1987; Abbeduto, Furman, & Davies, 1989; Abbeduto & Nuccio, 1991; Merrill & Jackson, 1992a; Merrill & Jackson, 1992b; Belva et al., 2012). This may be due to the fact that individuals with ID have reduced cognitive resources compared to typical peers (Kail, 1992; Koul & Clapsaddle, 2006). In areas such as health care, individuals with ID often face cognitive challenges in communicating their needs, understanding and adherence to recommendations or treatments (Ward, Nichols, & Freedman, 2010). Given the communicative challenges faced by individuals with ID, it stands to reason that the most effective ways to communicate with these people may be different from the ways in which information is routinely communicated with persons who do not have ID.

In order to determine the most appropriate interventions and approaches to communication with an individual with ID, it is necessary to understand the degree of communicative impairment that exists for that individual. Recent studies have shown that while a general trend can be observed in which those with more severe ID tend to possess fewer communicative skills (Cascella 2004), there exists significant heterogeneity in the communicative abilities among those with severe ID (Carlesimo, Marotta, & Vicari, 1997; McLean, Brady, & McLean, 1996; McLean et al., 1999; van der Meer et al., 2011). Among those with mild ID, some are relatively unimpaired and effectively fall within what may be considered the normal range of communicative function. These individuals have even been included within normative samples of standardized speech-language tests (Cascella 2006).

An individualized functional approach has been used successfully to devise alternative communication methods to improve information exchange with individuals with locked-in syndrome, another group for whom communication often poses significant challenges (Soderholm, Meinander, & Alaranta, 2001). Functional assessment research has become an important component in treating challenging behaviors in individuals with ID (Matson et al., 2011a), with inherently communicative functions such as attention, and demands being incorporated into the functional assessment (Matson et al., 2011). Functional communication training has also exceeded criteria as a well-established treatment for addressing problem behavior in children with ID and has been characterized as likely, though not proven, to be efficacious with adults (Kurtz et al., 2011).

Subjective Well-Being

Over the past two decades, researchers have drawn attention to the importance of the quality of life of people with intellectual disabilities. Subjective well being and feelings of happiness are considered as key components of quality of life. Subjective well being refers to the global experience of positive reactions to one's life (Diener & Lucas, 2000).

Researchers in the intellectual disability field have focused on improving people's objective and external conditions such as the services they are offered, their physical conditions, their employment or political advocacy and others. Such improvements may not lead to enduring well being in people with intellectual disabilities (Dykens, 2006). The concept of well being has been applied to people with intellectual disabilities. Several studies have found that levels of subjective well being in people with intellectual disability are similar to those in people who do not have intellectual disability (Cummins, 2001; Shephard-Jones, 2005; Emerson & Hatton, 2008).

Functional life skills such as social abilities, communication, affective skills and emotional competence together make up the ability to adapt with everyday life (Gumpel, 1994; O'Reilly, 2004; Smith & Matson, 2010). Deficiencies in these skills can curb people with intellectual disability to live up to their personal and professional potentials. It might cause lower well being and happiness. Intellectually disabled people have more limited social and emotional adaptive skills (Arthur, 2003; La Malfa, 2009).

Families Having a Person with Intellectual Disability

Literature review focuses on data collected from various countries and consist of perceptions given by primary caregivers, mostly mothers. The overall aim of society, through government policy and community services, is to enable the child with a disability to function as effectively as possible, and also to enable parents and other siblings to function effectively, and wherever possible, live lives of quality (Brown & Brown, 2003). Family is the environment which enables an individual to develop and grow effectively. The issue is not just the child with an intellectual disability but also the family and the interaction of disability in the family which matters as a whole. Thus, it is important to know as to how disability affects those in the family who are not disabled and how can we develop ways of improving these negative effects in order to make each member function optimally.

Researchers (e.g., Andrews, 1974) have recognized for a long time that perceptions are a major driving force of human behaviour, that is, what is perceived and believed affects how the individual or, in this case family members behave. This includes how a family is affected by its belief and value system, the nature of disability services, whether they are private or public; health and the satisfaction of health in the family, and so on. There are often pressing challenges, for the disability of one member of the family negatively influences the behaviour or resources of the family as a whole, for example, when a mother has to give up her job to look after her child.

It seems plausible that intervention and support in one key area is likely to improve other aspects of family functioning and therefore overall family satisfaction. Key areas differ to some extent from family to family, or over time in the same family, arguing for an individual approach to support. There are families where internal aspects of family life are positive and the challenges largely arise from outside the family, e.g., community reaction, lack of support, and lack of appropriate respite when required. These challenges necessitate careful and considered observation, reflection, and flexibility on the part of policy and service personnel. Additionally, combining intervention and/or support in more than one domain, e.g., Family Health and support for the family in terms of enjoyment of life (Leisure and Recreation or Career Preparation) is likely to have greater and possibly wide-ranging effects on a family's overall satisfaction and quality of life. This would need much close collaboration between different service groups and would require much greater coordination of policy between different departments and agencies. If such arguments are correct such an approach: (a) requires an accent on service and support across agencies; and (b) should have long-term economic savings, since such coordinated intervention might be expected to have holistic benefits, such as an increase in family overall health and economic viability. However, as stressed by Brown and Brown (2009), such intervention and coordination should critically involve the family perception of needs and choices.

Other children in the family also face the impact of a child with an intellectual disability in terms of studying and calling friends at home. Inviting guests or neighbours at home is also difficult because of major behavioural disturbances. This could also lead to decreased support from neighbours and other community members. All this results into the families and the person with intellectual disability being cut-off from the necessary support and community interactions. Such arguments raise important questions regarding why many organizations and individuals go to a great extent to advocate for inclusive policies (Brown & Brown, 2003).

Having a family member with an intellectual disability can have an effect on the entire family; the parents, siblings, and extended family members. It is a unique shared experience for families and can affect all aspects of family functioning.

On the positive side it can broaden horizons, increase family members' awareness of their inner strength, enhance family cohesion, and encourage connections to community. On the other hand, the time and financial costs, physical and emotional demands, and logistical complexities associated with caring for a disabled child/adult can have far-reaching effects. The impacts will likely depend on the type of condition and severity, as well as the physical, emotional, and financial wherewithal of the family and the resources that are available.

For families, caring for a disabled family member may increase stress, take a toll on mental and physical health, make it difficult to find appropriate and affordable child care, and affect decisions about work, education/training, having additional children, and relying on public support. It may be associated with guilt, blame, or reduced self-esteem. It may divert attention from other aspects of family functioning. The out-of-pocket costs of medical care and other services may be enormous. All of these potential effects could have repercussions for the quality of the relationship between family members, their living arrangements, and future relationships and family structure.

Families are telling us that one of the supports that they may need to enable them to continue to care for their family member at home are short breaks. Short Breaks give them a break from their role as carer and also provide their family member an opportunity to be with others and benefit from new experiences.

Thus, it is important to being a fundamental change in how we set the policies, administer disability services and then carry out practices at the managerial and frontline levels. It is also means that we need to bring a change in how we educate the personnel. It is essential to understand the lifestyle of families with children having intellectual disability and the major reasons of family disruption.

Elderly Person with Intellectual Disability

In recent years, aging has become an issue in the field of intellectual disability (ID), because longer life survival is resulting in increasing numbers of elderly adults with ID. Researchers investigating aging processes have generally found similar aging patterns for people with or without ID (Boyd & Tedrick, 1992); nonetheless, individuals with ID show some characteristics of premature aging resulting in a greater inclination to morbidity and deconditioning (Jacobson, Sutton & Janicki, 1986; Janicki & Jacobson, 1986 & Ashman & Suttie, 1996).

Demographic aging, which refers to the increasing numbers of elderly adults within the overall population, is currently presenting major challenges for both health and social care services and for the immediate families.

Traditionally, intervention for aging persons with disabilities has focused on chronic physical impairment, functional capacity, and mental condition. Several approaches have been used to try and minimize secondary conditions and reduce mortality rates. Comparative studies of elderly individuals, with and without ID, have raised several questions and have also revealed significant differences between the two groups.

The prevalence of various diseases (diabetes, hypertension), obesity, decrease of flexibility, and sedentary living can be used as indications of premature aging (Cousins, 1998). Individual aging changes are very diverse and behavioral changes in day-to-day lifestyle have a major role in aging (Nelson & Dannifer, 1992). The prevalence of physically debilitating symptoms in aging persons with ID increases the demands for active diagnostic and therapeutic services. Such conditions include moderate to severe hearing loss and visual impairment, a high incidence of balance and gait dysfunction, arthritis and urinary incontinence, obesity, and nonischemic heart disorders. Determination of premature aging may be indicated by a range of signs and symptoms. The evaluation and active screening of cognitive and functional capabilities are important in order to assess their specific needs and to determine appropriate rehabilitative and psychotherapeutic programs.

Aging is a process which is affected by various biological and social factors and is expressed very uniquely in each individual. Since longevity is increasing, this process of aging includes people with intellectual disability. The context of family is important when we consider the aging process as it plays a fundamental role in the care-giving for the older adults.

Researches conducted on families in the field of intellectual disability have usually focused on stress and burden associated with the care-giving process from a parental (maternal) perspective and the negative impact of disability on the family (Haley & Perkins, 2004; Hatton & Emerson, 2003). Research and literature also focuses on co-resident parents and adults with intellectual disability and need for future planning (Bigby & Balandin, 2004; Bigby, 2004). New policies need to be developed in order to bring a change in the care-givers role considering the changing demands (Hogg, Lucchino, Wang, Janicki, & Group, 2000).

Relations within the family keep changing and these remain an important source of support and provide a sense of belongingness. Family support and positive perceptions are aspects that seem to have a positive influence on the quality of life. Familial support and routine though being an integral part of the family relations, keeps varying from one family to another. Practical, emotional and/or financial aids are provided by and to various members of the family. For e.g. adult siblings provide emotional and practical support to aging parents. Many siblings will also likely carry on with familial support responsibilities for their brother or sister with a disability when parents are no longer able(Bigby, 1997; Dew, Llewellyn, & Balandin, 2004).Reciprocal support between parents and offspring with a disability may also occur regardless of living arrangement, as has been found in research involving co-resident families (Heller, Miller, &Factor, 1997). Furthermore, some parents anticipate their offspring with a disability may be a source of support, as they themselves age and need help with daily living.

Another important aspect of familial relations is routine. Routine seems to provide predictability and structure to familial contact and support. Depending on the family, routines can occur on a daily, weekly or seasonal basis. For e.g. parent going for grocery shopping while child is in school. Routines are also significant to older aged families of adults with a disability (Knox & Bigby, 2007). Family routines and rituals are, indeed, an important aspect of family life (Fiese et al., 2002) and maintaining some routines may better support families through various transitions (Zisberg, Young, Schepp, & Zysberg, 2007).

Measuring Quality of Life

Global quality of life (QOL) means the quality of a person's state of existence. Some people believe QOL to be multidimensional (Sloan, Loprinzi, Kuross, Miser, Mahoney, 1998) while other researches have found QOL to be about one single dimension like love (Proinin, 2000), ability to relate, or our fundamental sense of coherence (Antonovsky, 1985 & Antonovsky, 1987). The more spiritual and abstract the thinking about life is, the more QOL is about a single all-penetrating life-force, like God, the Great Spirit, or the great void (Sunya). The more materialistic the worldview, the more factors are believed to be of relevance. Modem biomedicine often presents the idea that illness and health are multi-dimensional phenomenon with multi-factorial causes. QOL has been described as well-being, life satisfaction, happiness, meaning of life, inner balance, self-actualisation, realisation of life's potentials, fulfilment of needs and abilities and functioning in general (Ventegodt, 1996). All these dimensions have been integrated into the theory of integrative quality of life (Ventegodt, Merrick & Anderson, 2003), which has been the basis of several QOL questionnaires like the SEQOL and the validated Quality Of Life-Q5 (QOL5) with only five items. QOL5 has been found to be a more valid tool for measuring of global QOL and efficient in documenting the effect of a therapeutic intervention on many different groups of patients (Ventegodt et.al, 2007). The interesting thing for us was, if we can expand this use into measuring the quality of life and treatment effect also of people with intellectual disabilities or other persons with insufficient language or communication skills. This can only be done if an obse1ver can fill in a QOL questionnaire on behalf of the person unable to conununicate. Basically the ability to read/understand, if another person is happy or unhappy is a precondition for successful parenthood. Therefore parents must be able to rate the QOL and mood of their child. We know this ability as empathy, the ability to feel the state of consciousness of other people. To our knowledge little research has been conducted into the degree of actual knowledge that comes from empathy. Is empathy a true source of knowledge of our fellow men? Are we able, through empathy, to know about other people's emotional and existential states, their thoughts and feelings, their degree of 1nental, spiritual and sexual development, and their global QOL as the total of all this? And even more interesting: Are we able to tell how the person would rate him or herself, if asked? This might be very different from our rating of the person, as we can use totally different standards, but maybe we even are able to sense the standard use for inner assessment of QOL and related issues? And are some people better to read people's minds than other? Do we know more about people we love than people we do not care for, meaning that a child that is more loved gets more parental reading and thus more fulfilment of its needs? Are people who chose to be healthprofessional more empathetic and better to guess than other people?

Direct interviewing approaches could be used for individuals with mild or moderate level of intellectual disability. Contemporary assessment tools include The Lifestyle Satisfaction Scale (Heal & Chadsey-Rusch, 1985), The Quality of Life Questionnaire (Schalock & Keith, 1993) among others. With people who have severe intellectual disability, direct interviewing is inappropriate. The validity and reliability of these assessments could be interrupted if these are used with individuals who have some verbal skills, acquiescence, inconsistency and last-option responding (Baroff, 1986; Felce & Perry, 1996; Heal & Sigelman, 1992; Matikka & Vesala, 1997). Such issues are exacerbated when an individual has atypical expressions, lacks formal communication skills, or tends to acquiesce (Matikka & Vesala, 1997). The validity of interview methods could be enhanced if the data is gathered from multiple interviews with familiar others (Heal & Sigelman, 1992).

To measure one's quality of life, one could be asked generally regarding how satisfied that person is with his/her life. This could be done in person, through the means of a questionnaire or by using a validated instrument or technique. Since quality of life is a concept which is a multidimensional, researchers usually seek to measure and assess it using multiple domains and indicators (Andrews, 1980; Brown, 1994; Cummins, 2000; Erikson & Uusitalo, 1987; Felce & Perry, 1996; Hughes, 1995; Parmenter, 1994, 1995; Sen, 1993; Solomon 1980; Zapf, 1987). Debate continues on whether subjective quality of life can or should be measured across multiple measures or whether a simple global measure is valid and achievable (Felce & Perry, 1996; Romney, 1994; Travers & Richardson, 1993).

Principles on assessment and measurement include the recognition and measurement of individual quality of life, which includes the recognition of valued personal experiences and circumstances, which reflect domains that contribute to a full and interconnected life.

Subjective and objective, both methods have been used to measure and assess quality of life. Objective methods include observable and quantifiable indicators whereas subjective methods use an individual's perceptions and qualitative assessments of happiness or satisfaction (Land, 1983; Lyons, 2000; Schussler & Fisher, 1985).

More instruments that measure QOL need to be developed and rigorously validated. This is especially the case for high-needs disability populations like those individuals that exhibit challenging behavior or have severe to profound ID, as it is questionable whether existing measures can be used with these populations.

Research on quality of life has played a role as a 'change agent' during the past few decades, primarily as a sensitizing notion, broadening to a conceptual framework for assessing quality outcomes and enhancing quality of life through understanding, support and intervention (Lyons, 2010; Schippers & Tubben, 2008). The very first criteria for research on quality of life is the use of a multidimensional approach which has several domains, with anticipated cross-cultural validity that allows research to be more clearly directed to specific areas.

Out of the various components of research, the first is conceptualization. It describes what quality of life is, namely a multidimensional construct, influenced by personal and environmental factors and their interactions (Schalock& Verdugo, 2002). These components are interrelated although, it is recognized that there is variability from person to person. They result from individual perception and choice, and change over an individual's life span (Brown & Brown, 2003).

The second component of application focuses on the enhancement of well being within the context of those involved, thus implying a wide variety of settings as well as a variety of individual and group purposes. Professional practices should reflect quality of life principles resulting in personally valued quality of life outcomes that are based on sound professional skills and methods such as observation and the measurement of choices that are important to the person (Brown, 2009; Brown & Brown, 2009). All the components need to be interactive. Working in any of the components requires effective assessment and feedback for adjustment to a total research or support program. It requires that the approach must be fully interdisciplinary from a research or a professional perspective. For example, what professionals learn from application often has an impact on measurement strategies and techniques and could result into re-conceptualization.

For effective research on quality of life, a criterion of creating a balance between qualitative and quantitative methods and triangulation of those methods, using assessment of both subjective (perceptual) and objective parameters. A systems perspective is also helpful which integrates the micro-level, meso-level and macro-level in which persons with disabilities live, so that predictors and causal factors in their lives could be identified (Lyons, 2010). Quality of life research requires active involvement of people with disabilities and their social network. Inter and Intra variability is critical in quality of life researches.

Evidence-Based Practices

Assessing the quality of life of people with intellectual disability is an essential part of managing these individuals. More important is to provide help to them on the basis of research evidence which would make us reach higher probabilities of being sure of treatment. There are two essential ideas in evidence-based practices: first, interventions should have clear empirical support and second, personal outcomes should be used to guide organizational change and quality improvement. The quality of life conceptual and measurement model can serve as a basis for evidence-based practices (Veerman & Van Yperen, 2007).It consists of four levels of evidence: descriptive, theoretical, indicative and causal.

Descriptive:

The essential elements of the intervention are made to be explicit and are summarized in program practices and standards as follows-

- A holistic, multi-dimensional approach
- A focus on the community and organizations being bridges to the community
- The use of best practices that are empirically based strategies that reduce the discrepancy (i.e., mismatch) between people and the environments through functional skill training, the use of assistive technology devices, accessing natural supports, and environmental modification/accommodation
- The use of individualized support strategies and their alignment with core quality of life domains
- The application of quality of life principles
- The use of quality of life-focused program practices as listed above
- The measurement of personal outcomes as a key component of evidence-based practices
- The demonstration of fidelity to the conceptual and measurement model
- The alignment of assessed support needs to quality of life domains
- The use of personal outcomes to guide organizational quality improvement

Theoretical

Here, the intervention has a plausible rationale which explains why it should work. It defines the concept operationally and establishes parameters for program planning and implementation. The theoretical rationale for why an emphasis on quality of life should work is found in the extensive international research (e.g., Brown & Brown, 2005; Cummins, 2005; Schalock et al., 2007) which suggests strongly that one's quality of life is: (a) is multi-dimensional and has the same components for all people; (b) influenced by personal and environmental factors; and (c) enhanced by self-determination, inclusion, individualized supports, and purpose in life.

Indicative

The indicative aspect includes intervention strategies which lead to the desired outcome. This level of evidence is reflected in: (a) studies (e.g., Bonham et al., 2004; Perry & Felce, 2005) which demonstrate that personal outcomes are enhanced when QOL principles and QOL-related program practices are employed; and (b) the publishing of service provider profiles that show longitudinal changes in quality of life outcomes for all service recipients (Keith & Bonham, 2005; State of Nebraska Health and Human Services, 2006).

Causal

This aspect states that either the outcome is caused by or related to the intervention or that there is clear evidence showing which component of the intervention are predictive of the outcomes. There has been considerable work determining the significant predictors of QOL-related outcomes for persons with ID/DD. Across a number of studies (Schalock et al.,2007; Schalock et al., 2008a, b), personal characteristics (such as IQ and adaptive behaviour levels), program practices (e.g., enabling choices, rights, self-determination, availability of transportation, and community inclusion), and setting characteristics (e.g., residential and employment status, setting size, and operational culture) are significant predictors of QOL outcomes.

CONCLUSION

People with Intellectual Disability are the most able individuals when they are brought up in families where they are given "Ownership" to perform their best with support from families and caregivers. Every experience ranging from the most difficult situation to the most achievable milestones in areas of Cognitions, social skills and emotional wellbeing is the essence of defining a Quality Life and Spiritual Well-being for each one of them and their families. Learning from others experiences helps families gather strength and reinforces positive living in enabling their Children with Intellectual Disabilities. Parent support groups and sharing of case studies about living dynamic changes of growth and development in areas of well-being with limited intellectual potential is the greatest rewarding experience on planet earth in terms of survival for these special Ones. It is important to keep engaging the inner soul with the external social environment so that there is no deprivation or depression coming in the way of quality living in them. Every new experience of pain and resistance when supported with care and love by the family members and caregivers gives a define meaning to the lives of individuals with intellectual disability.

In order to provide whatever is best suited for individuals with intellectual disability, one must be aware about their needs and requirements and how one can help them fulfill those. There are number of Government rules and regulations which are available for these individuals, only if family members and other significant people are aware about them. Applying different measures for young one and elderly will yield better outcomes as there are differences in terms of age related needs. Professional help is nowadays easily available but one should also make a choice in terms of what services one is availing. Following evidence-based practices and referring to recent researches is always the best way to go.

REFERENCES

Abbeduto, L., Furman, L., & Davies, B. (1989). Relation between the receptive language and mental age of persons with mental retardation. *American Journal of Mental Retardation*, *93*, 535–543. PMID:2706121

Abberley, P. (1987). The concept of oppression and the development of a social theory of disability. *Disability, Handicap & Society*, *2*(1), 5–19. doi:10.1080/02674648766780021

Abbey, A., & Andrews, F. M. (1986). Modeling the psychological determinants of life quality. In F. M. Andrews (Ed.), *Research on the quality of life*. Ann Arbor, MI: Institute for Social Research, University of Michigan.

Andrews, F. M. (1974). Social indicators of perceived life quality. *Social Indicators Research*, *1*(3), 279–299. doi:10.1007/BF00303860

Arthur, M. (1998). *Socio-communicative variables and behaviour states in students with the most severe and multiple disabilities: An observational study* (Unpublished PhD dissertation). Macquarie University, Sydney, Australia.

Belva, B. C., Matson, J. L., Sipes, M., & Bamburg, J. W. (2012). An examination of specific communication deficits in adults with profound intellectual disabilities. *Research in Developmental Disabilities*, *33*(2), 525–529. doi:10.1016/j.ridd.2011.10.019 PMID:22119701

Berry, P. B. (1972). Comprehension of possessive and present continuous sentences by nonretarded, mildly retarded, and severely retarded children. *American Journal of Mental Deficiency*, *76*, 540–544. PMID:5012135

Bickenbach, J. E. (1993). *Physical disability and social policy*. Toronto, ON: University of Toronto Press.

Bigby, C. (1997). Parental substitutes? The role of siblings in the lives of older people with intellectual disability. *Journal of Gerontological Social Work*, *29*(1), 3–21. doi:10.1300/J083v29n01_02

Bigby, C. (2004). *Ageing with a Lifelong Disability: A Guide to Practice, Program and Policy Issues for Human Services Professionals*. London: Jessica Kingsley.

Bigby, C., & Balandin, S. (2004). Issues in researching the ageing of people with intellectual disability. In E. Emerson, C. Hatton, T. Thompson, & T. R. Parmenter (Eds.), *The International Handbook of Applied Research in Intellectual Disabilities* (pp. 221–236). West Sussex, UK: Wiley. doi:10.1002/9780470713198.ch10

Bonham, G. S., Basehart, S., Schalock, R. L., Marchand, C. B., Kirchner, N., & Rumenap, J. M. (2004). Consumer-based quality of life assessment: The Maryland Ask Me! Project. *Mental Retardation*, *42*(5), 338–355. doi:10.1352/0047-6765(2004)42<338:CQOLAT>2.0.CO;2 PMID:15335259

Bowe, F. (1978). *Handicapping America: Barriers to Disabled People*. New York: Harper and Row.

Brown, I. (2006). *Family Quality of Life Survey: Main caregivers of people with intellectual or developmental disabilities*. Toronto: Surrey Place Centre.

Brown, I., & Brown, R. I. (2003). *Quality of Life and Disability: An Approach for Community Practitioners*. London, UK: Jessica Kingsley.

Brown, I., & Brown, R. I. (2009). Choice as an aspect of quality of life for people with intellectual disabilities. *Journal of Policy and Practice in Intellectual Disabilities, 6*, 10 17.

Brown, N., McLinden, M., & Porter, J. (1998). Sensory needs. In P. Lacey & C. Ouvry (Eds.), *People with profound and multiple learning disabilities: A collaborative approach to meeting complex needs* (pp. 29–38). London: David Fulton.

Brown, R. I. (1995). Measuring new dimensions through quality of life: The personal equation. *Evaluation Journal of Australasia, 7*(1), 14–23.

Brown, R. I. (1998). *Conceptualisation of quality of life: An overview*. Paper presented at the 1998 Australian Society for the Study of Intellectual Disability (ASSID) Conference: Conceptualisation of quality of life workshop, Flinders University of South Australia, Adelaide, Australia.

Brown, R. I., Bayer, M. B., & MacFarlane, C. (1989). *Rehabilitation programs: Performance and Quality of Life of adults with developmental handicaps*. Toronto: Lugus Productions.

Brown, R. I., & Brown, I. (2005). The application of quality of life. *Journal of Intellectual Disability Research, 49*(10), 718–727. doi:10.1111/j.1365-2788.2005.00740.x PMID:16162116

Butterfield, N., Arthur, M., & Linfoot, K. (1992). Meeting communication needs in communication programming for students with severe intellectual disability: The creating communicative contexts manual. *Special Education Perspectives, 1*(1), 35–43.

Carlesimo, G. A., Marotta, L., & Vicari, S. (1997). Long-term memory in mental retardation: Evidence for a specific impairment in subjects with Down's syndrome. *Neuropsychologia, 35*(1), 71–79. doi:10.1016/S0028-3932(96)00055-3 PMID:8981379

Carter, M., & Hook, J. (1998). Communication programming for students with high support needs: A model for deciding what to teach. *Special Education Perspectives, 7*(1), 42–55.

Cascella, P. W. (2004). *Receptive communication abilities among adults with significant intellectual disability*. Taylor & Francis Ltd.

Cascella, P. W. (2006). Standardised speech-language tests and students with intellectual disability: A review of normative data. *Journal of Intellectual & Developmental Disability, 31*(2), 120–124. doi:10.1080/13668250600681503 PMID:16782597

Cheslock, M. A., Barton-Hulsey, A., Romski, M., & Sevcik, R. A. (2008). Using a speech-generating device to enhance communicative abilities for an adult with moderate intellectual disability. *Intellectual and Developmental Disabilities, 46*(5), 376–386. doi:10.1352/2008.46:376-386 PMID:19090639

Cirrin, F. M., & Rowland, C. M. (1985). Communicative assessment of non-verbal youths with severe/profound mental retardation. *Mental Retardation, 23*(2), 52–62. PMID:3990553

Cummins, R. A. (1996). Assessing quality of life. In R. L. Schalock (Ed.), *Quality of life. Volume Conceptualization and measurement*. Washington, DC: American Association on Mental Retardation.

Cummins, R.A. (1996). The domains of life satisfaction: An attempt to order chaos. *Social Indicators Research, 38*, 303-28.

Cummins, R. A. (2005). Moving from the quality of life concept to a theory. *Journal of Intellectual Disability Research, 49*(10), 699–706. doi:10.1111/j.1365-2788.2005.00738.x PMID:16162114

Dew, A., Llewellyn, G., & Balandin, S. (2004). Post-parental care: A new generation of siblingcarers. *Journal of Intellectual & Developmental Disability, 29*(2), 176–179. doi:10.1080/13668250410001709520

Evans, D. R. (1994). Enhancing quality of life in the population at large. *Social Indicators Research, 33*(1-3), 47–88. doi:10.1007/BF01078958

Fabian, E. S. (1991). Using quality-of-life indicators in rehabilitation program evaluation. *Rehabilitation Counseling Bulletin, 34*(4), 344–356.

Feil, N. (1993). *The validation breakthrough.* Sydney: McLennan & Petty.

Felce, D., & Perry, J. (1996). Exploring current conceptions of quality of life. In R. Renwick, I. Brown, & M. Nagler (Eds.), *Quality of life in health promotion and rehabilitation: Conceptual approaches, issues, and applications* (pp. 51–62). Thousand Oaks, CA: Sage Publications.

Fiese, B., Tomcho, T., Douglas, M., Josephs, K., Poltrock, S., & Baker, T. (2002). A review of 50 years of research on naturally occurring family routines and rituals: Cause for celebration? *Journal of Family Psychology, 16*(4), 381–390. doi:10.1037/0893-3200.16.4.381 PMID:12561283

Fulcher, G. (1989). Disability: A social construction. In G. Lupton & J. Najman (Eds.), *Sociology of health and illness: Australian readings.* Melbourne: Macmillan.

Gleeson, B. (1995). Disability: A state of mind? *The Australian Journal of Social Issues, 30*(1), 10–23. doi:10.1002/j.1839-4655.1995.tb01023.x

Goode, D. A. (1994). *A world without words: The social construction of children born deaf and blind.* Philadelphia, PA: Temple University Press.

Goode, D. A., & Hogg, J. (1994). Towards an understanding of holistic quality of life in people with profound intellectual and multiple disabilities. In D. Goode (Ed.), *Quality of life for persons with disabilities: International perspectives and issues* (pp. 197–207). Cambridge, MA: Brookline Books.

Gustiatas, R., & Young, E. W. D. (1986). *A time to be born, a time to die: Conflicts and ethics in an intensive care nursery.* Reading, MA: Addison-Wesley.

Haley, W., & Perkins, E. (2004). Current status and future directions in family caregiving and aging people with intellectual disabilities. *Journal of Policy and Practice in Intellectual Disabilities, 1*(1), 24–30. doi:10.1111/j.1741-1130.2004.04004.x

Hatton, C., & Emerson, E. (2003). Families with a person with intellectual disabilities: Stress and impact. *Current Opinion in Psychiatry, 16*(5), 497–501. doi:10.1097/00001504-200309000-00002

Headey, B., & Wearing, A. (1992). *Understanding happiness: A theory of subjective well-being.* Melbourne: Longman Cheshire.

Health Commission of New South Wales. (1981). *Circular 81/8*. Sydney: Health Commission of New South Wales.

Heller, T., Miller, A., & Factor, A. (1997). Adults with mental retardation as supports to their parents: Effects on parental caregiving appraisal. *Mental Retardation*, *35*(5), 338–346. doi:10.1352/0047-6765(1997)035<0338:AWMRAS>2.0.CO;2 PMID:9339062

Hogg, J., Lucchino, R., Wang, K., Janicki, M. P., & Group, W. (2000). *Healthy Ageing: Adults with Intellectual Disabilities: Ageing & Social Policy*. Geneva: World Health Organization.

Hogg, J., & Sebba, J. (1987). Profound retardation and multiple impairment: Vol. 1. *Development and learning*. Rockville, MD: Aspen Publishers.

Keenan, B. (1992). *An evil cradling*. London: Vintage Press.

Keith, K. D., & Bonham, G. S. (2005). The use of quality of life data at the organization and systems level. *Journal of Intellectual Disability Research*, *49*(part 10), 799–805. doi:10.1111/j.1365-2788.2005.00755.x PMID:16162131

Knox, M., & Bigby, C. (2007). Moving towards midlife careas negotiated family business: Accounts of people with intellectual disabilities and their families "Just getting along with their lives together". *International Journal of Disability Development and Education*, *54*(3), 287–304. doi:10.1080/10349120701488749

Koul, R., & Clapsaddle, K. C. (2006). Effects of repeated listening experiences on the perception of synthetic speech by individuals with mild-to-moderate intellectual disabilities. *AAC: Augmentative & Alternative Communication*, *22*, 112–122. PMID:17114169

Kurtz, P. F., Boelter, E. W., Jarmolowicz, D. P., Chin, M. D., & Hagopian, L. P. (2011). An analysis of functional communication training as an empirically supported treatment for problem behavior displayed by individuals with intellectual disabilities. *Research in Developmental Disabilities*, *32*(6), 2935–2942. doi:10.1016/j.ridd.2011.05.009 PMID:21696917

Matson, J. L., Horovitz, M., Kozlowski, A. M., Sipes, M., Worley, J. A., & Shoemaker, M. E. (2011). Person characteristics of individuals in functional assessment research. *Research in Developmental Disabilities*, *32*(2), 621–624. doi:10.1016/j.ridd.2010.12.012 PMID:21211941

McLean, L. K., Brady, N. C., & McLean, J. E. (1996). Reported communication abilities of individuals with severe mental retardation. *American Journal of Mental Retardation*, *100*, 580–589. PMID:8735572

McLean, L. K., Brady, N. C., McLean, J. E., & Behrens, G. A. (1999). Communication forms and functions of children and adults with severe mental retardation in community and institutional settings. *Journal of Speech, Language, and Hearing Research: JSLHR*, *42*(1), 231–240. doi:10.1044/jslhr.4201.231 PMID:10025557

Merrill, E. C., & Mar, H. H. (1987). Differences between mentally retarded and nonretarded persons' efficiency of auditory sentence processing. *American Journal of Mental Deficiency*, *91*, 406–414. PMID:3812610

Murphy, B. (2000). Australian WHOQoL instruments: User's manual and interpretation guide. Melbourne, Australia: Australian WHOQoL Field Study Centre.

Nankervis, K. (1997). *Keynote Address*. Paper presented at the Annual Conference, Australian Society for the Study of Intellectual Disability, Hobart, Australia.

Oliver, M. (1996). *Understanding disability: From theory to practice*. London: Macmillan Press. doi:10.1007/978-1-349-24269-6

Perry, J., & Felce, D. (2005). Factors associated with outcomes in community group homes. *American Journal of Mental Retardation*, *110*(2), 121–135. doi:10.1352/0895-8017(2005)110<121:FAWOIC>2.0.CO;2 PMID:15762822

Sacks, O. (1995). *An anthropologist on Mars*. Sydney: Pan Macmillan Australia.

Schalock, R. L. (Ed.). (1990). *Quality of Life: Perspectives and issues*. Washington, DC: American Association on Mental Retardation.

Schalock, R. L. (1997). The concept of quality of life in 21st century disability programmes. In R. I. Brown (Ed.), *Quality of life for people with disabilities: Models, research and practice* (2nd ed.; pp. 327–340). Cheltenham, UK: Stanley Thornes.

Schalock, R. L. (1999, September). *The application of the concept of quality of life: IASSID Quality of Life Consensus Document: Discussion draft*. Paper presented at the 35th National Conference of the Australian Society for the Study of Intellectual Disabilities, Sydney, Australia.

Schalock, R. L. (2002, June). The concept of quality of life: What we know and do not know. Paper presented at the Inaugural IASSID Europe Quadrennial Conference, University College, Dublin, Ireland.

Schalock, R. L. (2004). Quality of life: What we know and what we don't know. *Journal of Intellectual Disability Research*, *48*(3), 203–216. doi:10.1111/j.1365-2788.2003.00558.x PMID:15025663

Schalock, R. L., Bonham, G. S., & Verdugo, M. A. (2008). The conceptualization and measurement of quality of life: Implications for program planning and evaluation in the field of intellectual disabilities. *Evaluation and Program Planning*, *31*(2), 181–190. doi:10.1016/j.evalprogplan.2008.02.001 PMID:18394704

Schalock, R. L., Gardner, J. F., & Bradley, V. J. (2007). *Quality of life for persons with intellectual and other developmental disabilities: Applications across individuals, organizations, communities, and systems*. Washington, DC: American Association on Intellectual and Developmental Disabilities.

Schalock, R. L., & Verdugo, M. A. (2002). *Handbook on quality of life for human services practitioners*. Washington, DC: American Association on Mental Retardation.

Schalock, R. L., Verdugo, M. A., Bonham, G. S., Fantova, F., & Van Loon, J. S. (2008). Enhancing personal outcomes: Organizational strategies, guidelines, and examples. *Journal of Policy and Practice in Intellectual Disabilities*, *5*(4), 276–285. doi:10.1111/j.1741-1130.2007.00135.x

Smyer, M. A., McHale, S. M., Birkel, R., & Madle, R. A. (1988). Impairments, handicapping environments, and disability: A life-span perspective. In P. S. Van Hasselt, P. S. Dtrain, & M. Herson (Eds.), *Handbook of developmental and physical disabilities* (pp. 9–20). New York: Permagon.

Söderholm, S., Meinander, M., & Alaranta, H. (2001). Augmentative and alternative communication methods in locked-in syndrome. Journal of Rehabilitation Medicine, 33, 235-239.

State of Nebraska Health and Human Services. (2006). *Nebraska developmental disabilities provider profiles*. Lincoln, NE: State of Nebraska Health and Human Services, Division of Developmental Disabilities.

Thompson, R. J., & O'Quinn, A. N. (1979). Developmental disabilities: Etiologies, manifestations, diagnoses, and treatments. New York: Oxford.

Turnbull, A. P., Brown, I., & Turnbull, R. H. (Eds.). (2004). *Families and people with mental retardation and quality of life: International perspectives*. Washington, DC: American Association on Mental Retardation.

Veerman, J. W., & Van Yperen, T. A. (2007). Degrees of freedom and degrees of uncertainty:A developmental model for the establishment of evidence-based youth care. *Evaluation and Program Planning*, *30*(2), 212–221. doi:10.1016/j.evalprogplan.2007.01.011 PMID:17689326

Ward, R. L., Nichols, A. D., & Freedman, R. I. (2010, November). Uncovering Health care Inequalities among adults with intellectual and developmental disabilities. *Health & Social Work*, *35*(4), 280–290. doi:10.1093/hsw/35.4.280 PMID:21171535

Wolfe, P. S. (1992). Challenges for service providers. In P. J. McLaughlin & P. Wejman (Eds.), *Developmental disabilities: A handbook for best practice* (pp. 124–141). Boston: Andover Medical.

Zapf, W., Glatzer, W., Noll, H. H., Habich, R., Berger-Schmitt, R., & Breuer, S. (1987). German social report: Living conditions and subjective well-being, 1978–1984. *Social Indicators Research*, *19*, 1.

Zisberg, A., Young, H., Schepp, K., & Zysberg, L. (2007). A concept analysis of routine: Relevance to nursing. *Journal of Advanced Nursing*, *57*(4), 442–453. doi:10.1111/j.1365-2648.2007.04103.x PMID:17291208

Chapter 8
Assessment and Management of ID in Childhood

Sumita P. Chowhan
Jain University, India

Plabita Patowary
Happiest Minds, India

ABSTRACT

Intellectual disability is a neurodevelopment disorder that affects the intellectual and adaptive functioning. The individual fails to meet standards of personal independence and social responsibility in one or more aspects of daily life, including communication, social participation, academic or occupational functioning, and personal independence at home or in community settings. There is an immense need to understand and be aware of the signs and symptoms of the disorder. This chapter focuses on the process of the assessment which is necessary to identify intellectual deficiency and also the issues that should be taken care of during the process. The various principles and tools of assessment, which can be used to measure IQ, are mentioned. It also focuses on the various challenging behaviors and functional analysis. It also focuses on recent and efficient management strategies that can be used to help the affected person cope and acquire new skills.

INTRODUCTION

ID is characterized by deficits in general mental abilities and these deficits result in impairments of adaptive functioning. The DSM V included the construct of adaptive behaviour in terms of three domains conceptual, social and practical domains. The conceptual (academic) domain involves competence in memory, language, reading, writing, math reasoning etc. The social domain involves awareness of others' thoughts, feelings, and experiences; empathy; interpersonal communication skills while the practical domain involves learning and self-management across life settings, including personal care, job responsibilities, money management, recreation, self- management of behavior, and school and work task organization, among others (DSM V,2013).

DOI: 10.4018/978-1-7998-1223-4.ch008

Intellectual disability shows limitations in two areas. These areas are:

- **Intellectual Functioning:** Refers to as IQ,which means ability to learn, make decisions and solve problems.
- **Adaptive Behaviours:** refers to skills require for day to day life such as being able to communicate effectively, interact with others and take care of oneself.

Signs of Intellectual Disability in Children

There are many different signs of intellectual disability seen during infancy stage, sometimes they may or may not noticeable until school age is reached. It depends on the severity of the problem:

- Delay in rolling over, crawling, siting or walking.
- Delay in speech or having trouble in talking.
- Delay in mastering skills like potty training, dressing, feeding oneself.
- Difficulty remembering things
- Inability to relate actions with consequences
- Behavior problems such as tantrums
- Difficulty in problem–solving or logical thinking.

In children with severe or profound intellectual difficulties, there may be other health issues such as seizures, autism, mood disorders, motor skills impairment, vision and hearing problem.

PSYCHOLOGICAL ASSESSMENT

Psychological assessment in children is a process to evaluate and understand the child's problems in different areas, ones capabilities, strengths and limitations. Four important questions to be answered from assessment are:

- Where is the impairment in the functioning & how is the child functioning impaired
- What are the consequences of the impairment & how it is impacting the normal functioning
- What are the other factors(social, motivational,) that contributing in the maintain of the impairment
- What interventions best suited for the impairment.

The factors complicate the process of assessment with intellectually disable children in obtaining the legitimate estimate of intellectual performance, Presence of severe sensory impairment for example vision, auditory, presence of severe emotional and behavioral disturbance, medication interfere with cognitive neurological functioning. Henceforth it becomes so important that the factors needs to be addressed while assessing for intellectual assessment.

The continuous research on intellectual disability, emphasized that the assessment of intellectual functioning must be evaluated within the context of individual's age and in relation to peer's performance of the same age(Tasseet al., 2011). Assessment also should cater for:

- Accuracy in assessment also relies on cultural and linguistic diversity as well as differences in communication, sensory motor and behavioral factors.
- Assessment should also give a picture of strengths the child possesses.
- Assessment should also list out the problem behavior and desirable behavior(Luckasson et al., 2002, p. 1)

Principles of Assessment

Based on the different intellectual deficient research association, American Psychiatric Association (APA) and the American Association of Mental Retardation (AAMR)the following principles applied to the process of assessment in children with intellectual disability. Initially ruling out psychiatric and non- psychiatric causes for problems of concern, the medical problems (Epilepsy, psychotic illness, vision issues, hearing problem etc.,) and then understanding the problems in expectations and supports and emotional turmoil, the social and emotional problems (parenting issues, social skills deficits etc.,). After ruling out certain aspects as mentioned above, it work towards identifying the problem by seeking information on actual level of functioning in cognitive (intellectual level through assessment tools), adaptive (level of independence in daily activities), including communication for instance, receptive and expressive language issues, and the presence of any comorbidity like ADHD, autism. Lastly but crucial in identifying level of support, the American Association on Intellectual and Developmental Disabilities (AAIDD) emphasized so much on identify levels of support which helps to understand usual level of functioning in areas of: self-care, interest/involvement in school or work, play/leisure activity, social participation, taking initiative in participating in various activities and level of supervision required.

Finally identifying behavioral issues (e.g., self-injurious behavior, stereotypies, obsessive thoughts,

The first step of identification of intellectual disability starts with taking case history, DSM and ICD criteria to assess then is to assess the delay in the milestones. However age range needs to be taken into consideration while screening the development delays in the milestone. During the process of taking the case history of the patient, first the chief complaints has to be noted down followed by the history of the illness. Family, social and developmental history should be also asked. To diagnose the case, MSE and appropriate assessments are also necessary (Ahuja, 2011).

To diagnose the intellectual developmental disorder, according to DSM V, three criteria that must be met are deficits in intellectual functions such as reasoning, problem solving etc, deficits in adaptive functioning which can result in failure to meet developmental and sociocultural standards for personal independence and onset of these deficits should be during the developmental period (DSM V, 2013).

Figure 1. Step wise pattern for identification and management of Intellectual Disability (Based on NIMH Protocol (Madhavan,Kalyan, Naidu.,Pashwarla, & Narayan, 1999)*

Identification/Screening of children with Intellectual Disability (ID):

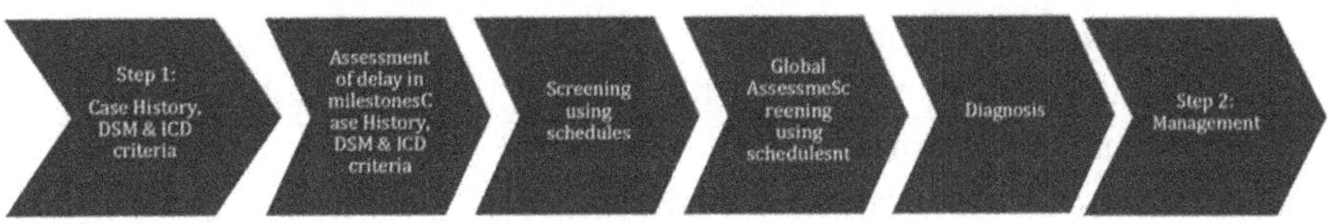

According to ICD, there should be reduced level of intellectual functioning resulting in diminished ability to adapt to demands of the normal social environment and they may have associated physical disorders like epilepsy or psychiatric problems (ICD 10, 1993)

Milestones

Growth and development of children follow a pattern. Universally every child passes through the stages of development/growth. These stages are called milestones of development. These milestones of development helps us to understand whether child have normal development or delayed development. The awareness of developmental milestones is important as it helps to identify children who show delayed development. Some of the normal milestones of development and its appropriate age range applicable to Indian situation are given below. However some discrepancies in attaining milestones is very much common, some children may skip few of the stages.

Several studies showed that there is a normal pattern of the milestones of a child's development. A child can smile at others, can hold head erect and put objects into mouth at 4 months. The child can roll from back to stomach at 6 months while he can stand by holding on to an object and holds objects with thumb and index finger at 10 months. By 18 months, the child can tell his own name and can show body parts when named at 24 months. When the child is 30 months old, he can speak in small sentences. The child can give meaningful verbal answers to simple questions ad differentiate big from small things at 36 months and can combs hair at 48 months. (Madhavan, Kalyan, Naidu.,Pashwarla, & Narayan (1999)

Assessment Tools

Secondly identification is made based on certain questionnaires or assessment schedules by screening out the child. The three schedules given by NIMH (1999), schedule 1for the children below 3 years, second for the children between 3- 6 years of age. The third one is for those children age from 7 and above (NIMH, 1999).

According to the American Association of Mental Retardation (AAMR), the criteria for diagnosis intellectual functioning is to consider both difficulties in intellectual functioning and difficulties in adaptive behavior. The psychological assessment plays a crucial role in diagnosing the presence and severity of mental retardation. To assess intellectual disability it is always essential that more than one assessment tool is used for diagnosing the case rather than using a single one to have a reliable and fair diagnosis. It is also important to have information on the individual's level of functioning including cognitive, adaptive, physical sensations, levels of receptive understanding and expressive language, social involvement (Bradley, Burke, Drummond, Korossy, Lunsky, Morris, 2010).

Important areas of assessment to be considered for diagnosing the children with intellectual disability:

- the developmental milestones, developmental schedules
- Assessment of overall Intellectual Functioning
- Assessment of Adaptive behavior
- Assessment of children's sensory & motor functioning, Language skills
- Assessment of behavioral functioning
- Assessment of children's strengths and weakness.

To develop a profile/case formulation, the importance of understanding the support needed based on the level of intellectual functioning needs to be emphasized, which helps to improve the global functioning of the children (Luckasson et al., 2002, p. 1).

Based on his or her level of language functioning as well as functioning in areas related to language and communication, including hearing,, speech production skills, cognitive level and emotional status, each individual's profile is unique and varied. Intervention considers coexisting strengths and needs in all areas to ensure individualized treatment and supports.

Tools Frequently used in the Area of Intellectual Disability Are Described Below

Weschler Intelligence Scale for Children (WISC): This IQ test is used for the children ages 6-16.This tests consists of various subtests. Overall it measures two areas i.e is verbal skill and performance skill. The verbal tests includes different substests such as Vocabulary, similarities, comprehension, math and informational knowledge. The performance tests include block design, picture completion and arrangement, object assembly and coding. MISIC is the Indian adaptation of Wechsler's Intelligence scale for children was used to assess the IQ of the children which gives scores on Verbal IQ, Performance IQ and full scale IQ. (Kohli, A. 2014)

Weschler Preschool and Primary Scale of Intelligence: The WPPSI test is designed for children aged 2 years 6 months to 7 years 3 months. It can be used to generate multiple sorts of intelligence scores like full IQ score, verbal IQ score, performance IQ score, processing Speed Quotient and general Language Composite The calculation of an IQ score for a child based on their test performance depends on their age. The WPPSI consists of 14 subtests, to be detailed below, with concrete examples. Young children, in the 2 years 6 months through 3 years 11 months age band, are typically administered only five of the subtests: Receptive Vocabulary, Block Design, Information, Object Assembly, Picture Naming. These are the Early Subtests. The other subtests are: Vocabulary, Picture Concepts, symbol search, word reasoning, coding, comprehension, picture completion and similarities . (Goerzel, 2013).

Binet-Kamat Test (BKT): It is a modified version of Stanford Binet Scale measuring intelligence of Indian children. The tasks of the tests are grouped into age levels extending from 3 years to superior adult level. Each age level consists of six tests. BKT include both verbal and performance tests. It is both power and speed test since some of the test items are timed. The test provides an estimate of MA& IQ. (Indian adaptation by Dr.V.V.Kamat, 1958) from 3-22yrs. Pattern analysis of the test items provide estimate of specific cognitive functions as, comprehension, memory, reasoning and other abilities. The test items are scored on an all-or- none basis. The basal age, i.e. the highest age level below which all test items are passed and 'ceiling age' at which all items are failed can be calculated as well as Mental Age (MA) has been calculated by adding partial credits to the basal age for every test passed beyond basal level.(Fathima,M. 2012)

Bayley Scale of Infant Development: These tests are used to assess the development of infants and toddlers ages 1-42 months. This test is also used for older children who are unable to take age appropriate tests. There are three sections: The first section include mental abilities. This includes tests of recognition memory, object permanence, shape discrimination, attention; Nonverbal communication and vocalization receptive and expressive language. The second section is motor abilities. This includes tests of gross and fine motor skills. The third is behavioural abilities. This includes tests of social and emotional behavior.

Developmental Screening Test: The test was developed by Bharath Raj to measure mental development of children from birth to 15 years of age. It consists of 88 items. Larger number of items at early age levels permits assessment of very young children. Italicized items on the schedule cover the speech and language development. Items represent development in various areas like social, behavioral, motor skills etc. in this test, a caretaker have to be present to report their observation regarding the development of the child. This test provides for a brief and fairly dependable assessment without requiring the use of performance tests (J, Bharath Raj; 2004)

Gesell Developmental Schedule: It is a drawing test which measures the "general" factor of intelligence. It helps in assessing the children's motor, adaptive, language and personal-social which helps to assess developmental disabilities, and to some extent intellectual disabilities. The child has to reproduce the geometrical drawings which are analyzed to give the percentile ranks to determine the intellectual functioning of the children (G, Arnold; 2011)

Seguin form Board: This test is based on a single factor theory of intelligence. It is devised by Seguin in 1907. Age group level is 3 to 15 years.It measures speed and accuracy by evaluating a child's eye-hand coordination, visual perception and cognitive ability. The child is asked to keep the ten geometrical shapes in their corresponding respective shapes in the wooden board.(J, Bharath Raj; 1971)

Coloured progressive matrices: It is devised by J. C Raven in the year 1936 which assesses nonverbal abilities. It can be administered at 5 through 11 years. This test consists of 36 items divided into three series (A, Ab, B) each made up of 12 items. The items have the form of incomplete matrices, where the children have to identify the missing part from the available options.

StanfordBinet Intelligence Test: SBIT was developed in 1916 revised bylewis M Terman from the Binet Simon scale and was later re revised in 1937, 1960 and 1986; 2003.it is a standardized test that measures the general intelligence of an individual. It can help to determine the level of intellectual functioning and the cognitive abilities and assist in the diagnosis of developmental delay, mental retardation etc. The test consists of 15 subtests and specific subtests are administered at different age level (2- 90 years). The subtests are grouped into 4 area scores: visual reasoning, verbal reasoning, quantitative reasoning and short term memory. The composite score evaluate the "general" intelligence score. Binetkamath test is the Indian adaptation of StandfordBinet intelligence test. This test consist of both verbal and performance test.

Bender gestalt test: Bender gestalt is developed by Lauretta Bender in the year 1938. It is a brief test of visual motor and perception test which provide information about an individual's development and also assess of any presence of neurological damage. It is suitable for 3 years and older. It has three sub test which are copy and recall test, motor test and perception test. Copying figure requires fine motor skills, the ability to discriminate between visual stimuli, the capacity to integrate visual skills with motor skills.

Benton's Visual Perception Test: It assesses visual perception, memory and visuoconstuctive abilities. This test is developed by Benton AL in 1998. It is used to assess children from 8 years and older. It is composed of 3 sets, or forms, of 10 designs which the individual is required to reproduce. It can be administered in five different ways. This test helps in identifying g any cognitive distortions, possible learning disabilities, dementia, Alzheimer's disease etc.

Gesell's Drawing Test: Gesell and his coworkers (Gesell, 1949) formed this test to assess the ability of the child to imitate or copy various forms like, circle, square, cross etc as an index of maturation as per the age norms. For eg., a 4 year old child can copy a cross. These forms can be usefully employed for a simple and reasonable accurate assessment of intelligence. These type of tasks are also included in BKT, Stanford binet test etc

Tests of Adaptive Functioning and Behavioural Functioning

Tests of adaptive functioning assess the social and emotional maturity of a child relative to his peers. They also help to evaluate life skills and abilities.

Vineland Social Maturity Scale: The Vineland social maturity scale consist of 89 items which assess social maturity and personal and social skills of an individual. It also helps in identifying the social deficits and assets which is good to locate the intellectual functioning of a growing child. It serves the purpose well as most of the clinical procedures of assessment and training are most often limited to the upper age limits of 15 years. It has 8 subscales which measure different skills in: general self-help ability, communication, locomotion, self-dressing abilities, self-eating abilities and socialization. It was originally devised by E.A Doll in 1935 and its Indian adapted version is devised by J Bharath Raj. This test is being used in many parts of the world and it proved itself to be uniquely useful instrument in measuring social maturity of children and young adults.

Vineland adaptive behavior Scale: This test measures the social skills of people from birth to 19 years of age. The test contains four sections These are communication; daily living skills; socialization; and motor skills. This test is not administered on children but it is given to primary caregivers and other familiar with child. This test is also used for children with behavioural disorders. (Early childhood measurement and evaluation, 2012).

Problem Behavior Checklist: Children's behavior checklist is used to detect emotional and behavioral problems in children and adolescents. Information is gathered from parents or the primary care taker. It is to be used with children aged 6 to 18 years. It consists of 113 questions, scored on a three point likert scale (0= absent, 1= occurs sometimes, 2= occurs often). The responses should be based on the past 6 months experiences. It has eight syndrome scales: Anxious, Depressed, Somatic complaints, Social problems, thought problems, Attention problems, Aggressive behavior, and Rule breaking behaviour. For identifying psychopathology in children and adolescents with mental retardation, The Aberrant Behaviour Checklist, a screening assessment tool is used widely (Achenbach&Rescorla, 2000).

As there are numerous tests which can assess IQ, selection of these tests should be proper, specially if the person has co morbid issues. There are specific different guidelines and adaptive measures of ID, which must be strictly adhered to.

Table 1.

Tests used in case of intellectual disability and other physical comorbid conditions			
Types of disability	Tests used for		
	Screening	Adaptive behavior	Global intelligence scale
Intellectual disability (ID)	DST	VSMS	BKT
ID and visual impairment	DST	VSMS	BKT; Prorate the IQ based on MISIC verbal scales
ID and hearing impairment	GDT and SFBT	VSMS	Prorate the IQ based on MISIC performance scales. BKT is not suitable because of high loading of verbal and language items
ID and cerebral palsy	DST and GDT	VSMS	BKT; profile analysis will help identify specific effect of motor deficits on test performance. prorate the IQ based on MISIC verbal scales.

Source: Kishore MT et. al. Clinical practice guidelines for assessment and management of intellectual disability.Indian Journal of Psychiatry (vol. 61, 2019). DST- developmental screening test; GDT- gesell's drawing test; VSMS- vineland social maturity scale, SFBT-seguin form board test, BKT-binet kamath test, MISIC- malin's intelligence scale for Indian children.

Intellectual assessment needs to be carried out using the age and culture appropriate instrument. The following tests are used based on levels of severity manifested in DSM V, ICD 10, screening tools of NIMH. The aforementioned tools would be administered based on levels of severity as indicated by screening tools, the diagnostic tools helps to understand the precise levels of functioning .The following diagnostic tools as shown in Table 2 would be selected based on age, education, culture, understanding of language and behavioral problems the child manifested. The Instruments helps to have a precise quotient of development (DQ), Intelligence (IQ), performance (PQ) social (SQ) and also the other sensation & motor issues and behavioral problems.

Global Assessment

Traditionally it was observed that only intellectual functioning is given importance. According to different diagnostic systems of classification, Mental retardation is defined as significantly subnormal intellectual ability that leads to deficits in functioning (DSM III, APA 1993). Later the construct of adaptive functioning is considered crucial. Recently the assessments not only look at intellectual deficit but also adaptive functioning and behavioral issues like appropriate & inappropriate behaviors are assessed in order to plan appropriate behavior modification programme. In recent trends the Global developmental delay concept has become crucial which refers to those children below 5 years who do not meet expected developmental milestone in several areas of intellectual functioning (Reynolds, Zupanick, Dombeck, 2013). In the recent trends the assessment on desirable behaviors is also emphasized to concentrate on motivations levels of children with intellectual disability.

Measuring Adaptive Functions

The Intellectual disability encompasses impairments of general mental abilities which in turn impact adaptive functioning. The impairment in adaptive functioning seem to in three domains, or areas. These domains determine includes different day to day tasks and how well an individual copes with those daily tasks

- The conceptual domain denotes skills related to language, reading, writing, reasoning, solving-maths problems, and Learning &memory, the ability to learn and remember.
- The social domain denotes interpersonal communication skills, the interpersonal ability the making and retaining friends, empathy, understanding others and social judgment.
- The practical domain refers to self-management in areas such as personal care, home activities money management, recreation, and consolidating school and work tasks and completingjob responsibilities. (DSM V, 2013)

The assessment and diagnosis to be made with respect to one's education, appropriate behavior and environmental factors. Before diagnosing the case with mental retardation understanding the socio economic status and cultural criteria and environmental conditions of the children plays an important role. Therefore these aspects to be considered with caution for diagnosis the case with intellectual disability.

DSM V (2013) has classified the adaptive characteristics of intellectually disabled individuals based on the level of severity. The three domains that each level of severity is discussed are: conceptual, social and practical domain. In mild severity level, conceptually, differences are found in school children and adults related to learning skills with support needed in one or more areas to meet age related expectation.

Executive functioning as well as STM is also impaired. In social domain, communication and language are more concrete or immature than expected for age. Individuals experience difficulties regulating emotions and behavior in age appropriate fashion. In practical domain, some individual may able to take responsibility of their own personal care even though they need support. Individual need support to perform a skilled vocation competently and to raise a family. In moderate level, conceptually, language and pre academic skills develop slowly. In social domain, individuals may not perceive or interpret social cues accurately. Social judgments are limited. In practical domain, extended period of training is required to make the individual learn to eat, dress, hygiene etc. in the severe level, little understanding is present of written language or of concepts involving numbers under conceptual domain. Socially and practically, spoken language is quite limited and speech comprises of single words or phrases and also requires support for daily living activities. Likewise, in the profound level, presence of motor and sen-

Table 2. Age wise classification of characteristics of Adaptive functioning in children with intellectually disability

Severity	Mild	Moderate	Severe	Profound
Pre school (3-19 years)	Characteristics are not overt from those normal people until late age, very minimal retardation	Communication and motor development are intact. Slight difficulties are observed in social	Difficulty in self- help behavior and motor development. The individual also	Needs help of caretaker in doing most of the tasks including activities of daily life.
	in sensory-motor areas.	awareness and executing day to day tasks for living but it can be developed and rectified if proper training is provided.	suffers from speech distortion and distorted communicative skills. Training does not provide a huge difference.	Distorted functioning in sensory motor areas is observed.
School age (6-20 years)	Appropriate social skills can be learned if training is provided and academic skills can be also acquired at least till 6th grade.	If proper training is provided to the individual, then appropriate social and occupational skills can be learned. Academic skills can be learned till 2nd grade. Child can also learn to travel	Child can acquire the skills to communicate and can be trained in elementary skills.	Very limited self- help skills are acquired.
		to the familiar nearby places alone. For example: to a nearby shop or park.		
Adult (21	Individual can	Self-help behavior	Self-help behavior	Motor and speech
and over)	achieve social and	can acquire properly	and self-help	development can be
	vocational skills in	after training is	protection skills	achieved. Self care
	adequate manner.	provided. Guidance	can be learned to a	needs can be
	Assistance is needed	is required when the	limited level in	achieved to a very
	when under social	individual is under	assisted	limited level.
	and economic stress.	mild social and economic stress.	environment.	

* Source DSM V, 2013

sory impairments can prevent functional use of objects in the conceptual level. In social and practical domain, individual experience limited understanding of symbolic communication and gestures. He is dependent on others for all aspects in day to day activities.

Based on the different research, Both the American Psychiatric Association (APA) and the American Association on Intellectual and Developmental Disabilities (AAIDD) practice use of severity codes as shown in table 4. These codes are used for diagnosis the case and categorizing intellectual disabilities into four levels mild, moderate, severe, profound. However, the meanings of the severity codes among two systems are seen differently. Previously APA used IQ scores to define severity. Recently these systems started concentrating on adaptive functioning to determine severity. However, the APA severity is based on categorizing levels of severity based on IQ and Adaptive functioning. In contrast, the AAIDD is based on the degree of support needed. This is called support intensity. The level of severity is assessed by the level of cognitive/intellectual functioning and the amount of support needed. The level of intellectual functioning is characterized by scores of approximately two standard deviations below the mean. The four levels of severity mild, moderate, severe and profound are classified as follows based on Intellectual functioning, support needed and mental age (Reynolds, Zupanick, Dombeck, 2013)

The recent trends follow the global functioning assessment process where in the developmental quotient (DQ), Intelligence quotient (IQ), performance quotient (PQ), social quotient (SQ), adaptive functioning) and also other sensory& motors kills, language& communication and also behavioral issues are assessed, both inappropriate and desirable behaviors are assessed to diagnose the case and to schedule the management plan (NIMH, 1990).

ISSUES IN ASSESSMENTS

Psychological assessment also should be viewed as sources of information and not as the endpoint of assessment. Different sources that can provide information which complements the psychological assessment process are: Clinical interview with the child, family and teacher, clinical & behavior observation of the child, school reports. Hence all the other sources of information needs to be considered rather than solely depending on psychological assessment especially when applies to children.

Since the child is in the developmental process, one should be extremely careful while interpreting the results. The examiner needs to be cautious and compassionate when analyzing and giving feedback to the parents. The examiner needs to be flexible in clinical analysis. For e.g., if the child is very shy and

Table 3. Different functioning and support needed in children with ID

Severity Level	Intellectual Functioning	Mental age	Support needed	Educational Functioning
Mild	55-69	8 -11 years	Intermittent (as needed basis)	Educable
Moderate	40-54	4-7 years	Limited(time limited training)	Trainable
Severe	25-39	2-3years	Extensive (long term home living support)	Trainable to self help
Profound	Below 20	2 years	Pervasive (life sustaining support)	Custodial

* Sources DSM, AAIDD

non- compliant then special procedures of psychological assessment should be used. There are several factors that can affect the child's performance in assessment.

- Child's ability to communicate
- Problems in comprehending the instructions
- Child's physical and mental health problems
- Low motivation levels
- Anxieties about being tested
- Difficulty level of the test items
- The rapport between the child and the examiner.
- Individual differences
- Latent possession of skills.

Enhance to the aforementioned points, the important point to be considered is the limitations of the test. Firstly, since it was always observed that the child performance can vary at different points, drawing conclusion solely based on testing can further complicate matters for the child.Secondly if assessments are used routinely, the significance of information is lost. Thirdly, the problem may not be based on test findings but on many factors in the child environment (Hirisave, Oommen, kapur 2002)

Hence the assessment results should not be taken as sole point of assessment but the alternative clinical information should be considered as a way of complementing the information obtained from other sources like by clinical interviews with the child and parents, and by naturalistic observation.

There are several problems observed specific to the assessment of children with intellectual disability such as

- The intellectual disability children have several motor and sensory impairment such as loss of vision, hearing impairment, and deficit in fine and gross motor functioning can leads to misinterpretation of results.
- Problems in expressive and receptive language because of which comprehending the instruction would become difficult and can also give rise to low score results.
- Cognitive problems like low attention and concentration and high distractibility hence shown difficulty in assessment
- Behavioral problem like hyperactivity, aggressive behavior and withdrawal, lack of motivation would cause difficulty in standardized psychological assessment.
- Social problem like shyness, scared to meet new people can also show discrepancies in assessment results.
- Even influence of socio-economic status, education, cultural issues influence the assessment of children with intellectual, these constructs should be taken as caution while diagnosis the case.

Hence forth it is always recommended to use more than one assessment tool and building up rapport is very crucial when assessing children with intellectual disability (Madhavan, Kalyan, Naidu.,Pashwarla, & Narayan (1999)

In addition to deficit in intellectual ability and adaptive behavior, some intellectual disabilities have medical problems or associated handicaps. Some of the most common medical problems encountered in the intellectual disability are epilepsy, hyperkinesis, physical handicap, nutritional disorders and psychiatric problems such as autism, psychosis and neurotic disturbances:

Epilepsy: About 40% of intellectual disabilities have convulsions of one type or other(Madhavan, Kalyan, Naidu.,Pashwarla, & Narayan (1999)

Conditions mistaken for Intellectual disabilities

1. Early infantile autism
2. Child with hearing impairment
3. Child with emotional disturbances
4. Cultural deprivation and lack of stimulation
5. Specific learning disabilities
6. Childhood psychosis
7. Child with visual handicap
8. Child with physical handicap

It is difficult to identify the intensity of each of the handicaps in a multiply handicapped person. It is also difficult to determine the ways in which the combinations of disabilities affect a person's behavior. Accurate assessment of the various handicaps is necessary in such children before a management plan is drawn out for them.

A NOTE ON THE ASSESSMENT TOOL USED

Children with special need have selective motivation and attention towards tasks that they involved with deem desirable and enjoy able task and it is contextual too. Other tasks that don't fit that given descriptions yield low levels of motivation, low levels of attention, fatigability and lead to greater chances of an aggressive-explosive episode. It is the role of the individual assessing the child to keep such factors under control but at times it could also be due to the inherent nature of the tool used.

In the light of the above information it becomes important that the tools and materials used for the assessment be appealing, attractive and inviting to the child to ensure optimal performance. This can be ensured by turning each of the sub tests into a series of games that the child deems as fun and rewarding. Some of the sub-tests in the battery like the block design test, picture completion test, the visual motor free test and the colour cancellation test were those that the children enjoyed performing. The use of colors and animated figures in a way that doesn't compromise on the nature of the test would help yield better performance. It is a known fact that children with special needs show high levels of motivation and low levels of distraction when performing tasks on the touch screen, which means having assessment tools with software application format in turn could result in optimal performance of the child in during the course of the assessment (Sharma &Chowhan, 2014)

INTERVENTION/MANAGEMENT PLAN

The management plan of the child depends on the severity levels of intellectual disability (mild, moderate, severity and profound) and their adaptive functioning and also associated conditions sensory handicaps such as vision, hearing, epilepsy, hyper kinesis, autism and inappropriate behavioral problems and desirable behaviors they exhibit. Based on the level of severity and associated conditions the management plan varies from infant stimulation, training in daily living skills and functional academics to prevocational and vocational skills. Apart from this the help is needed in speech problems, locomotion, management of problematic behavior and management of medical problem.

Research supports the provision of communication intervention to be very effective for individuals with ID (Sevcik & Romski, 2016; Snell et al., 2010). As indicated by a persons level of life functioning will improve if appropriate personalized supports are provided over a sustained period (The AAIDD (2013). The goal of communication Intervention treatment is to minimize the potential incapacitating effects of disabilities of both clients and their families and to maximize the probability of desirable outcomes.

The review of research describes the overview of behaviors commonly problematic in children population are sleep disturbances, agitated and aggressive behaviours, and self-injury behaviour. The general concepts which commonly applied to deal with the management of behaviour disorders seen in children and youth with an intellectual disability are seen as pharmacological form of treatment, however behavioral intervention is a more effective and better endured form of treatment, where the effect lasting longer (Ageranioti – Belanger, Brunet, D'Anjou and Gauthier, 2012). Similarly the results of the meta- analysis suggested that several risk markers could be identified for particular forms of challenging behaviour. Self-injury and stereotypy behaviour appeared to be more common amongst subjects with a severe/profound degree of ID. Self-injury behaviour (SIB) has been defined as a response that produces physical injury to the individual's own body. In children, it is most commonly reported in association with an ID (reported at rates ranging from 7% to 22%) (Berkson,.et. al, 2001). Mcclintock, Hall& Oliver (2003) propound that boys were considerably more likely to show aggression than girls. They also found that those with severe/profound degree of ID more likely to show self-injury and stereotypy behaviour than one with a mild/moderate degree of ID.

Regarding the intervention of challenging behavior, the recording of direct observations and baseline data about the frequency and duration of the behavior becomes crucial. Based on eventual context, the observed behaviour can be recorded on an ABC chart for subsequent analysis of the antecedents (A), behaviour (B) and associated consequences (C). In addition, questionnaires and rating scales may also be considered to gather information about the possible drive of the behaviour. Ideally, the formulation should lead to an intervention or a further period of assessment and analysis, including manipulation of the antecedents or consequences (Hanley et al 2003). Any interventions that are implemented will need to be evaluated for effectiveness and modified if necessary. Carr (1999) indicate that the meta-analysis has shown the importance of functional analysis in achieving a positive outcome of behavioural interventions for people with intellectual disability (Carr 1999).

The process involved in carrying out a functional analysis as indicated by Carr(1999) as follows

- To acquire a clear description of the behaviour
- To identify drives or factors that predict the occurrence of behaviour, will or will not occur
- To identify the drives or factors or consequences that maintain the behaviour
- To develop a hypothesis about the function of the behaviour
- To mark a direct observations that provide evidence supporting the hypothesis (O'Neill 1997)

Once the current level of functioning in all areas is obtained based on the level and severity of functioning the appropriated individualized management plan to be scheduled and executed. The systematic training and counseling session should to be planned to have structured programme to help children with intellectual disability to overcome their problems. Interventions for children and adolescents with ID focus primarily on either behavioral/ emotional issues or educational issues. To address problem behaviors, several techniques/programs are available across the developmental spectrum such as behavior chaining, secondary rewards, token economies (Handen, 1998).

Management Plan follows following steps:

- Systematic training of skills which they are lacking in.
- Behavior modification/Behaviour intervention
- Occupational training
- Parental Counseling

Systematic Skills Training

The training follows systematic procedure of task analysis, the skills should be divided into small, sequential steps. The training activity should be divided into small steps. The process of breaking down the skills into small steps is called task analysis. The child is given repeated training in each activity. The training follows systematic approach with regularity. Each component should be clearly titled so that persons using them have clear idea of how to use it. There must be no ambiguity in the components. Even systematic record keeping method and regular follow-up are important factors for an intervention programme to be successful. Strict guidelines for maintaining record is followed to ensure accuracy and uniformity in recording.(Madhavan, Kalyan, Naidu.,Pashwarla, & Narayan (1999)

Behavior Modification/Behavior Intervention

Behaviour Modification is the programme implemented to correct impairment in adaptive behavior. The problem exhibited in the children with intellectual disability as assessed by adaptive behavior checklist is divided broadly into two areas adaptive behavior (delay in motor development, self-help skills (NIMH, 1999) and secondly problem behaviors (tantrums, aggression, beating head bagging etc., (Ageranioti-Bélanger, Brunet, D'Anjou, Boivin,2012). The impairment in adaptive behavior would be in behavior deficit and behavior excess. The first choice of behavioral modification is the selection of reinforcement and extinction-based strategies. For children with behavior deficits the different positive schedules of reinforcement work very well. For behavior excess/inappropriate behaviour, the negative schedules of reinforcement and punishment needs to be executed to correct the behavior pattern.

Behavioral intervention programs have been very successful in targeting and altering problematic social, emotional, and behavioral concerns. The success of the behavioral programs can be associated with the mechanisms of program like focus on breaking down problem behaviors into component parts (simplicity) and to systematically shaping behaviors into more socially adaptive skills through contingency programs of management.(Mather &Goldstein(2015)

Children with intellectual disabilities shows deficits in self-help skills like inability to eat, speech deficit, unable to attend to bowel and bladder needs, inability to have eye-eye contact. These are called bevioural deficit. Children with intellectual disability shows excessive aggression, temper tantrums, mood swings. These are called behavioral excess. To develop effective functioning the deficits and excess needs to corrected or learnt through proper training.

Behavior modification works on the use of basic learning techniques, such as conditioning, positive and negative reinforcement, or aversion therapy, to teach simple skills or alter undesirable and problem behavior. Behavior modification is used to alter the impairment in adaptive behavior. It works on altering absence of adaptive behavior (self-help skills, language delay, and motor skill) and the presence of undesirable behavior (head bagging, beating, showing aggression).

According to (Madhavan, Kalyan, Naidu., Pashwarla, & Narayan (1999)in India, five major steps executed to alter undesirable problem and deficit behavior are identification of the problem, defining target behavior, behavior recording, functional analysis and treatment. They are implemented to correct the impairments in the adaptive behaviour. There are five major steps:

1. Identification of the problems, the first task of the therapist is to obtain the list of problem behaviour by using a behaviour check list or through observations.
2. Defining target behaviours, based on the severity of the problem, selecting targets behaviour. The behaviours to be modified first are called target behaviours. Target one task at a time by having clear treatment plan.
3. Behaviour recording, recording of target behaviours should be done on the basis of frequency, duration and time interval. Maintaining behaviour records is essential as well as evaluating the effectiveness of ongoing therapy.
4. Functional analysis, is a strategy for the assessment and treatment of behaviour problem. Specifically, functional analysis is a set of procedures that attempts to identify important contextual variables such as history and environment that help to cause and/or maintain problematic behaviours or the interaction between behaviour-environment. The goal of functional analysis is to effectively identify targets of intervention that are alterable such that appropriate treatments may be rapidly implemented and evaluated through concentrated intervention efforts.
5. Treatment procedures, techniques used for decreasing Inappropriate behavior

According to Reynolds, Zupanick,&Dombeck, (2013), there are various strategies that can be used as effective tool for intellectual deficit children which are:

1. One strategy is to break down one task into various small steps. Each sub task is introduced at a time. Once that sub test is mastered then the next step is introduced.
2. A second strategy is to modify the teaching approach. Instead of lengthy verbal directions, it can-teached by providing them performance task as the children learn more when the information is concrete and observed.
3. Thirdly, visual aids can be used to enhance the learning process. The children with ID understand better of what is expected of them with the help of charts, drawings etc.
4. The fourth strategy is to provide direct and immediate feedback. Individuals with ID require immediate feedback. This enables them to make a connection between their behavior and the teacher's response.

Behaviour Modification Techniques for Treating Undesirable /Inappropriate Behaviour (Carr, 2004)

- **Changing the Surroundings:** Challenging behavior can be diminished by altering the person's circumstances to make it less likely that the behavior will occur. For example: if a child cannot tolerate noisy public places, some soothing music can be provided to him and let him listen to the music in headphones.

- **Restructuring the Environment:** The occurrence of any behaviour is partly due to present or past antecedents. This is calls stimulus control. Eg. Child talking in class. Decreasing the behaviour by placing a screen around him
- **Extinction:** When behavior is followed by a reinforcer, it is strengthened or maintained. Without reinforcement, the behavior can eventually die out (extinguished). Initially, it can result in "extinction burst". When the person finds that the expected reinforcement is not coming, then he repeats the behavior number of time, expecting the occurrence of behavior. If the reinforcement is sternly withheld, no matter how repeatedly the behavior occurs, then the particular behavior lessens, slowly and gradually.
- **Punishment:** Consequences for a behaviour that reduces the future possibility of that behaviour. Common types of punishment are,
  - **Time-Out:** This means time-out from positive reinforcements. Mostly applied when behaviour are hazardous or self-injurious. Eg- the parents physically restrain the child when he/she beats others or punish by depriving him of positive reinforcements.
  - **Response Cost:** When undesirable behaviour occurs, a fixed numbers of tokens, stars or points are deducted from what the individual has already earned.
- **Time Out from Positive Reinforcement**: Time out from positive reinforcement is an option where the problem behavior happens when the person is already is in a reinforcing situation. Whenever the behavior occurs, the reinforcement is temporarily ceased. For example, earlier the child used to stay in her room alone aloof, without enjoying, so reinforcement is given every time she comes out of the room to play, interact and watch TV. But if the child started watching television excessively, a time out (for 5- 10 minutes) can be given when her favorite song or music appears in the TV.
- **Functional Communication Training:** Some children show problematic behavior which can be goal directed. It can be seen in them to gain attention or some tangible objects. These children can be taught the appropriate sign or the way to ask things and to express themselves. For example, if they want attention from the teacher to show their drawing, they can be trained to say "come here please" instead of exhibiting problematic behavior.
- **Stimulus Control:** Specific stimuli lead to specific associated response and this condition can be used to manage certain behavior. For example: a child has a habit of asking questions to his parents continuously and throw temper tantrums if not answered which create stress among the family. A sticker has been shown to the child and later the child has been trained not to ask questions until the sticker is not sticked to his shirt. Initially the sticker has been removed three times in one hour which gradually increased. It helped the child to be calm and wait for the appropriate time to ask questions.

Behaviour Modification Techniques for Increasing Appropriate Behavior (Madhavan, Kalyan, Naidu.,Pashwarla, & Narayan (1999):

By using reinforcement techniques, the desirable appropriate behaviors are encouraged. Reinforcement is defined as a consequence that strengthens ones future behaviour and also frequency of occurrence of behavior.

- **Token Programme:** A token economy rewards good behavior with tokens that can be exchanged for something desired.
- **Shaping:** Refers to gradually moulding or training an organism to perform a specific response (behavior) by reinforcing any responses that are similar to the desired response.
- **Prompting:** Initially physically guided, to understand the desirable behaviour and then this is reinforced. It is effectively used in teaching self -help skills.
- **Cueing:** Gestural cues, visual cues are given and prompting is effectively used in language training.
- **Fading Programmes:** When the reinforcement techniques are achieved, it shouldn't end abruptly as child gets dependent which could worsen the case. So it could be stopped with irregular intervals. It can make the child less dependable on the reinforcement.
- Altering the environment and graded change
- Chaining the task is broken into a number of small steps and each steps is taught to the child. Forward chaining and backward chaining. It was observed that backward chaining is found to be creating wonders in training children with ID.
- Steps in implementing reinforcement programme
    - Specify the goal. Eg. the child will look at the therapist's face and have eye to eye contact when the therapist calls his name and talks to him
    - Identify the reinforcer; Four important aspects should be followed while presenting a reinforcement:
        - Contingency
        - Immediacy
        - Consistency
        - Clarity
    - Teach the behaviour. Eg. When the child looks at the therapist even for some few seconds while the therapist is talking give the child a chocolate.
    - Fade out the reinforcement- e.g. Once the child learns to look more and more steadily into the therapist's eyes gradually fade out the edible reinforcer and use praise as rein forcers.

According to AAIDD (2013), a persons level of life functioning will improve if appropriate customized (as needed) supports are provided over a specific period till they learn the skills. The goal of treatment is to minimize the potential debilitating effects of disabilities on clients and their families and to maximize the likelihood of desirable outcomes.

There are many studies that assessing different modes of therapy and its efficiency on managing intellectual disabilities. Dialectical behavioral therapy can be very efficient in managing the challenging behavior of ID. DBT is a type of therapy the integrates the elements of CBT, ABA and strategies to address borad, lifelong regulatory deficits as it includes mindfulness, dialectical strategies, suicide protocol and offers a coping skills group (linehan, 1993) The treatment blends acceptance strategies (validation) and change strategies (e.g., behavioral strategies such as positive reinforcement, contingency management, and exposure) to simultaneously treat self- invalidation and reinforced patterns of escalating emotions, which are underlying factors associated with challenging behaviors . The adaptive Skills System is a altered emotion regulation skills curriculum designed for individuals with IDD (Brown, 2011)

Occupational Therapy (OT)

Occupational therapy work towards therapeutic practice of caring one self, ability to earn by doing some work, and entertainment activities to increase independent function, augment development, and prevent disability. Occupational therapy usually works towards accommodating any task or environment to achieve optimum independence and quality of life. Occupational Therapy includes assessment and treatment tasks to uphold the daily living and work skills of people with disability. These tasks can include grooming, bathing, toileting, dressing, eating, socializing, communicating, mobility, and sexual expression. Treatment begins by addressing the most basic self-care activities. Occupational therapy interventions focus on helping the client to adapt the environment, modify the task required through task analysis and by teaching the skill, and educating the client/family to increase participation in daily activities and performance of work activities among clients. (Hopkins and smith 1993 pp.04)

Parent Counselling

Initially, to impart the correct information of child with ID by being very professional and kind. The therapist should not hide anything. The counselling should help the parents to develop right attitude towards their child with ID, it happens that the parents either become overprotective or aggressive hence helping parents to develop right attitude is very crucial. The parents who accept the child's condition become overprotective and the parents who do not accept the child's condition become very critical.

Finally, to create awareness to parents regarding their in training the child to become self-reliant(. The major agenda and benefits of parental counselling in the present study are:

1. To provide psych education and awareness to the parents on mild level of intellectual disabilities in order help them better understand the problems of the child and provide appropriate assistance to them.
2. To provide support to the parents to deal with their emotional problems like frustrations, anxieties and hostilities so that they are better equipped to provide support to the child with Intellectual disability.

CONCLUSION

This chapter emphasized on the immense need to understand the signs and symptoms of the disorder. The chapter focuses on the detailed process of assessment to identify signs and symptoms of intellectual difficulties. The detailed assessment includes various assessment tools and different morbidity of disorders and also the issues related to be taken care of during the process. The chapter helps to understand the various levels of difficulties and the efficient management strategies to minimise the potential incapacitating effects of disabilities on clients and to maximise the likelihood of desirable outcomes. The chapter also discussions on challenging behaviour and its functional analysis and different management strategies and behavioural modification techniques.

REFERENCES

Achenbach, T. M., & Rescorla, L. A. (2000). *Manual for the ASEBA Preschool Forms & Profiles*. Burlington, VT: University of Vermont, Research Center for Children, Youth, & Families.

Ageranioti-Bélanger, S., Brunet, S., D'Anjou, G., Tellier, G., Boivin, J., & Gauthier, M. (2012). Behaviour disorders in children with an intellectual disability. *Paediatrics & Child Health, 17*(2), 84–88. doi:10.1093/pch/17.2.84 PMID:23372399

Ahuja, N. (2011). *A Short Textbook of Psychiatry.VII 01*. JP Brothers. doi:10.5005/jp/books/11464

American Association on Intellectual and Developmental Disabilities. (2011). *What is the AAIDD definition of intellectual disability?* Retrieved from http://www.aaidd.org/IntellectualDisabilityBook/content_7473.cfm?navID=366

American Association on Intellectual and Developmental Disabilities. (2013). *Definition of intellectual disability*. Retrieved from www.aaidd.org

American Psychiatric Association. (2013). *Diagnostic and statistical manual of mental disorders* (5th ed.). Washington, DC: Author.

Berkson, G., Tupa, M., & Sherman, L. (2001). Early development of stereotyped and self-injurious behaviors: Incidence. *American Journal of Mental Retardation, 106*(6), 539–547. doi:10.1352/0895-8017(2001)106<0539:EDOSAS>2.0.CO;2 PMID:11708939

Bharath Raj, J. (1971). AHSH Norms on seguin form board with Indian Children. *J. of AHSH, II*, 34–39.

Bharath Raj, J. (2004). *The developmental screening test manual.4th rd.* Mysore: SwayamsiddhaPrakashana.

Bradley, E., Burke, L., Drummond, C., Korossy, M., Lunsky, Y., & Morris, S. (2010). *Guidelines for managing the patient with developmental disability in the emergency room*. Retrieved fromwww.camh.net/Publications/Resources_for_Professionals/guidelines_manageclient_emerg2 003.pdf

Brown, J. (2011). The Skills System instructor's guide: An emotion regulation skills curriculum for all learning abilities. Bloomington, IN: IUniverse.

Carr, E. G., Horner, R. H., & Turnbull, A. P. (1999). *Positive Behavior Support for People with Developmental Disabilities: A Research Synthesis*. American Association on Mental Retardation.

Carr, J. (2004). *Understanding intellectual disability and health*. Retrieved from http://www.intellectualdisability.info/mental-health/behaviour-management

Dhanesh, K. G., & Karthikeyan, S. (2012). *Gender difference in level of intelligence and social quotient among children with autism spectrum disorders*. International Journal of Scientific and Research Publications.

Disability Information. (2013). *Department of communities and social inclusion*. Government of South Australia.

Dumont, M., & Beaulieu, C. (2007). Light exposure in the natural environment: Relevance to mood and sleep disorders. *Sleep Medicine, 8*(6), 557–565. doi:10.1016/j.sleep.2006.11.008 PMID:17383230

Fatima, M. (2012). *The effectiveness of computer –assisted exercise on certain cognitive variables among dyslexic children.* Retrieved from www.sodhgangainflibnet.ac.in

Goertzel, B. (2013). *The Wechsler Preschool and Primary Scale of Intelligence (WPPSI): A Brief Overview.* Retrieved from: http://goertzel.org/Preschool_IQ_Test_Overview.pdf

Hall, S., Oliver, C., & Murphy, G. (2001). Early development of self-injurious behavior: An empirical study. *American Journal of Mental Retardation, 106*(2), 189–199. doi:10.1352/0895-8017(2001)106<0189:EDOSIB>2.0.CO;2 PMID:11321609

Handen, B. L., & Gilchrist, R. (2006). Practitioner review: Psychopharmacology in children and adolescents with mental retardation. *Journal of Child Psychology and Psychiatry, and Allied Disciplines, 47*(9), 871–882. doi:10.1111/j.1469-7610.2006.01588.x PMID:16930381

Hanley, G. P., Iwata, B. A., & McCord, B. E. (2003). Functional analysis of problem behavior: A review. *Journal of Applied Behavior Analysis, 36*(2), 147–185. doi:10.1901/jaba.2003.36-147 PMID:12858983

Heather, S. (2013). Fighting the stigma caused by mental disorders: past perspectives, present activities, and future directions. World Psychiatric Association.

Hirisave, U., Oommen, A., & Kapur, M. (2002). Psychological assessment of children in the clinicalsetting - Introduction. In Psychological assessment of children in the clinical setting (pp. 1-5) Bangalore: NIMHANS.

Hopkins, H. L., & Smith, H. D. (1993). *Willard and Spackman's Occupational Therapy* (8th ed.). Philadelphia: J.B. Lippincott. Retrieved from http://www.sgh.org.sa/Portals/0/Articles/International%20Handbook%20of%20Occupational%20Thera py%20Interventions.pdf

Jan, J.E., Owens, J.A., Weiss, M.D., Johnson, K.P., Wasdell, M.B., & Freeman, R.D. (2008). Sleep hygiene for children with neurodevelopmental disabilities. *Ipsiroglu O.S Pediatrics, 122*(6), 1343-50.

Kahng, S., Iwata, B. A., & Lewin, A. B. (2002). Behavioral treatment of self-injury, 1964 to 2000. *American Journal of Mental Retardation, 107*(3), 212–221. doi:10.1352/0895-8017(2002)107<0212:BTOSIT>2.0.CO;2 PMID:11966334

Kishore, M. T., Nizamie, A., Nizamie, S. H., & Jahan, M. (2004). Psychiatric diagnosis in persons with intellectual disability in India. *Journal of Intellectual Disability Research, 48*(1), 19–24. doi:10.1111/j.1365-2788.2004.00579.x PMID:14675227

Kohli, A., Mahotra, S., & Kehra, N. (2014). Neuropsychological Profile of Children with Hyperkinetic Disorder. Journal. *Indian Association Child Adolescent Mental Health, 10*(3), 167–193.

Krutchzer, S., Deluca, J., & Caplan, B. (2012). Encyclopedia of neuropsychology. Academic Press.

Linehan, M. M. (1993a). *Cognitive behavioral treatment for borderline personality disorder.* New York, NY: Guilford Press.

Linehan, M. M. (1993b). *Skills training manual for treating borderline personality disorder.* New York, NY: Guilford Press.

Loewy, J., Hallan, C., Friedman, E., & Martinez, C. (2006). Sleep/sedation in children undergoing EEG testing: A comparison of chloral hydrate and music therapy. *American Journal of Electroneurodiagnostic Technology*, *46*(4), 343–355. doi:10.1080/1086508X.2006.11079593 PMID:17285817

Luckasson, R., Borthwick-Duffy, S., Buntinx, W. H. E., Coulter, D. L., Craig, E. M., Reeve, A., ... Tasse´, M. J. (2002). *Mental retardation:Definition, classification, and systems of supports* (10th ed.). Washington, DC: American Association on Mental Retardation.

Madhavan, T., Kalyan, M., Naidu, S., Pashwarla, R., & Narayan, J. (1999). *Mental retardation- a manual for psychologists*. Secunderabad, India: National Institute for the Mentally Handicapped.

Malin, A. J. (1949). Manual of Malin's Intelligence Scale for Indian Children. Lucknow: Indian Psychological Corporation.

Mather, N., & Goldstein, S. (2015). *Behaviour Modification in the classroom*. Retrieved from http://www.ldonline.org/article/6030/

Mindell, J. A., Kuhn, B., Lewin, D. S., Meltzer, L. J., & Sadeh, A. (2006). Behavioral treatment of bedtime problems and night wakings in infants and young children. *American Academy of Sleep Medicine Sleep.*, *29*(10), 1263–1276. PMID:17068979

O'Neill, R., Horner, R., & Albin, R. (1997). *Functional Assessment and Programme Development for Problem Behaviour: A Practical Handbook*. Brooks/Cole Publishing.

Review of Vineland Adaptive Behavior Scales-Second Edition (Vineland-II). (2012). *Early Childhood Measurement and Evaluation*. Retrieved from www.cup.ualberta.ca

Reynolds, Zupanick, & Dombeck. (2013). *Intellectual Disability and Severity Codes*. Retrieved from https://www.mentalhelp.net/articles/intellectual-disability-and-severity-codes/

Reynolds, T. B. A., Zupanick, C. E., & Dombeck, M. (2013). *Intellectual Diasability, Mentalhelp.Net. An American Addiction center resources*. Retrieved on 14 February 2019.Retrived from http://www.mentalhelp.net/articles/intellectual-functioning-mental-abilities/

Richdale, A., & Wiggs, L. (2005). Behavioural approaches to the treatment of sleep problems in children with developmental disorders. What is state of the art? *International Journal of Behavioral and Consultation Therapy*, *1*(3), 165–187. doi:10.1037/h0100743

Sevcik, R. A., & Romski, M. A. (Eds.). (2016). *Communication interventions for individuals with severe disabilities: Exploring research challenges and opportunities*. Baltimore, MD: Brookes.

Sharma, A., & Chowhan, S. (2014). *The Neuropsychological Components of Visual Processing and Learning in High and Low Functioning Children Exhibiting Autism Spectrum Disorder: A Comparative Study*. Unpublished manuscript.

Snell, M. E., Brady, N., McLean, L., Ogletree, B. T., Siegel, E., Sylvester, L., ... Sevcik, R. (2010). Twenty years of communication intervention research with individuals who have severe intellectual and developmental disabilities. *American Journal on Intellectual and Developmental Disabilities*, *115*(5), 364–380. doi:10.1352/1944-7558-115-5.364 PMID:20687822

Stuart, W., & Kingstone, M. (2018). The complexity of lifelong co morbidities with severe intellectual disability. *Journal of Intellectual and Developmental Disability*.

Tassé, M. J., Schalock, R. L., Balboni, G., Bersani, H., & Sharon, A. (2012). The Construct of Adaptive Behavior: Its Conceptualization, Measurement, and Use in the Field of Intellectual Disability. *American Journal on Intellectual and Developmental Disabilities*, *117*(4), 291–303. doi:10.1352/1944-7558-117.4.291 PMID:22809075

World Health Organization. (1992). *The ICD-10 classification of mental and behavioural disorders: Clinical descriptions and diagnostic guidelines*. Geneva: World Health Organization.

APPENDIX

Activities

Activity No. 1

In order to form concepts of various objects and things, various catalogues from various stores that could be interesting for the child. These catalogues could range from clothes, toys hunting fishing etc. One can make a collage out of it. The child could learn from the catalogues or from the pictures about the features of the specific objects which could help in forming the concepts of the objects. One can work on sorting with so many of these pictures. One can instruct the child to cut out the things and sort things that have wheels and things that have wings or sort the pants from the shirts. One can also cut out a child from a magazine and have the child dress them. For example: ask the child to find a *purple shirt* or have them put a hat *on top of* the boy's head.I

Can Target

- Categories & Sorting
- Vocabulary
- Basic Concepts (colors, prepositions)
- Life Skills

Activity No. 2

'Backward chaining' is a technique that which can help the child to learn a new skill. In this technique, the trainer will complete all the steps of the task except the last step. The child needs to complete the task. This continues as the trainer complete one less step and the child does one more. Until he can do the whole task on their own. The child receives motivation and confidence along with success. For example: when a child is taught how to put their shoes and socks, the first task is to break it into small steps and making him learn.

- Get shoes and socks from cupboard
- Bring socks and shoes over to chair
- Sit on chair
- Pull socks onto feet
- Slip shoes onto feet.

Chapter 9
An Overview on Issues Among Individuals With Intellectual Disability in India

Dorothy Bhandari Deka
Sarvodaya Healthcare, India

ABSTRACT

Intelligence is the general mental capacity that involves reasoning, planning, solving problems, thinking abstractly, comprehending complex ideas, learning efficiently, and learning from experience. Intellectual disability (previously termed "mental retardation") shows significant cognitive deficits (IQ score of below 70, i.e., two standard deviations below the mean of 100 in the population) and also significant deficits in functional and adaptive skills. Individuals with intellectual disability meet with various challenges in every span of life. The chapter tries to highlight some of the areas that are related to the concerns for the people with intellectual disability.

INTRODUCTION

Intellectual disability (intellectual developmental disorder) is a neuro developmental disorders is one of the conditions with an onset in the developmental period. This disability is characterized by inability to cope up with the mental abilities as per the child's chronological age (DSM V, 2015).

The common characteristics of intellectual disability are although uniqueness in every person, regardless of their IQ scores each individual has their own personality and areas of ability and difficulty. Generally a person with an intellectual disability has difficulty: learning and processing information as quickly as people without an intellectual disability. Grasping abstract concepts such as money and time, understanding the subtleties of interpersonal interactions, manipulating of the ideas and concepts is required for planning and organizing as compared to people without intellectual disability. The difficulties includes such as reasoning, problem solving, planning, abstract thinking judgment, academic learning, and learning from experience. This inability results in impairments of adaptive functioning, such as the individual fails to meet the ideals of a person's independence and social responsibility in one

DOI: 10.4018/978-1-7998-1223-4.ch009

or more aspects of daily life, that includes communication, social participation, academic or occupational functioning, and personal independence at home or in community settings. Diagnosis for intellectual disability includes an expected delay in developmental milestones that involves various areas of intellectual functioning (Ahuja, 2011).

The concept of 'intellectual disability' is that it is based on at least two different theoretical models of thought. Those advocating the use of the medical model state that intellectual disability is a 'trait' (it is something that one is born with and does not change over one's lifetime). Intellectual disability is thus seen as a physical impairment, the same as a deformed limb, or something that is deficient in an individual, and may well be innate (Spitz, 2006). The social model of disability asserts that although a person may have impairment (the deficit in cognitive and adaptive behaviour in the developmental period); it is society that disables people, not the impairment. The social model has gained recognition and strong support by those who are most affected by disability, including intellectual disability. The social model clearly influences the current thinking about the notion (Luckasson, et al.,1992). state "Mental retardation is not something you have, like blue eyes or a bad heart. Nor is it something you are, like being short or thin. It is not a medical disorder … Nor is it a mental disorder. Mental retardation refers to a particular state of functioning that begins in childhood and in which limitations in intelligence coexist with related limitations in adaptive skill.

Individual factors include personality, social and communication abilities, coping strategies and the presence of other disabilities (motor, social or sensory). The supports provided by family, friends and support staff are also crucial aspects of people's lives and have a profound influence on their confidence and function. Issues of access (including physical, social, communication, cognitive, financial access) to community based facilities and services also play a powerful role in either enabling or inhibiting opportunities for inclusion, participation and contribution and the ability of the individual to fulfill their community roles. (CDDH, 2015).

Presently, individuals with intellectual disability in India, majority of them are still excluded by the society irrespective of identified or unidentified. To fully understand the challenges that individuals with intellectual disability are facing within the Indian society, is by understanding that the barriers are primarily rooted in religious beliefs, cultural norms, and majorly lack of awareness regarding intellectual disability. India's rigid social structure within the society becomes a hurdle in inclusion and acceptance for individuals with intellectual disability.

Factors Influencing Intellectual Disability and its Comorbidities

Genetic factors play a major part in intellectual disability, numerous genetic causes may lead to intellectual disability. Genetic studies have been complicated for a long time by the extreme clinical and genetic heterogeneity. Genetic diagnosis can now be made in most patients with severe intellectual disability. Severe intellectual disability is mostly caused by a de novo point mutation, an insertion or deletion, or a structural genomic variation (Vissers et.al, 2016). Down syndrome (trisomy 21) is the most common genetic cause of intellectual disability in the United States, occurring approximately once every 700 live births (Parker et al., 2010). Fragile X syndrome is the most common known inherited cause of intellectual disability, and it affects approximately 1 per 5,000 males (Coffee et al., 2009). More than 700 genes have been found to play a part in isolated intellectual disability and intellectual disability-associated disorders, and many more await discovery (Vissers et.al, 2016). Various environmental factors such as exposure to toxic substances, nutritional deficiencies, brain radiation, childhood brain infections, traumatic brain injury, and maternal infections can lead to intellectual disability. Also prenatal and postnatal complications such as complications of prematurity or complications during delivery such as forceps delivery may cause brain injury can lead to intellectual disability. (Gustafsson, 2003). Many cases of intellectual disability in the population still has unknown etiology.

Comorbidity is also found in cases with intellectual disability. Many neurodevelopmental, psychiatric, and medical disorders co-occur with intellectual disability such as learning disabilities, communication disorders, epilepsy, cerebral palsy and other numerous genetically transmitted conditions (APA, 2013). Estimates of the rates of psychiatric coexisting conditions vary. For many years there was an underestimation of the increased risk for development of comorbid conditions ("diagnostic overshadowing"). A research reported rates of 30 to 42 percent of psychopathology in children with "mental retardation" compared to 6 to 7 percent in children without the disability (Rutter et al., 1970). A study by Gillberg et al in the year 1986 reported that 57 percent of subjects with mild and severe "mental retardation" met diagnostic criteria for affective, anxiety, conduct, schizophrenia, and somatoform disorders and attention deficit hyperactivity disorder (ADHD). In general, at least 25 percent of persons with intellectual disability may have significant psychiatric problems, with the population experiencing, in particular, significantly increased rates of schizophrenia, depression, and ADHD (Bouras and Holt, 2007; Fletcher et al., 2007).

Prevalence of Intellectual Disability

Intellectual disability is an extremely stigmatizing condition and involves consumption of large public health resources, but most data about its burden is based on studies conducted in developed countries (Maulik et. al.,2011). Estimates of the prevalence of intellectual disabaility among children in the United States based on epidemiologic studies range widely, from 8.7 to 36.8 per 1,000 (Boyle & Lary, 1996; Camp et al., 1998). A major source of this wide range in prevalence is variation in the inclusion of mild intellectual disability (often defined to include individuals with IQs in the range of 50–70 and deficits in adaptive behavior). While the prevalence of serious intellectual disability (IQ <50 with deficits in adaptive behavior) in the United States and other developed countries is consistently found to be in the range of 2.5 to 5 per 1,000 children, that of mild intellectual disability ranges from as low as 2 to more than 30 per 1,000. The risk of mild intellectual disability is highest among children of low socioeconomic status (Durkin et al., 2007). From the evidence reviewed, disparities in the rates of intellectual disability by race and ethnicity are also reported. Socioeconomic status is a confounder for these disparities; however, there is also evidence that test bias and diagnostic bias contribute to these differences (Jencks & Phillips, 1998).

A meta-analysis study reported that across all 52 studies prevalence was higher among children/ adolescent compared to those on adults. Higher prevalence in low and middle group countries is of concern given the limitations in available resources in such countries to manage intellectual disability. The study states intellectual disability prevalence is 1% around the world (Maulik et. al., 2011). Similarly studies conducted in Taiwan reports prevalence of intellectual disability was 0.318 – 0.396% and men accounted for a higher percentage of cases than women in Taiwan. They also reported that this group requires more health care services as compared to the general population. Also in Serbia and Bulgaria estimated prevalence of intellectual disability is between 1 and 3% as in other south-east European countries. According to 2011 population census 1.5 million persons suffer from Intellectual disability out of which 0.9 are males and 0.6 are females. 57% of which are illiterate and 72% are unemployed. (2011, Disability Census)

Legal Services Provided for Individuals with Intellectual Disability

According to National Legal Services Authority (Legal Services to the Mentally Ill Persons and Persons with Mental Disabilities Schemes, 2010), there are few rights that are rendered to the individuals with intellectual disability. Rights provided to the individuals with intellectual disability such as, legal services to mentally retarded persons (MRs), appointment of guardians under the National Trust Act, 1999 for the their welfare in the society.

Matters to be considered while representing legal services to individuals with intellectual difficulty:

1. Individuals with Intellectual disability are not mentally ill individual
2. Legal services to Individuals with Intellectual disability.
3. Legal services for ensuring the health care.
4. Legal services for ensuring the fundamental rights of individuals with intellectual disability.
5. Right to education
6. Prevention of exploitation and abuse of individuals with intellectual disability.
7. Legal services for individuals with intellectual disability for owing and inheriting properties and to have financial rights.
8. Appointment of guardians under the National Trust Act, 1999
9. Need for setting up of a supported network
10. Creating awareness campaigns amongst the other school children
11. Awareness camps for educating the family members of individuals with intellectual disability.
12. Awareness programs for the general public
13. Sensitization Program for Judicial Officers and Lawyers

Also almost after a decade's wait, the Rights of Persons with Disabilities Act, 2016 came into effect on 30 December 2016. The Lok Sabha passed it on 17 December and the Rajya Sabha on 14 December. The Act will replace the Persons with Disability (PwD) Act of 1995.

The salient features of the Act are:

- Reservation in vacancies in government establishments has been increased from 3% to 4% for certain persons or class of persons with benchmark disability.
- Every child with benchmark disability between the age group of 6 and 18 years shall have the right to free education, framework for supporting institutional and social infrastructure, making accessible environment and provisions of punishment for violation of RPWD Act.
- District level committees will be constituted by the State Governments to address local concerns of PWDs.
- Special Courts will be designated in each district to handle cases concerning violation of rights of PWDs.
- Broad-based Central & State Advisory Boards on Disability are to be set up to serve as apex policy-making bodies at the Central and State level.
- Office of Chief Commissioner and those of the State Commissioners of Persons with Disabilities has been strengthened.
- The Act says that any person who "intentionally insults or intimidates with intent to humiliate a person with a disability in any place within public view" is punishable with imprisonment.

Challenges Faced by Parents and thc Individuals with Intellectual Disability during the Early Age

Intellectual disability in India is a major challenge which not only limits the capacity of the afflicted individual but at the same time also leads to the parent's vulnerability to the stressors (Jena et al, 2013).

There are multiple problems in families having a mentally retarded child. It has been found that one of the overwhelming, problems of these parents is related to the feeling of social ridicule for possessing a child with intellectual disability. As a reaction to this attitude, the parents may prefer to keep these children socially isolated. They often feel guilty and. hold each other responsible (Ryckman & Handerson, 1965).Parental acceptance depends upon the knowledge and the awareness of the parents along with the strength and the readiness to face all the challenges that they have to welcome with the growing age of the child. The parent's resources and the support also play an important role in the acceptance of the child. There is considered evidence to suggest that parents of children with intellectual disability experience greater stress than caregivers of children without intellectual disability. This stress tends to be chronic in nature and therefore persists over substantial period of time. Caring for children with intellectual disabilities drains out parent's economic, physical, mental and psychological resources. Behavioral problems which are frequently associated with intellectual disabilities add to parental stress (Jena et. al, 2013).

Parenting stress and adaptation depend upon the type of disability; the family's coping resources and formal and informal supports in the community (Breslau et al, 1982). Here the stress for the parents is that no matter what level of disability the child has in intellectual functioning, the actual stress is that the child cannot be cured by medicine it is a condition that will remain with the child till the last day of their life. The fact of this condition is more stressful for the parents rather than providing them the treatment so that their child can be healthy but here the parents also have to live with the condition of their child.

The parents coping with the fact depends upon the resources and formal and informal supports that are available in the community. The coping resources include "faith in God, self-determination, attitude and perception towards the situation, and the available resources such as support from family members, relatives, friends, neighbors, professionals, community and governmental policies and programs" (Peshawaria et al, 1998). There are two types of social support systems one is formal social supports which include services provided by professionals such as school programmes, parent education specialists, therapists, and government and non- government agencies. Another is Informal social supports encompass relationships between family members, relatives, neighbours, friends, and community groups. Proximal support from spouse and immediate relatives has been found to promote family adaptation and reduce stress (Gupta et al., 2012).

Parental stress in the lower socioeconomic status of the family can be associated with more stress because of less resource availability. Shortage of resources, including food, medication, durable medical equipment, and apparel can add to the stress of raising children with disabilities (Gupta et al, 2012). Parents of children with intellectual disability face financial burden and also diminished quality of life in social aspect (Khare, 2015).

In conditions of poverty, a child with a disability is regarded as a burden, an evil spirit, and an object of charity without rights, rather than as an unfortunate child (Gupta et al., 2012). Parenting issues usually depends upon the severity, visibility, unpredictability, and number of invasive procedures such as surgeries, and overall type of disability - behavioral, developmental or medical – rather than the medical diagnosis (Breslau et al, 1982).

Parental expressed emotions play a very important role in the child's growing age. The expressed emotions need to be balanced towards the child so that the child has a positive attitude towards their life. High expressed emotion is said when the family has a negative attitude towards the patient, thinks that the disability or the disorder is controllable but the patient is not choosing to get better. In family having high expressed emotions the members in the family thinks that family's problems are due to the disabled individual's mental illness, the individual with intellectual disability is blamed for it that the disabled individual has trouble problem solving within the family. The attitude towards the individual with intellectual disability is hostile when the expressed emotion is high. Low expressed emotion is when the family members are more reserved with their criticism. Findings support the theory that low to moderate levels of negative expression may be less beneficial or detrimental for children with ID compared to children without intellectual disability (Green & Bake, 2011).

High or low expressed emotion makes the disabled individual feel trapped, out of control and dependent upon others, feels that because of their problem everyone is facing difficulty and everyone in the home is being affected and raising the stress level for everyone in family (Barker et al., 2012).

Children with intellectual disability in the early age initially are not able to understand the condition they are going through but as they start maturing slowly they start realizing the fact of their life usually in the case of mild moderate level of intellectual difficulty children. They realize that they are not similar to their age appropriate friends and they are not able to perform the way their age group friends do. This can be seen in their behavior as the child starts being irritable, aggressive, at times shows stubbornness and some children also might show sad moods. Their understanding regarding the difficulty also leads to additional behavioral, emotional and social problem that the parents as well as the child face it (Lemay et al., 2003).

The process of understanding that the young individual will be limited in his learning abilities would be a difficult task for any parent to face (Brown & Randel, 2007). Parents having children with intellectual disability can have issues in preparing the child to overcome the present and the future challenges. Childhood challenges that is faced by the child with intellectual disability which is an early life concern for the parents is for their child's education, vocation and secondly peer group and social acceptance. Education and vocational training is one very important aspect for children with intellectual disability as it helps the child develop his/ her self-esteem along with a reason for survival, if they are motivated and supported by their surroundings, especially parents because as in the later stage when the child starts realizing that it's a condition that is never ending might be a cause for the onset of other mental health issues.

Presently in India, we are passing through a phase in the area of rehabilitation wherein efforts are being made to spread services and training programs, to raise awareness levels related to mainstreaming and provision of equal rights and opportunity for the individuals with intellectual disability (Peshawaria et al, 1995)

Vocational Training and Employment for Individuals with Intellectual Disability

The ultimate aim of any education and training is for a gainful employment and it is one of the most critical aspects of independent living. This is true with every individual including the individuals with intellectual disability. Individual with intellectual disability are more likely to be unemployed and generally earn less than other disability areas even when they are employed. Individual with intellectual disability are rarely employed, probably due to the stigma attached to individual with intellectual disability (Abidi, 1999).

There are three major areas where the individuals with intellectual disability can be employed. One of them is Sheltered Employment, here the person with intellectual disability is trained in an occupation and employ him in the workshop itself. Another one are of employment is Open Employment, here the routine job is successfully performed by individuals with intellectual disability with initial support from the trainer. The individual with intellectual disability can work gainfully provided has developed social competence. The third area is Self Employment; it can be successful when the family of the individual with intellectual disability provide him with appropriate training and support (Narayan & Kurani, 1990).

Though individuals with intellectual disability are able to do complex tasks, if given a structured situation and adequate preparation (Gold,1972). But it needs the training for the same. The assumption of work roles in competitive or non -competitive work environment for the individuals with intellectual disability calls for three types of assistance: first is simplicity of environment so that they can respond promptly and efficiently, second formation of work personality through specific preparation for the tasks comprising the position where she /he is going to be employed. Third is development of supporting roles for them in the family and community (Narayan & Kurani, 1990).

Employment and income are also affected by the severity of disability .There is a 3 per cent quota for persons with disabilities (PWD act 1995). As such there is no separate quota out of the said 3 per cent for individuals with intellectual disability. The major issues identified in this area are:

1. Identification of Jobs & Reservation Clause of The Disability Act: The Disability Act 1995 provides for a 3% reservation in "identified posts" for people with disabilities in all categories of jobs. The posts were meant to have been identified soon after the Act coming into force and updated every 3 years. The initial identification of posts at the Central Government level was not completed until 2001 and no formal expansion of identified posts has been completed subsequently.
2. Repeated Medical Examination of Disabled Employees: Disabled employees get certain benefits like higher transport allowance; preference in the allotment of government accommodation etc. Every time a person applies for availing these benefits, she/he is asked to get a Medical Test done. The authorities do not accept the Disability Certificate, as an authentic proof of disability.
3. Accessibility: It is a major issue in Government offices there are not much facilities are for individuals to make the work environment more conducive to work.
4. Discrimination: An important legal right for persons with disabilities is the right to live free from discrimination in employment. Discrimination may normally take different forms. Some employers use pre-employment physicals to identify individuals with disabilities and to refuse their job applications. Some employers deny training, promotions and fringe benefits to employees with disabilities. Employees have been downgraded, discharged or harassed when an employer learns of the existence of a disability, or thinks that an employee is disabled (Employment of Persons with Disabilities in Public Sectors in India- Emerging Issues and Trends 2008).

Just as normal adults work to earn their livelihood, persons with intellectual disability also have the potential to work and earn if they are provided with the necessary training, placement and other supports. At present, many of them are idle, work in sheltered workshops or work for a few hours every week. Their earnings do not reflect their capabilities. To make employment a realistic option for people with intellectual disability, appropriate jobs from the open market need to be identified. Simple jobs that require minimum supervision needs to be selected for successful training and placement of individuals with intellectual disability. Vocational rehabilitation helps individual with intellectual disability to hold on to a job (Abidi, 1999).

Health Issues in Individuals with Intellectual Disabilities

Individuals with intellectual disabilities are prone to a wide range of medical conditions that can affect the person physically as well as their mental health.

The most common physical health problems are epilepsy, mobility problems, and sensory problems. Health problems often occur in people with genetic syndromes. A small, general practice database study found that a quarter of people with intellectual disabilities and epilepsy were seizure-free and a third had poorly controlled seizures Oral health is often poor, and toothache may manifest as challenging behavior. Gastro-esophageal reflux disease often remains unnoticed (Henry et. al, 2008). Family members and care givers of individual with intellectual disability also come for receiving lifelong contraception or to have surgery to regulate fertility of the person with intellectual disability. The reproductive health, rights and contraceptive needs of women with intellectual disabilities have been the subject of extensive legal, ethical and health care deliberations in the United States (Paransky & Zurawin, 2003). The concerns of parents and care givers regarding pregnancy and menstrual management have in some cases led to women being surgically sterilized or undergoing hysterectomy. The women's capacity to make autonomous decisions and to care for children is not always clear, and the rights and wishes of the individual women have to be protected as far as possible (Diekema, 2003). Newer medical options, including hormonal implants, permit less invasive and reversible management of fertility and menstruation (Paransky & Zurawin, 2003).

Individuals with intellectual disability not just have physical health issues along with it there are also barriers present that hinders in their good health care such as missing out on health information in magazines, books and public health campaigns due to limited literacy. Cognitive difficulties might hinder in understanding the significance of maintaining the healthy diet, lifestyle choices, and disease screening. Social and communication difficulty in various circumstances may lead to hindrance in health monitoring. In order to improve the scenario of barrier for health issues among the individuals with intellectual disability strategies can be used. For fulfilling the purpose of the strategies very firstly the health professional and care givers need to be equipped with training and knowledge regarding their behaviour, exchange of response, comprehending capabilities, and how much the person with intellectual disability is able to do things on their own. People with intellectual disability often rely on health management and the barriers that prevent the identified health needs are being met with the help of support staff and healthcare staff (Tracy & McDonald, 2015).

Sexual Knowledge: Feelings and Needs of Individual with Intellectual Disability

Important changes in public policies and attitudes have resulted in improved opportunities for people with mental disabilities. Unfortunately, societal attitudes have not changed much with regard to their sexual needs. Even today, society at large refuse to acknowledge that all people have sexual feelings, needs, and desires, regardless of their physical and/or mental abilities .Making good decisions about sexuality is a critical part of adulthood, but sometimes people with intellectual disabilities don't get the support or education they need to navigate this complex aspect of life (Walker–Hirrch, L. 2007). Sex education is a central issue for all the community integration of people with intellectual disability, yet they are greatly disadvantaged in this the nature of their disability as they are likely to experience difficulty when dealing with such subtle and complex issues. The development of appropriate sexual skills is easier said than done, because sex education is such a vexed topic, particularly in the area of disability. In order to avoid confronting sexual issues, some parents and care- givers deny that people with intellectual disabilities are sexual beings (Marita et al., 1996).

People with intellectual disability as mentioned may be denied as sexual being this may be true for individuals with severe or profound disability and is certainly not true for individuals with mild intellectual disability as people with intellectual disability might have less or no experience in sexual relationship unlike other individuals of their age but they might have positive feelings towards sexual needs and feeling (UNICEF, 2005). Consequently providing training for daily life and teaching them the basic life and social skills for their survival in is very important for the child to learn and adapt with the society and along with it sex education is also one of the very important aspects that the individuals with intellectual disability need to be know about as because adolescents with intellectual disability are the vulnerable ones. They are usually exploded not by strangers rather mostly by their own relatives or neighbours or friends. Therefore educating them right from the gender difference, puberty, their safety at home and at public places, unusual touch by relatives or strangers, knowledge about sex and its process and the appropriate age and social norms related to it would help the individual to have a better idea and reason to protect themselves. This will also help them in understanding the society in a more matured way so that they can lead a simple but a safe and secured life. As the WHO-UNFPA Guidance Note says, "The sexual and reproductive health of persons with disabilities is not a unique, complex, or highly specialized issue. It is, however, an issue that needs more attention and greater creativity, and it needs more attention now.

Marriage and its Consequence for Individuals with Intellectual Disability

Global human rights laws grant all individuals with disabilities, including individuals with intellectual disabilities, the right to marry and have families. The key issue in marriage among individuals with intellectual disability is not the marriage itself, but the awareness and consent of the individual with disability to enter into the institution of marriage on their own free will. According to the laws, the disabled person have the right to go through the same marriage ceremony and celebration as the other young people in the family goes through and those in their social circles but the concern is that how much will they understand about the longer term implications of living within a new family structure, as well as the rights and responsibilities that marriage entails and the added responsibility of being sexually active and to have children. Therefore individuals with intellectual disability, in the middle age of their life; it is important for them to know about the institution of marriage and the responsibilities that come with it. It is the duty of the parents to make them aware of the process of marriage and its responsibilities as that will help the individual with intellectual disability to understand the overall picture of marriage and take a better decision by the individual for the their future (Groce et al., 2014).

The importance to educate the individual is important to make them aware of the responsibility so that if the parents are willing that their child should marry and start a new life with a partner, the individual with intellectual disability can give their own views and consent for their own future. Forcing the individual with intellectual disability to marry without consent will be an injustice for the individual as well as for the person with whom the individual will marry. It is difficult to answer the question as to why parents of adults with intellectual disability would encourage or force their children into marriages if their children are reluctant to wed or if they are frightened, confused or unable to understand the roles and responsibilities expected of them in marriage (Groce et al, 2014). But if given a thought the parents of individual with intellectual disability might think their child's marriage would secure their child's future and also probably someone who can look after their child after their parents grow old and weak to look after their child with the condition.

In case marriage takes place, it is important that the family and the partner are well aware of the condition of the disability of the individual before they marry. It is an illegal action if the parents of individual with intellectual disability do not inform the would be partner and their family about the condition and the marriage is taken place. Responsibility of parents increases as their child reaches the appropriate age of marriage, to educate them, help them take an insightful decision if they want to enter the institution of marriage and very importantly the whole process of marriage should be done in a lawful way rather than in deception (Nambi, 2005)

Quality of Life of Individuals with Intellectual Disability

Quality of life (QOL) in general terms is the overall well-being of an individual. It is basically the comfort experienced by an individual in their life. Quality of life has a wide range of contexts that include the fields of international development, healthcare, politics and employment. The standard indicators of the quality of life include not just wealth and employment it also includes the built environment, physical health and mental health both, education, recreation and leisure time, and social belongings.

Quality of Life is a universal concept as everybody has a quality of life and the quality of life of people with disabilities has the same components as the quality of life of people without disabilities (Interim report, 2003). The issue that the concept addresses is the lives of persons and ensuring that citizens with intellectual disability, experience the same human rights and a life of quality as any other member of society. To this end, the quality of life concept reflects the following four principles:

1. Quality of life is composed of the same factors and relationships for all people;
2. Quality of life is experienced when a person's needs are met and when the individual has the opportunity to pursue life enrichment in major life activity settings;
3. Quality of life has both subjective and objective components; and
4. Quality of life is a multidimensional construct, influenced by individual and environmental factors (Navas et al, 2012)

The field of intellectual disability is strongly influenced by the Quality of Life paradigm; the framework supports the equality of persons, which is reflected in concepts such as self-determination, liberation, inclusion, and empowerment. In daily practice the concepts are translated into tangible actions, professionals are often challenged with difficulties to apply the quality of life principles for individuals with intellectual difficulty.

The application of principles of quality of life, which should in ideal conditions should lead to positive outcomes with regard to social participation, independence, and well-being seems to be at risk, as accounts from professionals indicate that empowerment is sometimes replaced by actions solely aimed at "controlling," "dominating and excluding" clients with intellectual disability and co-occurring mental health problems (Morisse et al, 2013). In this respect, adequate support is a challenge and because of this complexity, the application of the QOL paradigm is not self-evident, although there seems to be consensus about the fact that the same domains are relevant for all persons, including this specific subpopulation. The policy of deinstitutionalization was based on the proposition that quality of life of individuals with intellectual disabilities will improve as a result of being moved from institutions to community-based care settings.

Old Age and Individuals with Intellectual Disability

Ageing adults with intellectual disabilities are at particular disadvantage and risk. Older adults with severe and profound impairments are disregarded or institutionalized. Older adults with mild and moderate intellectual disability can be trained and educated so that they can look after themselves and lead a normal life like others but the same cannot be done with elderly person with severe and profound intellectual disability.

The highest priorities for the majority of people with intellectual disabilities in less developed countries generally include basic health care, adequate nutrition and housing, education, human rights, and political, social and economic stability (WHO, 2000).

In case of elderly individual housing is often inadequate and health provision is usually neglected. Nowadays the immediate family members are seen to ignore the older individuals with or without intellectual disability. Elderly people if kept in old age home or even at home can manage with their basic needs but elderly ones with intellectual disability if ignored by their family members they usually face a lot of problem. Communication and behavioral difficulties are generally observed. Speech and motor impairments may serve as barriers to communicate when no immediate family member is available with individuals with intellectual disability when need to deal with health services provision. Behavioral issues such as fear, confusion, and aggressiveness among adults with intellectual disabilities may have difficulty cooperating with health services provisions (Henny, 2008).

In both women and men, proper nutrition, exercise, and access to preventive health care can increase health and longevity. Women with intellectual disabilities generally receive less preventive health care than women generally, just as women receive less preventive health care than men. In developing countries, women with intellectual disability may be affected more frequently by malnutrition than are men. In many nations, older women with intellectual disabilities experience challenges that are particular to their sex. Their specific needs are often overlooked or dismissed. Older adults with co-morbid conditions experience particular problems and their compound physical and/or mental health conditions not addressed (WHO, 2000).

Older adults with impairments should be provided with rehabilitative services, vocational opportunities, and quality old-age services, which are not adequately provided. Government in developing countries should provide the disabled elderly people with adequate legal rights and also economical schemes can help them become independent. Shelter including food and stay along with basic skill training and adequate health and economic support from the government can make better changes in developing countries for older people with intellectual disability.

A study in the year 2010 by Strydom and collegues, examined health-related literature on aging and intellectual disabilities with specific focus on age-associated health risk factors, such as cardiovascular, gastrointestinal, and musculoskeletal system health issues, and age-related oral health and lifestyle health risks, primarily the contributions to overweight or obesity. The review revealed varying differences in the prevalence of health risk factors, significant evidence is emerging that cardiovascular disease is as prevalent among people with intellectual disability and is as common a cause of death as in the general population. The study also revealed that a growing body of work on health risk factors, such as overweight and obesity, which are often linked to the onset of a variety of diseases and impairing conditions. Thus healthier lifestyles, better nutrition and more exercise, and greater surveillance of health risks were seen as ways to improve the health status of aging adults with ID.

Studies revealed that by the age 60, about 1 of every 16 adults with intellectual disability gets affected by some form of dementia. This rate increases as the population ages. People with Down syndrome are 3 times more likely to have Alzheimer's or Dementia than other adults with intellectual disability. Both men and women with intellectual disability tend to experience decreased bone density at younger ages than people without intellectual disability that increases risk for osteoporosis. Adults with intellectual disability have a similar risk for falling as the elderly population, but at much younger ages (Heller, T. et al, 2010).

Attitude of Society Towards the Individual with Intellectual Disability

Attitudes towards disability are not the same within countries, communities, or even families. Different types of impairments carry different levels of stigma, as does the severity of the impairment and how it was acquired. People with intellectual disabilities, severe mental health conditions, albinism, and sensory disabilities are often more stigmatized than people with physical disabilities. People with disabilities who can participate in their communities experience fewer stigmas than those with more severe disabilities. Females who are disabled are doubly disadvantaged, due to the stigma associated with gender as well as disability. Socio-economic status can affect attitudes towards disability. People with disabilities in rural areas may experience more harmful practices than in urban areas (Rohwerder, 2018).

The social system plays a major in the acceptance of the individuals with intellectual disability and the support from the society can actually bring changes to the lives of the children with intellectual disability. In country like India, although in most of the places in the country is aware of the conditions but still the acceptance and support is not available from the society. Government has provided immense support to the children with intellectual disability for the well fare of the child as well as for the family. Social acceptance of the individual with intellectual disability is one major factor that can bring change to the social scenario and this can be a support to the immediate family and the child's mental health. Although deinstitutionalization and inclusive education, community integration has increased, still public attitudes continue to pose a potential barrier to the full social inclusion and equal rights of people with intellectual disability (Sheriden & Scior, 2013).

Disability stigma includes lack of understanding and awareness regarding the causes of disabilities and their resulting characteristics is a key factor in the stigma experienced by people with disabilities. Misconceptions about the cause of disabilities often result from cultural or religious beliefs. Disability is often believed to be the misdeed of ancestors, parents, of the person with disabilities or because of some supernatural forces such as demons/spirits, witchcraft or punishment or fate from God. As a result people with disabilities may be thought to be not quite human or a source of shame, which has serious consequences for how they are treated. Misconceptions about the nature and abilities of people with disabilities, including their inability to contribute financially or to have a normal relationship, will not be able to report sexual abuse, their disability is contagious or they bring bad luck, their bodies have magical powers or that they are witches, also contribute to the stigma and discrimination they experience. Discriminatory legislation and policies reinforce prejudice and discrimination, while the isolation of people with disabilities perpetuates negative stereotypes (Rohwerder, 2018).

Society's attitude towards the individuals with intellectual disability might lead to socials comparison among the children with intellectual disability and the ones who do not have any disability. Such comparisons might affect the individual's attitude towards self. Individuals with intellectual disability might develop low self-esteem, lack of self-confidence which might later cultivate into social withdrawal behavior or depression in the individual.

IMPLICATIONS, MANAGEMENT AND PREVENTION FOR FUTURE IMPROVEMENT FOR INDIVIDUALS WITH INTELLECTUAL DISABILITY

Every individual is unique. Intellectual ability provides a guide as to how quickly a person is able to process new information grasp abstract concepts and manipulate ideas. The facts that will help understanding and managing people with intellectual disability could be majorly focused on their learning ability and information processing. It is required to understand that they are slow learners and the processing of information is slow as compared to others without intellectual disability. It is also important to understand that they have difficulty with abstract concepts such as money, time and the subtleties of interpersonal interactions (CDDH, 2015).

Individuals with intellectual disability require the kind of support and assistance is depended on their cognitive ability and the expectations on them in and within particular environments. We also need to be careful that whether they have other associated developmental disabilities such as cerebral palsy, autism or sensory impairments so that needs can be fulfilled accordingly for the individual with intellectual disability. Every one of us has areas of ability and other areas of function that we find difficult(CDDH, 2014) Subjective categories of mild, moderate, severe and profound levels of intellectual disability, defined on the basis of IQ 'scores', provide an escort to the level and types of support an individual might require.

Individuals with a mild intellectual disability that is according to ICD 10, 2007 individual with an IQ of 50- 69 may learn to read and write (depending on educational opportunities). Most people with mild intellectual disability have important relationships in their lives and participate in a variety of activities and do contribute to their families and their communities. Some of them live and travel independently while others require support and assistance in using public transport, managing money, and planning and organizing their lives. Most individuals with mild intellectual disability can work, and some of them can hold a job, with or without a level of personal or employment support. Many individuals do form intimate relationships and some do marry and raise children with various levels of social support such as from family, friends and the service system. People with mild intellectual disability do have trouble with academic learning and so reading, writing and numeral might remain at a basic level. Many people find the subtleties of interpersonal relationships and social rules difficult to comprehend (particularly as adolescents) and may unintentionally disobey social boundaries.

Individuals with a moderate intellectual disability, according to ICD 10, 2007 individual with an IQ of 35 – 49, do have important relationships in his/her life and will usually enjoy a variety of activities with families, friends and paid support workers and form valued and lasting friendships. With specific travel training many people learn to use public transport on familiar routes, but may have difficulty in management of money and issues while problem solving when unexpected events occur. Most people do learn to recognize some words in context (such as Ladies/Gents/Exit). People with adequate vision will benefit from visual prompts to clarify meaning, such as daily timetables and pictures used in communication systems. People with a moderate intellectual disability might need lifelong support in managing finances, and planning and organizing their lives and activities (CDDH, 2014) People with moderate level of intellectual disability, their ability to be independent in personal care tasks, such as toilet hygiene, dressing and bathing, will depend on what kind of opportunities do they get to learn and practice with these tasks also depends on their level of cognitive ability, and the presence or absence of other developmental disabilities such as cerebral palsy or any physical disability or any health issues.

According to ICD 10, 2007, individuals with a severe intellectual disability (IQ 20 – 35) or profound intellectual disability (IQ <20), usually recognizes familiar people and has strong relationships with key people in their lives. Most will have little or no speech and will rely on facial expression and body language and gestures to express their needs or feelings and those interacting with and supporting them must be active and keen observers in interpreting changes in a person's behavior. Communication systems for people with severe and profound level of disability generally rely on photographs or objects to facilitate understanding, example a picture of a cup, or the cup itself, may be used in conjunction with the spoken question, "Would you like a drink?" People with severe/profound disabilities will require lifelong assistance in personal care tasks, communication and support in accessing community facilities/ services (CDDH, 2015).

For the management of individuals with intellectual disability expertise training is required in order to know how to manage such individuals. Training should be provided to the facilitators in hospitals, schools, rehabilitation centers in various areas in order to deal with the individuals with intellectual disability. Training in various areas such as:

- Understanding the person's needs and behavior.
- Being non-judgmental and empathetic with the person.
- Ways of communication with the person.
- How to understand their potential and channelized them accordingly.
- How to respond to their emotions.

Expert training can facilitate positive development in the area of intellectual disability. But along with the intensive training for the facilitators to manage people with intellectual disability, awareness about intellectual disability is also important. Providing education and awareness in various parts of our country might help parents to support their child with intellectual disability.

Rehabilitation is one very important spectrum that helps in progress of the individuals with intellectual disability. In a disability report by WHO, 2011, rehabilitation is defined as "a set of measures that assist individuals who experience, or are likely to experience, disability to achieve and maintain optimal functioning in interaction with their environments". Rehabilitation enhances the potential of the individuals with intellectual disability. Rehabilitation also helps in behavioral modification of the people. The enhancement in potential can lead the individual with intellectual disability develop a better picture of their own self in the society with increased self-confidence and an accepting self-image.

Along with managing individuals with intellectual disability, parental stress also needs to be managed so that children with intellectual disability are not hampered due to the stress bust out of parents. Parents having children with intellectual disability needs to be trained not only for how to look after and take care of their child with intellectual disability also for training is required for the parents so that they know how to manage their own stressors. Teaching parents to manage the stressors of their own is important so that their own physical health and mental health is in a good condition which will facilitate them to work for their own child with intellectual disability in a productive manner. On the other hand it will also help the parents not to blame or have stress outburst in front of their child which may lead to deterioration in the child's condition.

There are methods that can be taught to the parents regarding how they can manage their stress for their own good physical health and mental as well as their child's also. The techniques are: firstly for mothers having children with intellectual disability are taught self-help and language skill training. Secondly cognitive training such as cognitive restructuring or enhancing problem solving skills can be taught in order to deal with distortions, misconceptions and unrealistic expectation that contribute to the parental stress in children with intellectual disability. Thirdly relaxation can be taught for self-monitoring of stress and physiological reaction to self. Fourthly cognitive behavioral therapy can be used for parents in order to help them deal with and reduce issues such as self-blame and guilt in parents of children with intellectual disability. Cognitive behavioral techniques such as coping, communicating, problem solving skills can be taught. Such methods can help parents of children with intellectual disability in managing with the stressors and prevention in deteriorating the condition of their own physical and mental health as well as of their child. Singer et al. (2007) carried out a systematic review and meta-analysis of the impact of various interventions on parental distress (depression and related variables) even when the primary focus of the intervention may not have been stress reduction (i.e., behavioral parent training). Seventeen studies were included in the review, and results showed that cognitive behavioral interventions (CBT), behavioral parent training, and multi-component interventions all reduced parental distress. Larger reductions in distress were found for multi-component interventions (e.g., parent training, plus CBT, plus case management and/or respite care). However, only five studies included comparison against an active control intervention or an attention control condition. Given the lack of resources available to support families in several contexts (e.g., rural communities, low and middle income countries), parent-to-parent support models (parents trained to offer psychological/counseling support to other parents) are especially interesting. In a randomized waiting list control design effectiveness study (i.e., focused on support groups already established), Singer et al. (1999) found that those parents receiving support reported increased family strength and more progress towards meeting their current needs.

Teaching the care givers the ability to cope up with their stressors and awareness regarding the needs and basic understanding for the individuals can be done by arranging mental health programs in both urban and rural areas of the country, programs in schools and educational institute will also help develop understanding the concept and have a better outlook for the individuals with intellectual disability. Posters and useful advertisements regarding where and how facilities for the individuals with intellectual disability is available can help the parents as well as the individual for wellbeing in future. (WHO, 2003). Psychoeducation is one very important spectrum that the health care facilitators need to provide to the parents and caregivers of the person with intellectual disability. This will facilitate the parents and the caregivers to focus on every concern areas for the person with intellectual disability so as to have a smoother life ahead with the person and managing the issues related to the disability.

Education and awareness will not any facilitate the immediate members of the individual with intellectual disability but also will lead to change in attitude and mind set of the society towards the intellectual deficient people. The more understanding, acceptance and change in attitude will bring progress in our country as well.

CONCLUSION

In developing countries, for future improvement and development, individuals with intellectual disability should be provide with proper health and skill training facilities starting from the early age. Programs for educating intellectually disabled individual regarding the society and its needs and norms along with awareness about substance use and abuse and sexual exploitation should be arranged so that, this particular lot is not exploited and misused.

Awareness programs for parents and immediate family members should be provided regarding the issues and difficulties faced by the disabled person. Family members should also be educated regarding expressed emotions towards the individual with intellectual disability. Parents especially, should be trained to motivate and train individuals with intellectual disability for basic skill learning and if possible educate the disabled individuals till the grade they can cope up with.

Society also needs to be made aware about the issues and difficulties that the individuals with intellectual disability face so that the society can accept them socially. Societal acceptance could provide motivation and mental support to the individuals with intellectual disability.

People working in health, education and rehabilitation sector should be trained so that they know how to manage individuals with intellectual disability. Disabled individual usually have difficulty in communicating their needs and requirement and expressing their emotions in socially accepted way. Therefore training the people and parents in such areas would make the relation smoother between them.

Providing legal and economic rights to the individuals with intellectual disability gives them independence and free from exploitation and importantly provides support when family members are not present. Constitution provides them with rights to be the part of the society but the society either do not accept them or misuses the rights. Our aim should be to equip the individuals sufficiently so that they are able to survive along with the acceptance of the existing society

The issues concerned do come in various ranges on the basis of the categories but the responsibility doesn't just end here after discussing the concerned issues regarding the individuals with intellectual disability. India as a developing country needs to put immense effort for the individuals with intellectual disability. Future research should build on this foundation of the primary need from spreading awareness, where the care givers and family members are empowered to use the constitutional rights given to the people with mental retardation. A lot has been talked about their vocation needs but employment is still an issue future researches should emphasis on the available opportunities for people with mental retardation. India is a country where discussion of sexual needs is a taboo but it leads to the abuse of the people with mental retardation. Hence it is an important area which is worthy of future exploration in order to sustain their life with harmony.

REFERENCES

Abidi, J. (1999). Current status of employment of disabled people in Indian industries. *Asia Pacific Disability Rehabilitation Journal*, *10*(2).

Ahuja, N. (2007). *Short Text Book of Psychiatry*. Academic Press.

American Association on Intellectual Developmental Disabilities. (2010). *Intellectual disability: Definition, classification, and systems of supports*. Washington, DC: AAIDD.

American Psychiatric Association. (2013). *Diagnostic and statistical manual of mental disorders* (5th ed.). Washington, DC: APA.

American Psychological Association. (2015). Diagnostic and Statistical Manual of Mental Disorder: Publication manual of the American Psychological Association (5th ed.). Washington, DC: Author.

Barker, E. T., Greenberg, J. S., Seltzer, M. M., & Almeida, D. M. (2012). Daily Stress and Cortisol Patterns in Parents of Adult Children with a Serious Mental Illness. *Journal of Health Psychology*, *31*(1), 130–134. doi:10.1037/a0025325 PMID:21895369

Bhat, A.M., Sharma, V. & Jena, S.P. (2013). Managing stress in parents of children with intellectual disability. *Indian Journal of Health and Well-Being, 4*(9), 1790-1793.

Bouras, N., & Holt, G. (2007). *Psychiatric and behavioural disorders in developmental disabilities and mental retardation*. Cambridge, UK: Cambridge University Press.

Boyle, C.A. & Lary, J.M. (1996). Prevalence of selected developmental disabilities in children 3-10 years of age: The Metropolitan Atlanta Developmental Disabilities Surveillance Program, 1991. *Morbidity and Mortality Weekly Report.*

Breslau, N., Staruch, K. S., & Mortimer, E. A. (1982). Psychological distress in mothers of disabled children. *American Journal of Diseases of Children*, *136*, 682–686. PMID:6213143

Brown & Randel. (1997). *The Individual with Intellectual Disabilities and Sex Education: Perspectives of Involved Adults.* Presented at the *7th Annual Meeting of the International Society for the Study of Human Subjectivity*, Columbia.

Camp, B. W., Broman, S. H., Nichols, P. L., & Leff, M. (1998). Maternal and neonatal risk factors for mental retardation: Defining the "at-risk" child. *Early Human Development*, *50*(2), 159–173. doi:10.1016/S0378-3732(97)00034-9 PMID:9483389

Coffee, B., Keith, K., Albizua, I., Malone, T., Jowrey, J., Sherman, L., & Warren, T. (2009). Incidence of fragile X syndrome by newborn screening for methylated FMR1 DNA. *American Journal of Human Genetics*, *85*(4), 503–514. doi:10.1016/j.ajhg.2009.09.007 PMID:19804849

Diekema, D. (2003). Involuntary sterilization of persons with mental retardation: Ethical analysis. *Mental Retardation and Developmental Disabilities Research Reviews*, *9*(1), 21–26. doi:10.1002/mrdd.10053 PMID:12587134

Durkin, M., Schupf, N., Stein, Z., & Susser, M. (2007). Mental retardation. Stamford, CT: Appleton & Lange.

Employment of Persons with Disabilities in Public Sectors in India -Emerging Issues and Trends. (1995). *An Evaluation Study with Special Reference to Persons with Disabilities Act*. Commissioned by Planning Commission, Government of India.

Fletcher, J., Loschen, E., Stavrakaki, C., & First, M. (2007). *Diagnostic manual-intellectual disability: A textbook of diagnosis of mental disorders in persons with intellectual disability*. Kingston, NY: NADD.

Gillberg, C., Persson, E., Grufman, M., & Themner, U. (1986). Psychiatric disorders in mildly and severely mentally retarded urban children and adolescents: Epidemiological aspects. *The British Journal of Psychiatry, 149*(1), 68–74. doi:10.1192/bjp.149.1.68 PMID:2946351

Gold, M. W. (1972). stimulus factors in skill training of retarded adolescents on a complex assembly task: Acquisition, transfer, and relation. *American Journal of Mental Deficiency, 76*, 517–526. PMID:5012132

Green, S., & Bake, B. (2011). Parents emotion expression as a predictor of child's social competence: Children with or without intellectual disability. *Journal of Intellectual Disability Research, 55*(3), 324–338. doi:10.1111/j.1365-2788.2010.01363.x PMID:21241394

Groce, N., Gazizova, D., & Hassiotis, P. (2014). Forced Marriage among Persons with Intellectual Disability. *Journal of Intellectual Disabilities.*

Gupta, V.B., Mehrotra, P. & Mehrotra, N (2012). *Parental Stress in Raising a Child with Disabilities in India*. Academic Press.

Gustafsson, C. (2003). *Intellectual disability and mental health problems: Evaluation of two clinical assessment instruments, occurrence of mental health problems and psychiatric care utilization.* Retrieved from: https://uu.divaportal.org/smash/get/diva2:163146

Hassall, R., Rose, J., & McDonald, J. (2015). Parenting stress in mothers of children with an intellectual disability: The effects of parental cognitions in relation to child characteristics and family support. *Journal of Intellectual Disabilities, 49*(6), 405–418. doi:10.1111/j.1365-2788.2005.00673.x PMID:15882391

Heller, T. (2010). Age-related Health Issues in People with Intellectual Disability. *Impact, 23*(1).

Henny, M. J., Schrojenstein, L. V., & Walsh, P. N. (2008). Managing Health Problems in People with Intellectual Disabilities. *British Medical Journal, 337*, 1408–1412. PMID:19064601

Jencks, C., & Phillips, M. (1998). The Black-White Test Scope Gap: Why It Persists and What Can Be Done. *The Brookings Review, 16*(2), 24–27. doi:10.2307/20080778

Khare, S. (2015). Impact of quality of life in parents of mentally retarded children: Research findings in a regional centre. *Innovation Journal of Nursing and Healthcare, 1*(3), 171-178.

Lemay, J. F., Herbert, A. R., Dewey, D. M., & Micheil, A. I. (2003). A rational approach to the child with mental retardation for the paediatrician. *Journal of Paediatrics and Child Health, 8*(6), 345–356. doi:10.1093/pch/8.6.345 PMID:20052328

Maulik, P. K., Mascarenhas, M. N., Mathers, C. D., Dua, T., & Saxena, S. (2011). Prevalence of intellectual disability: A meta-analysis of population-based studies. *Research in Developmental Disabilities, 32*(2), 419–436. doi:10.1016/j.ridd.2010.12.018 PMID:21236634

Morisse, F., Vandemaele, E., Claes, C., Claes, L., & Vandevelde, S. (2013). Quality of Life in Persons with Intellectual Disabilities and Mental Health Problems: An Explorative Study. *The Scientific World Journal*, 8.

Murthy, R. S. (2010). *Mental Health Care in India –Past*. Present and Future.

Myers, J. S. (1962). Education and Rehabilitation. *Journal of Education, 145*, 1, 3–34.

Nambi, S. (2005). Marriage, Mental health and the Indian legislation. *Indian Journal of Psychiatry, 47*(1), 3–14. doi:10.4103/0019-5545.46067

Narayan, J., & Kurani, D.R. (1990). *Vocational training and employment of persons with mental retardation.* Academic Press.

National Legal Services Authority. (2010). *Legal services to the mentally ill persons and persons with mental disabilities: Scheme Sheet.* Author.

Navas, P., Verdugo, M. A., Gómez, L. E., & Schalock, R. L. (2012). The concept of quality of life and its role in enhancing human rights in the field of intellectual disability. *Journal of Intellectual Disability Research, 56*(11), 1036–1045. doi:10.1111/j.1365-2788.2012.01585.x PMID:22672317

Paransky, O., & Zurawin, R. (2003). Management of menstrual problems and contraception in adolescents with mental retardation: A medical, legal and ethical review with new suggested guidelines. *Journal of Pediatric and Adolescent Gynecology, 16*(4), 223–235. doi:10.1016/S1083-3188(03)00125-6 PMID:14550386

Peshawaria, R., Menon,, D.K., Ganguly, R., & Roy, S., RajanPillay, P.R.S., & Gupta, A. (1998). A study offacilitators and inhibitors that affect coping in parents of children with mental retardation in India. *Asia Pacific Disability Rehabilitation Journal, 9*(1).

Peshawaria, R., Menon, D.K., Ganguly, R., Roy, S., Rajan Pillay, P.R.S., Gupta, A., Kumar V, Giri, R.S., & Ayub, L. (1995). *Understanding Indian Families, having persons with mental retardation.* Academic Press.

Population Census. (2011). Retrieved from: www.census2011.co.in/disability.php1802-2019

Quality of life of young people with an intellect disability in Ireland: Interim Report. (2003). Retrieved from: https:// www.fedvol.ie

Rohwerder, B. (2018). *Disability stigma in developing countries.* Institute of Development Studies.

Rutter, M., Graham, J., & Yule, W. (1970). *A neuropsychiatric study in childhood.* London: Heinemann Medical Books.

Ryckman, D. B., & Henderson, R. S. (1965). The meaning of a retarded child for his parents—A focus for counsellors. *Journal of Mental Retardation., 3*(4). PMID:14342622

Sexuality and Disability in the Indian Context. (2010). TARSHI.

Sheridan, J., & Scior, K. (2013). Attitudes towards people with intellectual disabilities: A comparison of young people from British South Asian and White British backgrounds. *Research in Developmental Disabilities, 34*(4), 1240–1247. doi:10.1016/j.ridd.2012.12.017 PMID:23417129

Singer, G. H. S., Ethridge, B. L., & Aldana, S. I. (2007). Primary and secondary effects of parenting and stress management interventions for parents of children with developmental disabilities: A meta-analysis. *Mental Retardation and Developmental Disabilities Research Reviews, 13*(4), 357–367. doi:10.1002/mrdd.20175 PMID:17979202

Singer, G. H. S., Marquis, J., Powers, L. K., Blanchard, L., Divenere, N., Santelli, B., ... Sharp, M. (1999). A multi-site evaluation of Parent to Parent programs for parents of children with disabilities. *Journal of Early Intervention, 22*, 217–229. doi:10.1177/105381519902200305

Siperstein, G. N., KeerthiSugumaran, D., Bardon, J.N., & Parker, R.C. (n.d.). *Attitudes of the Public in India towards People with Intellectual Disabilities*. Retrieved from: https://www.media.specialolympics.org

Strydom, A., Haveman, M., Heller, T., Lee, L., Maaskant, M., & Shooshtari, S. (n.d.). *Major Health Risks in Aging Persons With Intellectual Disabilities: An Overview of Recent Studies.* . doi:10.1111 /j.1741-1130.2010.00248

The Centre for Developmental Disability Health Victoria (CDDH). (2015). *Working with people with intellectual disabilities in healthcare settings: Fact Sheet.* Retrieved from: www.cddh.monash.org

Tracy, J., & McDonald, R. (2015). Health and Disability: Partnerships in Health care. *Journal of Applied Research in Intellectual Disabilities, 28*(1), 22–32. doi:10.1111/jar.12135 PMID:25530571

Violence against Disabled Children: A summary report. (2005, July 28). UNICEF at the United Nations.

Vissers, L., Gilissen, C., & Joris, A. (2016). Genetic studies in intellectual disability and related disorders. *Nature Reviews. Genetics, 17*(1), 9–18. doi:10.1038/nrg3999 PMID:26503795

Walker-Hirsch, L. (2007). *The Facts of Life...and More Sexuality and Intimacy for People with Intellectual Disabilities.* Brookes Publishing Co.

World Health Organisation. (2003). *Caring for children and adolescents with mental disorders.* WHO.

World Health Organisation. (2007). International Classification Diseases (10th ed.). Geneva: WHO.

World Health Organisation. (2009a). *Mental health aspects of women's reproductive health. A global review of literature.* WHO.

World Health Organisation. (2009b). *Promoting Sexual and Reproductive Health for People with Disabilities.* WHO.

World Health Organization. (2000). Ageing and Intellectual Disabilities - Improving Longevity and Promoting Healthy Ageing: Summative Report. Geneva, Switzerland: WHO.

World Health Organization. (2011). *Rehabilitation. World report on disability.* WHO.

Chapter 10
Awareness Towards Intervention for Individuals With Intellectual Disability

Palak Upadhyay
Dayanand Medical College and Hospital (DMC&H), India

Jyoti Mishra
GMCH 32, India

ABSTRACT

Intellectual disability is sub-average intellectual functioning with impaired adaptive functioning. The limitations in their adaptive skill hampers the ability to cope with stressful life events. There are many issues which require attention while dealing with them like parental level, peer groups, schools, presence of comorbid conditions, etc. Interventions at right stage under efficient supervision can lead to healthy and smooth functioning of cases with ID and with good outcomes. Difficulties like lack of human resources, quality training of clinical psychologists in India, scarcity of effective clinical guidelines, conflicts among the team approach, acceptance in the family and society requires attention in current scenario. There are many things that can be offered but what we need is their acceptance in our society and awareness towards Intervention. This chapter aims at acknowledging these issues to create awareness amongst the responsible caregivers. Timely recognition of treatable causes of intellectual disability can be very rewarding and prevent a lifelong disability.

INTRODUCTION

In the prehistoric period, individuals with intellectual disability (then known as 'feeble mindedness'), was posed by an advocate W.E. Fernald as 'a section who lived happily in institutions and got segregated from mainstream society; hence, what else they look or want'. This perspective further took various folds in terms of being sensitive and providing much deserved helping approach to this section. The World Health Organization defines Disability as "an umbrella term, covering impairments, activity limitations,

DOI: 10.4018/978-1-7998-1223-4.ch010

and participation restrictions." Impairment is a problem in body function or structure; activity limitation is a difficulty encountered by an individual in executing a task or action; participation restriction is a problem experienced by an individual in involvement in life situations. Thus disability is a complex phenomenon, reflecting an interaction between features of a person's body and features of the society in which she or he lives. Intellectual disability (ID) means disability in the cognitive capacity of an individual. Although there is a great variability in development, there are earlier and a later limit to what is considered 'normal/ typical' development. Statistically, children with intellectual disability are those who develop at a rate significantly below average-the lowest 3% on the normal, bell-shaped curve distribution- indicating why ID is called a "developmental disability". In simple terms, whatever a mentally normal child can do within a particular frame of time the mentally sub-normal child is either unable to do or will take longer period of time to complete. The learning of particular skill will also depend upon the complexity of the task or on the rate of learning. The delay of learning also depends upon the severity of intellectual disability. It is very obvious and natural that the parents of developmentally disabled child will wonder what will be the future of their child. Will she / he be normal? Will she / he be able to get job? Will the child be able to live independently? Will the child be accepted in the society and family? These are the few questions which will haunt the society in general and the caregivers in particular and thus awareness towards intervention is required for better outcome.

Intellectual disability can be defined as impairments of general mental abilities that impact adaptive functioning in three domains, or areas. These domains determine how well an individual copes with everyday tasks:

- The conceptual domain includes skills in language, reading, writing, math, reasoning, knowledge, and memory.
- The social domain refers to empathy, social judgment, interpersonal communication skills, the ability to make and retain friendships, and similar capacities.
- The practical domain centres on self-management in areas such as personal care, job responsibilities, money management, recreation, and organizing school and work tasks.

These mental abilities are measured by Intelligence Quotient (IQ) tests. A score of two standard deviations below average represents significant cognitive deficit and would occur in about 2.5% of total population signifying that 97.5% of people of the same age and culture would score higher. The test used to measure IQ must be standardised and culturally acceptable. Intelletual Disability is defined at an IQ score of 70 or below. (DSM-5, APA, 2013).

It has been estimated that individuals with intellectual disability comprise from 1 percent – 3 percent of populations around the world. (WHO, 2001). The total number of disabled people in India are 26 million out of which 1.5 million have intellectual disability (Indian Census, 2011). A census reported by American bureau in the year 2015 that prevalence of receipt of special education services for ID in United States has declined from 2004 to 2012 after which they aggressively started to plan and execute schemes for this population (U.S.census bureau, 2015). IDs can be mild or more severe. Children with more severe forms typically require more support–particularly in school. Children with milder IDs can gain some independent skills, especially in communities with good teaching and support. Since, this disability demarcates such people from the normal individuals of the society they face various problems throughout their life due to stigma and discrimination. They don't get proper education, they require supervision, they cannot do job; they are isolated by the peer groups society.

In the medical model for definition of disability, individuals with certain physical, intellectual, psychological and mental impairments are taken as disabled. According to this, disability lies in the individual as it is equated with restrictions of activity with the burden of adjusting with environment through cures, treatment and rehabilitation. In contrast in the social model the focus is on the society, which imposes undue restrictions on the behaviour of individuals with impairment. In this, disability does not lie in individuals, but in the interaction between individuals and the society. The transition from an individual, medical perspective to a structural, social perspective has been described as the shift from a "medical model" to a "social model" in which people are viewed as being disabled by society rather than by their bodies. (WHO, 2011)

It is very unfortunate that the condition of the intellectually disabled population is very poor in India. In the Western countries the government has taken the responsibility of the mentally disabled population but in India the responsibility of those children is solely with the parents who do not have any other form of support whatsoever. Though the government has planed various schemes for this special population but majority of the population is unaware about these benefits and special schemes. Another important area of discussion is that, the benefit for the special population depends upon the level of severity of disability. To avail the benefits, the disability should be more than 40%. The question arises: What if the disability is less than 40%? Are they functionally maintaining so well that they are equivalent to normal population? They will face the same discrimination and isolation from society as other population of more than 40% disability faces.

Overall, this population including all categories of intellectual disability require special attention in all the aspects of their life from the family and society as a whole because their functional level also depends upon how others are responding to their disability. The fact cannot be denied that despite their limited intellectual capacity they have the ability to express their emotions, their needs and expectation from others. Notwithstanding the above facts our society becomes ignorant to them and to their existence. In many rural areas, this section has not been able to get the proper services regarding their diagnosis. Assessing individuals with ID requires precision and clinical acumen. Primary care givers in rural areas of India find it difficult to seek help from a professional which in turn helps in improving the condition of the client and care giver both. Thus apart from the behavioural management, it is also very important to be aware of other aspects of their life, be it education, parenting, life style, job perspectives and social life. The following paragraphs will throw light on various individuals, institutions and organizations that play significant role in the life of individuals with intellectual disability, the obstacles that they are facing and the recommendations which can help improve their overall outcome.

Awareness for Parents

A child is the most important part in parent's life. When parents come to know about the arrival of a new member in their life they start dreaming about the future and healthy life of the child. However this dream shatters when they become aware about the intellectual disability of the child. Parents are often the first to notice that the child is having some problem. Initially there comes the phase of denial when it is very difficult for the parents to accept the bitter truth. They try to ignore the truth and convince themselves that it is not true and this just cannot happen to their children. However with time, they gradually come to terms with the bitter truth about their child being intellectually disabled and then start asking themselves: Why me? Why my child? Then they start blaming themselves for being responsible for their child's mental condition. Slowly they accept the fact. The important part is whether the acceptance is positive or negative? If it is a positive acceptance than it becomes very healthy for the parents to cope with the unpleasant situation. However, if the acceptance is negative then the situation becomes very adverse. Sad part of the story is that fathers hardly play a role and mostly blame mothers for being responsible for the mental condition of their children. It is a common scene in psychiatry and psychology clinics that mostly the disabled child is accompanied by mother only. Is she the only person in the family who is responsible for the child? Everyone can be careless towards the intellectually sub-average child but a mother cannot. It was reported in a study mothers of developmentally delayed children reported that their infants presented substantial parenting difficulties, but at the same time, self-reports of stress associated with parenting were not different from normative levels (Moran, Pederson, Pettit, & Krupka, 1922). Many times both parents are equally worried and tensed about their kids and they take it as a joint responsibility. In a study it was seen tha parents of children with developmental delays experienced greater levels of stress, and had children with higher maladaptive behaviour than children without delays. Despite differences in reported stress, parents of children with delays were using similar amounts and styles of coping as parents of children without delays (Lopez, Clifford, Minnes, & Kuntz, 2008).

As we know that intellectual disability requires continuous training and supervision. Individuals with ID may experience challenges in acquiring the skills necessary for independent living and achieving success in postsecondary education/training programs, employment settings, and social situations. Parents often lack patience, want immediate and permanent cure. When they fail to achieve the results they lose their patience and because of that they frequently change their doctors. At the end they lose their hope of improvement. In such cases assurance, proper and planned management becomes very essential as parents are the most important participators in therapy as they hold the most knowledge about their child. They are the one who spend most of their time with the child, much more than a therapist can spend. Parents become the best doctor available for the child. Targeting them for the behavioural management can result in significant improvement in the child. With proper parental counselling the therapist should make them aware that though they can take second or multiple opinions, there is no need to frequently change doctors. Parents must be counselled that though it is not a completely reversible condition, they must move ahead with positive hope. They must be explained that changes would be slow. Proper awareness training program, psycho-education and parental counselling plays a very important role.

It is natural for parents to wonder what the future will hold for their child. Will the child be able to obtain a job and will she/he be able to live independently? In the early years of life, it is often impossible to answer these questions. It is important to remain optimistic about the child's progress, yet realistic when the problems are severe. This is often a difficult balance to achieve. All children, however, continue to learn and as adults they will also continue to develop new skills. Each new learned skill contributes to the growing child's scope for functionality and participation and contribution in society. It is very important to celebrate the child's achievements throughout their life. If the parents have any concerns, they must have authentic institutions/professionals with whom they can feel free to discuss core issues concerning the child's care. Parents often report feeling of loneliness and isolation and have a notion that others will not understand what they are going through. Families often find it very helpful if they find another family having a similarly affected member who are going through, or have been through, similar experiences. Parents report that other parents have been their best source of information and support.

Another important point while counselling of parents is that both the parents should be present in the session. The counselling should first focus on how to make the parents positively accept their child's mental condition. Only then would they work together towards the betterment of the child with optimistic state of mind. Sometimes it so happens that one parent gives up hope. This is the crucial period when the other parent becomes a strong and positive support and makes other more hopeful towards the child. In parenting sessions it is very important to tell the parents to have patience and to emphasize that there would be no dramatic sudden changes. The effort has to be continuous and sustained to see positive results. It is very important to know that parental counselling should not only be restricted to the parents of the affected child. At community level through the help of media, awareness should be spread among all families, even those who do not have affected children at their home. All this to reemphasize those children with ID have equal rights as their own children. They should not be discriminated on any ground and not treated as untouchables. The parents must also fight for their child's right. Parents can be the best doctor for their intellectually disabled child with the support of good professional guidance.

Awareness for Comorbid Conditions

Special guidance should be given to parents or caregivers regarding the proper assessment and management of other comorbid conditions like hearing difficulty or visual problem, behaviour problem, self injurious behaviour (SIB) etc. Care givers often assume that the patient lacks eye contact (as in case of autism) when they might be looking slightly off-axis due to some visual difficulty (Kiani & Miller, 2010). Therefore, helping the client with assessment of other conditions related to speech, language, hearing or visual difficulty is required at early stage would be beneficial. Family members find it difficult to look beyond their cognitive impairment. All such areas are left out while parents are struggling hard to meet daily needs of an individual with ID. For SIB, proper therapeutic management like behaviour therapy is required because it is often ignored or is left untreated. Other conditions like physical deformity (if any) or episodes of seizure (epilepsy) are also very commonly found in such cases. Early assessment and suitable interventions regarding all these comorbid conditions must be readily available within reach.

Role of Siblings

Siblings can play a crucial role in improving the quality of life for people with ID. A study has revealed that a significant support role is carried out by the siblings for individuals with ID when their parents are no longer able to do so (Griffiths & Unger, 1994). Often such tasks like helping in household tasks, basic financial management, vocational training and social life skills can be taught by siblings in absence of parents (Heller & Caldwell, 2006). Stewart et al. (2001) revealed that relationship among siblings are more positive and they grow closer as they become older. There is a significant role of gender differences among siblings in providing care and support to this population. Since sisters easily initiate, healthily maintain the contacts and offer support to their siblings in comparison to brothers (White & Riedmann, 1992), therefore adult sisters can be of great help in rearing up such cases. Also a study held in 2002 by Erikson & Gerstel found men are less likely to help siblings with cleaning, doing laundry, making meals than women. A child would automatically pick up the repeated behaviour done by his sibling as every behaviour theory explains that every behaviour is learned. Social skills training via role playing with the help of siblings can yield fruitful results regarding improving the quality of life in cases with ID.

Awareness for Extended Family Members

The closely knit kinship systems in India have always cared for their members with intellectual disability. Institutionalisation, unlike in the West, has never been a major movement in India and a very small proportion of the population with intellectual disability lives away from home. Families generally take care of their needy relatives with compassion, because of a sense of duty. This does not mean that they do not suffer; studies have demonstrated that families experience high levels of stress because of the care burden upon family members, especially mothers (Girimaji et al, 1999). The term extended family is frequently used to describe a household in which parents and children live with close relatives or with whom the family has regular contact. These individuals may include grandparents, uncles, aunts and cousins. India is a country where large number of people lives together under a single roof. They share common rules, cultures and beliefs. The decision of the family related issues are taken together and mainly by the elders in the family and everyone is bound to follow the order or decision. In such families once the news of a child being mentally challenged is disclosed, there is huge emotional outburst. If grandparents and other members of the extended family show positive understanding and offer emotional support may positively impact the struggling mother and father. If grandparents and other members are critical and non-responsive, they may add to the parents' suffering and worsen the already existing challenging situation. This becomes a very big burden on the family. They blame the already depressed parents. The other children of the family ignore the affected child and also avoid playing with them. It is very sad that the parents of the developmentally disabled child are often isolated by their own family members, the reason being social status, stigma and fear of social rejection. If this would be the attitude of immediate family members then it would be farfetched to think about social acceptance of the child and parents. In a study it was seen that having a child with an intellectual disability can impose financial, social and physical stress on the family (Mak & Ho, 2007). Research also has shown that caregivers of children with disabilities experience greater stress than caregivers of children without disabilities (Hassall, Rose, & McDonald, 2005). If these initial obstacles are so difficult to overcome then it would be difficult to expect positive growth in the affected child. Thus talking about the intervention of the children with intellectual disability, the role of extended family and their impact becomes an important issue to deal with. It is difficult to expect all the members of the extended family to be there in the therapy sessions. In such cases, the head of the family should come for few sessions with the treating specialist so that she/he is made aware about the child's condition and make the significant and positive changes in the family in favour of mentally challenged child.

The extended family may perform many parental roles/duties. Cousins may be as close as siblings. Sometimes the proximity of the extended family may create problem for parents. For example, presence of extended family puts pressure on the other members to compare themselves to their relatives. The mother of the child with a disability who is surrounded by sisters, sister-in-law, mother-in-law and cousins whose children do not have disabilities may become upset by the constant reminder of her child being different from others. They sometimes intrude significantly in their personal affairs. Interestingly, many children with disability live with their grandparents who are their primary caregivers. These grandparents struggle with many of the same issues and challenges as other parents, including, depression, stress and other financial issues.

Proper awareness and training must be imparted to the extended members of the family. An endeavour must be made by the immediate family members to provide support, involvement, creating non discriminative environment and avoiding the feeling that the condition is a social stigma and against their social status. They should understand that this can happen to anyone. They may also provide financial support to the parents in terms of their child's special need and long term support. On the positive note, grandparents and other family members may contribute a great deal to the primary family unit and can increase its overall happiness.

Extended family has become a very important part in influencing intellectually disabled children and their parents. It has both positive as well as negative effect. Spreading awareness among them about ID and how their positive attitude, perception and emotional support can help the parents and affected children in coping with the conditions is important.

A special need and care is required for elderly population with ID. They appear to be burden in the families. They should be assessed well and tailor-made therapeutic plan should be framed for them. Family members should be counselled/ informed regarding their management plan. Excessive noise in the surroundings might lead to poor sleep, agitation, fearfulness, reduced ability to perform task properly (Wiese, 2018). One should foster their condition by making their locomotion smooth with oak wood surfaces and well illuminated surroundings which would have a positive effect in increasing the elderly individual's interaction with surroundings.

Awareness for Society

Human being is a social animal. Society has particular rules and norms and any deviance from that makes a human different from others and the society labels her/him as abnormal or insane. In this case it becomes very challenging for both the family as well as the mentally sub-normal individuals to live as per their expectations. Families of developmentally disabled population face various problems in their day to day activities no matter it is social, professional or personal life. No school is ready to take their children for education. Either no or very few number of organizations are there for their training, that too they teach for very few hours and charge enormous amount of money. The mentally challenged children are ignored by their peer groups and often bullied and looked down upon by the so called normal people. In such situations those children who are towards the higher functioning spectrum of the mental retardation category feel inferior. It is very surprising and really a matter of concern that even in educated societies, social marginalisation and exclusion of the mentally challenged children's families from social gathering is very common. They think that letting their children play with the intellectually challenged children will affect them adversely. It is very sad that the fear of acceptance in the society puts the families and care takers of ID population under immense pressure and it become a social stigma. Even the mentally normal siblings of the mentally challenged people have difficulty in getting married because of the social stigma attached with being a member of an affected family. Many families sometimes hide the fact that they have mentally challenged member in their family. They do not let the child go out from home and often they chain them in the home because of the social pressure. In India, women and girls face multiple forms of discrimination based on their gender, age, marital status, caste, tribe, and disability. Women with psychosocial or intellectual disabilities are among the most stigmatized and marginalized, and discrimination is done in every sphere of life whether personal or professional. A study in four districts of Gujarat found that people with disabilities were discouraged from attending weddings (UNNATI, 2004). Another study by Mohapatra and Mohanty (2004) in Orissa found that only 27 percent of women with intellectual disabilities leave their homes and 19 percent take part in social activities. Furthermore, only about one-third of women and girls interviewed had ever attended school prior to being admitted to institutions. Such negative attitudes towards women sideline them, preventing them from performing any of their societal roles to their full capacity and send them to social invisibility. If this would continue to be the condition of the developmentally disabled population then the future of this special population definitely looks very gloomy. In a national survey regarding hygiene (2013), it was revealed that females with ID were found in very poor conditions while they were menstruating and reason behind was that it brings double fold shame to the family. Society needs to accept the monthly cycle concept which can even exist with females with ID. They also need to be cared and trained well to maintain hygiene as a normal female is taught around her menarche.

Even in today's modern day society, because of the lack of understanding of intellectual disability and many misconceptions associated with such people, especially in rural areas, many people believe that intellectual disabilities are a result of past sins, a curse, or possession by a spirit. Worst part of the story is that many a times even the parents think that they would have done something bad in the past. In India, many parents of affected children come to the doctor as a last resort for their child's treatment. For them the role of the faith healers is more important than the mental health professionals because in India religion plays a very important role and it has a very significant impact on the thinking process of people. Interestingly, many of the faith healers are aware of the illness and retardation but they don't refer the case to the doctors. So, there should be a liaison between the faith healers/religious teachers and mental health professionals. Proper awareness should be given to the healers about symptoms and identification of the intellectual disability, so that they refer the cases directly to the professionals. For each proper timely referral they may be paid some remuneration or honorarium.

The society plays a very important role in an individual's life. So, it is society's duty to treat the ID population as an inseparable part of the society and not outcast the family of the intellectually disabled. Social awareness of intellectual disability is very essential and makes them aware that this is not a disease and anyone from the population can be affected by this. There are various causes of developmental disability and social involvement with others has nothing to do with this. There should be proper awareness programme on the community level. This can be done through organisation of plays and making the people, especially the youth of the country aware about intellectual disability. Acceptance of ID population as an inseparable part of the society will itself solve a lot many problems and will ease out much pressure from the families of children affected with ID.

Awareness for School Management

School is a primary institution of education. It gives hope and direction to the future of the students and the nation. However, providing education to intellectually disabled population in Indian society becomes difficult where social exclusion, stigma and discrimination of this affected population is very significant. Despite its importance, educational outcomes for children and adults with intellectual disabilities remain very poor. The current methods for getting admissions in normal schools show a very sad state of affairs. There is cut throat competition even at nursery level. There is a huge struggle among students for percentage. The higher the percentage of students, the higher chance of getting admission in school and also there are cases of bribery and donations to ensure seat in schools. In this race somewhere the disabled child is nowhere to be seen and is neglected. Neither can they vouch for higher percentages nor in most cases are the parents rich enough to give donations or huge admission charges. Though as per the government law disabled population have the right to get education in normal schools but no school is ready to take the intellectually disabled child in their schools. The head of such institutions think that having such children will affect other children in a negative manner. If this is the thinking of the so called intellectuals in a society then the future of education of ID children is bleak. This discrimination for education makes the disabled child more disabled and more dependent on their family. Education is the only source for better job and future. Education is recognized as a basic human right. The negligence from the normal schools gave rise to the NGO's to start special education program for disabled population. The knowledge and process of educating the disabled children or 'special education' as it is known now, came to India in the last two decades of the 19th century. Special education enables the teachers to focus on the needs of disabled children and these special schools are equipped with the resources that are required as per the needs of the disabled children. However, the major problems of these special schools are that they are very less in numbers in comparison to the intellectually disabled population. In addition to that, the resources such as funding for such organisations and special educators are also very few in numbers.

Another concern for parents is regarding the level of severity of intellectual disability. In the special school, the entire mental retardation category (mild, moderate, severe and profound mental retardation) study and get training together. Often grouping the categories together creates chaos in the training process. The mentally disabled children have different abilities and strengths as per the level of severity or mental retardation. The training module for mild mental retardation category will differ from the other mental retardation category and it is also very difficult for the special educators to manage all the categories together. This is a genuine concern of the parents. Every special school should have different sections as per the level of severity and as per the level of learning. Making individual category for all the four levels of severity will result in better outcomes in the overall development of affected children. It will also become easy for special educators to handle them without difficulty and make a specific plan for each category separately. Discriminating children on the basis of intellectual capability for imparting education is a crime. School is a place where all the race, religion and caste come together under a single roof without any bias or partiality. The school also should not discriminate children on the basic of their intellectual capabilities. Providing place in the school to the special population will give hope to the parents. The responsibility of the intellectually disabled population is not only of their caretakers and the government; it should be taken by all the members of the society specially the schools because education improves self esteem and makes the life of an individual more independent. The school authority should take this as an opportunity to provide education to intellectually disabled population. Another important step contributing in a big way could be by conducting surveys of school going children to identify children with disabilities to ascertain their specific needs and associated co-morbidities and to look for the extent to which these are being addressed.

A significant role of special educator took place in recent times. Rather than following a common teaching programme; an individualised education programme has taken place. Every special child has his/her separate manual which reflects her limitation and strengths along with all what he has achieved and what is he looking to achieve in future. Special visual aid and hearing aid while teaching can be used for better training in children with ID. A small number of special education teachers work with students with intellectual disability or autism, primarily teaching them life skills and basic literacy. However, the majority of special education teachers work with children with mild to moderate disabilities, using the education curriculum of normal children, or modifying it according to special child's individual needs. An informal functional assessment guide for all disabilities has been developed (NCERT, 1990) for use by teachers. There is no quota yet for persons with intellectual disabilities in government sector but for physically disabled there is 3% reservation. Children with mild to moderate intellectual disabilities could be benefited through courses under Modular Employable Scheme (MES) of the Ministry of Labour, Government of India. Special schools in India provide education up to 18 years, including pre-vocational and vocational training.

Managing school on the administration level and making the classroom free from prejudice and discrimination can open new vistas in planning the intellectually disabled children's future. The government of India recently endorsed the philosophy of inclusive education and has started the 'Education for all 6- to 14-year-olds' programme ('Sarva Shiksha Abhiyan'). This follows a zero-rejection policy, which means that all children – regardless of any type or degree of disability – should receive appropriate education, preferably within regular schools or through education at home from specially trained teachers. This programme has witnessed considerable growth in recent years.

Awareness for Education

A person with intellectual disabilities faces social stigma, bias and unable to exercise their fundamental human rights. Discrimination against people with intellectual disability is intensely rooted, widespread and creating obstacles in the way of positive change in intellectually disabled population. Without adequate education the intellectually disabled person will not be able to secure meaningful employment. If the person is unaware about this fundamental right of getting education, their life will be dependent on others, social exclusion will be there. All this put together will start the never ending vicious cycle of poverty and will add to the woes of already stigmatised and marginalised section of our society.

Education of children with disabilities has been a part of policy developments in India for the past few decades. The Individuals with Disabilities Act, 1995 and the Right to Education Act, 2009 have given a new thrust to the education of children with disabilities, as without including those the objectives of universalization of elementary education cannot be achieved. There are various other plans for supporting education for intellectually disabled population in India. They are as follows

1. Kothari Commission 1964-66,
2. National Policy on Education (NPE) 1986,
3. Centrally Sponsored Scheme of Integrated Education of Disabled Children (IEDC) 1974,
4. Plan of Action (POA) 1992,
5. Rehabilitation Council of India Act (RCI) 1992,
6. Salamanca statement and framework for action 1994,
7. Person with Disability (equal opportunity, production of right and full participation Act) 1995,
8. National Trust Act for the Welfare of individuals with autism, cerebral palsy, mental retardation and multiple disability 1999,
9. Sarva Shiksha Abhiyaan 2000,
10. Comprehensive action plan for inclusion in education of children 2005,
11. National Policy Individuals with Disabilities Act 2006,
12. Right of Children to Free and Compulsory Education Act 2009.

The Government of India's appreciation of the need to integrate children with disabilities came in 1974 when the Union Ministry of Welfare launched the centrally sponsored scheme of Integrated Education of Disabled Children (IEDC). All these acts were made to support education for special population. In 1992 Parliament of India enacted the Rehabilitation Council of India (RCI) Act, subsequently amended in 2000, to establish standardizing courses for the training of 16 categories of professionals required in the field of special education and rehabilitation of individuals with disability. Training of special educators and resource teachers that can offer support services to children with disabilities in regular schools is the responsibility of RCI. Even Plan of Action (POA) 1992 postulated that a child with disability who can be educated in a general school should be educated in a general school only and not in a special school. Even those children who are initially admitted to special schools for training in skills should be transferred to general schools once they acquire daily living skills, communication skills and basic academic skills. It provides educational opportunities for the disabled children in common schools, to facilitate their retention in the school system after they acquire the communication and the daily living skills at the functional level (Mondal & Mete, 2013). The initial focus of community-based rehabilitation (CBR) was on highly 'visible' impairments such as locomotor disability, blindness and deafness. However, within the past two decades intellectual disability has been included on the CBR agenda. The establishment of district disability rehabilitation centres (DDRCs) is one such example.

There is a false notion in society that intellectually disabled population cannot get education because of their poor intellectual capability. The fact is that based on the level of adaptive functioning in three domains: social, conceptual, and practical skills this population has been divided into four categories (ICD-10, 1992);

1. Mild mental retardation,
2. Moderate mental retardation,
3. Severe mental retardation,
4. Profound mental retardation.

The first mild mental retardation category has the ability to get primary education. Children falling in the category of moderate mental retardation can be trained in specific tasks like working in grocery stores, ration stores, stationery shops for helping the main shopkeeper, various housekeeping tasks like cleaning rooms, looking after hygiene and sanitation of an institute under someone's supervision. Their services can be utilised at airports and railway stations for helping passengers in loading and unloading of luggage.

The severe mental retardation category can do some work by prompting and supervision. Only the last category that is profound mental retardation needs lifelong support and care, however with some behaviour modification training and self help skill training they can learn many things of their day to day activities.

The question which arises is there enough number of institutions which are required for providing basic education and training to this group of people in India? The intellectually disabled population are spread all across the sub continent be it rural, semi-urban or urban but the special schools who teach these children are minuscule in number and that too only present in the metros. They charge huge money from the caretakers. Where would the poor and rural population go? It is a very sad state of affairs that only a very limited portion of population of intellectual disabled are fortunate enough to get these educational facilities. It is indeed very difficult to start special schools and vocational training centres for these especially abled children in each and every village and city of India. However all endeavours must be made that such children who require special education and training must be found out and not just left to be looked after by their parents who do not have any idea about what best can be done to improve the condition and functional level of their children. All efforts must be put to give them their fundamental right i.e., the right for education. Our government is promoting education all over India. Government has started mid-day meal plan to catch attention of parents to send their normal children for education. Such policies should also be extended for the intellectually disabled population.

The majority of families and care takers of intellectually disabled population don't think that it is important for their children to go to school. To top it up, most belong to very poor socio economic background.

They do not have money for even basic needs of food and clothes and shelter. Thus the core issue here is that this special population should not be just left to their families to be supported by. It should be the responsibility of the state or country at large to give them their basic human rights. The poor can't even afford education for their mentally normal children, so, how could they provide education for mentally challenged children. Thus the government must formulate plans and programs to promote education for this special population. The government can also start mid-day meal plan for special population, so that the parents and care takers can send their mentally sub-normal children to school. However, the question still remains that even if the government starts this mid-day meal plan how can we send all the mentally sub normal children to school as these special schools are very few in number. The solution is that, although the special schools are few in number but other schools for mentally normal children are everywhere in India run by the government and private organizations. As we know that every school has sections for every class. For example, standard one will have various sections like section-A, section-B etc. Adding one more section to particular standard for special children and placing one special educator can do wonders in providing education to majority of special population children. As all the schools have particular syllabus for particular class, the same can be done for developmentally disabled children. For example, standard one, section-E (ID children group) will follow a particular syllabus that can include basic education, self-help skill training etc.

Thus awareness among society regarding intellectually disabled children's right for education can give hope to the parents. This can at least provide some relief to the affected family.

Awareness for Government

The Government of India (GOI) has implemented various rehabilitation programs and schemes for intellectually disabled population. There are various other government schemes and programs like schemes offered by the national trust and other central government schemes like rail travel concession, income tax concessions etc. These acts and schemes offer equality of opportunity, regarding education, employment, freedom, right to property, right to enforce fundamental rights, right to live independently as others in the society, right to justice. The government has also focused on various aspects in terms of trained teachers/special educators, therapeutic services, special programs, providing learning material and promotion of non-government organizations (NGOs). Though the government has various plans and schemes in favor of intellectually disabled population, hindrances still exists in its full implementation. Are the members of the family of such population aware about all the programs, services and schemes? Surprisingly, even majority of mental health professionals are not aware of these government schemes and services, then, how can we expect that they will reach out to other people for creating awareness of all these services? It is very essential for the mental health professionals to be updated about whatever is happening in the field of intellectual disability. Majority of the population, guardians and caretakers of disabled person is unaware about the government facilities. It is very sad to know that often these parents and caretakers are not being informed about the services whenever they visit the professionals. The government should take more steps to make the society aware about the available services by the use of media like the news papers and television. Among all the resources media is a very powerful resource for spreading the awareness in the society. Apart from media, the special team of social workers specially prepared for the awareness campaign for the intellectually disabled population can also do wonders to make people aware about the services.

The government, despite of its various strict laws, is still facing various problems like dumping of patients in the government institutions, unawareness about the resources and government facilities, social discrimination, stigma and abuses. Shockingly, various incidents of sexual, emotional and physical abuse in the institutions and NGO's have been reported. These NGO's and institutions were considered to be a very safe and secure place for the treatment of the patient but surprisingly in today's scenario it is not like that. In various institutions and NGO's sexual, emotional and physical abuse are very common. It is very depressing that this special population are either ignorant of these abuses or even if they are aware of these assaults they don't know where and to whom they can go and can complain. Even if they complain these assaults to the police with someone's help, the police will not consider the statement of the victim because of their mental sub-normality. Many a times the institution tries to hide these incidents because the reputation of the institute is at stake. So, what is the use of these laws if not used when they are most required? Generally it is said that the home is the safest place for a person but the fact is that majority of the abuses take place at home by close family members and relatives and are never even reported. Even if the child or the abuse victim reports those incidents to the parents especially mother, then, he/she tries to hide the incidents because of the fear of social outcast and disrespect. A mentally disabled person is often sexually abused by the close relatives or cousins at home. The question is what step should be taken to stop these abuses against intellectually disabled population?

Another important point of concern about ID population is there is a mismatch between demand and supply of special institutions for these children, be it health care, educational support or vocational rehabilitation centers. Even if there are hospitals, they are in very limited numbers and out of them only few provide quality care. Parents of such children have to travel long distances to reach such hospitals, and after reaching the hospital they get only limited personal attention by the doctor in busy clinics. The point is simple: both the quality and quantity of such institutions need to be improved. The endeavor of the government should be to provide care at the doorstep. From each village a volunteer can be chosen who can identify population with intellectual disability and guide the family members on how to proceed about the care of the child, where to go for expert help, how to avail the government facilities. The volunteer can ensure regular follow up of the ID individuals at nearest health care centre.

The programs that already exist have various drawbacks, for example: lack of resources, have a very limited staff and absence of monitoring. The parents and caretakers of the disabled population lack information about the disabilities their child has and they do not know about the government-sponsored community services for their assistance. Due to the absence of the accessibility to government services, the families and caretakers find it difficult to cope with the demands of the intellectually disabled person. They have no guidelines to follow for their affected child, so they find it easy to admit their child in the hospital or institution for the intellectually disabled or they abandon the patient because they see them as a burden on their family. The government requires more efforts and plans to reduce these problems. The government requires facilitating the person with intellectual disability by providing health care services, rehabilitation, equal opportunity, accessible schools, acceptance in the society, independent living services. The government should have strict laws against those who sexually exploit or emotionally and physically abuse those affected with intellectual disability.

The policies and schemes that the government has started in favor of intellectually disabled population require more attention and awareness among society. The laws should be strictly followed in terms of the protection offered by them to target population. Strict laws by the government can stop many unwanted behavior and crime towards ID population.

Awareness for Mental Health Professionals

The role of mental health professionals in the field of intellectual disability is of utmost importance. They are the one who are at the core of the matter. They have authentic scientific knowledge about the mental illnesses and can contribute most by spreading more and more awareness about this much less talked about issue of concern in our society that is Intellectual Disability. As per 2011 Census, there are 26 million people with disabilities in India who constitute 2.7% of the total population. However, experts working in the field of developmental disabilities feel that prevalence of mental disability is much higher (Cavan & Rozatkar, 2013). The population affected is increasing but the resources to deal with these problems are very less.

In India the professionals working in the field of mental health are very few in numbers in comparison to the affected population. There is a huge demand supply mismatch. Perhaps, the reasons could be many like less number of institutions for training, less awareness about the courses running mainly in the area of psychology and psychiatric social work. Graduates and post graduate students are not aware about the possibilities available if they take up mental health as their subject. Thus less awareness can be a major reason for less numbers of clinical psychologists and psychiatric social workers. Interestingly one reason for less number of psychiatrists is that many of them choose Psychiatry as a last resort when they don't get seat in other specializations. In addition to that their family members fear that staying in contact with mentally ill patients may adversely affect the mental health of their own children and thus do no not support the decision of taking up psychiatry or mental health profession as their carrier choice. Surprisingly many also have this notion that those working in psychiatric mental institutions infamously referred to as "pagalkhana" in India will have difficulty in getting married. Also many parents are concerned about safety issues of their children opting for mental institutions as carrier opportunity. Sadly, the nurses working in those institutions often face various family problems especially when they go for night duties.

Mental health professionals while dealing with the intellectually disabled people and their family members must be very sensitive to their emotions. Involvement of family members in the therapeutic sessions is very important along with proper therapeutic plan and its implementation. The information that is provided to the parents and care takers should not be vague. If there is no visible improvement in the condition of the child then they should be referred to higher centres for more detailed evaluation and opinion of specialists. There may be associated co morbidities which might require investigations at higher centres. A very major issue is many doctors only prefer giving medicines and do not believe in behavioural/psychological management. This can hamper the proper management of the patients apart from being unethical.

Under section 19 of the Mental Health Act, family members and friends have the right to admit affected members in mental hospitals. Many a time these laws are misused by the family members just to get rid of from the responsibilities of mentally disabled person. In that case it becomes very important for mental health professionals to take the most appropriate decisions which might influence the management of the patient. While admitting the patients the doctor should make sure that whether the admission is required or not and if yes then make sure about the address they are giving and verify that address and phone number also in case if the doctor suspects that the patient might be dumped by the family members.

The mental health profession is a multidisciplinary profession. We should work as a team in the management of intellectual disability. In the field of mental health profession; the psychiatrist, the clinical psychologist and the psychiatric social worker all have their significant role in the management of intellectual disability. However we all know that in many setups the reality is different. They don't work as a team. Every stream try to overpower other's stream and put them on the superior platform. Is it really an ethical approach in dealing with intellectual disability? Are we alone capable of doing everything and can prevent or manage intellectual disability? We must all understand the importance of each other. We all are (psychiatrist, clinical psychologist, psychiatric social work) handicap without each other in dealing with intellectual disability. Researchers have shown that in dealing with mental illness, medicine and psychotherapy goes hand in hand. For proper management and outcome the role of medicine and therapy is fifty-fifty in terms of percentage. When we talk about intellectual disability this percentage increases towards behavioural management but it doesn't mean that medicine is not at all required. Apart from the role of clinical psychologist in the behavioural management, the role of psychiatric social work increases because they work at the community level. It was noticed that in working with people with ID that their care givers would perform the behaviour because of the task-focussed attitude. It would never involve or would have insufficient quality of the relationship by the care givers. More focus should be given to the interpersonal qualities, friendly attitude and normal social communication (without being agitated or disrespectful). They play a very important role in terms of primary intervention. Awareness training program on the community level, family psycho-education, making the family members aware about the plans and available resources of government and home visits are the activities that does wonders in terms of management and acceptance in the society. All the mental health professionals should work as a team in managing intellectual disability keeping the prejudices aside.

Awareness for Therapeutic Aspect

Managing a case of intellectual disability is a very challenging job and requires lots of patience. A very common issue which the mental health professional faces in clinical practice is to answer the questions of the parents and care takers of the intellectually disabled children. The parents often ask this question that whether their children will ever live the normal life like us? They also enquire that "suppose their child has a mild mental retardation category, subsequently, if they give proper practice and training to them, then whether their child will come under the average intellectual functioning or not?". Parents come to experts with lots of hope and expectations. Proper guidance and counselling to the parents and caretakers is very essential. The purpose of the clinical psychologist is first to set realistic goals in front of the parents. The expectations must never be too high and professional should never put forth false claims of magical improvement. Parents must be explained that rather than striving for curing the disability, our endeavour must be to make the child more functional. For this the clinical psychologist should convince the parents and caretakers to understand that they themselves are the real doctor of their children and having patience is of prime importance because the improvement of the ID children is very slow. Therefore, while dealing with this special population, the professionals should have proper management plan or module beforehand. However, the question arises that what should be the first step towards management. Every child has some qualities and strength in them. A clinician should explore those abilities in them and use them as a tool to make them more functional. These strengths and abilities can be assessed by using standard tools or a very good and reliable source of information could be parents and caretakers of the intellectually disabled children. While keeping this in mind we can start with the assessment and management plan for individuals.

There are many behavioural interventions in intellectual disability. What should be the primary step? In the mental health profession there are multiple levels at which one can intervene. It can be primary, secondary and tertiary intervention. Talking about primary intervention in the area of intellectual disability, the mental health professionals must identify what are the causes of ID and how can the causes itself be prevented from occurring. The best way would be doing various programs on the community level to prevent ID, for example awareness towards predisposing factors causing intellectual disability like "fetal alcohol syndrome". Alcohol consumption in female is common not only in urban areas but also it is very common in the rural areas. The focus of psycho-education and awareness should be more towards women and their mental & physical health in term of intellectual disability. We must identify other predisposing factors leading to intellectual disability so that we can stop them before its occurrence. Identifying chromosomal anomalies which are associated with mental retardation can be an important step towards primary prevention. Hypothyroidism is an important preventable cause of intellectual disability and all efforts must be made towards early identification of hypothyroidism. Neonatal screening for congenital hypothyroidism can go a long way in preventing intellectual disability in a large number of children, as also food fortification with iodine can help in prevention of acquired hypothyroidism. Secondary intervention means early identification of ID and appropriate intervention because the earlier the identification the better the prognosis. The other medical specialities should be an integral part of this prevention. As soon as they come across a child with intellectual disability, they should refer such patients to the mental health professionals and paediatricians so that they can start early assessment and intervention. Tertiary intervention means intervening at a stage where the focus is not on cure but to make the individual as functional as possible. It is very important to educate the parents that there is no permanent cure in intellectual disability but there is an immense scope of improvement. With proper management they can be made more functional and can also lead independent life after some vocational training. A therapist can even offer information, advice and support to parents and caretakers of a child with additional support through free phone helpline services. So, proper therapeutic module and required changes when it is needed can make a long term positive effect and make a good prognosis for this special population.

In recent times, apart from behaviour therapy and other family interventions, it was seen that music therapy has also been proven to be an effective measure in providing help to people with ID. A study revealed that elderly patients with ID who chose music listening intervention had significant improvement in anxiety reduction, reduced agitation and gave calming effect to the patients. Experience of listening music can be effective and is a straightforward intervention (Sakamoto, Ando & Tsutou, 2013). Also, Parent-Child Interaction Therapy combined (PCIT) with visual supports (VS) has found to be helpful in improving conditions of children with intellectual disability (Kathleen et al, 2014).

Awareness for Job Perspective

Intellectual disability makes a person disabled in many aspects of life. Throughout their life they are dependent on their family members or care takers for their basic needs. This dependency puts a lot of psychological and economical burden on the family members. Social stigma, no acceptance from schools for education, peer and social neglect and ignorance give rise to depressive symptoms in parents and care takers. Various NGO's are working in this field by making them independent and helping them to earn for themselves. They train them in making candles, cards, bags and many more such objects but very limited population is able to avail this training facility. If the government and private companies take the step to provide jobs for this special population as per their abilities, then every disabled individual will be able to earn bread for themselves and not be felt as a burden on family members.

A step by National Institute for the Mentally Handicapped (NIMH) in the Department of Adult Independent Living (DAIL) is working towards improving the quality of life of person with intellectual disability through vocational training and placement services. As part of these services, the individuals with intellectual disability are trained to acquire vocational and independent living skills. Independent living means living like anyone else with same limitations and same opportunities. Individuals with intellectual disability also observe the same style of living like other individuals of their society. The ability of individuals with intellectual disability to be productive was linked to social behaviour and practice and bore very little relationship to their intelligence (Cornelius, 2009). The role of Occupational Therapy is significant and cannot be overemphasised. The Comprehensive rehabilitation services based on life cycle approach are required to enhance quality of life of individuals with intellectual disability. Adult living skills enables individual to establish her/ his identity in the community. Vocational training is offered by nearly 60% of the 736 special schools in the country (Rao, Govinda, Shivakumar, 2003). The training strategies evolved are sheltered workshops, supported employment training; home based training and competitive employment training (Sivakumar & Kumar, 2004). Development and implementation of strategic partnership between occupational therapy and Human Resource (HR) Professionals/ agencies will promote inclusive employment. Trained individuals with intellectual disability can perform specific tasks independently. Human resource professionals develop and implement policies. Appropriate understanding by HR professionals about employability of individuals with intellectual disability is essential for inclusive employment (Berry & Kymar, 2012). So, a step towards job of the intellectually disabled population can make their future bright and independent and then no disabled person will be a burden on their family and caretakers.

RECOMMENDATIONS

Intellectual disability in a child is of concern for the nation. 'Neglect', 'discrimination', 'avoidance', 'stigma' and 'shame' are commonly used connotations for the intellectually disabled individuals and their families by the society. A society is so strong and powerful that it can make or break a family. Proper management, free and independent life, education and empowerment, space in the society are the few requirements of the intellectually disabled population. Intellectually disabled person should be kept in small-scale environment where they would have significantly more number of friends and frequent family contacts. This would directly impact on their social well-being and inclusion along with community involvement.

Use of computer based technology (e.g. iPad) and other effective means to teach relevant social skills and communication.(e.g., Bernard-Opitz, Sriram, & Nakhoda-Sapuan, 2001; Neely, Rispoli, Camargo, Davis, & Boles, 2013)

There are few recommendations for all those who are working for the intellectually disabled children and care for them and their families:

- Treat the intellectually disabled population as a member of the society. They have the same right to live in the society as the other normal individuals.
- Reduce the stigma and discrimination in the society against intellectual disability.
- Get authentic and detailed information about intellectual disability and spread correct knowledge and awareness in society.

- Every intellectually disabled person is different. They have different abilities and strengths. The plan of management should be as per the abilities of the individuals. An umbrella approach will not work. Proper management chart should be prepared and changes in the process should be done if required in the process of management.
- Improving the condition and the environment of the government institutions and NGO's in terms of infrastructure, living conditions, sufficient supply of water, food, clothes and medicine.
- Abuses against ID individuals are very common. Ensure proper security at required locations like schools, colleges, institutions, mental health hospitals and places of work. Even places where ID individuals are admitted and cared for can have people taking advantage of vulnerability of ID children. Thus, special care needs to be taken at such places where emotional, physical and sexual abuses in the institutions and NGO's may actually be a common thing not being disclosed by the institutions themselves. If any such case is reported, immediate legal step must be taken against the individual/ institution committing the crime. There should be a confidential complaint box, where the crime can be reported.
- Proper awareness training programs needs to be conducted. It will help in spreading the awareness regarding available government services to all those affected families who are unaware and unable to avail the services.
- It is also very important for the mental health professionals to be aware about the available government schemes and services and the related updates. It is a responsibility of all professionals working in the field of mental health to give correct and authentic information to the families and caretakers of the intellectually disabled individual.
- The government should provide adequate resources and funding to the institutions and NGO's working in the area of intellectual disability. Train more and more doctors, paramedical staff including psychiatrist, clinical psychologist, psychiatric social workers, counsellors and psychiatric nurses for better output. The more the strength, the better the outcome.
- There should be help-lines established for proper guidelines and detailed information regarding intellectual disability and even confidential complaints against any misdeed.
- Forced treatment and any kind of violence against intellectually disabled person should be strongly prohibited and stringent laws must be in place to prevent any crime against ID individuals.
- Prohibit discriminative practices and marginalization against intellectually disabled population and their families in the society. There should not be any discrimination and non-acceptance in the school. The door of education should be open to all the students disregarding cast, race and intellectual capacity. To employ trained teachers who are qualified in using sign language and Braille to facilitate training of special children will go a long way.
- Apart from the work in the sheltered workshops, they should have other job opportunities. Not only the government but all the private companies should provide jobs to the intellectually disabled population as per their abilities and in which they are vocationally trained.
- The special school for this special population should have separate sections as per the level of intellectual disability of the child. This will help in preparing proper management plan as per the level of their intellectual capacity.

FUTURE DIRECTIONS

Since much of the substantial work has already been done in this area of ID, we are still lagging behind on many prospects of making their lives more comforting and respectful with better living conditions. Public policy decisions and funding would be the driving force in bringing the change for this section. The gap between research and implementation of research in classrooms and therapy setup needs to be narrowed down. Next generation teachers or care givers should be well equipped in terms of advanced skills and innovative ideas. Evidenced based educational interventions must be shared to target the population. Effective collaboration of pharmacological, therapeutic and community involvement would only lead to reaching out to our established goals.

CONCLUSION

To conclude, intellectual disability is an important health issue which needs to be spoken about. Individuals with ID should be never discriminated on any ground. To create a society free of discrimination, there has to be comprehensive shifts in the manner in which our institutions and legal system works. However, it is the attitude of the society towards these differently abled children and families which needs to be changed. Children with ID are just like others with the only difference that they take more time than the so called "normal" people to complete or do any task. They have same emotions like others. Equal rights for children with ID requires not only provision of legal acts but also requires our society to change their thinking, attitude and perception towards the differently abled population. Awareness should be given to everyone in the society regarding their right for education, right for equality and the right to live a discrimination free life. Ensuring good job perspectives after education and to live their life as per their own wish and comfort should be the aim. There is a long way to go. We should remember that there is space for everyone; we just need to find the right space for the right person. There are many things that can be offered for individuals with ID in terms of management but what we need is acceptance in our society of people with ID and *Awareness towards Intervention.*

Everyone is a genius but if you judge a fish on its ability to climb a tree, it will live its whole life believing that it is stupid. ~ Albert Einstein

REFERENCES

American Psychiatric Association. (2013). *Diagnostic and statistical manual of mental disorders* (5th ed.). Retrieved from: http://www.dsm5.org/Pages/Default.aspx

Armstrong, K., DeLoatche, K. J., Preece, K. K., & Agazzi, H. (2015). Combining Parent–Child Interaction Therapy and Visual Supports for the Treatment of Challenging Behavior in a Child With Autism and Intellectual Disabilities and Comorbid Epilepsy. *Clinical Case Studies*, *14*(1), 3–14. doi:10.1177/1534650114531451

Baker, B., & Brightman, A. (2004). *Steps to independence: Teaching everyday skills to children with special needs* (4th ed.). Baltimore, MD: Paul H. Brookes.

Bernard-Opitz, V., Sriram, N., & Nakhoda-Sapuan, S. (2001). Enhancing social problem solving in children with autism and normal children through computer-assisted instruction. *Journal of Autism and Developmental Disorders, 31*(4), 377–384. doi:10.1023/A:1010660502130 PMID:11569584

Berry, B. S., & Kymar, K. R. (2012). Human resource professionals' perception on disability related barriers to employment of individuals with intellectual disability. *The Indian Journal of Occupational Therapy, 44*(2).

Census of India. (2011). *Central Statistics Office Ministry of Statistics & Programme Implementation Government of India.* Retrieved from: http://mospi.nic.in/Mospi_New/site/home.aspx

Chavan, B. S., & Rozatkar, A. S. (2014). Intellectual disability in India: Charity to right based. *Indian Journal of Psychiatry, 56*(2), 113–116. doi:10.4103/0019-5545.130477 PMID:24891695

Cornelius, D. J. K. (2009). *Vocational Training and Employment for Individuals with mental retardation to meet the needs of 21st Century.* Report of the National Seminar - Planning for Comprehensive Rehabilitation of Individuals with mental retardation, Chennai, India.

Disabled Individuals in India. (2002). *National sample survey 58th round.Ministry of statistics and programme implementation.* New Delhi: Govt. of India.

Eriksen, N., & Gerstel, N. (2002). A labor of love itself: Care work among adult brothers and sisters. *Journal of Family Issues, 23*, 836–856. doi:10.1177/019251302236597

Griffiths, D., & Unger, D. (1994). Views about planning for the future among parents and siblings of adults with mental retardation. *Family Relations, 43*(2), 221–227. doi:10.2307/585326

Hassall, R., Rose, J., & McDonald, J. (2005). Parenting stress in mothers of children with an intellectual disability: The effects of parental cognitions in relation to child characteristics and family support. *Journal of Intellectual Disability Research, 49*(6), 405–418. doi:10.1111/j.1365-2788.2005.00673.x PMID:15882391

Heller, T., & Caldwell, J. (2006). Supporting aging caregivers and adults with developmental disabilities in future planning. *Mental Retardation, 44*(3), 189–202. doi:10.1352/0047-6765(2006)44[189:SACAAW]2.0.CO;2 PMID:16677064

ICD 10. (1992). *Classification of mental and behavioural disorder: Diagnostic criteria for Research.* Author.

Kiani, R., & Miller, H. (2010). Sensory impairment and intellectual disability. *Advances in Psychiatric Treatment, 16*(3), 228–235. doi:10.1192/apt.bp.108.005736

Lopez, V., Clifford, T., Minnes, P., & Kuntz, H. O. (2008). Parental stress and coping in families of children with and without developmental delays. *Journal on Developmental Disabilities, 14*(2).

Mak, W. S., & Ho, S. M. (2007). Care giving perceptions of Chinese mothers of children with intellectual disability in Hong Kong. *Journal of Applied Research in Intellectual Disabilities, 20*(2), 145–156. doi:10.1111/j.1468-3148.2006.00309.x

Milani, D., Ronzoni, L., & Esposito, S. (2015). Genetic Advances in Intellectual Disability. *Journal of Pediatric Genetics*, *4*(3), 125–127. doi:10.1055-0035-1564438 PMID:27617122

Mohapatra, S., & Mohanty, M. (2004). Abuse and Activity Limitation: A Study on Domestic Violence Against Disabled Women in Orissa, India. *Indian. The Journal of Educational Research*, *2*, 56–67.

Moran, G., Pederson, D. R., Pettit, P., & Krupka, A. (1922). Maternal sensitivity and infant-mother attachment in a developmentally delayed sample. *Journal of Infant Behavior and Development*, *15*(4), 427–442. doi:10.1016/0163-6383(92)80011-I

Neely, L., Rispoli, M., Camargo, S., Davis, H., & Boles, M. (2013). The effect of instructional use of an iPad on challenging behavior and academic engagement for two students with autism. *Research in Autism Spectrum Disorders*, *7*(4), 509–516. doi:10.1016/j.rasd.2012.12.004

Rao, L., Govinda, & Sivakumar, T. C. (2003). Vocational Training of the mentally retarded. *EDUTRACTS*, *2*(10).

Sakamoto, M., Ando, H., & Tsutou, A. (2013). Comparing the effects of different individualized music interventions for elderly individuals with severe dementia. *International Psychogeriatrics*, *25*(5), 775–784. doi:10.1017/S1041610212002256 PMID:23298693

Sivakumar, T. C., & Kumar, R. (2009). *Selection and Training to develop adult independent living skills in the Indian context across socio cultural and economic levels*. Report of the National Seminar - Planning for Comprehensive Rehabilitation of Individuals with mental retardation, Chennai, India.

Stewart, R., Kozak, A., Tingley, L., Goddard, J., Blake, E., & Cassel, W. (2001). Adult sibling relationships: Validation of a typology. *Personal Relationships*, *8*(3), 299–324. doi:10.1111/j.1475-6811.2001.tb00042.x

UNNATI. (2004). *Understanding Disability: Attitude and Behaviour Change for Social Inclusion*. Retrieved from: http://www.unnati.org/pdfs/books/research-eng.pdf, 2.

U.S. Census Bureau. (2011). *National intercensal estimates (2000-2010): Table 1 Intercensal estimates of the resident population by sex and age for the United States: April 1, 2000, to July 1, 2010*. Retrieved from www.census.gov/popest/data/intercensal/national/nat2010.html

U.S. Census Bureau. (2015a). *Annual estimates of the resident population for selected age groups by sex for the United States, states, and counties, and Puerto Rico Commonwealth and municipios: April 1, 2010, to July 1, 2014*. Retrieved from http://factfinder.census.gov/faces/tableservices/jsf/pages/productview.xhtml?src=bkmk

U.S. Census Bureau. (2015b). *CPS table creator*. Retrieved from www.census.gov/cps/data/cpstablecreator.html

U.S. Census Bureau. (2014). *Total population by child and adult populations*. Retrieved from http://datacenter.kidscount.org/data/tables/99-total-population-by-child-and-adult-populations?loc=1&loct=1#detailed/1/any/false/35,18,17,16,15/39,41/416,417

U.S. Department of Education. (2013). *Thirty-fifth annual report to Congress on the implementation of the Individuals with Disabilities Education Act, Parts B and C. 2013: Part B data descriptions and data files.* Retrieved from http://www2.ed.gov/about/reports/annual/osep/2013/parts-b-c/part-b-data/index.html

U.S. Department of Education. (2014). *2012 IDEA part B child count and educational environments.* Retrieved from https://inventory.data.gov/dataset/2012-idea-part-b-child-count-and-educationalenvironments/resource/a68a23f3-3981-47db-ac75-98a167b65259?inner_span=True

White, L., & Riedmann, A. (1992). Ties among adult siblings. *Social Forces, 71*(1), 85–102. doi:10.1093f/71.1.85

Wiese, E. (2018). Improving the Quality of Life of Elderly with Intellectual Disability: A Literature Review on Environment and care. *Journal of Degenerative Intellectual and Development Disabilities, 1*(5).

World Health Organization (WHO). (2001). *The World Health Report 2001- Mental Health: New Understanding, New Hope*. Retrieved from: http://www.who.int/whr/2001/en/

World Health Organization (WHO). (2011). *World Report on Disability*. Retrieved from: http://www.who.int/whosis/whostat/2011/en/

Chapter 11
Attitude of General Public, Family Members, and Health Professionals Towards People With Intellectual Disabilities (PWID)

Mythili Hazarika
Gauhati Medical College Hospital, India

Sandamita Choudhury
151 Base Hospital, India

ABSTRACT

Attitude defines one's behavior towards the people with intellectual disability (PWID). History on PWID indicates influence of psycho-social, biological, religious, and educational factors for the existence of stereotypical attitudes. But since the early part of the 21st century efforts have been reported across countries in integrating the PWID in the community at large. Families of PWID undergo high levels of stress and emotional reactions which call for intervention. Families often adopt strategies to hide the existence of a disability, which delays the treatment and rehabilitation of PWID. Also, stakeholder attitudes towards them highly influences their rehabilitation and integration in the mainstream society. Hence, this chapter is an attempt to focus on the importance of attitude towards individuals with intellectual disability by general public, family members, teachers, students, employers, and health professionals and its implications and further recommendations for the betterment of their condition.

BACKGROUND

Intellectual disability (ID) is one of the most common disabilities across countries. Braddock and Parish (2002) have defined disability as socially determined interpretation of impairment by others. Therefore the whole concept of ID or how to define or categorize people with ID (PWID) has been always affected

DOI: 10.4018/978-1-7998-1223-4.ch011

by how people in different places, cultures at different periods of time have defined it and perceived it. Rehabilitation of PWID has largely been affected by changing concepts and attitudes. Attitudes are learned pre-dispositions to respond in a favorable or unfavorable manner to a particular person, behavior, event, thing, belief or situation in a direct or discreet manner. According to Charles Osgood, an attitude has three dimensions i.e. Moral (good or bad), potency (strong or weak) and activity (active or passive). These dimensions classify people's attitude towards ID. As relationships with significant others as well society are important determinants for the quality of life of individuals with ID our chapter is focused on attitudes towards them and their various dimensions of life which are significant factors for their adaptation and assimilation in the society.

The authors would focus on attitude towards persons with intellectual disabilities (PWID) worldwide and the review of literature will give an overall insight about this population. The terms mental retardation (MR) and intellectually disabled (ID) is used interchangeably in this chapter.

Attitudes Towards People with Intellectual Disabilities (PWID) in the Earliest Centuries

Egyptian Papyrus of Thebes in 1552 B.C. (Harris 2006) was the first to refer to ID. Attitudes in the earlier times were delimited by religious and spiritual explanations. The ancient Greeks and Romans before 18th century believed children with ID are the cause of curse by god who were allowed to die while some societies in Rome did allow some form of protection to children with ID who were born to the wealthy, by allowing them with right to property and also to have guardians (Beirne-Smith et al. 2006; Harris, 2006). Traditionally, in Indian context mental retardation (MR) or intellectual disabilities (ID) has been referred by Charaka and Susruta in Ayurvedaas as 'manasmandyam' (weak head) caused by genetic, nutritional and environmental factors and is influenced by 'Graha' (planetary influences). In the current scenario the past, present and future are attributed to supernatural powers and there is a strong belief in 'karma'. Hence, disabilities have been considered punishments for sins committed in a previous life by the individual or their family members (Schlossar, 2004). Interestingly before the 18th century, societies differed in conceptualization of intellectual disability. Those with mild ID who were socially competent never received special identification or treatment, and those with more severe conditions received protective care from their families or in monasteries while few societies believed people with more severe ID to be capable of receiving divine revelation (Beirne-Smith et al. 2006; Harris 2006).

Jean-Marc Itard in 1799, first developed systematic and documented program of intervention for ID in France. Seguin elaborated on Itard's methods and formulated a systematic program to educate the "feebleminded" at Salpetrière Hospital in Paris. Henceforth, the stakeholders in Europe worked towards educating PWID which received recognition and subsequently began to spread to other developed and developing countries. In the U.S., and other developed countries there was an initial optimism about rehabilitating, training, and reintegrating PWID into "normal" life. Positive attitudes prevailed and reformers like Dorthea Dix advocated improving treatment of people who were living in asylums, poorhouses, country homes, and almshouses in the mid-1800s. Samuel Howe in 1848 established the first public training facility in the U.S. for PWID and in the same year Hervey Wilbur established in his home the first private institution for PWID (Beirne-Smith et al. 2006) at Massachusetts. There were favorable attitudes during those times towards the PWID as mainstream education was the goal.

However, in the latter half of the 1800s US population became more urbanized and the early optimism about the curability of ID waned. It became highly apparent that people with more severe ID were less able than those without ID to adapt to a developing nation where employment depended on intellectual ability and less so on physical ability in most cases. Furthermore, the ideal of training, rehabilitation, and reintegration of PWID proved to be an illusion as with time it was noticed that people although learned skills but failed to attain "normalcy" as they couldn't pace themselves with the progressive society. Hence, eventually residential institutions were established after the systematic programs were not found to be quite effective. People's attitude towards ID became less favorable and they were called "feebleminded," and were blamed for the poverty, illness, and crime that accompanied urbanization creating a fearful and hostile attitude toward PWID. In those days again the anti-social behaviors and ID, as well as mental or psychiatric illness, tuberculosis, prostitution, and poverty were thought to be heritable. Negative attitudes prevailed to such an extent that great attention was focused on eliminating the possibilities for PWID and others to reproduce so as to control the undesirable heritable traits from passing on to their offspring (Beirne-Smith et al. 2006; Radford 1991; Reilly 1987).

The Eugenics movement started with the publication of the first book on *Hereditary Genius* in 1869 by Sir Francis Galton, a cousin of Charles Darwin, which established a theoretical basis for the heritability of ID (Beirne-Smith et al. 2006). The eugenists rightly concluded that only nature (not characteristics of nurture, like socio-economic status, education, nutrition) determined personality and intellect, so breeding had to be brought under supervision to prevent the degeneration of the human species (Radford 1991; Bachrach 2004). This social myth of heritability and ID was reinforced by the publication of two popular books in 1877 namely The Jukes: A Study in Crime, Pauperism, Disease and Heredity by Richard Louis Dugdale, and The Kallikak Family: A Study in the Heredity of Feeble-Mindedness in 1912 by Henry Goddard. Moreover, Goddard published from his research that many of the immigrants to the US were "*feebleminded*" (Beirne-Smith et al. 2006). Heritability factors in ID dominated the attitude towards them which was not favorable. This led to the belief among the supporters of the eugenics movement that medicine interfered with Darwinian natural selection and kept the weak alive and that people with MR and mental illnesses reproduced faster than intellectual and productive people (Bachrach, 2004).

Attitudes Towards People with Intellectual Disabilities (PWID) in the 20th Century

Following the Eugenics movement of the 19th century, US states like Indiana, Virginia, North Carolina, Georgia, and California enacted sterilization laws (Sofair and Kaldijian 2000). Indiana passed the nation's first sterilization law in 1907 for the "imbeciles" and they have been diagnosed as "unimproveable" (Reilly 1987). Between 1907-1944, more than 42,000 people in US and 22,000 people in 27 states were sterilized in an attempt to eliminate the presumed genetic sources of diseases including ID (Radford, 1991; Sofair and Kaldijian, 2000).In the UK, the Mental Deficiency Act of 1913 emphasized segregation of males and females over sterilization which was active till 1959. Unlike in the U.S., British practitioners preferred to implement educational programs for PWID and used a social definition of mental deficiency as "those individuals who could not fit in to the modern world" (Radford 1991; Reilly 1987). In Germany, compulsory sterilization law was passed during 1933, under which people with "congenital feeblemindedness" which was a very subjective diagnosis could be forcibly sterilized (Bachrach, 2004; Sofair & Kaldijian, 2000).

Further, the most common method of controlling reproduction by PWID was segregation in the U.S., Canada, and Great Britain, through limitations on marriage, immigration controls, sterilization, and, most importantly, custodial institutionalization (Joseph 2005; Radford 1991; Reilly 1987). The reason for the segregation was to protect the so-called "normal" people from the PWID and also to control their reproductive lives. "Custodial institutions were the means by which the feebleminded were removed from a society in which they were perceived as a genetic threat and they were placed in isolated environments, completely segregated by gender" (Radford 1991). Within institutions "feebleminded" men and women were kept strictly apart from each other and lot of them was forcefully sterilized. Medical literature supported sterilization in the 20th century. Unfortunately "euthanasia" of "idiot" children was advocated by some professionals in the US so as to avoid passing on their genes and thereby to reduce the burden on the society (Joseph 2005; Reilly 1987).

Attitudes Towards People with Intellectual Disabilities (PWID) in the Present Context

The 20th century marks the beginning for the search of the cause and cure of PWID in a scientific manner for which the psychological tests were developed leading to early identification of PWID. Tests identified mild intellectually disabled who were otherwise not been given a diagnosis (Beirne-Smith et al., 2006). Although there has been a positive transformation with the development of qualitative methods in social sciences in Britain and in the U.S. but institutionalizing them still continued (Radford, 1991).

Favorable attitudes towards PWID prevailed slowly when heritability as the only cause was refuted in 1928 by Penrose and contemporaries, when they revealed multiple etiologies for ID (Radford 1991). Various non-genetic factors such as metabolic disturbances or PKU (phenylketonuria) and environmental factors, such as infection, trauma, and endocrine disturbance, were recognized as having an association with ID. Though there were mixed reports about genes vs environment on the development of feeblemindedness still social policies reflected deterministic and largely inaccurate hereditarianism views of mental deficiency until after World War II (Radford 1991). Eugenic sterilization in Germany and in the U.S. was opposed by the Catholic churches and the Holocaust discredited eugenics practices (Bachrach 2004; Sofair and Kaldijian 2000; Reilly 1987).

By the early 1960s most state sterilization programs had ended in the developed countries (Reilly 1987).Legal rights, protection and services for PWID revolutionized the attitudes towards them in developed as well as in underdeveloped countries. In 1911, first time New Jersey mandated that education be provided for students with intellectual disabilities (Beirne-Smith et al., 2006).

With the formation of The National Association of Parents and Friends of Mentally Retarded Children in 1950 in US there was the transformation towards tolerance and compassion among the children and families with ID, along with the availability of financial support and formulation of new legislations and community services.

The world has undergone tremendous alterations in attitudes towards PWID in the last four decades with an increased focus on early intervention, community-based rehabilitation (CBR), definition and diagnosis, human rights, and legislation, with particular stress on deinstitutionalization leading to better quality of life and improved choice making (Beadle-Brown et al. 2007). The institutionalized ID population has declined at a significant rate in England, Canada, and Norway, and there is no report of anyone living in an institution in Sweden. Scandinavia was the first country to introduce the concept of "normalization" in 1950s, and suggested access to supports to ID so that they can experience patterns and conditions of everyday life that are as similar to those in the mainstream society (Beirne-Smith et al. 2006). In the US there has been an increase in the trend for individuals with ID to live in inclusive community settings, with appropriate supports to facilitate their experience. Since the 1980s the number of children diagnosed as intellectually disabled has dropped, partly as a result of increased early intervention, and also because of a more cautious professional outlook on definition and diagnosis (Beirne-Smith et al. 2006). The rate of institutions had declined in Australia and Ireland though both countries still have substantial portions of their PWID housed in institutions (Beadle-Brown et al. 2007). Though in Germany, Spain, the Netherlands, Greece, and Belgium deinstitutionalizing was but institutional care continued to dominate. Reports suggests that deinstitutionalization has just begun in countries like France, Poland, Romania, Hungary, and the Czech Republic while many PWID live in poor quality group settings (Beadle-Brown et al. 2007). Argentina continues to institutionalize a large proportion of its people with mental disabilities including ID (MDRI 2007) though mental health care providers are present unlike some developing countries like India where the mental health service providers for PWID in some states are absent.

Interestingly, according to a survey conducted by the World Health Organization's Atlas on 2007 among ID reported that institutional settings still continue to be prevalent in the middle income countries .It is insightful that though education, health, disability, and social welfare were the key governmental sectors involved in programs and policies related to ID, but the availability or the accessibility of such services were more widespread in high income countries with almost 90% reported of having high levels of access compared to only 10% of similar levels of access among low income countries. Special judicial laws for offenders with ID were prevalent in only half of the countries indicating under-development in many of the sectors

Though taxes accounted for the largest source of finances for services of the PWID but only 60% of such services were covered in low income countries compared to 90% in high income countries. Hence, the financial burden incurred for PWID is quite high in the societies of low income countries due to out of pocket expenditure with no favorable returns from PWID.

Across the world there has been a relentless effort for community care of the individuals with ID. Worldwide voluntary disability organizations have been providing community-based supports and services for decade, which are now evolving as 'mainstream disability specialists'. The intrinsic features which make the organizations a vital community resource include: they are naturally person-centered; they have specialist knowledge and skills; they can innovate and adapt to change; and they have forged strong connections both within communities and beyond (National disability survey, 2006). Social inclusion in the community requires active support to establish and maintain connections with family, friends, carers and community members. Successful campaigns carried out in Scotland and New Zealand influenced public attitudes towards PWID which involved a combination of strategies, like information, training and media portrayal (NSW Consumer Advisory Group). While in India and other developing countries the concept of community care needs a very different conceptualization because informal support is the norm and support by untrained non-professionals in non-institutional settings without any responsibility and accountability is apparent. The major program of the United Nations Development Programs (UNDP) is the community–based rehabilitation (CBR).In a very short time CBR has become very popular among the masses in India and integration of the people with ID into the societal mainstream has been the main focus. The goals of CBR would be fulfilled if people with disabilities, their families, and the local community join in this program and work together for realization of the goals (Dalal, 1998) but the efforts would fail if the attitude towards individual with intellectual disability is not favorable.

There has been a "strong awakening of interest in humane treatment of the mentally retarded" (Anastasi, 1982) in the 19th century in developing countries like but the common perception exists that intellectually disabled children are social outcasts, due to the stigmatizing consequences of the process of labeling

(Parekh and Jackson, 1997). Throughout the 1990's, the government of India has been developing acts and strategies, amendments and laws to cater to the various needs of the disabled people. Apart from the government, the Non-governmental organizations (NGO) too play a major role in supporting the inclusion of individuals with ID in various educational and occupational institutes. Though they have established orphanages, vocational training programs, parental organizations, half way homes, day care centers etc. to increase awareness and to empower individuals with ID there is still a huge gap between needs and services available for them.

The Multinational Study of Attitudes (2003) conducted in Brazil, China, Egypt, Germany, Ireland, Japan, Nigeria, Russia and USA showed cultural differences in the perception and attitudes toward PWID. Worldwide, the public perceives individuals with intellectual disabilities as more capable of engaging in simple activities such as sustaining friendships and washing and dressing, but less capable of complex activities such as understanding a national news event or handling emergencies. Across these countries, the public notion is that ID should "live with their family." In those countries that do not favor placement with the family, they believe that ID should live either in supervised apartments or independently.

Worldwide (more than 60% in the countries) people believe there are significant obstacles to the inclusion of individuals with intellectual disabilities in society. In particular, the public believes the lack of available supports (e.g., the lack of community services, job training and school resources), the negative attitudes of others and the negative attitudes of the media as major obstacles to inclusion. (Siperstein et al.2005)

In developing countries people perceive disability differently. In some studies they are considered as an object of pity, sympathy, and are isolated or rejected in the family and other social institutions while in others they have been looked as special people in need of love and affection. Interestingly in a few cases families regard their children with ID as "cursed" and a burden that they must deal with, which at times leads to their neglect, abuse and rejection; and often the child is hidden from the community as the family fears social rejection (Girimaji et al. 2001;Census Bureau, 2001). This leads to social isolation for which the community care fails to reach them. Despite advances in public policy and legislation, significant barriers towards people with ID exists while attitudes held by general public as well significant care givers especially parents are often cited as an important component of the "handicapping" environment by various researchers from time to time. The rigid social structure in India makes it extremely difficult to include individuals with ID into various occupations and institutes as they are perceived as fundamentally "flawed" having diminished capabilities, thereby placing them at the bottom of the social structure (Ghai, 2002).

Detection and identification of mild intellectual disabilities is not simply recognized and the benefits too do not reach them easily because unlike individuals who have genetic disabilities, those with mild ID, is often caused by environmental factors such as malnutrition and under stimulation, and they may have no anomalies in their physical features similarly with individuals with no disability (Reschly, 1996)

In conclusion there is not much change in the perception and acceptance of individuals with ID from earlier to modern times as the stereotypes are based on ignorance and families find it extremely difficult to disclose the presence of disability as they believe disability to be a 'loss of face'' which tarnish the family reputation. Hence, families often adopt strategies to hide the existence of a disability, which could be a source of delay in treatment and rehabilitation services and many times due to lack of knowledge about intellectual disability they do not seek for treatment services as well.

General Public Attitude Towards Individuals with ID

Every individual with or without ID is a part and product of his social environment so one's relationship, attitude and behavior patterns are vitally affected by the nature and extent of the harmony or disharmony of relationship with the family members, relatives, friends, community members, workplace colleagues and employers etc. Tragically enough, the persons with disabilities are comparatively less handicapped by their own disability than by the attitude of the society towards them (Silver, 1957; Shrivastava, 1970).

Moreover, they are not accepted by the society because people's attention is more focused on his/her disabilities rather than on his/her abilities and they are further victimized by the peculiar and irrational prejudice of the society. It has been a well-established fact that the able-bodied people tend to avoid interacting with people with disabilities, because they are uncertain about how to behave in their presence (Yamamoto, 1971; Thompson, 1982). Hence, the common attitudes towards individuals with ID range from curiosity, pity, mild dislike or embarrassment, repugnance, indifference, fear or sympathy.

There has been interesting facts from developing countries where services for ID are lacking. In 2003, Gary N. Siperstein et al. assessed the attitudes of the public in India towards PWID which included questions about perceptions of people with ID, knowledge of Special Olympics (SO) and beliefs about inclusion. Findings indicated that people in urban India were aware of ID as more than 70% had some type of contact with a person with ID like any other countries in the world. Also that people in India interacted with disabled people but majority i.e. more than 54% didn't have any knowledge about SO. United States and Ireland was estimated to have high levels of awareness and involvement with SO but India and all other countries lacked knowledge and were less involved in SO. Indians underestimated the capabilities of the people with ID and viewed them as severely impaired not only in complex independent living skills but also in simple self-help skills. This reinforced the stereotype that exists among the Indian public that individuals with ID as less capable than their non-disabled peers and are categorized as problematic comparable to other children (Ghai, 2002). Whereas in a few studies (Hazarika et al., 2014) it was seen that training in special schools helps in the development of self-help skills and social skills in children with ID like any other children without ID.

The importance of language in disability is very significant and so labeling disabled people with negative terms reflect negatively which is detrimental (Gorden and Rosenblum, 2001). Hence, the language used by general public to describe about disability and impairment affects the way society views them. Inappropriate language prove to be disempowering, humiliating and rude and often terms like victim, abnormal, defective, infirm, invalid, idiot, unsound expresses perceptions of helplessness and dependency on other individuals.

In a cross-cultural study, Benomir, Nicolson & Beail (2016) investigated attitudes to people with ID in Libya in the year 2011, and to compare the Libyan data with those for the UK. This study was the first to undertake quantitative analysis of attitudes to people with ID in Libya. The attitudes were in general less favourable than in the UK and other Western countries, but showed similarities with studies of attitudes to people with ID in Pakistan. The attitude of the general population towards people with intellectual disability (ID) provides important background for policy development. Furthermore, because of changes in attitudes across cultures, it is vital to ground policy development for each country in data from that country.

Murch, Choudhury, Wilson, Collerton, Patel, & Scior (2018) examined participants' attitudes towards individuals with intellectual disabilities with reference to participants' gender, age, level of education, frequency of contact and closeness.The results encourage more implicit-explicit attitude relationship research regarding disability. The associations between demographics, contact and implicit attitudes should be explored further. Research should question whether implicit attitudes reflect participants' true beliefs-denoting less importance to demographics-or whether they reflect wider societal values rather than individuals' attitudes.

Families and Parents' Attitude Towards their Children with ID

Some people in the neighborhood hate him. They never let their children to play with my son. Even if he tries to play with them their parents stop them. Others are kind, and tell me these children are blessings from God

Father of a 12 year old boy with intellectual disability in a study (Hamdani et al., 2014).

The attitude towards PWID is mixed but more towards negativity. Every child is special to a parent while some children have special needs and others do not and this determines the parental care and treatment services in the developmental stages of life (Ravindranadan, 2007). No parent would like his or her child to have any deficits in intellectual functioning. Intellectual disability typically reflects a misfit between the capabilities of an individual and the structure and expectations of the environment. All prospective parents look forward to a baby free from flaws, deformity and disability, but the birth of a intellectually disabled child comes as a traumatic experience involving strong negative reactions. Often terms such as " disabled", " impaired" or "abnormal" are interchangeably used for the child which itself profoundly influences the parent's opinions and attitudes towards their own children with intellectual disability. It has been noted that mothers undergo a more intense psychological trauma or emotional state as it involves adjustment of the notion of so called "perfect child" and the "death" of the child of parental expectation.

When a child is diagnosed to have ID the early parental reactions include ambivalence, anger, confusion, denial, self-pity, blame, feelings of helplessness, depression, disappointment, grief, guilt, mourning, rejection, shock, impulses to kill the child and suicidal impulses (McConachie, 1986; Mary, 1990; Ntombela, 1991). Parental reactions vary from experience of a state of shock at the initial disclosure with being unable to register or understand the news and thus withdraw. This is usually followed by a reaction stage, during which sudden emotions of denial, sadness, anger evolves and gradually parents enter an adaptation stage when they start inquiring and asking questions about what could be done for the future and finally enters a stage of reorganization when they would seek help and begin to plan ahead. But during all these stages love and sorrow, guilt, high expressed emotions of hostility, criticality, and over-protectiveness were reported. So the people working with individuals with ID need to know at which stage of adaptation the parents of ID are in for adequate treatment and rehabilitation of the child.

In a study by Hazarika et al., (2017) it was seen that though the parents of children with ID had love and acceptance towards their children but frustration, disappointment and overprotectiveness were significantly high which were considered to be deterrent factors in their growth and adaptive functioning in the society. Hence, the father of attachment theory (Bowlby, 1988) had rightly mentioned that the greatest loss and negative consequences of an ID child is lack of adequate nurturing relationship with parents. When parents are critical towards the child's immediate environment it negatively hampers the process of development. The way parents' react to a child with special needs partly depends on how they perceive it and the practical implications the disability or illness has on them (Chaturvedi, 1984). This in turn determines their attitude. Findings have been consistent about families experiencing high levels of stress and research has focused on parental dynamics. One view suggests that the presence of a child with special needs causes a crisis in the family. Hence, the environment in which a child is born and brought up has a huge impact on a child's psychological and physical well-being.

One very significant finding suggests that disability increases stress and negative emotions due to the manner by which they are informed of the child's disability that strongly influences initial reactions by parents (McConachie, 1986). Cunningham & Davis argued that parents who were informed 'well' reported feelings of sadness rather than of anger (as cited in McConachie, 1986). If there is a delay in the news about disability and is told in an impersonal manner than they are unlikely to accept the status easily (Ntombela, 1991).Though "there is no good way of letting parents know that their child is mentally handicapped, but there must be ways of not making a bad situation worse" (Hannam, 1975) and this is to be always kept in mind while dealing with children with ID and their parents for comprehensive management.

It has been suggested that negative reactions hampers ones emotionality with more of pessimistic and self -blaming attitude leading to family disharmony. Positive reaction combined with valued support, love, acceptance and contentment with one's own situation increases ones coping efforts. Problem focused coping strategies such as gathering information to deal with the underlying problem, planning, making decisions, resolving conflicts and making realistic goals acts as a booster to the psychological and physical resources during stress. Adverse consequences of stress further deteriorates the child's growth and development. (Gupta & Singhal, 2004)

In a study done by Lakhan & Sharma (2010) among 55,366 people on knowledge, attitudes and practices related to intellectual disability among families in Barwani, India it was found that a large number lacked knowledge and information about ID for which misconceptions and misperceptions were evident. Parents believed that birth of these children has taken place only due to sins of their previous life and not because of poor nutrition, improper delivery, or other birth related problems. This was reinforced by Persha and colleagues study in 2007 where in parents were convinced that their offspring could be cured if they could remove the effects of "God's punishment" by prayers. They paid money to faith healers to conduct worship rituals. However, many of these faith healers used practices like beating, burning on stomach, and not giving food for days in the name of treatment. In some studies the community believed that the intellectual disability is contagious, and can infect other children (Madhavan & Menon, 1988). Another belief was that marriage cures disability so many respondents wanted their disabled children to get married early in life (Peshawaria, 1994)

Grebler (1952) believes that the parent's attitude towards their child impacts greatly on the child's sense of self while Govender (1984) further mentioned the development of positive self-concept in disabled children if they are defined positively by their "significant others" and vice-versa. Thus the role of parents and siblings is of vital importance, especially for the mentally retarded child whose inter-personal experiences are mainly within the family context. Grebler mentioned in his study that the parents are immensely frustrated due to the elements present in the child's condition and external limitations as reported in most studies. Parent's personality determines the level of frustration and anxiety too. Parental reactions are interrelated to the attitude hence, if parents have feeling of guilt then ambivalence is mostly seen towards the child and if they condemn the external world for the child's status then they reject the child, and parents who don't blame anyone for the child's ID accept the child as he or she is. Parental unfavorable attitude cause behavior problems in these children which in turn prevent them from using their limited capacities. According to Ntombela (1991) emotional stress of parents is unavoidable due to the constant physical care, financial demands, restrictions placed lifestyles, the disappointment of having a handicapped child, the guilt feelings arising from their anger and rejection of the child and concerns about his/her. Another common attitude of parents i.e. Hyperpaedophilia,is reported in many studies which is the pathological over-attachment to the child. When this happens the parents love for the handicapped child develops into a grossly exaggerated devotion and over-protectiveness which negatively affects the life and needs of other members of the family as well as for adequate adaptation of the child to the mainstream society.

Attitudes of Siblings and Relatives Towards Individuals with ID

System theory suggests the importance of sibling sub-system as important determining factor for family homeostasis. Sibling relationships make up a child's first social network and are the basis for his or her interactions with people outside the family (Powell & Ogle, 1985). A child's temperament plays an important role in their response toward a sibling, including one with an ID. Although both positive and negative feelings exist in all sibling relationships, McHale and Gamble (1987) states "for school-age children and young adolescents, these relationships tend to be more positive than negative in their feeling tone. It is an interesting insight that children with disabled siblings appear to have more positive and fewer negative behavioral interactions than in those with non-disabled siblings". The positive aspects include higher levels of empathy and altruism, increased tolerance for differences, increased sense of maturity and responsibility, and pride in the sibling's accomplishments (Powell & Ogle, 1985). The attitudes of siblings are greatly influenced by the attitude of parents so if parental attitudes are positive then positive feelings in siblings follow and this is a very important observation to be aware of while giving psycho-education to parents of ID.

According to Ntombela (1991) siblings experience emotions range from jealousy, shame, guilt, to frustration. And it gets exacerbated by the material deprivation they experience due to the increased financial responsibilities towards the disabled child. Studies report shame leading to social isolation as they feel that they cannot invite their friend's home.

The siblings may feel victimized and feel frustrated due to the parent's restrictions concerning the kind of games and outings in which their disabled child and his/her siblings may be involved, so as to protect the child from social discrimination. The chores and responsibilities assigned to the siblings as a result of parent's involvement with the child with ID are matters of concern.

Attitudes of Teachers and Students Towards Individuals with ID

The educational experience of any student is influenced by teachers' attitude so if the attitude is negative then the impact is profound. Children with ID spend most of their time with teachers in schools and vocational institutes so their attitude matters a lot. Studies report mixed messages regarding the teacher's attitude.

Though the legal mandates declare children with ID to be included in the regular classrooms, but they don't ensure their acceptance or fair treatment in schools (Marks, 1997) and some studies also indicates that inclusion can fail to result in positive outcomes in these children (Genesi, 2000; Cook et al, 2000) if social comparison is upward and discrimination persists.

A study conducted by Efron & Efron (1967) revealed that special education class teachers expressed more favorable attitudes to the intellectually disabled than do teachers of ordinary children (Rawlins, 1983). But only a small minority of teachers is in favor of integrating the intellectually disabled-into regular classes (Gotlieb, 1975; Rawlins, 1983). Studies by Scruggs et al., (1996) gives an insight into the social desirability factor indicating that although in the educational fields teachers agreed with inclusive programs for children with ID, but in practice they expressed hesitancy. Intellectually disabled children were the most rejected children in twenty regular classes for their behavior in the classrooms, playground and outside the school environment and they were very seldom chosen as 'a best friend', irrespective of the organizational or integrated settings (Johnson, 1950; Rawlins, 1983). Several studies show that specific Inclusive Education (IE) training courses improve future teachers' attitudes and self-confidence (Glumbic, Kaljaca, & Brojcin, 2004; Stella, Forlin, & Lan, 2007), as well as their abilities and self-awareness regarding abilities of ID thus creating a more positive attitude (Cologon, 2012).

Davis, Tang, Oliver and Wu (2000) found that compared to a sample of Irish children, the Chinese children were more positive towards school integration and were more willing to have social interactions and form social relationships with people who were intellectually disabled.-While in Japan, a study (SO, 2004) among middle school students indicated underestimating the intellectually disabled and even hesitation to interact with them but North American students expressed their willingness to interact and had better perception of the competencies of the intellectually disabled. (Norins-Bardon et al., 2005). While, more than 516 studies stated that more the contact with people with intellectual disability, less was the prejudice. (Pettigrew et al., 2000; Hewstone, 2003) .

Students with higher marks or higher qualifications show better attitudes towards people with disabilities than those with lower marks and qualifications (Sharma, Forlin, Loreman, & Earle, 2006; Forlin et al., 2009).

Patel & Rose (2014) studied attitudes held by a British student population towards individuals with an intellectual disability. Students participated in focus groups addressing their attitudes, behaviours and perceptions of individuals with an intellectual disability. A lack of knowledge about intellectual disabilities was identified. Participants recognized exposure through the media as a tool to increase knowledge.

People's Attitude About their Education and Inclusion in the Mainstream

Education is the right of every child because it equips him to meet the challenges of life.

Inclusive Education (IE) or Mainstreaming as a type of education ensures the exercising of the right to a complete, and quality education for all, maximizing integration of the society and promoting diversity in knowledge sharing and experience (EADSNE, 2011). According to statistical data, Spain is one of the EU countries with the highest levels of IE. Only 0.4% of Spanish students with special educational needs (SEN) attend specific educational institutions (EADSNE, 2011; Chiner & Cardona, 2012) in contrast to 4% in Belgium, Denmark, Germany or Switzerland.

Some significant milestones in the field of education of the disabled are the Salamanca Statement and Framework for Action on Special Needs Education (UNESCO, 1994); the Declaration of Madrid in 2002; the UN Convention on the Rights of Persons with Disabilities (UN, 2006), which was signed by 147 countries and ratified by 97; and the 48th Session of the International Conference on Education "Inclusive Education: the way of the future" (UNESCO, 2008).

The policies of the government of India towards the education of children with disabilities have been reflected in the enactments, schemes and through institutions established for various relevant activities. According to the NSS 58th round (Jul.–Dec. 2008), 19.68% children with ID were enrolled in grades between 1st-5th, 8.62% were enrolled in grades between 6th-8th. Some of the major policies and legislature framework in India for education of the disabled in order to alter people's mind set and reduce discrimination are the constitutional safeguards provided by the Constitution (86th Amendment) Act 2002 declaring education as a fundamental right of all children in the age group of 6–14 years, adoption of the National Policy on Education (NPE) in 1986 whose objectives include integrating the physically and mentally handicapped with the general community as equal partners, to prepare them for normal growth and to enable them to face life with courage and confidence. Concept of special education, teacher's training to deal with ID, and importance of vocational enrolment was bought up in this policy. Policies like the Integrated Education of Disabled Children (IEDC) which is the centrally sponsored scheme of Integrated Education of the Disabled Children providing educational opportunities for the disabled children in common schools, to facilitate their retention in the school system, and also to place the children in special school to common schools after they acquire the communication and the daily living skills at the functional level. Another policy developed in 1992 is the Plan of Action (POA) which postulates that a child with disability who can be educated in a general school should be educated in a general school only and not in a special school. Even those children who are initially admitted to special schools for training in plus curriculum skills should be transferred to general schools once they acquire daily living skills, communication skills and basic academic skills. The Parliament of India enacted the Rehabilitation Council of India Act (RCI Act –1992) which was subsequently amended in 2000, to establish a statutory mechanism for monitoring and standardizing courses for the training of 16 categories of professionals required in the field of special education and rehabilitation of persons with disability. Persons with Disabilities (Equal Opportunities, Protection of Rights & Full Participation) Act, 1995: The most landmark legislation in the history of special education in India is the Persons with Disabilities (Equal opportunities, protection of rights & full participation) Act, 1995 involved with providing free education up to 15 years, integrating of disabled children with regular children and setting of special school in public and private sector and providing vocational training facilities. It is welcoming to note in the developing country like India that the Sarva Shiksha Abhiyan (SSA) has been operational since 2000-01 in partnership with state governments to achieve the goal of universalization of elementary education. This adopts a ZERO rejection policy and it covers the following components under education for children with disability. They are early detection and identification, functional and formal assessment, education placement, aids and appliances, support services, teacher training, resource support, Individual Educational Plan (IEP), parental training and community mobilization, planning and management, strengthening of special schools, removal of architectural barriers, research, monitoring and evaluation of females with disability.

Across the world the right of every child to education is proclaimed in the Universal Declaration of Human Rights (1948) and was strongly reaffirmed by the World Declaration on Education for All (1990). The UN Standard Rules on the Equalisation of Opportunities for Persons with Disabilities (1993) was an important resolution for improving the educational conditions of persons with disabilities which affirms, 'Those with special educational needs must have access to regular schools which should accommodate them within a child centered pedagogy capable of meeting these needs".

Though the mentioned legal policies and laws with few other policies have been mandatary in developed and developing nations but still there is a growing fear among parents and educationists that the children with ID would create discipline problems and decrease the growth and productivity of fellow students as a result cause hindrance to overall progress of the society. Hence, it is better to put them in separate special schools. This mind-set causes obstacles to the integrated education system. In a study among regular school teachers of Nigeria regarding inclusion of children with ID revealed that 57.4%

teachers could not cope with the children with ID because of their learning difficulties. Teachers with higher years of teaching experience were found to be more favorable to exclusion (Tolu.et al, 2014)

Moreover, just bringing a child into a mainstream classroom does not indicate integration if no other supports is in place. There are children who are integrated but very lonely as nobody plays with the child. These may lead to social exclusion, isolation and psychological problems in him/her. There is a lack of community resources like health and transportation, job training programs, lack of special teachers, and special learning aids to provide the supports necessary for their success in the inclusive workplace or schools. Need for social services is high but services are less and inclusion in the work and school environments has been extremely difficult due to the diversity that exists within some countries.

Four variables like general demographics, educational background, teaching experience and perceived competence to teach the disabled affect regular classroom teacher's (RCT) attitude towards mainstreaming. Teacher's cultural background, knowledge regarding intellectual disabilities that have been gained either with one's own personal experience or formal studies seems to be the factor towards building up of positive attitude. Perceived competence i.e. the RCT's perceptions of their ability to meet the academic and social needs of the disabled children, personality characteristics such as openness to experience, empathizing, conscientiousness, intuitive, good power of observation, even tempered and having received in service training appears to have a significant positive impact on attitude towards mainstreaming.

Alnahdi (2019) examined the attitudes of Saudi students towards peers with disabilities. It examined how these attitudes are related to age, attending a school that includes students with intellectual disabilities, and having a relative with a disability. The students presented positive attitudes towards peers with disabilities. Students in schools that included students with intellectual disabilities had more positive attitudes than other students. Older students were more likely to hold positive attitudes than younger students. Having a relative with a disability had no effect. The findings suggested that students generally hold positive attitudes towards children with disabilities. Moreover, including students with intellectual disabilities in schools associated with other students' awareness about students with differing levels of abilities. Expanding schools to include children with disabilities in society in general will probably help increase the likelihood that they will be accepted and diminish the stereotypes that follow them.

Attitudes of Employers Towards Individuals with ID and their Inclusion in Work

People with disabilities would be benefitted if they were employed in various skilled and unskilled tasks as it helps in skill development, increase income, decrease social isolation and leads to life satisfaction. But they face many challenges when integrating into the work force. Overcoming co-workers and employers' negative attitudes and perceptions is one such challenge. The employment rate of people with disabilities remains low despite efforts, legislation, and identified benefits of hiring people with disabilities (Stokes, 1990,Geng-qing & Qu, 2003; Ruggeri-Stevens & Goodwin, 2007;).

Despite rules and laws only 44% of intellectually disabled adults are in the labor force, either employed or looking for work, while just 34 percent are actually working, according to a survey by Special Olympics and conducted by Gallup and the University of Massachusetts at Boston. Studies by Rimrnerman, 1998 have shown that the attitudes of employers play a major role in determining the success of employing workers who have been labeled with mild and moderate intellectual disability. Employing such people reduces support and treatment costs of caring for these individuals, and allows them to pay taxes and improve their level of self-confidence and independence. Levy, Jones-Jessop, Rimrnerman

& Levy reported that larger companies have been found to be more positive in their attitudes towards hiring persons with disabilities than small companies (in Rimrnerman, 1998, p.246.)

People from the work-force who had prior experience with ID are positive towards their recruitment and less educated corporate executives place less emphasis on the educational accomplishments of persons with disabilities and are more favorable towards hiring them. People with ID who have vocational and social skills, had greater chance of employment while executives in many companies avoid hiring persons whose ID raises concerns about their ability to integrate into the workplace. But in another study coworkers of people with disabilities mentioned contagious excitement about the job as a positive experience while working with people with disabilities (Ruggeri-Stevens & Goodwin, 2007). It is also possible that public's underestimation is the result of the strongly held stereotype that exists among some people that individuals with ID are less capable than their non-disabled peers (Ghai, 2002).

In the United States, of the 43 million people classified as having disabilities, 56% are employed compared to 88% of people without disabilities (U.S. Census Bureau, 2007). Hence, discrimination against individuals with disabilities appears to continue as a serious problem all over the world. Many intellectually disabled people work in fast food joints, and retail chains such as Walgreens, Best Buy and Safeway have stepped up to hire them. Sheltered workshop is another platform which inculcates high self-esteem and sense of purpose in life, where about 30% of ID work but they face segregation from non-disabled workers in the basic task and outcome they perform. They can legally be paid less than the minimum wage under a 1938 federal law that allows wages to be based on comparing their productivity level with that of a non-disabled worker. But disability rights groups won a victory when President Obama signed an executive order raising the minimum wage to $10.10 an hour for federal contract workers. The order includes several thousand disabled workers at sheltered workshops run by federal contractors. In comparison to other countries surveyed, India is most comparable to South Africa in terms of where they believe individuals with ID should not work but countries like Japan, Ireland and the United States were extremely positive indicating that individuals with ID could work in skilled or unskilled work set-up.

In Columbia, the Rehabilitation Services Administration (RSA) is responsible for empowering individuals with disabilities to "maximize employment, economic self-sufficiency, independence, and inclusion and integration into society". By law, the local RSA would conduct a review and assess to determine eligibility and priority for services. Provision for supported employment, on-the-job training, and other experiences using supports and realistic work settings are also reported to be available and no individual is denied individual services based on disability. Once the local RSA determines that an individual is eligible for Vocational rehabilitation (VR) services, the VR specialist develops an Individual Plan for Employment (IPE). The IPE generally include among other things, the individual's employment goals and means to achieve them. (University Legal services report, Washington, 2010)

Some of the common barriers identified in inclusion of ID to employment are the perception that individual with ID lack the necessary skills to work in a competitive employment, belief that inclusion will have a negative consequence on the environment, such as lower the productivity of other workers and create safety problem for the individual himself and others, and the presence of external obstacles such as lack of services which prevent inclusion from happening and finally, inclusion is hindered by negative attitude harbored by many individuals.

Ineland & Hjelte (2019) analyzed how professionals from three welfare organizations describe quality in daily encounters with people with intellectual disabilities. Four hundred and twenty-one respondents participated in the study. Our empirical data consisted of written excerpts exclusively. Findings revealed that quality in encounters with people with intellectual disabilities was associated with personal attributes, pertinent knowledge, professional actions and ideological awareness. Findings also show differences in responses, both quantitatively (frequency) and qualitatively (content), which seem to be associated with organization. This reflects that human service organizations, as normative environments, underpin ideas about relevance and appropriateness in day-to-day situations, forming actions and perceptions among its members. They concluded that organizational context needs to be considered to enhance our knowledge on how different categories of professionals view quality and moral worth when working with people with intellectual disabilities.

Attitudes of Health Professionals Towards Individuals with ID

The trend towards deinstitutionalization and the movement towards community rehabilitation programs imply that more physician's are caring for mentally retarded patients in their daily practices. Medical students have positive attitudes towards people with intellectually disabled (Rutledge and Scatt, 1997) .A study on the systematic review on health care professionals and students attitude towards disability in New York indicated that one's experience with a person with disability, ones background with disability influences in becoming more comfortable with a challenging rehabilitation situation. Female health care students and professionals are found to be showing more positive attitude towards patients with disabilities then do their male colleagues (Satchidanand et al., 2009). Attitude of the medical students holds importance as they are the future professionals who would provide their service to the disabled. In a study conducted by Karl et al. (2013) to assess the effects of a clinical experience that involved caring for people with ID indicated favorable attitude among the medical students and they wanted to learn more about this group. A similar study by Khandelwal and Workneh (1986) to understand medical students' perceptions of, and attitudes towards, mental illnesses and ID, before the start of a 6-week psychiatric attachment indicated 92% regarded ID as an illness; 62% regarded it as very serious; 78% stated that they would have some problem in their family life.

Rose (1996) revealed that families are enormously affected by the perception of their health professionals' lack of information, support system and dissatisfaction with the services. In United States, a study by Doornbos (2002) suggested that 85% of the caregivers regarded communication problems with mental health professionals as the most non supportive aspect of a mental health care system, indicating that there lies incongruence between the collaboration and partnership between the two parties increasing iatrogenic burden for families. "Iatrogenic burden" was the term coined by Lefley (1996) to describe the stress felt by families from a system that most of the times reacts to them with indifference. Therefore, it is essential to generate collaboration between the health professionals and the families as often family is regarded as liability for the condition of the intellectually disabled, not that the population is unique and deserves special services themselves.

Mental health professionals clinical training programs should focus more on family coping, adaptation, and competence rather than family pathology (Mohr, Lafuze, & Mohr, 2000).Some of the barriers that prevent one from collaboration with the families include lack of insight about family stress, limited outreach to families, the lack of awareness of the needs of families, and continued exposure to a pathology.

A step was taken by National Association of the Mentally Ill (NAMI), Professional Provider Family Education Course (PPFEC) in United States which is a 10 week course developed for the purposes of educating, encouraging, and helping professional mental health providers to better understand the family's responses to mental illness and involve the family in the delivery of care, Physician's negative attitude towards individuals with ID will have deep detrimental effect on the delivery and outcomes of medical services and may influence the beliefs and attitudes of others who assist in this health care so the issue needs sensitive handling and management.

The experience that people with disabilities have with health care is a complex interaction between their medical condition and the social and physical environment. Attitudes of the nursing and healthcare staff affect the quality of care and people's adaptation to their disability, self-image and rehabilitation outcomes. Greek health and social care students showed poor attitudes towards people with physical and intellectual disability. When holding unfavourable attitudes, healthcare professionals become less involved with the peoplethey care for and they do not provide nursing care to the best of their abilities. Undergraduate and continuing education, along with workplace enhancements, should aim to provide high-quality health care to people with disabilities (Kritsotakis, Galanis, Papastefanakis, Meidani, Philalithis, Kalokairinou, & Sourtzi, 2017).

The age group, type of school, prior education regarding the disabled and the condition of caregiving to disabled people are factors influencing nursing students' attitudes towards people with disabilities. Attitudes of healthcare professionals are major factors in the rehabilitation and self-acceptance of people with disabilities. Consequently, it is important that nurses develop or maintain positive attitudes towards people with disabilities during their education (Uysal, Albayrak, Koçulu, Kan, & Aydın, 2014).

Yorke, Ruediger, & Voltenburg (2017) described the attitudes of doctoral physical therapy (DPT) students towards people with disability and examine predictive ability of demographic variables on those attitudes. Attitudes of DPT students over the course of their education did not change. Faculty should consider measuring attitudes and developing specific educational strategies to improve attitudes with the goal to improve patient care. Attitudes towards people with disability can impact their health care. Physical therapy students, in general, express positive attitudes towards people with disabilities and no differences in attitudes were determined in a group of Year 1 and Year 3 doctoral physical therapy students. Opportunities exist to intentionally thread educational strategies throughout a professional curriculum to facilitate further development of positive attitudes in doctoral physical therapy students.

Ryan & Scior (2014) reviewed of research on medical students' attitudes to people with intellectual disabilities. The attitudes of medical students warrant empirical attention because their future work may determine people with intellectual disabilities' access to healthcare and exposure to health inequalities. Results suggested that medical students' attitudes to people with intellectual disabilities were responsive to interventions. However, the evidence is restricted due to research limitations, including poor measurement, self-selection bias, and the absence of control groups when evaluating interventions.

Although recent studies suggest that health professionals hold positive attitudes towards people with ID, stigmatising attitudes may influence their efforts to serve people with ID in community healthcare practice. With respect to stigma, a lack of familiarity with and knowledge about people with ID was found. ID was considered as a stable condition not under personal control. Moreover, mainstream health professionals had either low or high expectations of the capabilities of people with ID. Professionals reported stress, lack of confidence, fear and anxiety, a tendency to treat people with ID differently and a lack of supporting autonomy. Stigmatising attitudes towards people with ID appeared to be present among mainstream health professionals. This might affect the ongoing challenges regarding inclusion in mainstream healthcare services. To facilitate inclusion in mainstream healthcare services, it is recommended to include contact and collaboration with experts-by-experience in education programs of health professionals. Future research should progress beyond descriptive accounts of stigma towards exploring relationships between cognitive, affective and behavioural dimensions as pointers for intervention. Finally, inclusion would benefit from an understanding of 'equal' treatment that means reasonable adjustments instead of undifferentiated treatment (Pelleboer-Gunnink, Oorsouw, Weeghel, & Embregts, 2017)

Ebuenyi, Rottenburg, Bunders-Aelen, & Regeer (2018) explored barriers and pathways to the inclusion of persons with mental and intellectual disabilities in technical and vocational education and training programmes in four East African countries, in order to pave the way to greater inclusion. Barriers and pathways to inclusion were found in the three interrelated components of the model. They are mutually reinforcing and are thus not independent of one another. Barriers regarding culture include negative attitudes towards persons with mental illnesses, structural barriers relate to exclusion from primary school, rigid curricula and untrained teachers and unclear policies. Culture and structure hence severely hinder a practice of including persons with mental disabilities in technical and vocational education and training programmes. Pathways suggested are aiming for a clearer policy, more flexible curricula, improved teacher training and more inclusive attitudes.In order to overcome the identified complex barriers, systemic changes are necessary. Suggested pathways for programme coordinators serve as a starting point. Implications for rehabilitation Clear and up-to-date information on mental disability is required to engender societal participation; especially that of stakeholders in technical and vocational education and training programmes. Affirmative action and policy implementations of national and international human rights legislations are required to address the challenges of enrolment in technical and vocational education and training programmes. Disability organisations and government should adopt a more open and strengths-based attitude, tailor-made curricula, specific teacher training as well as clearer policies to ensure better inclusion of persons with mental disabilities in technical and vocational education and training programmes.

Greek health and social care students showed poor attitudes towards people with physical and intellectual disability. Regarding intellectual disability nursing students had slightly less positive attitudes in "Similarity" but more positive attitudes in "Sheltering" subscales. Previous work and contact was related to more favourable and higher age to less favourable "Similarity" and "Sheltering" attitudes. Those who knew people with intellectual disabilities had less favourable "Empowerment" attitudes. Knowledge was related to more positive attitudes. When holding unfavourable attitudes, healthcare professionals become less involved with the peoplethey care for and they do not provide nursing care to the best of their abilities. Undergraduate and continuing education, along with workplace enhancements, should aim to provide high-quality health care to people with disabilities Kritsotakis, Galanis, Papastefanakis, Meidani, Philalithis, Kalokairinou & Sourtzi (2017).

Attitude towards sexuality of individuals with ID

"The world worries about disabilities more than disabled people do" – Warwick Davis

Sexuality is an innate part of each and every individual. Sexual behavior develops on three levels, biological, social and psychological (McLeod, 2008). Children and young people develop physically, mentally, emotionally and sexually through exploration, observation and processing the information gathered. Sexual development is not only physiological but also changes in sexual knowledge and behaviors.

Sexual needs or rather sexual health often becomes a neglected aspect of people with intellectual disability, although the biological needs that arises among human beings tends to be the same. Individuals with intellectual disabilities are no different in this respect, and express the need and desire to form relationships, engage in sexual contact, and acquire sexual knowledge (Kelly, Crowley, & Hamilton, 2009; Konstantareas & Lunsky, 1997; McCabe, 1999; Siebelink et. al, 2006).

Some of the essential skills in which PWID may require specific educative and/or medical management are in maintenance of hygiene, general gynecological care compliance, sexually transmitted infections (STI), abuse and knowledge about prevention of unwanted pregnancies

An efficacious way of protecting child's sexuality mostly during adolescents involves education in sexuality and gender mainstreaming. This could be provided by parents, teachers and friends. They could be taught in a disabled friendly language about the distinction between proper and improper touch, knowledge about private and public behavior, age appropriate sexual issues and teaching the importance of fulfilling sex life. Studies report that both males and females with ID react differently to the experience of sexual abuse. Findings suggest that females become passive in their later sexual relationships, make poor relational decisions and submit to physical, sexual and emotional abuse easily, while males are unable to understand the act and in turn internalize the action and become aggressive in their own relationship with others (Alplott, 1999; Block, 2000 ; Jobling et al.,2000 ; Griffth et. al., 2000; Trigler & Pfeiffer, 2001). The emotional impact of engaging in sexually inappropriate behaviors and/or being charged can include shame, guilt, fear, rejection, blame, stress, loss of trust and confusion. The physical impact can include bullying, isolation, STIs, pregnancy, a loss of job/home/money/freedom, risk of harm and injury. Inappropriate sexual (ISB) behavior at the earliest stage warrant redirection and depending on the behavior, age and impact to self or others can escalate to a situation whereby professional intervention is required

Education is the mechanism to promote the decision making abilities and empower the individuals with intellectual disability, thus reducing vulnerability and inappropriate sexual expression (Aylott, 2000; Black, 2000; Lumley & Scotti, 2001 ;Nirji,1972; Ward, et al.,2001).Vulnerability to abuse among intellectually disabled can be reduced by adequate social skills training, appropriate judgment skills, and provision of practical knowledge based training in formal sex education programs(Sobsey,1988;Sobsey &Varnhagen, 1988; Watson, 1984). Differentiating appropriate sexual behavior from inappropriate sexual behavior, relation to sexuality and protective behavior to individuals was addressed in a training program in People 1st Program (PIP), a project of Family Planning Western Australia (2009) which had favorable outcome.

Attitude of the Media Towards Individuals with ID

The role of media in promoting prevention, detection and rehabilitation of intellectual disabilities has been grim. There has been a noticeable lack of coordination between media professionals and those working for the disabled. There is a lack of moral responsibility to help in policy formulation and implementation by the media so there are very few media efforts to address disability needs and to promote disability awareness. There is general indifference to the cause of integration of people with disabilities into mainstream society by the media. Many times in various movies individuals with ID are projected with a touch of humor and sympathy which is both unethical and immoral while few of the films have also sought to enhance the sensitivity of society towards the needs, rights, sensibilities and potential of people with disabilities.

Although, there are few television and radio programs which telecast programs to promote assistive devices available for persons with disabilities as well as on integration of children with disabilities in normal schools but the main emphasis on early intervention in the management of disabled children is not often seen as the right target. Since stigma due to negative media coverage impedes the recovery process, triggers discrimination and prejudice, and creates barriers to seeking and finding decent housing, employment, and education, it is essential to make use of appropriate advertisement, share success stories and circulate appropriate facts about the condition to remove the stigma and dogmatization that lies among the population at large to create an aura of positivity and compassion towards PWID.

CONCLUSION

The general approach towards the care and rehabilitation of the individuals with ID reflects the confused state of mind of a person who wants to be emancipated and modern while preserving age-old traditions and cultural values. Though the Government policies, legislative actions, schemes and provisions, programs for the disabled give the impression of commitment to human rights and equal opportunities across countries but the ground reality is quite different in most of the developing countries.

There is not much work done to create awareness about disability in many countries so most people continue to believe that disability is either an irreversible medical condition or an act of fate. And in both the cases the onus of care rests with the family of the disabled and not on the community at large. Though various schemes have been offered for the welfare of this population, due to lack of adequate information among the stakeholders, the PWID, their families and organizations that work for them are either unaware or cannot avail of the provisions therein and many times it is seen that the process of availing the benefits of these schemes are very cumbersome as well as time-consuming.

There are significant myths and misconceptions about disability causing the disabled to be discriminated, isolated and marginalized. The legal definitions in many countries view disability strictly from the medical and/or psychometric perspectives that reinforce a medical model of intervention rather than the much-needed community-based rehabilitation. Very interestingly though the rehabilitation programs have received recognition but they are funded because of their activities rather than achievements and in reality they are not need based but fund driven so are very cost-intensive, lacking in real goal or long-term viability. Hence, these programs become counterproductive to the cause of development of rehabilitation services in the long run.

Overall, it is apparent that the general public of many countries lacks an appreciation of the range of capabilities of individuals with intellectual disabilities, and therefore has low expectations of what they can do. The world still believes that individuals with intellectual disabilities should work and learn in separate settings, apart from people without disabilities. The family is seen as the most appropriate living environment for individuals with intellectual disabilities, a function of both cultural values and availability of services. In thinking about the barriers to inclusion, there is unanimous recognition that the lack of resources and services in the community, employment and school are the major obstacles to inclusion. In addition, the world sees the negative attitudes of others, including the media, as standing in the way of inclusion.

People who perceive individuals with intellectual disabilities as more capable support inclusion in work and school, and believe that the existence of obstacles are not too large and expect few negative outcomes of inclusion.

The direct and indirect efforts made in many jurisdictions needs to be monitored on a continuous basis. These include efforts to ensure the substantive equality of people with disabilities in the field of employment, education, independent living and full societal participation. Hence, more research on this population is essential in all socio-economic levels for planning and program implementation. Also it is essential to translate research evidence into practice to bring about the change.

RECOMMENDATION

- Awareness and education programs are needed to educate the public about the capabilities of individuals with ID, and, that there is great variability that exists among people with ID. Further, it needs to be made clear that not all people with ID fall into the moderate to severely disabled category and that most people with ID are not physically distinguishable from their non-disabled peers.
- If education of the ID is to become a reality all over the World then the training of teachers has to become a top priority. The teachers need to be provided with intensive training to work with various disabilities. In-service teachers also need continued training to update their skills and knowledge of inclusive education strategies.
- It is important for the health professionals to focus more in the capabilities instead of the inadequacies in the assessment process in order to promote smooth functioning of the IEP that are to be maintained for the children .Also, ensuring that one's practice, clinic or hospital is open and welcoming to persons with intellectual disabilities, educating oneself and colleagues about the needs of individuals with intellectual disabilities, holding high health expectations for persons with intellectual disabilities and including them as partners in making decisions about their health are some steps towards a progressive mind-set.
- Specific organizations working for specific disability should develop advocacy program to sensitize the community and the administration to the needs of people with disability as a whole and not be involved in one or two specific disabilities only.
- Families and other stakeholders should be provided the necessary insight about their views and their attitudes towards their own children with ID.As families become more knowledgeable about the capabilities of their children with ID, they will begin to expect more from the community and take part in the community rehabilitation programs.
- A strong school and family partnership would ensure good planning taking into consideration of the student's needs and the school division's resources and policies. An effective way to attain that is to introduce self-help group of parents with intellectually disabled child. Thus parents with positive perception can help the other parents in the early stages of adjustment to develop positive and realistic expectation.
- There is a clear need to provide effective, timely, ongoing training for people responsible for the health and wellbeing of PWID. Provision of training to help parents, care givers and disability workers better identify inappropriate sexual behavior at its earliest stage may reduce the escalation, severity and repeated occurrence of behaviors that adversely impact lifestyle and opportunities of the PWID.
- In low income countries, disability is strongly linked to poverty so improving the quality of life of people with disabilities and their families should be the focus of the health care services as this would benefit a large disadvantaged section of the society.
- For the success of community based rehabilitation services, it is crucial that professionals learn from success in the developed countries, as well as from failures so need based programs should

be initiated which would be viable in the long run. The activities, mission and vision of any rehabilitation program should be clearly laid down and reviewed from time to time.

- Another strategy for promoting change in attitudes could be programs such as Unified Sports which provide a dynamic model for inclusion in the community by creating the opportunity for individuals with and without ID to participate in sports side-by-side in an effort to break down existing stereotypes.
- The current societal attitudes towards people with ID partially dictate the importance the government places on the issue. There is a need for legitimization of rights of the ID with acquiring of their basic services protesting against discrimination and injustice and acknowledging their richness and the diversity.
- Role of the media is crucial in changing the myths and superstitions about PWID and giving appropriate knowledge, responsible reporting, information about care, opportunities and rehabilitation of PWID to reduce prejudice and discrimination is the need of the hour

A positive change by general public, family members, teachers, students, employers and health professionals towards individuals with intellectual disability facilitate to improve overall quality of life, better inclusion to the society and adjustment and future works needs to be focused on ths.

Hindsight: There is no doubt that the dream for discrimination free and equal education for the people with intellectual disability may require a comprehensive change in the institutional arrangements and legal provisions but the most important change has to come in our mindset, in our thinking and attitude towards the disabled to bring about the larger change.

REFERENCES

Alderson, E. (2013). *Supporting People with Intellectual Disability to Express Appropriate Sexual Behaviors*. Retrieved from http://www.ndis.gov.au/sites/default/files/documents/5_Supporting_People_with_Intellectual_Disability_to_Express_Appropriate.docx

Alnahdi, G. H. (2019). The positive impact of including students with intellectual disabilities in schools: Children's attitudes towards peers with disabilities in Saudi Arabia. *Research in Developmental Disabilities*, 1–7. doi:10.1016/j.ridd.2018.10.004 PMID:30388506

Arendt, S. W., & Paez, P. (2014). Managers' Attitudes Towards Employees with Disabilities in the Hospitality Industry. *International Journal of Hospitality & Tourism Administration*, *15*(2), 172–190. doi:10.1080/15256480.2014.901065

Bachrach, S. (2004). In the name of public health – Nazi racial hygiene. *The New England Journal of Medicine*, *351*(5), 417–420. doi:10.1056/NEJMp048136 PMID:15282346

Beirne, S. M., Patton, J. R., & Kim, S. H. (2006). *Mental retardation: An introduction to intellectual disabilities*. Upper Saddle River, NJ: Pearson Merrill Prentice Hall.

Benomir, A. M., Nicolson, R. I., & Beail, N. (2016). Attitudes towards people with intellectual disability in the UK and Libya: A cross-cultural comparison. *Research in Developmental Disabilities*, *51-52*, 1–9. doi:10.1016/j.ridd.2015.12.009 PMID:26773692

Block, P. (2000). Sexuality, fertility and danger: Twentieth-century images of women with cognitive disabilities. *Sexuality and Disability, 18*(4), 239–254. doi:10.1023/A:1005642226413

Bowlby, J. (1988). *A secure base: Parent-child attachment and healthy human development*. New York: Basic Books. Retrieved from http://www.psychology.sunysb.edu/attachment/online/inge_origins.pdf

Braddock, D., & Parish, S. L. (2002). *An institutional history of disability*. Washington, DC: American Association of Mental Retardation.

Braithwaite, D. O., & Thompson, T. L. (1999). *Handbook of Communication and People With Disabilities: Research and Application*. Retrieved from https://books.google.co.in/books?isbn=1135675805

Brown, B. J., Mansell, J., & Kozma, A. (2007). Deinstitutionalization in intellectual disabilities. *Current Opinion in Psychiatry, 20*(5), 437–442. doi:10.1097/YCO.0b013e32827b14ab PMID:17762584

Chaturvedi, S. K., & Malhotra, S. (1984). A follow up study of mental retardation focussing parental attitudes. *Indian Journal of Psychiatry, 26*(4), 370–376. PMID:21966015

Chiner, E., & Cardona, M. C. (2012). Inclusive education in Spain: How do skills, resources, and supports affect regular education teachers' perceptions of inclusion? *International Journal of Inclusive Education, 17*(5), 526–541. doi:10.1080/13603116.2012.689864

Cologon, K. (2012). Confidence in their own ability: Postgraduate early childhood students examining their attitudes towards inclusive education. *International Journal of Inclusive Education, 16*(11), 1155–1173. doi:10.1080/13603116.2010.548106

Cook, B. G., Tankersley, M., Cook, L., & Landrum, T. (2000). Abstract of Teachers' Attitudes toward their included students with disabilities. *Exceptional Children, 67*(1), 115–135. doi:10.1177/001440290006700108

Dalal, A. (1998). CBR in Action - Some Reflections from the Sirathu Project. *Asia Pacific Disability Rehabilitation Journal, 9*(1), 29–31.

Davis, C., Oliver, C., Tang, C. S., & Wu, A. (2000). Chinese children's attitudes towards mental retardation. *Journal of Developmental and Physical Disabilities, 12*.

Doornbos, M. M. (2002). Predicting family health in families of young adults with severe mental illness. *Journal of Family Nursing, 8*(3), 241–263. doi:10.1177/107484070200800306

Ebuenyi, I. D., Rottenburg, E. S., Bunders-Aelen, J. F. G., & Regeer, B. J. (2018). Challenges of inclusion: A qualitative study exploring barriers and pathways to inclusion of persons with mental disabilities in technical and vocational education and training programmes in East Africa. *Disability and Rehabilitation, 6*, 1–9. doi:10.1080/09638288.2018.1503729 PMID:30398073

European Agency for Development in Special Needs Education. (2011). *Mapping the implementation of policy for inclusive education - An exploration of challenges and opportunities for developing indicators*. Retrieved from http://www.european-agency.org/publications/flyers/mipie /MIPIE-summary-of-proposalsEN.pdf/view

Forlin, C., Loreman, T., Sharma, U., & Earle, C. (2009). Demographic differences in changing pre service teachers' attitudes, sentiments and concerns about inclusive education. *International Journal of Inclusive Education, 13*(2), 195–209. doi:10.1080/13603110701365356

Frey, G. C., & Temple, V. A. (2008). Health promotions for Latin Americans with intellectual disabilities. *Salud Pública de México, 2*, 167–177. doi:10.1590/S0036-36342008000800010 PMID:18470345

Genesi, D. (2000). *Disability Discrimination against students in the classroom.* Retrieved from http://www.cedarville.edu/academics/education/classes/edsp202/examples/literature_review_genesi.htm

Geng-qing, C., & Qu, H. (2003). Integrating persons with disabilities into the workforce: A study on employment of people with disabilities in foodservice industry. *International Journal of Hospitality & Tourism Administration, 4*, 59–83. doi:10.1300/J149v04n04_04

Ghai, A. (2002). Disabled Women: An excluded agenda of Indian feminism. *Hypatia, 17*(3), 49–66. doi:10.1111/j.1527-2001.2002.tb00941.x

Girimaji, S., Zahman, S., Wijetunja, P. M., Pejarasangharn, U., & Nagpal, J. (2001). *Mental Retardation: From Knowledge to Action.* Retrieved June 24, 2005 from http://whqlibdoc.who.int/searo/2001/SEA_Ment_119.pdf

Glumbic, N., Kaljaca, S., & Brojcin, B. (2004). The attitude of future special educators towards inclusive education of children with mild intellectual disability. *Journal of Intellectual Disability Research, 48*, 505–505.

Gordon, B. O., & Rosenblum, K. E. (2001). Bringing Disability into the Sociological Frame: A comparison of disability with race, sex, and sexual orientation statuses. *Disability & Society, 16*(1), 23–44.

Govender, N. (2002). *Attitudes of Parents towards their Mentally Retarded Children: A Rural area Examination.* Academic Press.

Grebler, A. M. (1952). Parental attitudes towards mentally retarded children. *American Journal of Mental Deficiency, 56*, 475–483. PMID:14902885

Gupta, A., & Singhal, N. (2004). Positive Perceptions in Parents of Children with Disabilities. *Asia Pacific Disability Rehabilitation Journal, 15*(1). Retrieved from http://english.aifo.it/disability/apdrj/apdrj104/positive-perceptions.pdf

Hamdani, S., Atif, N., Tariq, M., Minhas, F., Iqbal, Z., & Rahman, A. (2014). Family networks to improve outcomes in children with intellectual and developmental disorders: A qualitative study. *International Journal of Mental Health Systems, 8*(1), 7. doi:10.1186/1752-4458-8-7 PMID:24485093

Hannam, C. (1975). *Parents and Mentally Handicapped Children.* London: Penguin.

Harbour, C. K., & Maulik, P. K. (2010). History of Intellectual Disability. *International Encyclopedia of Rehabilitation.* Retrieved from http://cirrie.buffalo.edu/encyclopedia/en/article/143/

Hazarika, M., Das, S., & Choudhury, S. (2017). Parents' attitude towards children and adolescents with intellectual developmental disorder. International journal of child development and mental health, 5(1), 11–21.

Hewstone, M. (2003). Inter-group contact: Panacea for prejudice? *The Psychologist, 12*(7), 352–355.

Ineland, J., & Hjelte, J. (2019). Knowing, being or doing? A comparative study on human service professionals' perceptions of quality in day-to-day encounters with clients and students with intellectual disabilities. *Journal of Intellectual Disabilities, 22*(3), 246–261. doi:10.1177/1744629517694705 PMID:30134782

International Labour Office. (2003). *Employment of People with Disabilities: The impact of Legislation.* India Country Profile. Retrieved March, 17, 2005 from http://www.ilo.org/publi/english/employment/skills/disability/download/ cpindia.pdf

Jacobson, J. W., Mulick, J. A., & Rojahn, J. (2007). Handbook of Intellectual and Developmental Disabilities. Academic Press. doi:10.1007/0-387-32931-5

Jobling, A., Moni, K., & Nolan, A. (2000). Understanding friendship: Young adults with Down syndrome explore relationships. *Journal of Intellectual & Developmental Disability, 25*(3), 235–245. doi:10.1080/13269780050144299

Joseph, J. (2005). The 1942 'euthanasia' debate in the American Journal of Psychiatry. *History of Psychiatry, 16*(2), 171–179. doi:10.1177/0957154X05047004 PMID:16013119

Karl, R., McGuigan, D., Withiam-Leitch, M. L., Akl, E. A., & Symons, A. B. (2013). Reflective impressions of a precepted clinical experience caring for people with disabilities. *Intellectual and Developmental Disabilities, 51*(4), 237–245. doi:10.1352/1934-9556-51.4.237 PMID:23909585

Kelly, G., Crowley, H., & Hamilton, C. (2009). Rights, sexuality, and relationships in Ireland: "It'd be nice to be kind of trusted. *British Journal of Learning Disabilities, 37*(4), 308–315. doi:10.1111/j.1468-3156.2009.00587.x

Kelly, G., & Parry, A. (2008). Managing Challenging Behaviour of People with Acquired Brain Injury in Community Settings: The first 7 years of specialist clinical service. *Brain Impairment, 9*(3), 293–304. doi:10.1375/brim.9.3.293

Khandelwal, S. K., & Workneh, F. (1986). Perception of mental illness by medical students Indian. *Journal of Psychological Medicine, 9*, 26–32.

Konstantareas, M. M., & Lunsky, Y. J. (1997). Socio-sexual knowledge, experience, attitudes, and interests of individuals with autistic disorder and developmental delay. *Journal of Autism and Developmental Disorders, 27*(4), 397–413. doi:10.1023/A:1025805405188 PMID:9261666

Kritsotakis, G., Galanis, P., Papastefanakis, E., Meidani, F., Philalithis, A. E., Kalokairinou, A., & Sourtzi, P. (2017). Attitudes towards people with physical or intellectual disabilities among nursing, social work and medical students. *Journal of Clinical Nursing, 26*(23-24), 4951–4963. doi:10.1111/jocn.13988 PMID:28771877

Lakhan, R., & Sharma, M. (2010). A study of Knowledge, Attitudes and Practices (KAP) Survey of Families towards their Children with Intellectual Disability in Barwani, India. *Asia Pacific Disability Rehabilitation Journal*, 21.

Madhavan, T., Menon, D. K., & Kalyan, M. (1988). *Mental Retardation: A Manual for Village Rehabilitation Workers*. National Institute for the Mentally Handicapped.

Mary, N. L. (1990). Reactions of black, hispanic, and white mothers to having a child with handicaps. *Mental Retardation*, *28*(1), 1–5. PMID:2308509

McCabe, M. P. (1999). Sexual knowledge, experience, and feelings among people with disability. *Sexuality and Disability*, *17*(2), 157–170. doi:10.1023/A:1021476418440

McConachie, H. (1986). *Parents & Young mentally handicapped children: a review of research issues*. London: Croom Helm.

McHale, S. M., & Gamble, W. C. (1987). Sibling relationships and adjustment of children with disabled brothers and sisters. In F. Fuchs Schachter & R. K. Stine (Eds.), Practical concerns about siblings: Bridging the research-practice gap (pp. 131-158). New York: Haworth Press.

McLeod, S. A. (2008). *Erik Erikson/Psychological Stages*. Retrieved from www.simplypsychology.org/Erik-Erikson.html

Mencap. (2007). *Death by indifference*. Mencap.

Mental Disability Rights International (MDRI). (2007). *Ruined Lives: Segregation from Society in Argentina's Psychiatric Asylums*. Washington, DC: Mental Disability Rights International.

Mondal, A., & Mete, J. (2011). *Education of Children with Disabilities in India: Concern and Policy Perspective*. Academic Press.

Morris, J. (2005). *Citizenship and disabled People, Disability Rights Commission*. London: DRC.

Murch, A. J., Choudhury, T., Wilson, M., Collerton, E., Patel, M., & Scior, K. (2018). Explicit and implicit attitudes towards people with intellectual disabilities: The role of contact and participant demographics. *Journal of Applied Research in Intellectual Disabilities*, *31*(5), 778–784. doi:10.1111/jar.12429 PMID:29168267

Norins-Bardon, Matsumoto, & Siperstein. (2005). *US students attitudes to students with intellectual disabilities*. Global Youth Summit, Nagano, Japan. Available at www.specialolympics.org

Nowicki, E. A. (2006). A cross-sectional multivariate analysis of children's attitudes towards disability. *Journal of Intellectual Disability Research*, *50*(5), 335–348. doi:10.1111/j.1365-2788.2005.00781.x PMID:16629927

Ntombela, T. (1991). *The family of a mentally retarded child* (Vol. 1). Social Work Practise.

Patel, M., & Rose, J. (2014). Students' attitudes towards individuals with an intellectual disability. *Journal of Intellectual Disabilities*, *18*(1), 90–103. doi:10.1177/1744629513511355 PMID:24196840

Pelleboer-Gunnink, H. A., Oorsouw, V., Weeghel, V. J., & Embregts, P. J. C. M. (2017). Mainstream health professionals' stigmatising attitudes towards people with intellectualdisabilities: A systematic review. *Journal of Intellectual Disability Research*, *61*(5), 411–434. doi:10.1111/jir.12353 PMID:28198094

Persha, A., Arya, S., & Nagar, R. K. (2007). Biological and Psychological Predictors of Developmental Delay in Persons with Intellectual Disability: Retrospective Case- File Study. *Asia Pacific Disability Rehabilitation Journal, 18*(1), 93–100.

Peshawaria, R., Menon, D. K., Ganguly, R., Roy, S., Pillay, R.P.R.S., & Gupta, A. (1995). *Understanding the Indian Families Having Persons with Mental Retardation.* NIMH. Retrieved from http://nimhindia.gov.in/Understanding%20Indian%20Families.pdf

Pettigrew, T. F., & Tropp, L. R. (2000). Reducing prejudice and discrimination. *The Claremont Symposium on Applied Social Psychology*, 93-114.

Powell, T. H., & Ogle, P. A. (1985). *Brothers & sisters: A special part of exceptional families*. Baltimore, MD: Paul H. Brookes Publishing.

Radford, J. P. (1991). Sterilization versus segregation: Control of the 'feebleminded', 1900-1938. *Social Science & Medicine, 33*(4), 449–458. doi:10.1016/0277-9536(91)90327-9 PMID:1948159

Ravindranodan, S., & Raju, V. (2007). Attitudes of parents of children with mental retardation. *Journal of the Indian Academy of Applied Psychology, 1*, 137–141.

Rawlins, R. C. A. (1983). *Attitudes to Mental retardation: a cross cultural study* (MA Counseling Psychology Thesis). Pietermaritzburg: University of Natal.

Reilly, P. R. (1987). Involuntary sterilization in the United States: A surgical solution. *The Quarterly Review of Biology, 62*(2), 153–170. doi:10.1086/415404 PMID:3299450

Reschly, D. J. (1996). Identification and Assessment of Students with Disabilities. *The Future of Children Special Education for Students With Disabilities, 6*(1). Retrieved from https://www.princeton.edu/futureofchildren/publications/docs/06_01_02.pdf

Rimmerman, A. (1998). Factors relating to attitudes of Israeli corporate executives towards the employability of persons with intellectual disability. *Journal of Intellectual & Developmental Disability, 23*(3), 245–254. doi:10.1080/13668259800033731

Ruggeri-Stevens, G., & Goodwin, S. (2007). "Learning to work" in small businesses: Learning and training for young adults with learning disabilities. *Education + Training, 49*(8/9), 745–755. doi:10.1108/00400910710834139

Rutledge, M. S., & Scott, M. H. (1997). Students' attitudes towards people with mental retardation. *Academic Medicine, 72*(4).

Ryan, T. A., & Scior, K. (2014). Medical students' attitudes towards people with intellectual disabilities: A literature review. *Research in Developmental Disabilities, 35*(10), 2316–2328. doi:10.1016/j.ridd.2014.05.019 PMID:24952372

Satchidanand, N., Gunukula, S. K., Lam, W. Y., McGuigan, D., New, I., Symons, A. B., ... Akl, E. A. (2012). Attitudes of healthcare students and professionals toward patients with physical disability: A systematic review. *American Journal of Physical Medicine & Rehabilitation, 91*(6), 533–545. doi:10.1097/PHM.0b013e3182555ea4 PMID:22596075

Schlossar, S. (2004). *Opening Doors. Multicultural Disability Advocacy Association of NSW*. Retrieved on June. 13.2015 from http://www.mdaa.org.au/publications/ethnicity/indian/IndianOpenDoors.pdf

Scott, M. H., & Rutledge, C. M. (1997). Students' attitudes toward people with mental retardation. *Academic Medicine*, *72*(4), 246–247. doi:10.1097/00001888-199704000-00005 PMID:9125936

Scruggs, T. E., & Mastropieri, M. A. (1996). Teacher perceptions of inclusion/ mainstreaming, 1958-1995: A research synthesis. *Exceptional Children*, *1996*, 59–74. doi:10.1177/001440299606300106

Shrivastava, S. P. (Ed.). (1970). Social Work and the Rehabilitation of the Physically Handicapped, The Journal of Rehabilitation in Asia, 11(1).

Siebelink, E. M., de Jong, M. D. T., Taal, E., & Roelvink, L. (2006). Sexuality and people with intellectual disabilities: Assessment of knowledge, attitudes, experiences, and needs. *Mental Retardation*, *44*(4), 283–294. doi:10.1352/0047-6765(2006)44[283:SAPWID]2.0.CO;2 PMID:16834465

Silver, H. (1957). *The Physically Handicapped, Social Work Year Book*. Academic Press.

Singal, N. (2009). *Education of children with disabilities in India*. Retrieved from http://unesdoc.unesco.org/images/0018/001866/186611e.pdf

Siperstein, G. N., Hardman, M. L., Wappett, M. T., & Clary, L. (2001). *National Evaluation of the Special Olympics Unified Sports Program (Final Report for Special Olympics, Incorporated)*. Boston: University of Massachusetts, Center for Social Development and Education.

Siperstein, G. N., Sugumaran, K., Bardon, J. N., & Parker, R. S. (2001). *Attitudes of the Public in India towards People with Intellectual Disabilities*. Retrieved from www.specialolympics.org/uploadedfiles/.../india_full%20report.pdf

Sofair, A. N., & Kaldijian, L. C. (2000). Eugenic sterilization and a qualified Nazi analogy: The United States and Germany, 1930-1945. *Annals of Internal Medicine*, *132*(4), 312–319. doi:10.7326/0003-4819-132-4-200002150-00010 PMID:10681287

Special Olympics. (2004). *A Study of Youth Attitudes about Intellectual Disabilities*. Retrieved from http://www.specialolympics.org

Special Olympics. (2005). *Multinational Study of Attitudes towards Individuals with Intellectual Disabilities*. Retrieved from www.specialolympics.org/...Studies.../Multinational_Attitudes_Study.asp

Stella, C. S. C., Forlin, C., & Lan, A. M. (2007). The influence of an inclusive education course on attitude change of pre-service secondary teachers in Hong Kong. *Asia-Pacific Journal of Teacher Education*, *35*(2), 161–179. doi:10.1080/13598660701268585

Stokes, S. (1990). Restaurant supervisors: Don't discount the disabled. *The Cornell Hotel and Restaurant Administration Quarterly*, *30*(4), 14–17. doi:10.1177/001088049003000405

Tervo, R. C., Azuma, S., Palmer, G., & Redinius, P. (2002). Medical students' attitudes toward persons with disability: A comparative study. *Archives of Physical Medicine and Rehabilitation*, *83*(11), 1537–1542. doi:10.1053/apmr.2002.34620 PMID:12422321

Tolu, E.A., Temitayo, & Kofoworola, A. (2014). Exclusion of Children with Intellectual Disabilities from Regular Classroom: Nigeria Perspective. *African Journal for the Psychological Study of Social Issues*, *17*, 99-109. Retrieved from http://ajpssi.org/index.php/ajpssi/article/view/94/pdf_65

United Nations Educational, Scientific and Cultural Organization. (1994). *The Salamanca Statement and framework for action on special needs education.* Paris: Author.

United Nations Educational, Scientific and Cultural Organization. (2008). *Inclusive education: The way of the future*. 48th session of the International Conference on Education, Genova.

United Nations Educational, Scientific and Cultural Organization. (2008). *Defining an Inclusive Education agenda: Reflection around the 48th session the International Conference on Education*. Retrieved from www.ibe.unesco.org/.../48th.../Defining_Inclusive_Education_Agenda_2

University Legal Services. (2012). *The Work Option for Individuals with Intellectual Disabilities: The Obstacles and the Possibilities*. Retrieved from www.ulsdc.org/Employment%20Report_FINAL.pdf

U.S. Census Bureau. (2007). *American with disabilities act: July 26*. Author.

Uysal, A., Albayrak, B., Koçulu, B., Kan, F., & Aydın, T. (2014). Attitudes of nursing students toward people with disabilities. *Nurse Education Today*, *34*(5), 878–884. doi:10.1016/j.nedt.2013.09.001 PMID:24080269

Werner, D. (2006). *Disabled Village Children: A Guide for Community Health Workers, Rehabilitation Workers, and Families*. Berkeley, CA: Hesperian Foundation.

Williams, J. R., & Algozzine, B. (1979). Teachers' Attitudes toward Mainstreaming. *The Elementary School Journal*, *80*(2), 63–67. doi:10.1086/461173

Wilson, A. S. (2007). *Caregiver Attitude of Sexuality of the Intellectually Disabled Population*. Proquest Theses & Dissertation.

World Health Organization. (2007). *Atlas: global resources for persons with intellectual disabilities.* Geneva: World Health Organization. Retrieved from http://www.who.int/mental_health/evidence/atlas_id_2007.pdf

York, A. M., Ruediger, T., & Voltenburg, N. (2017). Doctor of physical therapy students' attitudes towards people with disabilities: A descriptive study. *Disability and Rehabilitation*, *39*(1), 91–97. doi:10.3109/09638288.2016.1140830 PMID:26883300

Chapter 12
Emotional Intelligence in Individuals With Intellectual disability

Priyadharshini Sivasubramanian
Gujarat Forensic Sciences University, India

ABSTRACT

This chapter is aimed to draw attention to the integrated understanding of an individual with intellectual disability. It is very well known that intellectual disability is described as significant inefficiency in cognitive skills like learning, reasoning, problem solving, and in adaptive behavior, but this is not all when the individual is considered as a whole. This is where emotional intelligence comes in to help the individual cope with the cognitive disability. This chapter will discuss emotional intelligence in people with intellectual disability and how understanding of this will lead to better management plans for individual with intellectual disability, which will in turn lead to better empowerment. Further, this chapter will discuss the research gaps in this area and future study scope.

INTRODUCTION

Intellectual disability, historically referred to as mental retardation, is characterized by significant impairments in intellectual functioning and limitations in adaptive behavior that begin prior to the age of 18 (Schalock et al. 2007). Conceptual, social, and practical skills such as personal care, use of the telephone, and managing money are examples of adaptive behaviour. The impact of intellectual disability can range from mild (e.g., a person can engage in meaningful conversation and carry out simple occupational skills) to profound (e.g., a person is completely dependent on others for personal care and has minimal verbal abilities) impairment. In the year 2011, U.S president Barack Obama signed a law called as Rosa's law, in which the term mental retardation was replaced by Intellectual disability. Therefore, in DSM V the term used is intellectual disability. Individuals having this condition are not addressed as retards they are addressed as individual with intellectual disability. This was done keeping in mind that cognitive

DOI: 10.4018/978-1-7998-1223-4.ch012

disability solely does not define an individual. An individual is an integration of cognitive abilities, emotional abilities and spiritual ability. To be precise, see the definition given by DSM V (2013):

Intellectual disability or intellectual developmental disorder is a disorder with onset during the developmental period that includes both intellectual and adaptive functioning deficits in conceptual, social and practical domains. The following two criteria must be met:

Deficits in intellectual functions, such as reasoning, problem solving, planning, abstract thinking, judgment, academic learning, and learning from experience, confirmed by both clinical assessment and individualized, standardized intelligence testing.

Deficits in adaptive functioning that result in failure to meet developmental and socio-cultural standards for personal independence and social responsibility. Without ongoing support, the adaptive deficits limit functioning in one or more activities of daily functioning such as communication social participation and independent living, across multiple environments, such as home, school, work and community.

In this chapter among the two deficits, focus will be on adaptive functioning. According to DSM V, adaptive functioning is how well a person meets community standards of personal independence and social responsibility. A simpler explanation of adaptive functioning is how a person responds to the given environment in a given time. The adaptive functioning is categorized into 3 domains: Contextual domain, Social domain and Practical domain.

The contextual domain involves competency in memory, language, reading, writing, math reasoning, and acquisition of practical knowledge, problem solving, and judgment in novel situations.

The social domain involves awareness of others thoughts, feelings and experiences, empathy, interpersonal communication skills, friendship abilities and social judgment among many others.

The practical domain involves learning and self management across life, which includes personal care, job responsibilities, money management, recreation, self management of behavior, school and work task organization among many others (DSM V).

This chapter aim to focus on the working status of emotional intelligence in individual with intellectual disability and how training in this area will enhance and improve the other domains. At the beginning let's start with understanding what emotional intelligence is?

Emotional Intelligence

According to salovey and mayer (1990), "Emotional intelligence is the ability to manage self and other people from the aspect of feeling and emotion, is able to distinguish the two terms apart and able to use the information to guide one's thinking and action." It is also defined as the ability of an individual to express, appraise and understand the emotional expressions in others and ability to regulate one's own emotions. Keeping this in mind, Goleman in 1998 proposed two main domain in which emotional intelligence is categorized for understanding: Recognition of emotion and regulation of emotion.

To be effective performer, the cognitive process has to be under control of the emotional process. Therefore, Goleman (1998) clubbed many researches and came up with 4 components for effective use of emotions. They are:

- **Self Awareness:** Knowing one's emotion. Ability to know what one is feeling at a given moment of time and at a given situation. In 1994 John Mayer called it as meta-mood an affective analogue for meta-cognition.

- **Emotional Self Management:** It is the ability to regulate distressing affects like anxiety and anger and to inhibit emotional impulsivity. It is mainly emotional self control which includes delayed gratification and controlling impulsivity. It regulates motivation for goal directed behavior.
- **Social Awareness:** It involves recognizing other's emotions. This characterizes the ability to keep oneself in other's shoes. Thinking what this person would have undergone if the situation happen to oneself. This fundamental "people skill' is called empathy. People who are empathetic are attuned to the subtle social signals that indicates what others need and want. Empathy builds in altruism which is the basis for social morality.
- **Relationship Management:** Ability to attune ourselves or influence the emotions of other person.

What is Emotions?

The word emotion is derived from the word "Emovere" which means to move. Its root word is Movi whose meaning indicates movement i.e. set in motion. According to Damasio (1998) emotions are an execution of a very complex program of action. Actions which denotes movement. Some actions are gross physical movement like facial expression in fear. Some are the internal movements that happens in heart or gut and some movement that is not necessarily muscular but rather release of molecules for example release of hormones from endocrine system to the blood stream. All these are movements which can be the potential emotional response. The emotions are differentiated into three categories. They are: 1)Background emotions- which are induced internally and mainly its focus is the general welfare of the individual. Emotions like well being, calmness etc comes under this categories. 2) Primary or universal emotions- It involves distinct neural and chemical circuits. There are six emotions under this category. Fear, anger, disgust, sadness, surprise and happiness. These six emotions are also given by Ekman in the year 1990. 3) Social Emotion- In this category, emotions which are not only biological but also socially learned are involved like sympathy, compassion, pride, guilt, embarassment, shame, jealousy, envy, gratitude and admiration (list of emotion as given by Damasio 2000).

Frijda (1988) defines emotions as subjective experiences, whose core is the pleasure or the pain, and describes them through laws. This description implies two assumptions: emotions exhibit regularities which arise from the causal mechanisms that generate them and human beings do not create or control what they want to feel, they obey the emotions laws. Ekman (1992) and Davidson (2000) consider that emotions recruit physiological changes necessary for the body to respond in an evolutionarily adaptive manner, where each specific emotion prepares the body for a set of actions. They modify the cognitive activities by sometimes making cognition difficult and sometimes by promoting it. Emotions also provide affective information since being aware of our feelings enables us to make value judgments and take decisions based on what we feel. Furthermore, they also organize the subjective, behavioral and physiological components of the emotional process and have particular functions like interpersonal functions since they report others about our motivations pushing them to act.

William James proposed one of the first theories to emotion which related emotion and an individual's physiological function. It was in the successive researches and theories, the relationship between neuronal network of the brain and emotion was studied. It was found that sub-cortical structure called as limbic system plays a major role in expression of emotion. A part in limbic system which is involved in the recognition of the emotion in stimuli and responding to it is amygdala. Other than the structure, it is also seen that monoamine system is also involved in the regulation of emotion and they are: dopamine, nor epinephrine and serotonin. Therefore, both bio-physiological system and environmental circumstance interact together to regulate the emotion of the individual. In order to understand more of emotion, it is necessary to discuss about the characteristic manifestation of different primary or universal emotion.

Happiness is a sense of joy and a pleasant feeling of contentment (Izard, 1991). It can occur both as a result of pleasurable circumstances in the environment or by the stimulation internally (for example feeling good after an exercise). Researches done on 50's and 60's give an ample evidence of fundamental hedonic brain system responsible for pleasure and happiness. Finding say that there is an overlap in the brain system which is involved in fundamental pleasure like food and sex with those of higher order pleasures like altruism, musical etc. To be more precise, "liking" is stimulated by interlinking of nucleus accumbens and ventral pallidum, "wanting" is stimulated by mesolimbic dopamine transmitters and cortical regions like orbito-frontal, cingulate, medial-prefrontal and insula are involved in the anticipation, appraisal, experience and memory of pleasurable stimuli (Kringelbach, 2005). This shows that the pleasure areas in the brain is anatomically distributed but are liked to each other for the manifestation of the emotion happiness.

There are number of neurological evidences which shows that there is a separate neural system which plays in arousal and recognition of negative emotion like sadness, fear and anger than those play in the processing of happiness. A study done on an individual whose had a bilateral damage to amygdala was seen to have poor emotional arousal to negative emotion and also poor understanding of the negative stimuli. This shows that amygdala is the major part of brain which is involved in appraisal of primary negative emotion and recognition of the emotion in the stimuli (Adolph, 1999). This may be the reason why an individual sometimes can feel sadness and happiness at the same time, for example A mother feels sad that her child is going out of house for studies at the same time she feel happy for her child's accomplishments (Lane,1997).

Overall view of functional neuroanatomy of emotion involves the given area: 1) medial prefrontal cortex for general emotional processing. this involves some cognitive ability; 2) Fear specifically stimulates the amygdala. This does not have a cognitive demand. The reaction is purely universal; 3) Sadness is associated with the subcallosal cingulate; 4) Induction of emotion activated by the occipital cortex and amygdala; 5) Anterior cingulate and insula is associated with emotional recall and imagery; and 6) emotional tasks with cognitive demand also involved anterior cingulate and insula (Phan, et.al. 2002).

In conclusion it can be seen that the emotional processesing can happen without much cognitive demand. The research finding show that manipulation of emotion can lead to change or new learning of behavior for example application of reward system to increase the desirable behavior and application of punishment to decrease the undesirable behavior (Gordon, 2018).

Emotional Development

From birth to death, emotions are central to human functioning and growth. It is so pervasive that we often forget its important role in our life. They help us make the most important decisions, lies at the heart of all social relationships and is central to socialization and cultural processes. Core aspects of emotions are inherited and universal. The whole of emotional development surrounds around three aspects of experiencing, expressive emotional responses and recognition. In which regulation and coping is also involved. The development ranges from simple reading out of internal states in early to increasing differentiation in expressive emotion and the actual internal states in as early as 3 years of age (Lewis, 2008; Dion, 2011).

Saarni (2008) described emotional development in childhood taking into account functionalist theory and dynamic systems theory. According to him development is divided into 7 age period. They are 1) Infancy (0 to 12 months); 2)Toddler (12 months to 21/2 years); 3) Pre-school (2-5years); 4) Early elementary school (5-7 years); 5)Middle Childhood (7-10years); 6) Pre-Adolescence (10-13 years); and 7) Adolescence (13+years).

During the infancy period the child synchronizes with others through expression, understands differences in others emotions, expressive responsiveness increases. These children regulate their emotions by self soothing and learning to modulate reactions, gives attention to coordinated actions and reliance on caregivers under stress situations. They use social games, social referencing through which infants come to learn the world around them and instrumental social signal use like faking a cry to draw attention (Saarni, 2011). At this stage the primary emotions differentiates into happiness, anger, sadness, surprise, shame and fear (Papalia et.al. 2001). Children learn relationship between emotion and behavior.

In the toddler period which ranges from 12 months to 2 1/2 years, children develop emotions like shame and pride as a result of developing self evaluation and self consciousness. They can start using words to describe their affective states and there is a increase in verbal comprehension. In this period, emotions are regulated by being self aware of their emotional response and getting irritated when not allowed for their need for autonomy. Children develop early forms of empathy and pro-social actions. Overall they understand that they are separate entity from other person and objects (Saarni, 2011).

At the age two top five which is also called preschool period, an individual start pretending emotional expression in play and teasing and also understand the false facial expression can conceal the actual feelings to others. By this time children starts using some cognitive strategies, for example they understand that a symbol can represent a completely different object. This symbolic aspect facilitates emotional regulation. But, the regulation of emotion is dominated by the behavior strategies. In this period their communication with others helps them to understand social interaction and their corresponding behavioral expectations (Izard, 2004; Estrada, 2008 & Saarni, 2011).

In early childhood period and the middle childhood period, the coping of emotion involves seeking help but increases in situational problem solving, then towards middle childhood preferred coping strategy is problem solving if control from the care giver is moderate. They also learn distancing as a coping strategy if control is minimal. There is also a change in concept of emotions. Older children give greater importance to internal mental states. Increase in social relationship enhancing strategies like keeping cool emotional expression in front of peers and smiling when approaching a friend (Harris, 1981; Saarni, 2011).

During preadolescence stage, they become capable of generating multiple ways of coping to stressful situations and understand the realistic control in stressful situations. They start to make distinction between genuine expression given to a friend and a persona put on for others. Increase in the social sensibility is seen. Children also begin to self evaluate without anybody's appraisal (Saarni, 2011; Cristina, 2013).

In adolescence and early adulthood, an individual by now is adequate in exercising insightful coping by being aware of one's own emotional cycles. Here, they enter into the process of forming their distinct identity and their own distinct moral principles to get forward with life. They learn to develop a skillful presentation of themselves so that they can make an impression. Individual in this stage begin to understand that the most important thing in management of a good relationship is mutual and reciprocal communication and understanding (Saarni, 2011 ; DeLoache, 1994).

When it comes to understanding of emotional development in individual with intellectual disability, there is very minimal research in this area to give detail light on it. The researches which have been done shows that there is developmental delay in emotional system, such as 'affect differentiation', 'anxiety' and 'aggression regulation', although not as severe as cognitive delay. It is also seen that people having combined conditions like autism with intellectual disability have lower levels of emotional development than the individual having only intellectual disability (Sappock, et.al., 2013).

Cognitive Intelligence vs. Emotional Intelligence

History of emotional intelligence dates back to the year 1920, when Edward Thorndike first spoke about "social intelligence". It is defined as "the ability to understand and manage men and women and boys and girls to act wisely in human relations." Psychologist Nicholas Humphrey believes that it is social intelligence than quantitative intelligence, which defines us of who we are as humans. After Thorndike, in 1940 David Wechsler, who is known as the father of IQ discussed the "Non-intellective aspects" of intelligence. At a meeting of American Psychological Association, he reiterated that factor analysis of his IQ assessment did not explain nearly all of the variance and his belief was that non intellective factors contributed to the residual variance. Leuner in the year 1966 published paper on Emotional Intelligence and emancipation. According to him there is a significant relationship between understanding emotions and verbal memory and verbal fluency which is a cognitive ability. He found no significant relationship between cognitive abilities and perceiving, using and managing emotions. Trait emotional intelligence correlated with better language performance in children characterized by low or medium cognitive ability but not in people with high cognitive ability. After leuner, Claude Steiner in 1974 published his first article on emotional literacy. In 1983, Howard Gardner in his work of multiple intelligence included non intellective factors such as interpersonal, intrapersonal and naturalistic intelligence, apart from his 5 other cognitive factors. He gave these personal factors a separate status of intelligence (Sparrow, & Knight, 2006).

Wayne Payne used the first phrase "emotional intelligence" in the year 1986. His thesis went unpublished. He spoke about the importance of emotional intelligence in mental health of an individual. The term emotional quotient was introduced by Keith Beasley in 1987. By the year 1990, there were many scattered published article on emotional intelligence in different journals and books. Peter Salovey and Jack Mayer bought these entire scattered articles and combined it into a landmark article "Emotional Intelligence" published in the journal Imagination, Cognition and Personality. He proposed that emotional intelligence is a process different from cognitive intelligence. It starts from appraisal and expression of emotion of self and others, regulation of emotion in self and other and ultimately utilization of emotion (Knight, & Sparrow, 2006).

Researches in affective neuroscience posit that there is a difference between emotional intelligence and cognitive intelligence. As cognitive intelligence involves capacity that are purely neo-cortical and emotional intelligence are those that integrate neo-cortical and limbic circuitry. It gives a top down approach to brain evolution. The tertiary affects and neocortical awareness functions involves cognitive executive functions which is the main cause of thought and planning residing in frontal cortex, emotional ruminations and regulations that resides in medial frontal regions and free will involving higher working memory functions (Intention to Action). The secondary process affect involves learning via basal ganglia. Under this comes the classical conditioning helped by baso-lateral and central amygdala, instrumental and operant conditioning i.e. seeking via nucleus accumbens and behavioral and emotional habits which is largely unconscious involving dorsal straitum. Then, the primary process, basic pre-mordial affective states are majorly subcortical. This involves sensory affects e.g. pleasurable and unpleasurable/disgust feelings, homeostatic affect involving brain body interoceptors e.g. hunger, thirst etc., and emotional affect involving emotion action system. The primary affects are universal whatever may be the condition. Secondary affect is in the more evolved mammals and tertiary affect is majorly for cognitively evolved humans. This is where higher cognitive functions come into play (Panksepp, et.al., 2010).

Emotional quotients are found to be more important the standard IQ ability as it was observed that as an individual goes higher in the organization, emotional intelligence becomes more important (Golman, 1999). Darwin believed that its emotional intelligence that helps an individual adapt to dynamic environment and eventually survive.

From the above theory, it can be hypothesized that an individual with intellectual disability will only have difficulty in the area where cognitive ability is involved but emotional processing in secondary and primary affects are preserved. Few research on the importance of emotional development indicates that emotional development is crucial in the overall development of human beings (Cote & Miners, 2006; Frederickson & Fumham, 2004; Panksepp, et.al., 2010).

Emotion Regulation in Intellectually Disabled Populations

Emotion Recognition

When the term "intellectual disability" is combined with "emotion" there are very few identified articles. Among them. the majority of studies pertaining to emotion regulation for persons with intellectual disability address the early part of the regulatory process, emotion recognition. Research indicates that individuals with intellectual disability can reliably identify their own emotions (Lindsay et al., 2004; Lindsay, Michie, Baty, Smith, & Miller, 1994; Rose & West, 1999). In general, people with mild to moderate intellectual disability can also recognize and accurately label facial expressions in others (Moore, 2001) and improve this skill with training (Rydin-Orwin, Drake, & Bratt, 1999; Stewart & Singh, 1995). Moore's (2001) review and the few studies on this topic published after his review specifically conclude: (1) The ability to discriminate pleasant versus unpleasant emotions is equally accurate for individuals with and without intellectual disability. However, intellectually disabled individuals have more difficulty labeling specific emotions. (Owen, Browning & Jones, 2001); (2) Individuals with intellectual disability are able to label some emotions more easily than others. Across several studies, it appears that happiness is more easily identified (Matheson & Jahoda, 2005; Moore, 2001; Owen, Browning & Jones, 2001; Wishart, Cebula, Willis, & Pitcairn, 2007). On the other hand, identification of a neutral face that does not portray an emotion is more difficult than identification of a positive or negative emotional expression (Moore, 2001). Two additional studies have examined the relationship between aggressiveness and facial recognition ability. The first study (Matheson & Jahoda, 2005) examined the difference in emotion recognition between aggressive and non-aggressive individuals with intellectual disability and found happiness, sadness, and anger were the easiest emotions for all participants to identify regardless of whether they frequently engaged in aggressive behaviour. Furthermore, the aggressive and nonaggressive groups demonstrated comparable abilities for labeling emotions. However, the aggressive group had more difficulty recognizing the emotion when contextually complex emotional photos were presented. The second study (Jahoda, Pert, & Trower, 2006) found that aggressive participants were able to recognize facial affect or take another person's perspective just like their non-aggressive counterparts. These findings contradicted the researcher's hypothesis that a deficit in emotion recognition is a significant factor in underlying aggression. Additional research is needed to understand the relationship between emotion recognition and aggression in intellectually disabled populations.

Self and Behavioural Regulation

Baurine and Nader (2012) tried to find the difference and similarities between individual with and without Intellectual disabilities. The finding of the study showed that similar frequencies of socio-emotional behaviors, including behavior toward social rules, emotional expressions and adaptation of emotions, in both groups of children. The children with intellectual disabilities expressed and adapted to their emotions in the same way as their counter group (joy, sadness, frustration and anger) and they did not moderate their externalized behavior less than the typically developing children. Concerning verbal and non-verbal modalities of socio-emotional regulation, the results showed that there was no difference in the way verbal modality was used to express and regulate their emotions between individuals with and without intellectual disability. These results correspond to observations about preschoolers who have the ability to modify and control the intensity of their emotional expressions according to the situation and social rules (Saarni, 1999), and who use language as a strategy to regulate their emotions (Cole et al., 1994), notably to distract themselves in frustrating situations (Stansbury and Zimmerman, 1999). When verbal expression and non verbal expression is compared then nonverbal is more stronger in people with intellectual disability as they have general delay in linguistic area (Rondal, 1985).

The children with intellectual disabilities seem to develop their abilities in socio-emotional regulation more slowly, but they do not display any difference of development compared with younger typically developing children. It contrasts with the observation of a deficit in emotion regulation in two other studies in a limited sample of children with intellectual disabilities (Brun and Mellier, 2004). Baurine posited that people with intellectual disabilities had less social behavior (socio-extravert behavior) than the typically developing group. Although the people with intellectual disabilities used language to express and to regulate their emotions, they used the verbal modality less in their social behaviors than the group consisting of individual without intellectual disability. Serafica (1990), emphasized that, in children with intellectual disabilities, their low cognitive abilities underlying their social skills slow down their initiation and maintenance of exchanges with their peers. According to Guralnick (1999), children with intellectual disabilities have altered social capacities, including difficulties in establishing a relationship of friendship with their peers. Individual with intellectual disabilities evoke less negative emotions than their counter parts. therefore, when peer interaction in preschool is strong, they develop a high level of social skills, allowing them to decrease their level of negative emotions (Fabes et al., 1999). Positive links have been highlighted between their emotion regulation examined in other play contexts (*e.g.* in pretend play with peers or parents) and their interactions with others (peers or parents) (Adams Dillon, 2009, Fabes et al., 1999, Galyer and Evans, 2001, Lindsey and Colwell, 2003). According to Galyer and Evans (2001), a deficit in emotion regulation has been associated with common emotional and behavioral difficulties, including poor adjustment to school, poor peer relationships and poor social competence. Graziano et al. (2007) also reported that children with better skills in emotion regulation had a slightly more positive relationship with their teachers and were less likely to have behavioral disorders.

Now coming to the intensity of emotions in children, this changed depending on the context, with greater intensity being displayed in competitive and cooperative contexts with peers: the children expressed their emotions more intensively when they were in interaction with peers than in a neutral context with an adult. In terms of positive emotions, smiling offers the possibility of maintaining exchanges (Brun, 2008). Furthermore, cooperation between children is based on social interactions during problem-solving and is characterized by emotionally expressive and positive exchanges and reflecting more expressions of joy (smiling and laughter) (Herbé et al., 2007).

Intervention In Individual with Intellectual disability

Sheydaei, Adibsereshki, & Movallali (2015) aimed to investigate the effect of emotional intelligence training on the communication skills of students with intellectual disabilities. The findings show, the emotional intelligence training enhanced the communication skills of the students with intellectual disabilities. To further enhance the evidance, the role of emotional intelligence training on the communication skill for the medical students was seen positive in the study done by Fletcher et al. (2009). Alagheband et al. (2002) in their examination of the relationship between the emotional intelligence and the communication skills of high school students found that except for empathy and responsibility, there was a significant correlation between the different dimensions of emotional intelligence and communication skills. It seems that there is a close relationship between emotional intelligence and communication skills, and that these skills can be considered as part of the overall structure of emotional intelligence. This means that someone who has the ability to understand others' mood changes can accurately identify, control and manage their own and others' emotions. Hassani et al. (2011) also examined the relationship between emotional intelligence and interpersonal problems, with results indicating a significant relationship between the majority of the EI components and interpersonal problems. The different components of emotional intelligence could predict some aspects of interpersonal difficulties. Emotional intelligence, with mental health supports, reduced interpersonal problems and improved the quality of social and interpersonal relationships. In fact, the ability to recognize facial expressions and emotional responses to these expressions and emotions is essential for people's interactions; individuals with intellectual disabilities are generally deficient in these skills specifically verbal expression. Nichols et al. (2013) studied communication problems in children with autism, and concluded that these children have problems in emotion recognition, and that they can be treated with emotional intelligence training. Emotional intelligence training teaches students how to have effective communication skills and to be able to communicate with others without problems. During training, students could evaluate their capabilities through activities such as role playing, games and the use of flash cards, which aimed to teach them these skills and increase the interaction between them. Usually, emotional intelligence training can improve the communicative functions of students by acquainting them with interpersonal skills, social skills, and basic knowledge of the components of verbal and nonverbal communication. The intervention process of emotional intelligence can help design the management plan for the individual with intellectual disabilities. People with intellectual disabilities show similar ability of recognition of emotion compared to their counterparts. This shows that they do have the ability to recognize, express and understand basic emotions but because of their underlying low cognitive ability they face problem in recognizing, expressing and understanding more complex emotions (Sarafice 1990). Through emotional intelligence training these individuals can be helped to improve their abilities. In turn, they will be able to live up to their roles in life.

FUTURE DIRECTION

The body of literature on emotion and emotion regulation is rapidly expanding. Understanding of these concepts and their applications to intellectually disabled population are lagging far behind. Many questions remain unexamined, much less unanswered. What is the normative emotional development process for infants and children with intellectual disability? How does emotion regulation develop in persons with intellectual disability? Do emotion regulation abilities develop later in the lifespan than they do for children without intellectual disability? How do people with intellectual disability utilize language to regulate their emotions? When language abilities are impaired, do other modes of intelligence serve an emotion regulating role? How can emotion regulation be enhanced in children and adults with intellectual disability? How can families' best facilitate effective emotion regulation development for persons with intellectual disability? While effective treatments have been demonstrated for challenging behaviors in this population, the question remains as to what the underlying mechanism is that prompts these gains (Willner, Brace, & Phillips, 2005). Directing research efforts toward the proposed dimensions of emotion regulation (Gratz & Roemer, 2004) may prove fruitful. In order to lay the foundation to be able to answer some of these questions, some articles have recommended the following:

Researchers can begin by replicating the many important emotion and emotional regulation studies that have already been conducted in non-intellectually disabled populations. Observational studies can aid in our understanding of the normative process of developing emotion regulation abilities. In addition, future experimental studies should employ matched control groups whenever possible. (Baurein and Nader, 2012).

The development of reliable and valid tools for assessing the components of emotion regulation in persons with intellectual disability is essential. This represents an overall need as measures assessing emotion regulation in the general population is limited (Gratz & Roemer, 2004). This will require multiple modalities, and researchers are encouraged to be creative in developing assessment tools that individuals will engage with and understand. Some measures should also be quick and easy to re-administer to allow researchers the ability to observe improvements over time. Measurement tools should also address or be applicable to a variety of different emotions, as in the case of anger, where tools that reliably assess this emotion are lacking (Taylor, 2002). In particular, researchers need to be aware of the differential emotion recognition abilities for more neutral emotions versus more intense emotions.

Case studies and brief reports can be very useful tools for researchers and clinicians. Valuable research can be conducted on small samples as well as with qualitative or simple quantitative methods. Clinicians need this information to be disseminated in order to provide the best treatment possible (Taylor, 2002).

REFERENCES

Adolphs, R., Russell, J. A., & Tranel, D. (1999). A role for the human amygdala in recognizing emotional arousal from unpleasant stimuli. *Psychological Science*, *10*(2), 167–171. doi:10.1111/1467-9280.00126

Agnoli, S., Mancini, G., Pozzoli, T., Russo, P. M., Baldaro, B., & Surcinelli, P. (2012). The Interaction Between Emotional Intelligence and Cognitive Abilities in Predicting Scholastic Performance in School Aged Children. *Journal of Personality and Individual Differences*, *53*(5), 660–665. doi:10.1016/j.paid.2012.05.020

Alaghband, M., Tavakoli, S., & Alaghband, L. (2002). The relationship between communication skills and emotional intelligence of female high school students. *Research in Social Psychology*, *2*(6).

Allen, L. B., McHugh, R. K., & Barlow, D. H. (2008). Emotional disorders: A unified protocol. In D. H. Barlow (Ed.), *Clinical handbook of psychological disorders: A step-bystep treatment manual* (4th ed.; pp. 216–249). New York, NY: Guilford Press.

American Psychiatric Association. (2012). *Diagnostic and statistical manual of mental disorders (5th. text revision)*. Arlington, VA: Author.

Aqil, Z., & Ahmed, E. (2014). A comparative study of IQ and EQ in physically disabled and abled adults. *International Journal of Scientific Engineering and Research*, 2347-3878.

Benson, B. A., & Fuchs, C. (1999). Anger arousing situations and coping responses of aggressive adults with intellectual disability. *Journal of Intellectual & Developmental Disability*, *24*(3), 207–214. doi:10.1080/13668259900033991

Black, L., Cullen, C., & Novaco, R. W. (1997). Anger assessment for people with mild learning disabilities in secure settings. In B. S. Kroese, D. Dagnan, & K. Loumidis (Eds.), *Cognitive-behaviour therapy for people with learning disabilities*. London: Routledge.

Browder, D. M., Wood, L., Thompson, J., & Ribuffo, C. (2014). *Evidence-based practices for students with severe disabilities* (Document No. IC-3). Retrieved from University of Florida, Collaboration for Effective Educator, Development, Accountability, and Reform Center website: http://ceedar.education.ufl.edu/tools/innovation-configurations/

Campbell-Sills, L., & Barlow, D. H. (2007). Incorporating emotion regulation into conceptualizations and treatments of anxiety and mood disorders. In J. J. Gross (Ed.), *Handbook of Emotion Regulation* (pp. 542–559). New York: Guilford Press.

Campos, J. J., Campos, R. G., & Barrett, K. C. (1989). Emergent themes in the study of emotional development and emotion regulation. *Developmental Psychology*, *25*(3), 394–402. doi:10.1037/0012-1649.25.3.394

Chapman, R. A., Shedlack, K. J., & France, J. (2006). Stop-think-relax: An adapted self control training strategy for individuals with mental retardation and coexisting psychiatric illness. *Cognitive and Behavioral Practice*, *13*(3), 205–214. doi:10.1016/j.cbpra.2005.08.002

Cole, P. M., Michel, M. K., & Teti, L. O. (1994). The development of emotion regulation and dysregulation: A clinical perspective. *Monographs of the Society for Research in Child Development*, *59*(2/3), 73–102. doi:10.2307/1166139 PMID:7984169

Dahl, A., Joseph, J., & David. (2011). Emotional action and communication in early moral development. *International Society for Research of Emotion*, *3*, 147. doi:10.1177/1754073910387948

DeLoache, J. S., & Burns, N. M. (1994). Symbolic functioning in preschool children. *Journal of Applied Developmental Psychology*, *15*(4), 513–527. doi:10.1016/0193-3973(94)90020-5

Fabes, R. A., Eisenberg, N., Karbon, M., Troyer, D., & Switzer, G. (1994). The relations of children's emotion regulation to their vicarious emotional responses and comforting behaviors. *Child Development, 65*(6), 1687–1693. doi:10.2307/1131287 PMID:7859549

Fletcher, I., Leadbetter, P., Curran, A., & O'Sullivan, H. (2009). A pilot study assessing emotional intelligence training and communication skills with 3rd year medical students. *Patient Education and Counselling, 76*(3), 376-9.

Gratz, K. L., & Roemer, L. (2004). Multidimensional assessment of emotion regulation and deregulation Development, factor structure, and initial validation of the difficulties in emotion regulation scale. *Journal of Psychopathology and Behavioral Assessment, 26*(1), 41–54. doi:10.1023/B:JOBA.0000007455.08539.94

Gross, J. J. (2007). Preface. In J. J. Gross (Ed.), *Handbook of emotion regulation* (pp. xi–xiv). New York: Guilford Press.

Gross, J. J., & Muñoz, R. F. (1995). Emotion regulation and mental health. *Clinical Psychology: Science and Practice, 2*(2), 151–164. doi:10.1111/j.1468-2850.1995.tb00036.x

Gross, J. J., & Thompson, R. A. (2007). Emotion regulation: Conceptual foundations. In J. J. Gross (Ed.), *Handbook of emotion regulation* (pp. 3–24). New York: Guilford Press.

Hasani, G., & Tedadi, Y. (2011). The relationship between emotional intelligence and interpersonal problems. *Research in Health Psychology, 2*(4).

Hayes, S. C., Wilson, K. G., Gifford, E. V., Follette, V. M., & Strosahl, K. (1996). Experiential avoidance and behavioral disorders: A functional dimensional approach to diagnosis and treatment. *Journal of Consulting and Clinical Psychology, 64*(6), 1152–1168. doi:10.1037/0022-006X.64.6.1152 PMID:8991302

Jahoda, A., Pert, C., & Trower, P. (2006). Socioemotional understanding and frequent aggression in people with mild to moderate intellectual disabilities. *American Journal of Mental Retardation, 111*(2), 77–89. doi:10.1352/0895-8017(2006)111[77:SUAFAI]2.0.CO;2 PMID:16466287

Joseph, L., & Ittyerah, M. (2015). Recognition and understanding of emotions in persons with mild to moderate mental retardation. *Journal of Psychosocial Rehabilitation and Mental Health, 2*(1), 59-66.

Kringelbach, M.L., & Berridge, K.C. (2010). The functional neuroanatomy of pleasure and happiness. *HHS Author Manuscripts, 9*(49), 579-587.

Lane, R. D., Reiman, E. M., Ahem, G. L., Schwartz, G. E., & Davidson, R. J. (1997). Neuroanatomical correlates of happiness, sadness and disgust. *The American Journal of Psychiatry, 154*(7), 926–933. doi:10.1176/ajp.154.7.926 PMID:9210742

Lindsay, W. R., Allan, R., Parry, C., Macleod, F., Cottrell, J., Overend, H., & Smith, A. H. W. (2004). Anger and aggression in people with intellectual disabilities: Treatment and follow-up of consecutive referrals and a waiting list comparison. *Clinical Psychology & Psychotherapy, 11*(4), 255–264. doi:10.1002/cpp.415

Lindsay, W. R., Michie, A. M., Baty, F. J., Smith, A. H. W., & Miller, S. (1994). The consistency of reports about feelings and emotions from people with intellectual disability. *Journal of Intellectual Disability Research, 38*(1), 61–66. doi:10.1111/j.1365-2788.1994.tb00348.x PMID:8173224

Linehan, M. M. (1993). *Cognitive-behavioral treatment of borderline personality disorder*. New York: Guilford.

Masi, G. (1998). Psychiatric illness in mentally retarded adolescents: Clinical features. *Adolescence*, *33*(130), 425–434. PMID:9706328

Matheson, E., & Jahoda, A. (2005). Emotional understanding in aggressive and nonaggressive individuals with mild or moderate mental retardation. *American Journal of Mental Retardation*, *110*(1), 57–67. doi:10.1352/0895-8017(2005)110<57:EUIAAN>2.0.CO;2 PMID:15568967

McClure, K. S., Halpern, J., Wolper, P. A., & Donahue, J. J. (2009). Emotional regulation and intellectual disability. *Journal of Developmental Disabilities*. Retrieved from http://www.researchgate.net/publication/263763300

Moore, D. G. (2001). Reassessing emotion recognition performance in people with mental retardation: A review.bn. *American Journal of Mental Retardation*, *106*(6), 481–502. doi:10.1352/0895-8017(2001)106<0481:RERPIP>2.0.CO;2 PMID:11708935

Morgan, H. (1992). An analysis of Gardner's Theory of Multiple Intelligence. *Roeper Review*, *18*(4), 263–269. doi:10.1080/02783199609553756

Owen, A., Browning, M., & Jones, R. P. (2001). Emotion recognition in adults with mild moderate learning disabilities. *Journal of Learning Disabilities*, *5*(3), 267–281. doi:10.1177/146900470100500309

Panksepp, J., Asma, S., Curran, G., Gabriel, R., & Greif, T. (2010). The philosophical implications of affective neuroscience. *Journal of Consciousness Studies*, *19*(3-4), 6–48.

Pardellar, S., Frajo-Apor, B., Kemmler, G., & Hofer, A. (2017). Emotional Intelligence and cognitive abilities - association and sex difference. *Psychology Health and Medicine*, *22*(8), 1001–1010. doi:10.1080/13548506.2016.1255766

Pereira, C.M.G., & Faria, S.M.M. (2013). Emotional development in children intellectual disability - A comparative approach with "normal" children. *Journal of Modern Education Review*, *2*(2), 120-135.

Phan, K. L., Wager, T., Taylor, S. F., & Liberzon, L. (2002). Functional neuroanatomy of emotion: A meta-analysis of emotion activation studies in PET and fMRI. *Journal of Neuroimage*, *16*(2), 331–348. doi:10.1006/nimg.2002.1087 PMID:12030820

Rose, J., & West, C. (1999). Assessment of anger in people with intellectual disabilities. *Journal of Applied Research in Intellectual Disabilities*, *12*(3), 211–224. doi:10.1111/j.1468-3148.1999.tb00078.x

Rydin-Orwin, T., Drake, J., & Bratt, A. (1999). The effects of training on emotion recognition skills for adults with an intellectual disability. *Journal of Applied Research in Intellectual Disabilities*, *12*(3), 253–262. doi:10.1111/j.1468-3148.1999.tb00081.x

Saarni, C. (2011). Emotional development in childhood. *Encyclopedia on early childhood development*, 24-29.

Sappock, T., Budczies, J., Bohe, S., Dziobek, K.I., Dosen, A., & Diefenbacher, A. (2013). Emotional development in adults with autism and intellectual disabilities: A retrospective clinical analysis. *Journal Plus One*. . doi:10.1371/journal.pone.0074036

Schalock, R. L., Luckasson, R. A., Shogren, K. A., Borthwick-Duffy, S., Bradley, V., & Buntinx, W. H. E. (2007). The renaming of mental retardation: Understanding the change to the term intellectual disability. *Intellectual and Developmental Disabilities*, *45*(2), 116–124. doi:10.1352/1934-9556(2007)45[116:TROMRU]2.0.CO;2 PMID:17428134

Sheydaei, M., Adibsereshki, N., & Movallali, G. (2015). The effectiveness of emotional intelligence training on communication skills in students with intellectual disabilities. *Iranian Rehabilitation Journal*, *3*(3).

Singh, N. N., Lancioni, G. E., Winton, A. S. W., Adkins, A. D., Singh, J., & Singh, A. N. (2007). Mindfulness training assists individuals with moderate mental retardation to maintain their community placements. *Behavior Modification*, *31*(6), 800–814. doi:10.1177/0145445507300925 PMID:17932236

Sovner, R., & Hurley, A. D. (1986). Four factors affecting the diagnosis of psychiatric disorders in mentally retarded persons. *Psychiatric Aspects of Mental Retardation Reviews*, *5*(9), 45–49.

Sroufe, L. A. (1979). The coherence of individual development. *The American Psychologist*, *34*(10), 834–841. doi:10.1037/0003-066X.34.10.834

Steiner, C. (2003). *Emotional Literacy; Intelligence with a Heart*. Retrieved from Http://dgek.de/wp-content/uploads/2015/09/steiner-emotional-literacy.pdf

Stewart, C. A., & Singh, N. N. (1995). Enhancing the recognition and production of facial expressions of emotion by children with mental retardation. *Research in Developmental Disabilities*, *16*(5), 365–382. doi:10.1016/0891-4222(95)00024-H PMID:8532916

Taylor, J. L. (2002). A review of the assessment and treatment of anger and aggression in offenders with intellectual disability. *Journal of Intellectual Disability Research*, *46*(s1), 57–73. doi:10.1046/j.1365-2788.2002.00005.x PMID:12031019

Thompson, R. A. (1991). Emotional regulation and emotional development. *Educational Psychology Review*, *3*(4), 269–307. doi:10.1007/BF01319934

Weschsler, D. (1950). Cognitive, Conative and Non-intellective Intelligence. *American Psychological Association*, *5*(3), 78-83.

Whitaker, S. (2001). Anger control for people with learning disabilities: A critical review. *Behavioural and Cognitive Psychotherapy*, *29*(3), 277–293. doi:10.1017/S1352465801003022

Willner, P., Brace, N., & Phillips, J. (2005). Assessment of anger coping skills in individuals with intellectual disabilities. *Journal of Intellectual Disability Research*, *49*(5), 329–339. doi:10.1111/j.1365-2788.2005.00668.x PMID:15817050

Wishart, J. G., Cebula, K. R., Willis, D. S., & Pitcairn, T. K. (2007). Understanding of facial expressions of emotion by children with intellectual disabilities of differing etiology. *Journal of Intellectual Disability Research*, *51*(7), 551–563. doi:10.1111/j.1365-2788.2006.00947.x PMID:17537169

Chapter 13
Psychosocial Interventions for Individuals With Intellectual Disability

Rajesh Jay Sharma
Sunrise Behavioural Health Pty Ltd, Australia

Jahirul Mullick
Monash University, Australia

ABSTRACT

People with intellectual disabilities are prone to various challenges in relation to self-care, emotional regulation, and decision making. Sometimes due to their cognitive and adaptive skill limitations, they display challenging behavior that further impacts on their quality of life. This chapter presents the concept of applied behavior analysis (ABA) and a discussion on the principles of applied behavior analysis (ABA) in prevention and treatment of challenging behaviors of individuals with intellectual disability. Functional behavior analysis (FBA) and its stages are described with examples for the future practitioners. As ABA has a major contribution in the treatment of challenging behaviors in individuals with intellectual disability, research supported treatment strategies are presented. This chapter also explained strategies for improving the adaptive behaviors of individuals with intellectual disability.

INTRODUCTION

In the recent years, there has been an increased interest and focus on improving the quality of life of individuals with disabilities. In the year 2006, the United Nations drafted the Convention on the Rights of the Persons with Disabilities (CRPD) aimed at securing and protecting the human rights of persons with disabilities. As of now, about 160 countries have become signatories of this convention and many countries are working towards making legislations consistent with the CRPD to protect the human rights of individuals with disabilities (UN Convention on the Rights of the Persons with Disabilities, 2015). Among the developed nations, Australia has made it illegal to discriminate people based on their

DOI: 10.4018/978-1-7998-1223-4.ch013

disabilities in 1992 by enacting disability discrimination act (DDA), people with a disability must be treated on the same basis as people without disabilities (Basser, & Jones, 2002). The DDA (1992) has shown positive impact on the lives of people with disabilities particularly in accessing school education (Dempsey, 2003).

Individuals with intellectual disabilities often face increased challenges in self-care, emotional regulation and decision making due to their cognitive and adaptive skill limitations, which further impacts on their quality of life (Emerson, 2001a). A large proportion of population with intellectual disability display several forms of challenging behaviours including aggressive behaviours, self-harm, stereotypical behaviours and sexual misconducts (Crocker, Mercier, Lachapelle, Brunet, Morin & Roy 2006; Emerson et al., 2001b; Poppes, Putten, & Vlaskamp, 2010). Poppes et al. (2010) found a prevalence of self-harm and stereotypical behaviour in 82% of their participants with profound intellectual and multiple disabilities (PIMD) and 45% of their study participants displayed aggressive and destructive behaviours. Challenging behaviour appears to be a central theme in intellectual disability and its treatment. Applied Behaviour Analysis is considered the most science-based prevention and treatment of challenging behaviours as well as improving the adaptive behaviours of individuals with intellectual disability.

Applied Behaviour Analysis and Challenging Behaviours

Applied Behaviour Analysis (ABA) is the practice of applying behaviourism, which focus on principle of stimulus-response, in a systematic way to solve challenging behaviours and teach functional life skills. ABA considers that all behaviours are learned through interaction with the environment. It is science concerned and backed by the principle that behaviour can be explained without the internal mental states or consciousness. Cooper, Heron and Heward (2007) defined ABA as, ''Applied behaviour analysis is a scientific approach for discovering environmental variable that reliably influence socially significant behaviours and for developing a technology of behaviour change that takes practical advantage of those discoveries". In a nutshell, the ABA practitioners are interested in discovering the functional relationships between behaviour and environmental variables rather than searching for causes of challenging behaviours in intra-psychic or other abstract mental concepts such as, mental conflict, ego, unconscious forces, self-concept or self-esteem. Baer, Wolf, and Risley (1968) proposed seven dimensions of ABA. These seven dimensions are considered as the defining features of ABA (Cooper et al., 2007).

1. **Applied:** The 'applied' dimension of ABA refers to commitment of the discipline of ABA to improve the socially significant behaviours to enhance the quality of life of people
2. **Behavioural:** 'Behavioural' dimension seeks to stay focused on what the individual does rather what he or she thinks or feels. Behaviours are seen as physical or environmental events that can be measured in terms of frequency, duration, latency, and intensity or other physical measurement.
3. **Analytic:** 'Analytic' dimension seeks to establish a predictive and functional relationship between independent and dependent variable; presence or absence of independent variable reliably determines the changes in dependent variables
4. **Technological:** 'Technological' dimension of ABA requires that all interventional procedures are to be identified and described with optimal details to facilitate an easy use or replication of the intervention procedures by readers or other practitioners and get the same or similar results when intervention procedures are implemented with integrity.

5. **Conceptually Systematic:** Conceptually systematic dimension asserts that ABA interventions are not merely a set of tricks; rather the intervention strategies are derived from decades of applied research and behavioural principles.
6. **Effective**: Effective dimension asserts that an intervention is considered effective only when it produces a socially significant behavioural change of practical value.
7. **Generalization of Behaviour Change:** Generality dimension seeks to extend the behavioural change beyond the original treatment setting to other settings, and untargeted related behaviours.

In addition to these seven characteristic dimensions of ABA, Wolf (1978) added the eighth dimension of ABA i.e., Social Validity. Wolf (1978) emphasized that the behavioural change outcome must be socially valid / socially valued, and methods of behavioural change must not be viewed as punitive or restrictive but rather viewed as socially acceptable positive strategies of behaviour change by society. These characteristic dimensions are worth emulating for behaviour analysts and other related practitioners of helping professions in their practice to deliver effective treatment for clients (Baer et al., 1968). As evident in the research literature the treatment strategies derived from the ABA have demonstrated effectiveness in reducing the various forms of challenging behaviours in individuals with disabilities (LaVagina & Willis, 2012; Tarbox, Wallace, Tarbox, Landaburu, & William, 2004; Britton, Carr, Kellum, Dozier, & Weil, 2000; Jones, Drew, & Weber, 2000; Fisher, Adelinis, Thompson, Worsdell, & Zarcone 1998; Didden, Duker, & Korzilius, 1997; Hanley, Piazza, & Fisher, 1997; Lalli, Casey, & Kates, 1997; Grace, Thompson, & Fisher 1996; Homer, & Day, 1991; Piazza, Hanley, & Fisher, 1996; Iwata, Pace, Cowdery, & Miltenberger 1994). It is important to mention that sometimes ABA is considered as single type of intervention for a specific population i.e., people with autism. This is a narrow perception about ABA. ABA is, rather, a branch of science that apply basic principles of behaviour (e.g. stimulus-response) to solve socially important challenging behaviours. In order to support a person who is engaged in challenging behaviours, it is important to identify the reasons why s/he may be engaged in challenging behaviours. Behaviours are not repeated, if they do not serve a purpose or function for the person.

Functional Behaviour Assessment

Identifying functions of challenging behaviours is a critical component of a sound behavioural intervention. Functional behaviour assessment (FBA) is a systematic approach that identifies the type and sources of reinforcers or reinforcing events maintaining the challenging behaviours. The reinforcers could be positive or negative, automatic, or tangible items. Challenging behaviours often attract more and quicker attention than non-problematic behaviours often in the form of social or positive reinforcement such as smile, attempts to soothe or calm, attempts to distract, advice or suggestion, reprimands, and tangible reinforcers such as access to preferred items. Similarly, many individuals engage in challenging behaviours such as self-harm, aggression, tantrums, non-compliance to delay or escape the non-preferred demands, requests, or activities, these behaviours are understood to have been getting negative reinforcement or social negative reinforcement. All problem behaviours are not necessarily maintained by the positive, negative or tangible reinforcements. Some of the behaviours are maintained simply because those behaviours produce their own reinforcing value or reinforcement. The FBA helps to generate the hypothesis about the functions of challenging behaviours; the hypothesis can be tested using Functional Analysis Methodology (Cooper et al., 2007 pp 501-504). O'Neill, Horner, Albins, Sprague, Storey and Newton (1997) have delineated three stages of functional behaviour assessment, including –

Stage 1: *Indirect Assessment* - includes conducting interviews with family members and caregivers, and gathering information about the problem behaviours using questionnaires, scales, and checklists;

Stage 2: *Direct Observation* involves observing the client's naturally occurring behaviours in his / her natural environment or context. Usually clinicians use A-B-C event / narrative recording or A-B-C checklists, and scatterplots to assist with direct observations; and

Stage 3: *Functional Analysis* involves intentionally manipulating the independent variable (such as attention or escape which is hypothesized to maintain or reinforce the problem behaviour) and to examine its reinforcing value or strength on the target challenging behaviour.

The stages are elaborately discussed in the next section with examples. See **Appendix A** for 'FBA Process Checklist,' which included ten steps breakdown of conducting FBA.

Indirect assessment

Functional behaviour assessment often begins with interviewing client's family members and other caregivers to identify the behaviours of concern and the circumstances under which the client engages in those behaviours such as where, when, with whom, how long, how often. It is equally important to review the files of client's reports such as diagnostic assessment, past treatments including medical and non-medical interventions, school records, behavioural incident reports, and behavioural data. File reviews and interviewing provides broad-based information about the problem behaviours. However, information gleaned may be incomplete and inaccurate or partially accurate (Feenley & Jones, 2006). Many authors have developed rating scales, questionnaires and checklists to identify the functions of behaviours. For example,

- Motivation Assessment Scale (Durand & Crimmins, 1988),
- Functional Analysis Screening Tool (Iwata & DeLeon, 1996),
- Functional Analysis Interview Form (O'Neil, Horner, Albin, Storey, & Sprague, 1990),
- Problem Behaviour Questionnaire (Lewis, Scott, & Sugai, 1994),
- Functional Assessment Checklist for Teachers and Staff (March et al, 2002),
- Functional Assessment Informant Record for Teachers-Preschool version (Dufrene, Doggett, Henington, & Watson, 2007),
- Questions About Problem Behavioural Function (Matson & Vollmer, 1995).

Most of these assessment tools require minimum amount of training to administer them and these rating scales, questionnaires, and checklists are often useful in identifying the maintaining factors associated with challenging behaviours. However, the responses captured by these rating scales, questionnaires and checklists could be misleading and not revealing the true functions of the problem or target behaviour. Therefore, it is important to include direct observational assessment.

Direct Observational Assessment

Direct observational assessment gathers information about three occurrences including – a) what happened right before the targeted behaviour, b) what was the targeted behaviour looks like, and c) what happened after the targeted behaviour. There are a number of direct observation methods available and two of them are very popular. They are scatterplots and Antecedent-Behaviour-Consequence (A-B-C) chart (Mayer, Sulzer-Azaroff & Wallace, 2014).

Scatterplots

Scatterplot recording is also one of the descriptive (direct) functional behaviour assessment tools to identify the time segment associated with the presence and absence of problem behaviours. Scatterplot is a data collection sheet containing time intervals and these intervals are blocked within and across successive days depending upon the frequency and duration of the target behaviours. Touchette, McDonal and Langer (1985) divided the observation day into a series of 30 minutes time intervals and used designated symbols to mark the low and high frequency of problem behaviour on the scatterplot sheet. Often information gathered from the scatterplot is useful in planning and conducting further analysis during the time periods associated with the higher frequency problem behaviours (Cooper et al., 2007 pp 509). The following example (Figure 1) shows the targeted behaviour occurred during each observation day.

The findings presented in the above figure did not indicate towards any significant trends in behaviour pattern. The bassline data shows whenever the preferred activity is interrupted with NO by adults the tantrum behaviour occurred.

A-B-C Chart

The A-B-C event recording was originally developed by Bijou, Peterson, and Ault (1968). The A-B-C event recording also known as ABC narrative recording is a direct observational method used most often in clinical settings. Observation of client's behaviour is made in his or her natural setting and real-time data is recorded. The A-B-C data recording is completed only when the target behaviour occurs. The data collector or observer uses a form containing five columns i.e. date, time (duration of the behaviour), antecedent, behaviour, and consequences. The observer is required to note down the date of observation, day, time (how long the target behaviour lasted), precisely write down what preceded the target behaviour

Figure 1. Occurrence of targeted behaviour during observations

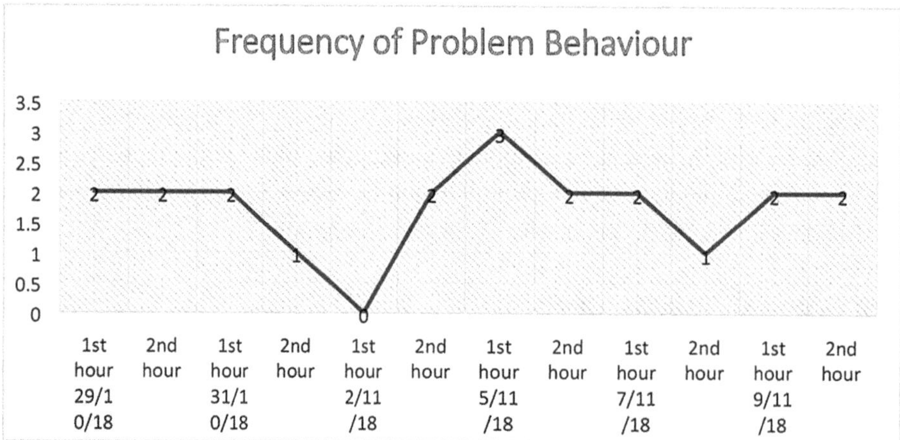

(antecedent), and what happen immediately after the occurrence of the target behaviour (consequence). Each occurrence of the behaviour of concern (target behaviour) is recorded and analysed in the A-B-C format (Kozlowski & Matson, 2012). Clinicians often modify or adapt the existing A-B-C recording form to capture the target behavioural event to suit their own research or clinical needs.

ABC Narrative Recording often helps to operationalise the definition of target behaviour and assists in developing hypothesis about the functions of problem behaviour (Lanovaz, Argumedes, Roy, & Duquette, 2013). A-B-C event recording form can also be used for continuous recording of naturally occurring events. A-B-C narrative recording can potentially help identify several antecedent stimuli and their predictive relations to the target problem behaviours as well as commonly occurring consequences to the problem behaviours. Lalli, Browder, Mace and Brown (1993) have identified and coded antecedent stimuli and its behavioural responses and similarly codified the consequences as a part of their descriptive assessment during classroom activities. In A-B-C continuous recording, the natural occurring behaviours are documented for an extended period of time in the A-B-C format irrespective of the occurrence of target problem behaviours. A-B-C continuous recording conducted in natural settings often suggests a predictive relation between antecedent event and the target problem behaviour as well as problem behaviour and its consequences (i.e. escape form demand). A-B-C continuous recording is often time consuming whereas, ABC Narrative Recording is less time consuming because the data is documented only when the target problem behaviour occurs (Cooper et al., 2007 pp. 506-509). It is important for clinicians to exercise caution while interpreting the A-B-C recordings. Thompson and Iwata (2007) noted in their study that descriptive assessment (A-B-C recording) overestimated the attention as a reinforcing or maintaining factor of problem behaviour.

A-B-C chart

In this example, Jack is already tired and annoyed which could have easily set him up for angry outbursts. On the top of that, his mother seemed to have unintentionally ignored him which is not typical of her behaviour. Jack's mother's speaking to someone else on the phone could have possibly made it even worse experience of deprivation of social attention. Having heated arguments with his sister at 5:00 pm might have also increased Jack's need for more positive social attention. Jack's perception of loss of positive social attention from his mother seemed to have triggered an angry response from Jack in the form of slamming bedroom door and saying, 'you need to shut up now'. In fact, through these behaviours, Jack is clearly demanding social positive attention from his mother but unfortunately in a highly socially inappropriate manner. Jack's mother seemed to unintentionally be reinforced the aggressive behaviour by immediately providing him a sympathetic/ social attention. As evident in the example, analysis of setting

Table 1.

Date, time & settings	Antecedents	Behaviour	Consequences
29/10/18 7:00 pm Jack at home, appeared tired after a long day at school and a tense argument with his sister at 5:00 pm	Jack's mother is cooking dinner and speaking to her sister over her phone softly. She didn't acknowledge Jack's presence.	Jack slammed the bedroom door and yelled at his mother "you need to shut-up now"	Mother immediately disconnected the phone and asked Jack if he was okay.

events tends to identify 'what could occasion the problem behaviours in slow motion?' and antecedent event tells us 'what could trigger the problem behaviours?' and whereas the consequence or the event that follows the problem or target behaviour inform us 'what could maintain, strengthen or reinforce the target or problem behaviours?'. When planning interventions, the clinician would need to conduct a thorough analysis of setting events, antecedent analysis, and consequence analysis in relation to the frequency, duration and intensity of the problem behaviours. Usually fifteen to twenty records of ABC in a variety of contexts could help identify antecedent and consequent events closely related to onset and maintenance of the problem behaviours.

Functional Analysis

Functional Analysis is a standard assessment methodology in ABA. The term 'functional' is frequently used, as behaviours are not repeated unless they serve a function. Therefore, the purpose of a behaviour is known as function and behaviour can occur to fulfil many different functions. There are four functions of behaviour i.e., SEAT.

Functional analysis enables the clinicians to determine the functional relations between the challenging behaviours and environmental events. Mayer, Sulzer-Azaroff and Wallace (2014) suggest, "Technically the term functional implies the lawful manner in which the rate, form, or other pattern with which the behaviour is repeatedly relates to how the consequences of that behaviour have influenced it previously" (p.). Iwata, Dorsey, Slifer, Bauman, and Richman (1994;1982) & Hanley (2012) had initially developed the procedures for conducting functional analysis involving test conditions of Alone, Contingent, Attention and Escape from Demands, to pinpoint the source of reinforcement such as social positive reinforcement (e.g., attention), social negative reinforcement (e.g., escape from demand), and automatic reinforcement (e.g. sensory stimulations) maintaining the challenging behaviour. Hagopian, Wilson and Wilder (2001) determined in their study that their research participants' challenging behaviours such as aggressive, disruptive and self-harming behaviours were maintained by an access to tangible item. Tangible items were not included as test conditions in the studies by Iwata et al. (1994; 1982) standard procedures. A 'Tangible Condition' was later included in the functional analysis designed to test the socially mediated positive reinforcement. Vollmer, Marcus, Ringdahl, & Roane (1995) were among the first few researchers using the standardized tangible condition in their studies. Hanley, Iwata and McCord (2003) noted in their review on functional analysis of problem behaviours that functional analysis procedures are varied and often have been adapted to meet the clinical assessment needs of the clients

Table 2.

S Sensory	Provides Sensory experience; Looks good, feels good, smells good
E Escape	Removes unwanted activities and interaction; From loud noise, incident
A Attention	Offers access to people or interaction; attention from adults, peers
T Tangibles	Provides desired items or activities; access to food, iPad, toys etc.

or contexts. However, most of the functional analyses continue to share the characteristics as pioneered by Iwata et al. (1994; 1982).

Clinicians often choose the relevant test conditions for experimental or functional analysis based on the descriptive assessment results. The functional analysis is conducted either in an analogue condition (resembling the natural setting) or during the naturally occurring events such as, regular ongoing instruction in the classroom (trial based functional analysis). Generally, 'Alone' condition examines whether the problematic behaviour is maintained by automatic reinforcement such as self-stimulations. Under this condition, the client is left alone in a room, and observer records the frequency of the target behaviours occurring most often, without having been seen by the clients directly. The purpose of the 'Attention' test condition is to examine whether the problematic behaviour is maintained by the attention. The clinician actively ignores the client's appropriate behaviours to gain attention, by appearing busy in some task and waits for the occurrence of the problematic behaviour, once the target behaviour is displayed, the clinician or experimenter immediately provides contingent attention in the form of reprimand, request or suggestion relevant to the problematic behaviour such as, 'Don't hit yourself', 'You are hurting yourself, it is painful'. The frequency of the target behaviour (self-injurious behaviours) is documented. 'Demand Condition' aims to test whether the problematic behaviour is escape maintained. The client is presented with an age appropriate task of moderate difficulty level depending upon the skills level of the client. If the client engages in the target problem behaviour, then the client is allowed to escape or leave the situation briefly for about thirty seconds. The experimenter or clinician notes down the frequency of the occurrence of the target problem behaviour on the data sheet. Finally, the client is placed in the 'Control' condition. The 'Control' (play) condition provides an engaging and enriching environment for the client. The clinician or experimenter does not provide any consequences for engaging in problematic behaviour, however, the experimenter redirects the client and counts the frequency of target problem behaviour. The client is offered attention at least every thirty seconds. The data from this condition (play) serves as a baseline score for comparison purposes for all test conditions. The test conditions are alternated over a number of days and data is collected using a frequency measure. Each test condition must last at least 10 minutes in length. Data is often plotted on a graph for visual analysis to identify a causal link between the test conditions (such as attention, demand, alone) and the problematic behaviours. Functions of behaviours are determined by the elevation of the frequency of problem behaviour on the graph. For example, if elevated problem behaviour is observed under the 'attention' condition, this suggests that the problematic behaviour is maintained by social positive reinforcement such as attention. Similarly, elevated problematic behaviours under the 'demand' condition indicate that the target behaviour is escape maintained. It is often observed that under control / play condition, problem behaviour may not surface altogether or might occur in low frequencies. It is possible that the problematic behaviour might occur in higher frequencies in more than one test condition such as, 'attention' and 'demand'. However, the functional analysis is considered inconclusive or invalid if the frequency of problem behaviour is higher across all conditions including 'control/ play' condition (Mayer et al., 2014 pp 197; Cooper et al., 2007 pp 504-505; Iwata et al., 1994; 1982)

TREATMENT STRATEGIES

Applied Behaviour Analysis as a discipline has a major contribution in the treatment of challenging behaviours in individuals with intellectual disability (Matson & Coe, 1992). Didden et al. (2007) noted that the treatment based on identified functions of behaviours consists of strategies to modify the motivating operations, modifying antecedents, changing or removing the reinforcing or consequent events, and teaching replacement behaviours; adaptive and functional skills.

Modifying Motivating Operations

Motivating operations (MO) is a term used for establishing operations (EO). Keller and Schoenfeld (1950) introduced the term EO. Jack Michael reintroduced the term in 1982 with its current meaning, i.e. an environment or events that change the value of a stimulus as a reinforcer as well as frequency of behaviour that has been maintained or reinforced by that stimulus (Cooper et al., 2007; Michael, 2000; 1982).

Hagopian et al. (2001) found in their study that the research participant's challenging behaviour was maintained by escape and tangible item. The researchers could ameliorate the challenging behaviour providing the identified tangible item non-contingently frequently, using Non-Contingent Reinforcement procedure (NCR) and teaching the research participant to request for break when needed. The researchers noted a decrease of 96% in the challenging behaviours.

Simó-Pinatella, Font-Roura, Planella-Morató, McGill, Alomar-Kurz, & Giné, (2013) conducted a systematic research literature review of modification of MOs and their impact on challenging behaviours. Their review included 31 published research articles from eight leading behavioural and special education research journals. The research participants (fifty-five) in these selected studies were school children with intellectual disability. Simó-Pinatella et al. (2013) concluded that modification of MO (either increasing or decreasing the value of reinforcers by temporary deprivation or satiation) usually has treatment effect on the challenging behaviours.

Modifying Antecedents

Antecedent based strategies aim to alter or modify the stimuli just before the individual engages in a challenging behaviour (Kern, Choutka & Sokol, 2002). This involves identifying the antecedents of disruptive behaviour through functional behaviour assessment and then working actively to change them prior to a challenging behaviour. Feeley and Jones (2006) outlined 4 antecedent-based strategies: Offering choices; Using high probability requests (with which the individual is more likely to comply) paired with reinforcement and followed by a low probability request; Collaboration and Using preferred item as a distractor.

Horner et al. (1991) conducted two studies to investigate the effect of high probability requests on aggression and self-injury of participants whose behaviour was maintained by escape/ avoidance. Results from both studies indicated that high probability interspersed requests were effective in reducing aggression and self-injury and increasing participants' responsiveness to instructions.

Changing or removing the reinforcing or consequent events

Reinforcers and consequences are used in ABA to facilitate the learning of the desired behaviour and decrease undesirable and challenging behaviour. The reinforcing and consequent events can be altered through the use of various differential reinforcement procedures such as, DRO (differential reinforcement of other behaviour), DRA (differential reinforcement of alternative behaviour), and DRI (differential reinforcement of incompatible behaviour) and extinction.

When using DRO, the therapist delivers a reinforcer when the problem behaviour has not occurred during specific times, i.e. reinforcement is contingent on problem behaviour not occurring. In DRA, delivery of reinforcement is contingent on an appropriate alternative to the inappropriate response. The alternative response to be reinforced should be functional for the individual. For example, if the function of engaging in aggressive behaviour for a client is to get attention, s/he can be taught to raise their hand instead by reinforcing that behaviour. DRI is used to deliver reinforcement upon the occurrence of a behaviour that is incompatible with the behaviour selected for reduction (Deitz & Repp, 1983). For example, sitting still and rocking back and forth are incompatible behaviours. The two cannot be performed simultaneously. The desired behaviour is reinforced (sitting still) and not the other behaviour (rocking back and forth).

These differential reinforcement procedures are often used in conjunction with the extinction procedure. Extinction involves withholding reinforcement for a previously reinforced behaviour following the occurrence of challenging behaviour (Lerman & Iwata, 1996). Consistency is very important in the use of extinction. Inconsistent extinction may actually maintain behaviour and make the behaviour resistant to extinction. The appropriate behaviours should also be reinforced consistently. Repp and Karsh (1994) used DRA and extinction in dealing with participants with developmental disabilities using tantrums to get attention. The challenging behaviour decreased substantially post-intervention and the results were maintained at one-year follow-up.

Teaching Replacement Behaviours

Teaching communicative behaviours that replace the disruptive and challenging behaviour is very helpful for individuals with disability as it provides them an avenue to communicate their needs and express themselves in a socially appropriate manner. Functional communication training (FCT) is a replacement strategy, used to teach the individual an appropriate communicative response that serves the same function as the problem behaviour (Carr et al., 1994). For example, for children who run away to escape a task can be taught to raise their hand to excuse themselves from the task. FCT is a specific type of DRA (Fisher, Kuhn, & Thompson, 1998). It has been used extensively with positive outcomes for individuals with disability (Brooks, Todd, Tofflemoyer & Horner, 2003; Carr et al., 1999; Hagopian, Fisher, Sullivan, Acquisto, & LeBlanc, 1998; Derby et al., 1997; Didden, Duker, & Korzilius, 1997; Hall, Neuharth-Pritchet and Belfiore, 1997).

TEACHING FUNCTIONAL SKILLS TO INDIVIDUALS WITH INTELLECTUAL DISABILITY

Functional skills are skills that are vital for an individual to function in society (Lerner, 2003). These include daily living and self-care skills, such as self-hygiene, toileting, reading, cooking, communication skills, academic skills and community participation skills (Mesibov, Shea, & Schopler, 2004). Individuals with disability are often limited in their ability to carry out tasks related to everyday living. Teaching functional skills to individuals with intellectual disability is thus very important to help them increase their ability to live as autonomously as possible.

ABA based strategies such as Imitation, shaping and chaining are often utilized to help individuals with disabilities to acquire new skills and behaviours (Mayer, Sulzer-Azaroff & Wallace, 2014 p.p. 248-

294). Similarly, Cooper et al., 2007 (Pp 413) have emphasized the significance of imitative skills to help acquire social and communication skills quickly as well as develop other new behaviours and skills. Some young children with developmental disabilities particularly individuals with autism spectrum disorders fail to acquire the imitative repertoire (Rogers, Hepburn, Stackhouse, Wehner, 2003). Therefore, these individuals need to be taught the imitation skills first. Holth 2003, has provided a detailed behavioural analytic description of the term 'Imitation' that description has been further precisely refined by Cooper et al., 2007 (Pp 413), they have defined imitation as a 'behaviour-environment relations' and physical movement are considered to have predictive value to function as a model for imitation. Model as an antecedent stimulus is capable of evoking imitative behaviours. The model must control the occurrence of the imitative behaviour. The definition has an emphasis on the immediacy of the initiation of behaviour of the organism (the imitative behaviour must be initiated within 3 to 5 seconds following the presentation of model). It is important that the imitative behaviour and the model resemble each other and share the same sense mode i.e. auditory, visual, tactile etc. (Holth, 2003)

Cooper et al., 2007 (Pp 415) have suggested some pre-requisite skills imitation training such as learner's capacity to stay seated and hands in lap, orienting his/ her attention on the model / teacher or object etc. For implementing the imitation skill training, Cooper et al., 2007 (Pp 417), have recommended some guidelines such as an emphasis on active and brief training sessions, reinforcing both prompted and imitative behaviours initially and gradually fading out the prompts and eventually reinforcing only those imitative behaviour occurring within 3 to 5 seconds of the presentation of the model and without prompts. Cooper et al., 2007 (Pp 417) have also suggested to combine verbal praise, attention with tangible reinforcers, as the client makes progress clinician can slowly fade out the edible reinforcers and strengthen the verbal praise and attention. However, if the data does not show continuous progress or displays deterioration in skill acquisition, the clinician may re-consider the prompting hierarchy, ratio and variety of reinforcers or other contextual variables such as difficulty task or other environmental distractions.

Imitation and modelling have their origin in social learning theory (Bandura, 1977), which suggests that people learn through observing other people's behaviour and outcomes of those behaviours. New behaviour can be learnt more rapidly by observational learning than by shaping alone (Bandura, 1969). Attention and motivation are of utmost important for observational learning to take place. Modeling refers to learning that occurs after the observation of the behavior of a model. It is a type of learning that occurs as a result of observing and retaining behavior of others. For learning to take place, observer merely needs to watch the behavior of the model and does not need to engage in overt responses or receive any consequences. Imitation, on the other hand involves learning by copying or replicating the behavior exhibited by the model. For example, imitation can be used to teach children to tie shoelaces by copying exact steps of a model doing the same. This can also be used in conjunction with chaining and reinforcement.

Models are usually individuals that are observed, but they can also be symbolic (presented via TV, books, movies and videos). Video modeling (i.e. demonstration of desired behavior through video) is very popular and has been found to be effective in teaching a range of self-care, social- communication and daily living skills to children with disabilities (Kellems & Edwards, 2015; Allen, Wallace, Renes, Bowen & Burke, 2010; Cihak, Fahrenkrog, Ayres & Smith,2009; Bellini & Akullian, 2007; Delano, 2007; Keen, Brannigan & Cuskelly, 2007; Shipley-Benamou, Lutzker & Taubman, 2002; Wert & Neisworth, 2003).

Shaping is another technique that is used to teach new skills or develop a new behaviour that are not yet present in a person's behavioural repertoire. It is a systematic process of reinforcing successive approximations of target behaviour. Each time an approximate desired behaviour occurs it is reinforced, whereas other behaviours that are not approximations of target behaviour are not reinforced. Responses that resemble the target response or that include components of that response are reinforced (Kazdin, 2012). For example, to teach a child to eat food (target behaviour), any response related to eating such as, sitting on the table, being near the plate, touching food etc. will be reinforced. When using shaping it is very important to define the target behaviour and to know when to deliver and withhold reinforcement (Wolfgang, 2001). Many researchers have used shaping successfully to teach self-help skills to individuals with developmental disabilities (Azrin & Foxx, 1971; Watson, 1968; Bensberg, Colwell & Cassel, 1965).

Chaining procedures can be used to teach functional skills to individuals with intellectual disability. Chaining is a technique used in ABA to teach complex tasks to individuals with a disability by breaking them down into discrete and simple steps. The chain/task is broken down into links/steps, using task analysis. Three types of chaining procedures are used (Cooper et al., 2007): Forward chaining is a chaining procedure in which the teaching progresses from the first task in the chain to the next and so on. The behaviour is taught in its naturally occurring order. Each step in the chain must be mastered before progressing to the next step. For example, to teach a child to wash hands, the task first needs to be broken down into steps (task analysis)-Turn on water, wash hands, put soap on hands, rub palms together, rinse hands, turn off water, take towel, dry hands, and put towel down. The forward chaining of this task will begin with the first step, i.e. turning on water, and move to the next step with the mastery of each step. A backward chaining procedure is the reverse of the forward chaining procedure, in that the teaching process moves from the last step in the chain to the first step. In the washing hands example, the teaching will begin with the last step, i.e. putting towel down and move to the first step, turning on water, after all the steps in between are mastered. Backward chaining is used when the individual can complete most steps at the end of the chain. It provides immediate satisfaction to the learner and can operate as a natural reinforcer. In total task chaining, the individual is taught entire behaviour chain at each presentation. Unlike forward and backward chaining procedures, total task chaining does not require the learner to master steps before progressing to the next one. Total task training is often used when the learner knows many of the tasks but needs to learn how to do them in sequence. Using the example above, the child will be given prompts and assistance as needed to wash hands in the natural order.

Chaining procedures can also be taught through the use of videos, pictures and computer-based multimedia. Video and computer-based teaching procedures have been found to be effective in teaching self-care (Norman, Collins, & Schuster, 2001;Tiong, Blampied, & Le Grice, 1992), and daily living skills (Kagohara et al., 2013; Graves, Collins, Schuster, & Kleinert, 2005; Mechling, Gast, & Barthold, 2003; Rehfeldt, Dahman, Young, Cherry, & Davis, 2003) to individuals with disability.

PROGRAMS FOR PARENTS AND FAMILIES

Parents of children with intellectual disabilities face many challenges including feelings of guilt, frustration, disappointment, uncertainty, worry, sadness, and grief (Zupanick, 2019). They also face difficult-emotions in relation to an acute social stigma and feeling of loss of their dreams, hopes, and aspirations for their child. These challenges are ongoing, and parents and families need to learn how to cope with these wide range of issues. Although parents and caregivers often report feelings of stress, anxiety and depression (Blacher, Neece, & Paczkowski, 2005) in dealing children with intellectual disability, they want to interact positively and help their children on a regular basis. Parents and family members often get frustrated without delay while dealing with their children with intellectual disability, because they do not know how to support their children and how they can reduce their stress level. Nowadays, many different programs and interventions are available to help parents and families in their caregiving roles. Mindfulness-based stress reduction (MBSR) training is one such program that has been effectively used with parents and caregivers of individuals with developmental disabilities in order to reduce parent stress and depression, improve life satisfaction and happiness and decrease behaviour problems in children (Neece, 2014; Singh et al., 2014; Bazzano et al., 2013; Singh et al., 2010; Singh et al., 2007; Singh et al., 2006).

A number of parent training programs have also been developed to help parents to deal more effectively with their child behaviour. These programs also support in build positive parent-child relationships. Stepping Stones Triple P (SSTP) is designed specifically for parents of children with disabilities (Sanders, Mazzucchelli & Studman, 2003). The program aims to improve the knowledge, skills, and confidence of parents to deal with a range of behavioural and developmental issues of children (Sanders, Mazzucchelli & Studman, 2004). SSTP is based on the Triple P model of multi-level intervention, with five different levels of intensity, where parents can choose a level more appropriate to their needs (Sanders et al., 2004). The program has been found to be effective in improving child's behaviour, parenting styles, parenting satisfaction and efficacy, parental adjustment, and parental relationships (Roux, Sofronoff, & Sanders, 2013; Tellegen & Sanders, 2013; Sofronoff, Jahnel & Sanders, 2011; Whittingham, Sofronoff, Sheffield & Sanders, 2009; Plant & Sanders, 2007).

The Incredible Years Parent Training Program (IYPT; Webster-Stratton, 2001; 2000) is another popular parent training program designed for typically developing children with behaviour problems. The program includes training parents in use of strategies such as praise, limit setting, and reinforcement to teach acceptable social behaviour and treat challenging behaviours in children (Reid, Webster-Stratton & Hammond, 2007). McIntyre (2008) adapted the IYTP for parents of children with developmental delays. The intervention consisted of 12-weekly 2.5-hour group sessions, including topics such as, play, praise, rewards, limit setting, and handling challenging behaviour. The researcher concluded that the program was effective in reducing negative parenting and child maladaptive behaviour. Parents also reported high program satisfaction.

Parent-Child Interaction Therapy (PCIT; Eyberg, Boggs & Algina, 1995) has also been used successfully with families of children with disabilities. Like other parent training programs mentioned earlier, the PCIT also aims to teach skills that parents can use to build a nurturing and positive relationship with their child and deal effectively with their child's behaviour. The therapy involves two phases – a) Child-Directed Interaction phase, and b) Parent-Directed Interaction phase. In both the phases, therapists provide active coaching to parents to help them master the parent-child interaction skills. The program has demonstrated positive outcomes on parent-child interactions, child behaviour, parenting stress and parent perceptions of child behaviour (Solomon, Ono, Timmer & Goodlin-Jones, 2008; Bagner & Eyberg, 2007). Zupanick (2019) suggests that supportive psychotherapies can be beneficial, as psychotherapy supports parents and members of the family who work through difficult emotions that arise when caring children with disabilities. Family support group membership which would offer community feeling through understanding and supporting each another is also very effective in coping with these challenges of life time.

CONCLUSION

Applied Behaviour Analysis and Intellectual Disability share a long-term relationship with each other. The development of the discipline of applied behaviour analysis (ABA) had led to better treatment outcomes and improved quality of life measures for individuals with developmental disabilities (Remington 1998). More than forty years of cumulative applied behaviour analytic peer reviewed scientific research has been constantly refining the behavioural technologies. Today ABA enjoys the reputation of being the most research evidence-based approach in the disability sector particularly for treating the challenging behaviours and improving the quality of life by teaching self-help, communication, pre-vocational, vocational, academic, social skills etc. Positive Behaviour Support approach has become a preferred approach to support people with developmental disabilities such intellectual disability and autism spectrum disorders presenting challenging behaviours (Emerson & Einfeld 2011). However, there is a severe shortage of professionals trained in ABA partly due to a fewer universities offering the undergraduate and post graduate programmes in ABA (Rethink Autism Provides Distance BCBA Supervision…., 2010). Dillengburger (2012) argued for an extensive use of ABA technologies for teaching children with intellectual disabilities both academic and non-academic skills rather than wasting time in developing a newer teaching methodology. Dissemination of knowledge and skills of ABA among helping professionals such as teachers, psychologists, social workers, nurses, and people employed in the disability sector may need to be prioritized over other treatment and teaching methodologies. A systematic supervision by credentialed behaviour analysts can potentially offer better learning opportunities for the supervisees and an assurance of quality behavioural services to the public. It is equally important that more institutions of higher learning such as colleges and universities should offer programmes in behavioural psychology or applied behaviour analysis. It may also be helpful to include courses in ABA in the general education as well as in the special education programmes to prepare well-trained education professionals who would be able to support these students in the least restrictive environments by providing them high quality educational and behavioural services.

Applied Behaviour Analysis is a rapidly growing discipline, and it still needs to catch up with several issues. Remington (1998) noted that almost half of studies published in Journal of Applied Behaviour Analysis (a flagship journal of ABA) were focused on treatment of severe problematic behaviours, aggression, stereotypy, and language / communication. Other important areas of intellectual disability such as self-care/ daily living skills, leisure skills etc remained under represented. Most behaviour analysts or behaviour specialists take a consultative role. Data collection and treatment implementation is generally carried out by others such as teacher aid, disability support staff etc. Most of ABA programme implementers have limited college / university educational experience in ABA. Many concepts and procedures in ABA look deceptively easy without a working knowledge of ABA and work experience. The A-B-C analysis often gets misinterpreted and at times inappropriate behaviours do get reinforced unintentionally by less experienced staff. The treatment outcome most often depends on how well the procedural and treatment integrity were maintained. The success of behavioural interventions often requires a strong commitment from parents, care givers and disability support staff. At times parents/ carers fail in their commitment or drop out of the programme prematurely due to funding issues or other concerns. It is recognized that parenting or caring for an individual with intellectual disability or other developmental disability brings in considerable amount of psychological distress to the family members (Yamaoka, Tamiya, Moriyama, Felipe Alfonso Sandoval Garrido, Sumazaki & Noguchi (2015). Psychological counseling support to the parents / caregivers of children with developmental disabilities may help parents to stay motivated and resilient.

REFERENCES

Allen, K. D., Wallace, D. P., Renes, D., Bowen, S. L., & Burke, R. V. (2010). Use of video modeling to teach vocational skills to adolescents and young adults with autism spectrum disorders. *Education & Treatment of Children*, *33*(3), 339–349. doi:10.1353/etc.0.0101

Azrin, N. H., & Foxx, R. M. (1971). A rapid method of toilet training the institutionalized retarded. *Journal of Applied Behavior Analysis*, *4*(2), 89–99. doi:10.1901/jaba.1971.4-89 PMID:16795291

Baer, D. M., Wolf, M. M., & Risley, T. R. (1968). Some current dimensions of applied behavior analysis. *Journal of Applied Behavior Analysis*, *1*(1), 91–97. doi:10.1901/jaba.1968.1-91 PMID:16795165

Bagner, D. M., & Eyberg, S. M. (2007). Parent–child interaction therapy for disruptive behavior in children with mental retardation: A randomized controlled trial. *Journal of Clinical Child and Adolescent Psychology*, *36*(3), 418–429. doi:10.1080/15374410701448448 PMID:17658985

Bandura, A. (1969). *Principles of Behavior Modification*. New York: Holt, Rinehart and Winston.

Basser, L. A., & Jones, M. (2002). The Disability Discrimination Act 1992 (Cth): A three-dimensional approach to operationalising human rights. *Melb. UL Rev.*, *26*, 254.

Bazzano, A., Wolfe, C., Zylowska, L., Wang, S., Schuster, E., Barrett, C., & Lehrer, D. (2013). Mindfulness based stress reduction (MBSR) for parents and caregivers of individuals with developmental disabilities: A community-based approach. *Journal of Child and Family Studies*, *24*(2), 298–308. doi:10.100710826-013-9836-9

Beavers, G. A., Iwata, B. A., & Lerman, D. C. (2013). Thirty years of research on the functional analysis of problem behavior. *Journal of Applied Behavior Analysis*, *46*(1), 1. doi:10.1111/j.1365-2788.2006.00948.x

Bellini, S., & Akullian, J. (2007). A meta-analysis of video modeling and video self-modeling interventions for children and adolescents with autism spectrum disorders. *Exceptional Children*, *73*(3), 264–287. doi:10.1177/001440290707300301

Bensberg, G. J., Colwell, C. N., & Cassel, R. (1965). Teaching the profoundly retarded self-help activities by behavior shaping techniques. *American Journal of Mental Deficiency*, *69*, 674–679. PMID:14286827

Bijou, S. W., Peterson, R. F., & Ault, M. H. (1968). A method to integrate descriptive and experimental field studies at the level of data and empirical concepts. *Journal of Applied Behavior Analysis*, *1*(2), 175–191. doi:10.1901/jaba.1968.1-175 PMID:16795175

Blacher, J., Neece, C. L., & Paczkowski, E. (2005). Families and intellectual disability. *Current Opinion in Psychiatry*, *18*(5), 507–513. doi:10.1097/01.yco.0000179488.92885.e8 PMID:16639109

Britton, L. N., Carr, J. E., Kellum, K. K., Dozier, C. L., & Weil, T. M. (2000). A variation of noncontingent reinforcement in the treatment of aberrant behavior. *Research in Developmental Disabilities, 21*(6), 425–435. doi:10.1016/S0891-4222(00)00056-1 PMID:11153827

Brooks, A., Todd, A. W., Tofflemoyer, S., & Horner, R. H. (2003). Use of functional assessment and a self-management system to increase academic engagement and work completion. *Journal of Positive Behavior Interventions, 5*(3), 144–152. doi:10.1177/10983007030050030301

Carr, E., Horner, R., Turnbull, A., Marquis, J., McLaughlin, D., & McAtee, M. (1999). *Positive behavior support for people with developmental disabilities: A research synthesis.* Washington, DC: American Association on Mental Retardation.

Carr, E., Levin, L., McConnachie, G., Carlson, J., Kemp, D., & Smith, C. (1994). *Communication-based intervention for problem behavior.* Baltimore, MD: Paul H. Brookes.

Cihak, D., Fahrenkrog, C., Ayres, K. M., & Smith, C. (2009). The use of video modeling via a video iPod and a system of least prompts to improve transitional behaviors for students with autism spectrum disorders in the general education classroom. *Journal of Positive Behavior Interventions.* doi:10.1177/1098300709332346

Cooper, J. O., Heron, T. E., & Heward, W. L. (2007). Applied Behavior Analysis (2nd ed.). Academic Press.

Crocker, A. G., Mercier, C., Allaire, J., & Roy, M. (2007). Profiles and correlates aggressive behaviour among adults with intellectual disabilities. *Journal of Intellectual Disability Research: JIDR, 51*(10), 786–801. doi:10.1111/j.1365-2788.2007.00953.x PMID:17803497

Deitz, D. E., & Repp, A. C. (1983). Reducing Behavior through Reinforcement. *Exceptional Education Quarterly, 3*(4), 34–46. doi:10.1177/074193258300300410

Delano, M. E. (2007). Video modeling interventions for individuals with autism. *Remedial and Special Education, 28*(1), 33–42. doi:10.1177/07419325070280010401

Dempsey, I. (2003). The impact of the Disability Discrimination Act on school students with a disability in Australia. *Austl. & NZJL & Educ., 8*, 35.

Didden, R. (2007). Functional analysis methodology in developmental disabilities. In P. Strumey (Ed.), *Functional analysis in clinical treatment: Practical resources for mental health professional* (pp. 65–86). San Diego, CA: Elsevier Academic Press. doi:10.1016/B978-012372544-8/50005-7

Didden, R., Duker, P. C., & Korzilius, H. (1997). Meta-analytic study on treatment effectiveness for problem behaviors with individuals who have mental retardation. *American Journal of Mental Retardation, 101*(4), 387–399. PMID:9017085

Dufrene, B. A., Doggett, R. A., Henington, C., & Watson, T. S. (2007). Functional assessment and intervention for disruptive classroom behaviors in preschool and head start classrooms. *Journal of Behavioral Education, 16*(4), 368–388. doi:10.100710864-007-9048-8

Durand, V. M., & Carr, E. G. (1991). Functional communication training to reduce challenging behavior: Maintenance and application in new settings. *Journal of Applied Behavior Analysis, 24*(2), 251–264. doi:10.1901/jaba.1991.24-251 PMID:1890046

Durand, V. M., & Crimmins, D. B. (1988). Identifying the variables maintaining self-injurious behavior. *Journal of Autism and Developmental Disorders, 18*(1), 99–117. doi:10.1007/BF02211821 PMID:3372462

Emerson, E. (2001). *Challenging behaviour: Analysis and intervention in people with severe learning disabilities* (2nd ed.). Cambridge, UK: Cambridge University Press. doi:10.1017/CBO9780511543739

Emerson, E., & Einfeld, S. (2011). *Challenging Behaviour*. Cambridge, UK: Cambridge University Press. doi:10.1017/CBO9780511861178

Emerson, E., Kiernan, C., Alborz, A., Reeves, D., Mason, L., Mason, H., & Hatton, C. (2001). The prevalence of challenging behaviors: A total population study. *Research in Developmental Disabilities, 22*(1), 77–93. doi:10.1016/S0891-4222(00)00061-5 PMID:11263632

Eyberg, S. M., Boggs, S. R., & Algina, J. (1995). Parent–child interaction therapy: A psychosocial model for the treatment of young children with conduct problem behavior and their families. *Psychopharmacology Bulletin, 31*(1), 83–91. PMID:7675994

Feeley, K., & Jones, E. (2006). Addressing challenging behaviour in children with Down syndrome: The use of applied behaviour analysis for assessment and intervention. *Down's Syndrome: Research and Practice, 11*(2), 64–77. doi:10.3104/perspectives.316 PMID:17048800

Fisher, W. W., Adelinis, J. D., Thompson, R. H., Worsdell, A. S., & Zarcone, J. R. (1998). Functional analysis and treatment of destructive behavior maintained by termination of "don't" (and symmetrical "do") requests. *Journal of Applied Behavior Analysis, 31*(3), 339–356. doi:10.1901/jaba.1998.31-339 PMID:9757579

Fisher, W. W., Kuhn, D. E., & Thompson, R. H. (1998). Establishing discriminative control of responding using functional and alternative reinforcers during functional communication training. *Journal of Applied Behavior Analysis, 31*(4), 543–560. doi:10.1901/jaba.1998.31-543 PMID:9891393

Friedman, D., Holmbeck, G. N., Jandasek, B., Zukerman, J., & Abad, M. (2004). Parent functioning in families of preadolescents with spina bifida: Longitudinal implications for child adjustment. *Journal of Family Psychology, 18*(4), 609–619. doi:10.1037/0893-3200.18.4.609 PMID:15598166

Grace, N. C., Thompson, R., & Fisher, W. W. (1996). The treatment of covert self-injury through contingencies on response products. *Journal of Applied Behavior Analysis, 29*(2), 239–242. doi:10.1901/jaba.1996.29-239 PMID:8682739

Graves, T. B., Collins, B. C., Schuster, J. W., & Kleinert, H. (2005). Using video prompting to teach cooking skills to secondary students with moderate disabilities. *Education and Training in Developmental Disabilities, 40*, 34–46.

Hagopian, L., Fisher, W., Sullivan, M., Acquisto, J., & LeBlanc, L. (1998). Effectiveness of functional communication training with and without extinction and punishment: A summary of 21 inpatient cases. *Journal of Applied Behavior Analysis, 30*, 229–237. PMID:9652101

Hagopian, L. P., Wilson, D. M., & Wilder, D. A. (2001). Assessment and treatment of problem behavior maintained by escape from attention and access to tangible items. *Journal of Applied Behavior Analysis, 34*(2), 229–232. doi:10.1901/jaba.2001.34-229 PMID:11421317

Hall, A. M., Neuharth-Pritchett, S., & Belfiore, P. J. (1997). Reduction of aggressive behaviors with changes in activity: Linking descriptive and experimental analysis. *Education and Training in Mental Retardation and Developmental Disabilities, 32*, 331–339.

Hanley, G. P. (2012). Functional assessment of problem behavior: Dispelling myths, overcoming implementation obstacles, and developing new lore. *Behavior Analysis in Practice, 5*(1), 54–72. doi:10.1007/BF03391818 PMID:23326630

Hanley, G. P., Iwata, B. A., & McCord, B. E. (2003). Functional analysis of problem behavior: A review. *Journal of Applied Behavior Analysis, 36*(2), 147–186. doi:10.1901/jaba.2003.36-147 PMID:12858983

Hanley, G. P., Piazza, C. C., & Fisher, W. W. (1997). Noncontingent presentation of attention and alternative stimuli in the treatment of attention-maintained destructive behavior. *Journal of Applied Behavior Analysis, 30*(2), 229–237. doi:10.1901/jaba.1997.30-229 PMID:9210303

Holth, P. (2003). Generalized imitation and generalized matching to sample. *The Behavior Analyst, 26*(1), 155-158.

Horner, R. H., Day, H. M., Sprague, J. R., O'Brien, M., & Heathfield, L. T. (1991). Interspersed requests: A nonaversive procedure for reducing aggression and self-injury during instruction. *Journal of Applied Behavior Analysis, 24*(2), 265–278. doi:10.1901/jaba.1991.24-265 PMID:1890047

Iwata, B., Dorsey, M., Slifer, K., Bauman, K., & Richman, G. (1994). Toward a functional analysis of self-injury. *Journal of Applied Behavior Analysis, 27*, 197-209.

Iwata, B. A., & DeLeon, I. (1996) The functional analysis screening tool. Gainesville, FL: The Florida Centre on Self-Injury, The University of Florida.

Iwata, B. A., & Dozier, C. L. (2008). Clinical application of functional analysis methodology. *Behavior Analysis in Practice, 1*(1), 3–9. doi:10.1007/BF03391714 PMID:22477673

Iwata, B. A., Pace, G. M., Cowdery, G. E., & Miltenberger, R. G. (1994). What makes extinction work: An analysis of procedural form and function. *Journal of Applied Behavior Analysis, 27*(1), 131–144. doi:10.1901/jaba.1994.27-131 PMID:8188555

Jones, K. M., Drew, H. A., & Weber, N. L. (2000). Noncontingent peer attention as treatment for disruptive classroom behavior. *Journal of Applied Behavior Analysis, 33*(3), 343-346. doi:10.1901/jaba.2000.33-343

Kagohara, D. M., van der Meer, L., Ramdoss, S., O'Reilly, M. F., Lancioni, G. E., Davis, T. N., ... Sigafoos, J. (2013). Using iPods® and iPads® in teaching programs for individuals with developmental disabilities: A systematic review. *Research in Developmental Disabilities, 34*(1), 147–156. doi:10.1016/j.ridd.2012.07.027 PMID:22940168

Kahng, S., Iwata, B. A., Fischer, S. M., Page, T. J., Treadwell, K. R., Williams, D. E., & Smith, R. G. (1998). Temporal distributions of problem behavior based on scatter plot analysis. *Journal of Applied Behavior Analysis, 31*(4), 593–604. doi:10.1901/jaba.1998.31-593 PMID:9891396

Kazdin, A. E. (2012). *Behavior modification in applied settings.* Waveland Press.

Keen, D., Brannigan, K. L., & Cuskelly, M. (2007). Toilet training for children with autism: The effects of video modeling. *Journal of Developmental and Physical Disabilities, 19*(4), 291–303. doi:10.100710882-007-9044-x

Kellems, R. O., & Edwards, S. (2015). Using Video Modeling and Video Prompting to Teach Core Academic Content to Students With Learning Disabilities. *Preventing School Failure*, 1–8.

Keller, F. S., & Schoenfeld, W. N. (1950). *Principles of psychology: A systematic text in the science of behavior.* New York: Appleton-Century-Crofts. doi:10.1037/11293-000

Kern, L., Choutka, C. M., & Sokol, N. G. (2002). Assessment-based interventions used in natural settings to reduce challenging behaviors: A review of the literature. *Education & Treatment of Children, 25*, 113–134.

Kozlowski, A. M., & Matson, J. L. (2012). Interview and observation methods in functional assessment. In J. L. Matson (Ed.), *Functional assessment for challenging behaviour* (pp. 105–124). New York, NY: Springer New York. doi:10.1007/978-1-4614-3037-7_7

Lalli, J. S., Browder, D. M., Mace, F. C., & Brown, D. K. (1993). Teacher use of descriptive analysis data to implement interventions to decrease students' problem behaviors. *Journal of Applied Behavior Analysis, 26*(2), 227–238. doi:10.1901/jaba.1993.26-227 PMID:8331019

Lalli, J. S., Casey, S. D., & Kates, K. (1997). noncontingent reinforcement as treatment for severe problem behavior: Some procedural variations. *Journal of Applied Behavior Analysis, 30*(1), 127–137. doi:10.1901/jaba.1997.30-127 PMID:9103988

Lanovaz, M. J., Argumedes, M., Roy, D., Duquette, J. R., & Watkins, N. (2013). Using ABC narrative recording to identify the function of problem behavior: A pilot study. *Research in Developmental Disabilities, 34*(9), 2734–2742. doi:10.1016/j.ridd.2013.05.038 PMID:23787117

LaVigna, G. W., & Willis, T. J. (2012). The efficacy of positive behavioural support with the most challenging behaviour: The evidence and its implications. *Journal of Intellectual & Developmental Disability, 37*(3), 185–195. doi:10.3109/13668250.2012.696597 PMID:22774760

Lerman, D., & Iwata, B. (1996). Developing a technology for the use of operant extinction in clinical settings: An examination of basic and applied research. *Journal of Applied Behavior Analysis, 29*(3), 345–382. doi:10.1901/jaba.1996.29-345 PMID:8926226

Lerner, J. (2003). *Learning disabilities: Theories, diagnosis, and teaching practices* (9th ed.). Boston, MA: Houghton Mifflin Company.

Lewis, T., Scott, T., & Sugai, G. (1994). The problem behaviour questionnaire: A teacher- long-term effects of functional communication training in home settings. *Journal of Applied Behavior Analysis, 30*, 507–531.

Mactavish, J. B., & Schleien, S. J. (2004). Re-injecting spontaneity and balance in family life: Parents' perspectives on recreation in families that include children with developmental disability. *Journal of Intellectual Disability Research, 48*(2), 123–141. doi:10.1111/j.1365-2788.2004.00502.x PMID:14723655

March, R. E., Horner, R. H., Lewis-Palmer, T., Brown, D., Crone, D., Todd, A. W., & … . (2000). *Functional Assessment Checklist: Teachers and Staff (FACTS)*. Eugene, OR: Educational and Community Supports.

Matson, J. L. (2012). Functional assessment for challenging behaviors. New York, NY: Springer. doi:10.1007/978-1-4614-3037-7

Matson, J. L., & Coe, D. A. (1992). Applied Behaviour Analysis: Its impact on the treatment of mentally retarded emotionally disturbed people. *Research in Developmental Disabilities*, *13*(2), 171–189. doi:10.1016/0891-4222(92)90023-Y PMID:1574625

Matson, J. L., & Vollmer, T. R. (1995). *User's guide: Questions About Behavioral Function (QABF)*. Baron Rouge, LA: Scientific Publishers, Inc.

Mayer, G. R., Sulzer-Azaroff, B., & Wallace, M. (2014). *Behavior analysis for lasting change* (3rd ed.). Cornwall-on-Hudson, NY: Sloan Publishing.

McIntyre, L. L. (2008). Adapting Webster-Stratton's incredible years parent training for children with developmental delay: Findings from a treatment group only study. *Journal of Intellectual Disability Research*, *52*(12), 1176–1192. doi:10.1111/j.1365-2788.2008.01108.x PMID:18671808

Mechling, L. C., Gast, D. L., & Barthold, S. (2003). Multimedia computer-based instruction to teach students with moderate intellectual disabilities to use a debit card to make purchases. *Exceptionality*, *11*(4), 239–254. doi:10.1207/S15327035EX1104_4

Mesibov, G. B., Shea, V., & Schopler, E. (2004). *The TEACCH approach to autism spectrum disorders*. Springer Science & Business Media. doi:10.1007/978-0-306-48647-0

Michael, J. (1982). Distinguishing between discriminative and motivational functions of stimuli. *Journal of the Experimental Analysis of Behavior*, *37*(1), 149–155. doi:10.1901/jeab.1982.37-149 PMID:7057126

Michael, J. (2000). Implications and refinements of the establishing operation concept. *Journal of Applied Behavior Analysis*, *33*(4), 401–410. doi:10.1901/jaba.2000.33-401 PMID:11214018

Neece, C. L. (2014). Mindfulness-based stress reduction for parents of young children with developmental delays: Implications for parental mental health and child behaviour problems. *Journal of Applied Research in Intellectual Disabilities*, *27*(2), 174–186. doi:10.1111/jar.12064 PMID:23813562

Norman, J. M., Collins, B. C., & Schuster, J. W. (2001). Using an instructional package including video technology to teach self-help skills to elementary students with mental deficiency. *Journal of Special Education Technology*, *16*(3), 5–18. doi:10.1177/016264340101600301

O'Neill, R. E., Horner, R. H., Albin, R. W., Sprague, J. R., Storey, K., & Newton, J. S. (1997). *Functional Assessment and Program Development for Problem Behavior* (2nd ed.). Pacific Grove, CA: Brooks/Cole.

O'Neill, R. E., Horner, R. H., Albin, R. W., Storey, K., & Sprague, J. R. (1990). Functional Analysis of Problem Behavior: A Practical Assessment Guide. *Sycamore Publishing, Sycamore, IL.* of challenging behaviours in individuals with mild mental retardation: meta-analysis of single- subject research. *American Journal of Mental Retardation*, *111*, 290–298.

Passey, J., & Feldman, M. (2004). Descriptive analysis of parent–child interactions in young children with or at risk for developmental delay. *Behavioral Interventions*, *19*(4), 233–246. doi:10.1002/bin.164

Piazza, C. C., Hanley, G. P., & Fisher, W. W. (1996). Functional analysis and treatment of cigarette pica. *Journal of Applied Behavior Analysis*, *29*(4), 437–450. doi:10.1901/jaba.1996.29-437 PMID:8995829

Plant, K. M., & Sanders, M. R. (2007). Reducing problem behavior during care-giving in families of preschool-aged children with developmental disabilities. *Research in Developmental Disabilities*, *28*(4), 362–385. doi:10.1016/j.ridd.2006.02.009 PMID:16781115

Poppes, P., van der Putten, A. J. J., & Vlaskamp, C. (2010). Frequency and severity of challenging behaviour in people with profound intellectual and multiple disabilities. *Research in Developmental Disabilities*, *31*(6), 1269–1275. doi:10.1016/j.ridd.2010.07.017 PMID:20728304

Prevalence and types of aggressive behaviour among adults with intellectual disabilities. (n.d.). *Journal of Intellectual Disability Research, 50*(9), 652-661. doi:10.1111/j.1365-2788.2006.00815.x

Rehfeldt, R. A., Dahman, D., Young, A., Cherry, H., & Davis, P. (2003). Teaching a simple meal preparation skill to adults with moderate and severe mental retardation using video modeling. *Behavioral Interventions*, *18*(3), 209–218. doi:10.1002/bin.139

Reid, M. J., Webster-Stratton, C., & Hammond, M. (2007). Enhancing a classroom social competence and problem-solving curriculum by offering parent training to families of moderate-to-high-risk elementary school children. *Journal of Clinical Child and Adolescent Psychology*, *36*(4), 605–620. doi:10.1080/15374410701662741 PMID:18088218

Remington, B. (1998). Applied behaviour analysis and intellectual disability: A long-term relationship?1. *Journal of Intellectual & Developmental Disability*, *23*(2), 121–135. doi:10.1080/13668259800033631

Repp, A. C., & Karsh, D. (1994). A hypothesis-based interventions for tantrum behavior of person with developmental disabilities in school settings. *Journal of Applied Behavior Analysis*, *27*(1), 21–31. doi:10.1901/jaba.1994.27-21 PMID:8188561

Rethink autism provides distance BCBA supervision to candidates seeking certification in behavior analysis. (2010). PR Newswire.

Rogers, S. J., Hepburn, S. L., Stackhouse, T., & Wehner, E. (2003). Imitation performance in toddlers with autism and those with other developmental disorders. *Journal of Child Psychology and Psychiatry, and Allied Disciplines*, *44*(5), 763–781. doi:10.1111/1469-7610.00162 PMID:12831120

Roux, G., Sofronoff, K., & Sanders, M. R. (2013). A Randomized Controlled Trial of Group Stepping Stones Triple P: A Mixed-Disability Trial. *Family Process*, *52*(3), 411–424. doi:10.1111/famp.12016 PMID:24033239

Sanders, M. R., Mazzucchelli, T. G., & Studman, L. J. (2003). *Practitioner's manual for standard Stepping Stones Triple P*. Brisbane: Triple P International Pty. Ltd.

Sanders, M. R., Mazzucchelli, T. G., & Studman, L. J. (2004). Stepping Stones Triple P: The theoretical basis and development of an evidence-based positive parenting program for families with a child who has a disability. *Journal of Intellectual & Developmental Disability*, *29*(3), 265–283. doi:10.1080/13668250412331285127

Shipley-Benamou, R., Lutzker, J. R., & Taubman, M. (2002). Teaching daily living skills to children with autism through instructional video modeling. *Journal of Positive Behavior Interventions*, *4*(3), 165–175. doi:10.1177/10983007020040030501

Singh, N. N., Lancioni, G. E., Winton, A. S., Fisher, B. C., Wahler, R. G., Mcaleavey, K., ... Sabaawi, M. (2006). Mindful parenting decreases aggression, noncompliance, and self-injury in children with autism. *Journal of Emotional and Behavioral Disorders*, *14*(3), 169–177. doi:10.1177/10634266060140030401

Singh, N. N., Lancioni, G. E., Winton, A. S., Karazsia, B. T., Myers, R. E., Latham, L. L., & Singh, J. (2014). Mindfulness-Based Positive Behavior Support (MBPBS) for mothers of adolescents with autism spectrum disorder: Effects on adolescents' behavior and parental stress. *Mindfulness*, *5*(6), 646–657. doi:10.100712671-014-0321-3

Singh, N. N., Lancioni, G. E., Winton, A. S., Singh, J., Curtis, W. J., Wahler, R. G., & McAleavey, K. M. (2007). Mindful parenting decreases aggression and increases social behavior in children with developmental disabilities. *Behavior Modification*, *31*(6), 749–771. doi:10.1177/0145445507300924 PMID:17932234

Singh, N. N., Lancioni, G. E., Winton, A. S., Singh, J., Singh, A. N., Adkins, A. D., & Wahler, R. G. (2010). Training in mindful caregiving transfers to parent–child interactions. *Journal of Child and Family Studies*, *19*(2), 167–174. doi:10.100710826-009-9267-9

Sofronoff, K., Jahnel, D., & Sanders, M. R. (2011). Stepping Stones Triple P seminars for parents of a child with a disability: A randomized controlled trial. *Research in Developmental Disabilities*, *32*(6), 2253–2262. doi:10.1016/j.ridd.2011.07.046 PMID:21871779

Solomon, M., Ono, M., Timmer, S., & Goodlin-Jones, B. (2008). The effectiveness of parent–child interaction therapy for families of children on the autism spectrum. *Journal of Autism and Developmental Disorders*, *38*(9), 1767–1776. doi:10.100710803-008-0567-5 PMID:18401693

Sturmey, P. (2007). Functional analysis in clinical treatment. Amsterdam: Academic Press.

Tarbox, J., Wallace, M. D., Tarbox, R. S. F., Landaburu, H. J., & Williams, W. L. (2004). Functional analysis and treatment of low rate problem behavior in individuals with developmental disabilities. *Behavioral Interventions*, *19*(3), 187–204. doi:10.1002/bin.158

Tellegen, C. L., & Sanders, M. R. (2013). Stepping Stones Triple P-Positive Parenting Program for children with disability: A systematic review and meta-analysis. *Research in Developmental Disabilities*, *34*(5), 1556–1571. doi:10.1016/j.ridd.2013.01.022 PMID:23475006

Thompson, R. H., & Iwata, B. A. (2007). A comparison of outcomes from descriptive and functional analyses of problem behavior. *Journal of Applied Behavior Analysis, 40*(2), 333–338. doi:10.1901/jaba.2007.56-06 PMID:17624074

Tiong, S. J., Blampied, N. M., & Le Grice, B. (1992). Training community-living, intellectually handicapped people in fire safety using video prompting. *Behaviour Change, 9*(2), 65–72. doi:10.1017/S0813483900006379

Touchette, P. E., MacDonald, R. F., & Langer, S. N. (1985). A scatter plot for identifying stimulus control of problem behavior. *Journal of Applied Behavior Analysis, 18*(4), 343–351. doi:10.1901/jaba.1985.18-343 PMID:4086416

United Nations. (n.d.). Conventions on the Rights of the Persons with Disabilities. *Treaty Series, 2515*, 3. Retrieved November 17, 2015, from UN Treaty Collection website: https://treaties.un.org/Pages/ViewDetails.aspx?src=TREATY&mtdsg_no=IV-15&chapter=4&lang=en

Van Houten, R., Axelrod, S., Bailey, J. S., Favell, J. E., Foxx, R. M., Iwata, B. A., & Lovaas, O. I. (1988). The right to effective behavioral treatment. *Journal of Applied Behavior Analysis, 21*(4), 381–384. doi:10.1901/jaba.1988.21-381 PMID:3225255

Vollmer, T. R., Marcus, B. A., Ringdahl, J. E., & Roane, H. S. (1995). Progressing from brief assessments to extended experimental analyses in the evaluation of aberrant behavior. *Journal of Applied Behavior Analysis, 28*(4), 561–576. doi:10.1901/jaba.1995.28-561 PMID:16795882

Watson, L. S. Jr. (1968). Application of behaviour-shaping devices to training severely and profoundly mentally retarded children in an institutional setting. *Mental Retardation, 6*, 21–23. PMID:5705586

Webster-Stratton, C. (2000). The Incredible Years Training series. Office of Juvenile Justice and Delinquency Prevention Bulletin Review, 1–24.

Webster-Stratton, C. (2001). *The Incredible Years: Parents, teachers, and children training series, leader's guide*. Seattle, WA: Author.

Wert, B. Y., & Neisworth, J. T. (2003). Effects of video self-modeling on spontaneous requesting in children with autism. *Journal of Positive Behavior Interventions, 5*(1), 30–34. doi:10.1177/10983007030050010501

Whittingham, K., Sofronoff, K., Sheffield, J., & Sanders, M. R. (2009). Stepping Stones Triple P: An RCT of a parenting program with parents of a child diagnosed with an autism spectrum disorder. *Journal of Abnormal Child Psychology, 37*(4), 469–480. doi:10.100710802-008-9285-x PMID:19023654

Wolf, M. M. (1978). Social validity: The case for subjective measurement or how applied behavior analysis is finding its heart. *Journal of Applied Behavior Analysis, 11*(2), 203–214. doi:10.1901/jaba.1978.11-203 PMID:16795590

Wolfgang, C. H. (2001). *Solving discipline and classroom management programs: Methods and models for today's teachers*. New York: John Wiley.

Yamaoka, Y., Tamiya, N., Moriyama, Y., Sandoval Garrido, F. A., Sumazaki, R., & Noguchi, H. (2015). Mental health of parents as caregivers of children with disabilities: Based on Japanese nationwide survey: E0145200. *PLoS One*, *10*(12), e0145200. doi:10.1371/journal.pone.0145200 PMID:26692344

Zupanick, C. E. (2019, May 26). Support & Help for Families With Intellectually Disabled Children [Weblog post]. Retrieved from https://www.mentalhelp.net/articles/support-amp-help-for-families-with-intellectually-disabled-children/

APPENDIX

FBA Process Checklist

Step 1. Review the available client's records

- Referral information
- Prior health & allied health reports
- Current FBA/BSP/treatment plans Restrictive practice data
- Incident reports
- Reports from other external sources

Step 2. Meet with the family/ the carers' team

Apprise the family and other clinicians (program manager & team leader) of your involvement. Clarify the role, purpose, engagement, & expectations.

Step 3. Define the behaviours of concern

- In observable and measurable terms

Step 4. Indirect Assessment

- Interviews (using FBAI form) with parent(s), guardian(s), & staff(s)
- Use rating scale, questionnaires, checklists/screening tools Document anecdotes (if any)
- Seclusion/ restraint data
- Activities of daily living (if relevant)
- Reinforcer surveys

Step 5. Direct Observation /Assessment (meeting with participant)

- Scatter plot/ routine assessment
- A-B-C data
- Data on frequency, duration, latency etc. Preference/ reinforcer assessment
- Ecological assessment (if appropriate)

Step 6. Review the operational definitions of behaviour of concern (if needed)

Step 7. Graphing and data analysis

- Identify setting events
- Identify antecedents
- Graph the data on frequency, duration, latency etc.
- Graph A-B-C data
- Identify when the behaviour of concern is more likely to occur
- Identify when the behaviour of concern is least likely to occur
- Identify the consequences that follow the behaviours of concern

Step 8. Conduct additional behavioural assessment (if needed)

- Antecedent analysis
- Functional analysis
- Trial-based functional analysis

Step 9. Summarise findings for each behaviour of concern

- Setting events/routine
- Antecedents
- Consequences
- Functions of behaviour

Step 10. Prepare a formal FBA report and discuss with relevant team members
(To inform the development of treatment plan or positive behaviour support plan)

Chapter 14
Reflecting on Crime and Legal Issues in People With Intellectual Disabilities:
Theory, Perspectives, and Future Approaches

Vaitsa Giannouli
Aristotle University of Thessaloniki, Greece

ABSTRACT

This chapter discusses research findings on intellectual disability (ID), criminal law, and the different forms of aggressive behavior such as sexual violence, homicide, theft, arson, and alcohol-drug abuse. ID is a generalized neurodevelopmental disorder, characterized by significantly impaired and varying intellectual-adaptive functioning. Given that a number of legal issues have been raised over the past decades regarding individuals with ID and civil as well as criminal law, particular attention will also be given to neuropsychological research regarding civil law and the most common problems for individuals with ID, such as financial capacity and capacity for medical consent. Finally, there will be a section for the most important issues regarding the trial and conviction for individuals with ID, and a presentation of a research on attitudes toward ID and legal issues. The chapter concludes with suggestions for reform of the law relating to ID and the need for further research.

INTRODUCTION

The chapter is an attempt to present the latest information regarding crime and legal issues among individuals with Intellectual Disability (ID). The widespread adoption of a changed construct and of a new term, which replaces mental retardation by renaming it in DSM 5 (Schalock, Luckasson & Shogren, 2007), and the legislatively mandated changes in terminology (Stavrakantonaki & Johnson, 2018), can not clarify and examine in depth the significance of ID for a number of legal issues. As scientific lit-

DOI: 10.4018/978-1-7998-1223-4.ch014

erature indicates the theme of legal issues turns out to be particularly salient for ID worldwide (Levine, Proulx & Schwartz, 2018). Researchers in psychology and law (legal psychology and forensic psychology) become more interested in examining aspects of individuals with ID, who may play the role of suspect or victim according to the criminal law (Carr et al., 2016; McCarthy et al., 2019), or the role of the person who claims civil capacities according to the civil law. As a result, this chapter will be an in-depth introduction, which will be focused on a variety of relevant themes, which are selected in order to include key terms and information on law and ID.

Individuals with ID and Criminal Law

There is a general tendency to consider individuals with ID as a group of people who are more likely to commit a crime (New South Wales. Law Reform Commission, 1994), a belief that is based on the fact that individuals with ID may be over-represented in the criminal justice system (Baroff, Gunn & Hayes, 2004; Hayes, 1996; Holland, Clare, & Mukhopadhyay, 2002; Jones, 2007; Søndenaa, Rasmussen, Palmstierna, & Nøttestad, 2008). Given the intellectual and other psychosocial disadvantages which they experience and their incapacity to evade arrest, the level of offending behavior in this group is found to be strikingly low (Holland et al., 2002), because much criminal activity of individuals with ID goes undetected or unreported, and as a result scientific research can only investigate data and individuals who are already involved with the criminal justice process. Individuals with ID are not overrepresented in prisons in most western countries (Boer et al., 2018; Gulati et al., 2018; Murphy & Mason, 2014). For example, the likelihood of conviction for a man with ID in a European country, such as Sweden is as high as for a man without disability (Hodgins, 1992). It is of special interest that in a research from Denmark convicted individuals with ID, who had been admitted to psychiatric hospitals were found to have an increased risk of committing various kinds of crimes in comparison with individuals with ID without a previous admission history (Hodgins et al., 1996).

Individuals with ID are usually seen as potential suspects for crimes worldwide and this is due to a general misunderstanding and bias of different societies and communities (Lyal, Holland & Collins, 1996; McNulty et al., 1995; Vaughan, Pullen & Kely, 2000). Studies using IQ as a continuous variable indicate that significantly below-average intellectual ability is an independent predictor of future offending (Holland et al., 2002), but the studies which adopt an IQ-based concept of ID show lower rates of offending than those which use wider definitions (e.g. attendance at special schools). There is also evidence coming from a systematic review by Simpson and Hogg (2001) for believing specifically that the prevalence of arson and sexual offences may be higher relative to other kinds of crimes for individuals with ID than for other offenders (Barron, Hassiotis & Bannes, 2002; Simpson & Hogg, 2001), but there exist contradictory evidence for that (Murphy & Mason, 2014). For example, studies support that individuals with ID do not engage predominantly in any one form of criminal behavior, and that their readily identifiable characteristics do not set them apart from offenders without a diagnosed disability (Salekin, Olley & Hedge, 2010). Intellectually disabled offenders start offending at an early age [ID youth, aged under 18 may demonstrate delinquent behavior as other individuals who are not of legal age, and who commit acts considered to be rule violations, which according to legal definitions, include such acts as robbery, assault, property damage, drug possession, and other similar crimes (Salkind, 2002)], and these same young offenders usually have a history of multiple offences. This finding could be explained by impulsivity that is a general characteristic during the teenage years even in healthy youths (Stoyanova & Giannouli, 2018a). In addition to that, frustration, lack of social skills in dealing with provocative situations, and aggression associated with poor self-concept, are all factors influencing behaviors linked to violent offences (Jahoda et al., 1998). Specifically, offenders with ID are considered to be a group with complex needs who may pose a recurrent risk to the public (Barron, Hassiotis & Bannes, 2002). Individuals with ID and forensic involvement are those who may also have a diagnosis of borderline to mild IQ and psychopathology (psychotic disorder), are also more likely to have previously used drugs or alcohol, and have significantly longer prior lengths of stay in psychiatric hospitals (Raina & Lunsky, 2010). A recent study found that offenders, as indicated from police data, grew up in large and unstable multi-problem households and had psychosocial problems, while offenders with mild to borderline ID displayed externalizing behavior before the age of 12, were susceptible to peer pressure, had low social-relational skills, and committed more violent property crimes than offenders without ID (Segeren et al., 2018).

Individuals with ID: Exploring Violence and Crime

A number of studies support that offenders have impaired cognitive abilities, yet it is unclear if cognitive dysfunction per se contributes to aggressive antisocial behaviors (Wallinius et al., 2019). According to a review, over half of the ID population engages in some form of aggression, but only a small number is responsible for frequent or severe acts with serious legal implications, although ID is associated with psychosocial adversities and psychiatric comorbidities (Benson & Brooks, 2008; Gopalan, Sharma & Unnikrishnan, 2014). More specifically, individuals with ID are at increased risk for both violent and sexual victimisation as well as offending (Fodgsen et al., 2016). Although individuals with ID are significantly less likely to have an official record of victimisation and offending, as is supported for Australia, their rates of violent and sexual victimisation and offending were significantly higher (Fodgsen et al., 2016). The presence of comorbid mental illness considerably increases the likelihood of victimisation and offending. Thus, the presence of comorbid mental illness aggravates the risk of offending and victimization (Fodgsen et al., 2016). The relative prevalence of aggressive behavior is found to be higher among institutionalized persons compared to those living in group homes or other community-based facilities (as data from Australia indicate: Sjigafoos et al., 1994). In the same study of institutionalized individuals with ID and aggressive behavior, a higher percentage of males were described as functioning in the severe/profound or moderate range of intellectual disability with one-third having no intelligible speech capacity (Sjigafoos et al., 1994). The current aggression levels for an individual can be predicted by many factors such as gender, level of mental retardation, and history of previous institutional placement, and the strongest predictor is proposed to be the personal history of aggression (Davidson et al., 1994), but without evidence or research until now supporting the possible link between adult criminality and testosterone levels in ID.

The aggressive behavior may take many forms, with the most frequent in order: property damage, verbal, self-oriented and physical aggression, and sexually aggressive behavior, most of which is characterized as mild in severity. Of course, there is only a minority of individuals displaying aggressive behavior leading to injury of the victim and there are few or none recorded gender differences (Crocker et al., 2006). In contrast to the above, a possible rapid increase in arrests during adolescence in tandem with a relatively rapid decline during adulthood, which is called the 'age-crime curve', has not yet been empirically proven to be true for the ID population mainly due to the lack of existing research. Finally, it is claimed, based on empirical evidence, that the relationship between moral reasoning and illegal behavior may be curvilinear, such that lower moral reasoning and higher moral reasoning relates to lower rates of illegal behavior and possible inappropriate conduct. It seems that individuals with ID are reasoning at a lower moral stage than their peers, and it is proposed that some people with intellectual disabilities may actually be less likely to engage in illegal behavior, because they are reasoning at an earlier moral stage. Individuals with 'borderline' intelligence would be more likely to engage in illegal behavior, something that suggests that the relationship between moral reasoning and illegal behavior is moderated by intelligence (Langton Clare & Murphy, 2011).

ID and Sexual Violence

Sexual violence refers to any sexual act or attempt with the aim of abusing by violence or coercion someone else or even a group of others (Giannouli, 2018a). Research on forensic issues and ID come mainly from the USA and UK, and as a result conclusions have to be confined to these countries only (Søndenaa, Rasmussen & Nøttestad, 2008). There is an old tendency in the scientific literature that rapists tend to be of low intelligence (Day, 1994), while other researchers claim that low IQ is not more frequent in sexual violence, and is equally found in individuals who commit aggressive non-sexual crimes (Vera, Barnard & Holzer, 1979; Ruff et al., 1976). Although attitudes toward sexuality and ID are not thoroughly investigated in different countries (Cuskelly & Bryde, 2004), children with disabilities are 3.4 times more likely to be maltreated than their nondisabled peers (McClean et al., 2017; Sullivan & Knutson, 2000) or adults experience sexual assault at a rate seven times that of nondisabled people (Harris, 2019). This makes the states to show a strong interest in finding ways to plan and protect adults and children with disabilities from abuse and neglect (Harris, 2019). Sexual abuse is proven to be a significant variable in the history of future sexual offenders, while physical abuse seems a significant variable only in the life history of nonsexual offenders (Lindsay et al., 2001). One major cognitive factor contributing to sexual violence demonstrated by individuals with ID is the problem of understanding the laws relating to sexuality (O'Callaghan & Murphy, 2007). About the sex of sexual offenders with ID, it seems that female offenders show similar characteristics to their male offenders with ID, but there are higher levels of mental illness, higher levels of prior sexual abuse and lower levels of re-offending for the female sexual offenders (Lindsay et al., 2004). For the male sexual offenders a high prevalence of family psychopathology, psychiatric illness, minor physical disabilities, sexual experience, impaired relationship skills and sexual recidivism are found (Day, 1994). Among individuals with ID, women are more likely to have a diagnosis of mood disorder and sexual abuse history, while men are more likely to be diagnosed with substance abuse diagnosis, legal issues, and documented past destructive behavior (Lunsky et al., 2009). Finally, based on the finding that emotion dysregulation is linked to sexual offending, as well as reoffending, across a number of different theories, current interventions, such as biofeedback, focus primarily on improving emotion regulation in sexual offenders with ID (Gray, Beech & Rose, 2019).

ID and Homicide

There is little systematic attention on examining murders committed by individuals with ID, which paradoxically are the most well-known non-suicidal dangerous behavior among individuals with ID (Day, 1993). Typically 0.5 – 1.5% of prisoners worldwide are diagnosed with intellectual disabilities (range 0% to 2.8% across studies), something that makes the number of prisoners with ID considerable and this condition as one with important implications for policy and practice (Fazel, Xenitidis & Powell, 2008). But are all murderers mentally ill? Some researchers claim that ID murderers are not as common as murderers coming from the general population, but female murder defendants are more likely to receive a diagnosis of ID (Dwyer & Frierson, 2006). There may be a link between the severity of ID and violent behaviors toward third parties. According to self-report measures, individuals who reported low self-concept also reported high levels of depression, but mildly mentally retarded individuals were more likely to report anger against others than severe/moderately retarded persons (Benson & Ivis, 1992).

ID and Theft

The taking of another person's property without that person's permission or consent may be an act that can be prosecuted as a crime for individuals with ID. They may commit such an act, because they may not understand what these acts really are (their legal consequences), and they may not identify themselves as illegal or 'bad' when committing this sort of crime. In addition to that, there are many forms of theft (burglary, embezzlement, larceny, looting, robbery, shoplifting, library theft, and fraud), but there is no research on the characteristics of the persons who commit these specific acts or the factors that may lead an individual with ID to such acts (Parry & Drogin, 2007).

ID and Arson

Fire-setting behavior may be expressed as arson attempts in individuals with ID, and although there is evidence that the prevalence of arson may be higher relative to other kinds of crimes for people with ID in UK (Simpson & Hogg, 2001), these ID individuals are also over-represented, according to data, in the criminal justice system in Australia (Curtis, McVilly & Day, 2014). Unfortunately, there is no large-scale systematic research on the characteristics of the individuals with ID and this type of behavior. A study from UK supports that the most common reasons for setting fires for individuals with ID are: the feeling of being angry, wanting revenge, and excitement around fires. External factors that may play an important role is a precipitating argument or wanting to move to different accommodation (Orchard, 2013). In addition to that, according to another study from the UK the most common reason for arson is revenge, closely followed by suggestibility, while the majority of offenders with ID have an associated diagnosis of personality disorders along with an Axis I psychiatric diagnosis. Other factors include large family size, history of childhood psychiatric disorders, abuse, homelessness, unemployment and relationship difficulties (Devapriam et al., 2007). Finally, fire setting is claimed to be associated with significant psychopathology (e.g. psychosis and personality disorders), but not all of the convicted individuals with ID have a formal arson conviction. Fire setters according to that are more likely to have a violence conviction, and criminal sections/restriction orders (Alexander et al., 2015).

ID and Alcohol-Drugs Abuse

Substance use disorder in patients with ID and mental health disorders admitted to psychiatric hospitalisation are prevalent (Salavert et al., 2018), but this is not found in other studies that examine young adults with mild to moderate ID from the general population, who are less likely to use substances than their non-disabled peers (Robertson et al., 2018). Thus, prevalence of alcohol use disorders is low in adults with ID (Williams, Kouimtsidis & Baldacchino, 2018), but some studies report contradictory evidence for alcohol and drug use in this population (Huxley et al., 2018). Individuals with mild ID who are involved with the criminal justice system regularly consume alcohol and use illicit drugs (Lindsay,

Tinsley & Emara, 2012), and this implies that there may be a possible link between substance abuse and offending behavior in this population. Although they may be just (ab)users of illegal substances, they may participate in groups of dealers as well. Individuals who had offended reported greater use of both legal and illicit drugs than their non-offending counterparts and many reported that they had been under the influence of alcohol or illicit drugs at the time of committing the offence (McGillivray & Moore, 2001). Alcohol and cannabis are the commonest drugs of abuse in the English ID population, while cocaine, stimulants and opiates are abused by a small, but significant number of ID offenders (Plant et al., 2011). The history of alcohol abuse for individuals with ID is associated with alcohol-related offences and theft, and there are higher rates of alcohol problem history which are associated with histories of a number of offences, psychiatric disturbance in adulthood, psychiatric disturbance in childhood, and experiences of childhood adversity (Lindsay et al., 2013). Drug-involved inmates with high intellectual abilities are less motivated to enter substance abuse treatment compared to those with average and low intellectual abilities-characterized as individuals with ID (Vandevelde et al., 2005). The risk of reoffending, that is the recidivist rate for individuals with ID is related with the variables of unemployment, substance abuse and a psychiatric history (Klimecki, Jenkinson & Wilson, 1994), but there are no relevant studies focusing on individuals with ID and illegal acts that are committed prior to and for drug and alcohol use, as well as recommended systematic psychotherapeutic approaches (Ivanova & Giannouli, 2017).

Individuals with ID and Crime: The Influence of Other Variables

In the relationship between different forms of crime and ID, we may hypothesize the existence of a series of confounding variables, such as the socioeconomic status, the gender, and the educational qualification of the individual with ID. For example, a Norwegian research supports that the socio-economic status does have a relationship with ID, since parents of children with severe mental retardation seem to have a higher socioeconomic level than parents of children with mild mental retardation, something that holds true only for the identification of the children and only for this specific country and sample of participants (Strømme, & Magnus, 2000). More specifically, when examining adolescents and adults with ID and anti-social behavior, a lower socio-economic status and the existence of mental health problems are claimed to be associated with the actual expression of any form of anti-social behavior (Dickson et al., 2005; Lund, 1990; Timms & Goreczny, 2002). Although sexual crimes are claimed not to be overrepresented among ID individuals, there are more reported cases of individuals with ID who are men and who are charged with sexual offenses, rather than women. This does not really give us a clear picture, because much criminal offending goes undetected and unreported. Because of that studies can only investigate and include in the counting of individuals those already involved with the criminal justice process (Holland et al., 2002). In addition to that, the data usually come from individuals who are already in prison for their offenses, and ending up in prison may be related to the fact that men with mild ID and a history of sexual offending have significantly lower expressed general empathy for their own and other victims, something that may involve them in similar illegal activities and exposure to the police (Hockley & Langdon, 2015). Finally, no research so far presents a clear conclusion regarding the relationship concerning the type and the duration of previous education for ID offenders and the type and/or severity of the committed crime.

Legal Issues Related to Financial Matters and Medical Consent for Individuals with ID

Civil law refers to non-criminal law. It includes a wide array of issues concerning capacity for medical consent, capacity for sexual consent, financial capacity, testamentary capacity, driving capacity, and capacity for independent living (American Psychological Association, 2005; 2006). Individuals with ID may not have the capacity to decide for actions with legal implications, such as their own wedding (Reed, 1997). So, legislation in EU countries and USA is clear, when capacity is in doubt, it might be necessary for the individual to be referred to a competency hearing or/and may need the appointment of a guardian. Within the context of current legislation (mainly in western countries) relating to mental capacity in adults, elders is the most examined group, but individuals with ID should also come to the center of attention (Carey, 2010; Demakis, 2011). Although in the United States the capacity to make legal/financial decisions is considered through legal surrogate decision-making processes, until now little has been done for this new and at the same time old medico-legal topic in Europe, with the exception of the introduction of the Mental Capacity Act in the UK. Two forms of legal capacity are presented in detail below: financial capacity and capacity for medical consent.

ID and Financial Capacity

Individuals with (even) mild ID have problems in financial capacity and more specifically in decision making for everyday financial issues (Suto et al., 2005). Individuals with ID as all other cognitively impaired groups of patients face difficulties regarding the decision making process (Giannouli & Tsolaki, 2014; 2016), since they have problems in identifying the decision to be made, gathering relevant information, identifying alternatives, weighing evidence, choosing among alternatives, describing verbally how to take relevant action and reviewing decision and consequences (Giannouli & Tsolaki, 2011; 2015). Any difficulty even in one of the above steps of the decision making process may lead the individual to decisions that are harmful to himself/herself or others and to actions that are considered by contemporaries as illegal (e.g. receiving or giving goods-property that is acquired in an illegal way, participating in illegal activities and fraud etc.) (Giannouli, Stamovlasis & Tsolaki, 2018).

ID and Capacity for Medical Consent

Consent for medical treatments and procedures may result to serious legal outcomes. Individuals with mild or moderate ID are characterized as incapable to provide informed consent to hypothetical treatment scenarios-vignettes (Ho et al., 2018; Morris, Niederbuhl & Mahr, 1993). While adults with ID as a group show consent deficits, many may attain consent capacity scores comparable to those of 'normals' (Fisher et al., 2006). Most adults with mild and no mental retardation and almost half of adults with moderate mental retardation in a study were characterized as able to make and justify treatment choices and fully or partially understand treatment information. Most adults without mental retardation, 50% with mild, and 18% with moderate mental retardation are able to partially appreciate relevance of treatment choice to patient's situation and weigh treatment risks against benefit (Cea & Fisher, 2005). As a conclusion, clinicians and legal experts should always consider the wide range of individual differences (Giannouli & Tsolaki, 2019).

ID, Trial and Conviction

There are some basic questions for trial and conviction: Should offenders with ID be treated and held accountable-responsible for their actions in the same way as nondisabled citizens? (Glaser & Deane, 1999). ID does not necessary eliminate that someone has the ability to appreciate right from wrong, but this condition causes some unique difficulties for the person. Individuals with ID according to their families are significantly disadvantaged when they come into contact with the justice system, and more specifically with the criminal justice system personnel and jurors who are likely to fail to identify defendants with ID. For this reason it is argued that offenders with ID must be supported by legal representation from the earliest stages of the legal process (Cockram, Jackson & Underwood, 1998), and be dealt with differently from the general population (Jones, 2007). As a consequence, several states in the USA have laws that exempt persons who have ID from the death penalty and other severe sentences under the criminal code (Borromeo, 2001; Olvera, Dever & Earnest, 2000; Polloway, 2015).

Another question to be answered: Should individuals with ID who have been victims or witnesses or even responsible themselves of a crime be given limited access to the criminal justice system, often on the basis of assumptions about their incapacity to be interviewed by the police, and to give evidence in court? (Gudjonsson, Murphy & Clare, 2000). In general, the trial of a person with or without ID is the same as for 'normal' individuals regardless of country or legal system, but there is a tendency to consider individuals with ID as people who face barriers, due their cognitive-emotional-behavioral problems such as possible difficulties in oral language development, deficits in memory skills (Kebbell, Hatton, & Johnson, 2004), difficulty in learning social rules, difficulty with problem solving skills, delays in the development of adaptive behaviors, such as self-help or self-care skills and lack of social inhibitors, which determine the way they get involved with the legal system (Daily, Ardinger & Holmes, 2000). The above deficits can also be exacerbated by an ignorance of the current law.

Do the cognitive deficits of individuals with ID influence the procedures in civil and criminal law matters? Individuals with ID may have problems during criminal proceedings with the confession and waiver, proceeding to trial and functioning at trial (Appelbaum & Appelbaum, 1994). They are found to be less able to comprehend their rights in legal procedures, they are significantly more likely to respond to suggestive questioning, confabulate more and change more frequently their answers than normal individuals (Clare & Gudjonsson, 1993; Everington & Fulero, 1999; Perske 2008; 2011; Ridley, Gabbert & La Rooy, 2012). Interrogative suggestibility may have higher rates in children and adults with ID than in normal children and adults, because of their much poorer memory, but differences in suggestibility are only partly explained by poorer memory scores as false confessions do happen (Schatz, 2018). Age may play a significant role alongside the existence of ID, since children with ID are more susceptible to altering their answers under pressure than are adults with ID (Beail, 2002; Gudjonsson & Henry, 2003). Individuals with ID in the USA face special problems in the process of interrogation and confession, particularly with regard to the understanding of the information of the Miranda rights or also called Miranda warning (Fulero & Everington, 1995), and by being suggestible and acquiescent on interviews and making 'unwise' decisions (Murphy & Mason, 2014). Individuals with ID are thought to be incompetent witnesses in courts, although a relevant research claims that there is available evidence that they can provide accurate accounts of witnessed events. Of course, the accounts are usually less complete than those provided by the general 'normal' population and are greatly influenced by the methods of questioning. The available evidence suggests that cross-examination methods may lead to memory distortion, and that the use of closed, complex, and leading questions and the absence of aids to recall may have a particularly adverse effect on people with mental retardation (Kebbell & Hatton, 1999).

So, individuals with ID may be arrested and accused of crimes for which they often receive discriminatory treatment, are falsely convicted and punished (even with serious punishments, such as death penalty in the USA) (Lorenzo, 1991). Although experts raise doubts concerning the death penalty, which is characterized as a cruel and unusual punishment [Atkins v. Virginia, 536 U.S. 304 (2002)], still each American state and court has the responsibility to define who is mentally retarded or as we now call Intellectually Disabled. For example, Georgia as a state with the 1988 statute is prohibiting the execution of persons with intellectual disability, but there is a growing criticism as minimal specification regarding adjudication is not clarified yet (Ricciardelli & Jaskyte, 2019). Police and other criminal justice personnel often misunderstand the responses that people with ID make to them. Their main characteristics often include an inordinate desire to please authority figures, an inability to abstract from concrete thoughts, observation of interrogators for clues regarding responses, a longing for friends, a pleasant facade, abhorrence of the term "mental retardation", memory gaps, impaired judgment, and problems with receptive and expressive language skills. In addition, they often lack understanding of rights, court proceedings, and/or punishment. Therefore, they may confess to crimes they did not actually commit and receive sentences of capital punishment (Perske, 1991; Perske, 2005), but we have to keep in mind that the above lack of competence may not be true for every individual with ID (Bonnie, 1990).

ID and Forensic Neuropsychological Assessment

From the facts considered arise a number of questions about law and ID. Two main questions to be answered are: 'What information do the lawyers and the court need?' and 'How information which will serve as proof of limited intellectual functioning in ID are gathered and examined by mental health experts and presented to legal experts?'.

Following the tendency in modern criminology, we have moved from the study of the clues (19th century Scotland Yard approach) to a focus on the specific crime to the study of the person-criminal. Because of that, court-ordered and independent forensic neuropsychological examinations are necessary and in our days there is a growing number of cases when criminal offendants at some point of the legal procedure are claiming ID or civil cases for which a neuropsychologist's opinion and consultation is required for clarifying the above (Heilbronner, 2004; Larrabee, 2005; Sweet et al., 2002). This rapidly increasing need for neuropsychological expert witness' input in both civil and criminal legal proceedings is due to the vital question of the current capacity to stand trial and/ or the capacity to form criminal intent at the time of the offense (insanity) and/or the risk for future dangerous acts related to violence and re-offending, which can only be thoroughly assessed by forensic neuropsychologists by examining not only the cognitive capacities, but also the case of malingering-feigned ID (Boone, 2007). Since brain damage is not itself an adequate basis for legal decision making, the scope of neuropsychological assessment and investigation is the systematic and objective exposition of the nature, extent, and course of the individual's brain dysfunction and an explanation of its behavioral consequences relative to the psychological issue at hand (Martell, 1992). The diagnosis of a lifelong condition affecting cognitive and social development needs many sources of information and each neuropsychological evaluation may not only focus on the diagnosis and recording of deficits, but also on the future rehabilitation planning (Jakab, 1990).

The forensic neuropsychologist determines the procedure(s) which are required to answer the question(s) posed by the retaining party. A request may be made by the retaining party to administer certain tests, but the neuropsychologist is obliged to explain and support scientifically if different or additional measures-tests should be used (Bush, 2005; Hounsome et al., 2018). There are a variety of neuropsychological tests which could be used for the assessment in civil and criminal settings. More specifically, the classic standardized neuropsychological tests are widely used for the examination of civil capacities (Giannouli & Tsolaki, 2011), and there are a lot of areas to be addressed with caution during a neuropsychological examination: language, current intellectual level-IQ, verbal and visuo-spatial memory, attention/concentration, executive functioning, and emotional adjustment (McKinlay & McGowan, 2003). The decision making capacity seems to be really important for all civil cases and there are is a variety of new specific tests for that in different cultural and legal settings (Giannouli, 2014; Giannouli & Tsolaki, 2015), but neuropsychological information regarding competence follow the continuous paradigm of variation in degrees and by function, unlike the civil proceedings for which an absolute value of yes or no (competent-incompetent) must be answered (Schoenberg & Scott, 2011). Another frequent question in civil courts is whether the individual understands what he has done in cases of civil law (e.g., making a will and excluding his/her family members or making decisions with direct and indirect financial/legal consequences). In this respect the collected data during the evaluation may be used during the proceedings, by changing for example the way that the verbal material is presented.

The above findings for possible deficits could be included in medico-legal reports along with data from the individual/relatives interviews, and information coming from records on their functional capacity in various social settings and their health background. The forensic neuropsychologist must then answer the specific question at hand, for example in the case of criminal acts, whether the individual was before the commission, at the time and now (in)capable of doing a criminal act. In this case the forensic neuropsychologist can do that by providing a complete assessment of dangerousness based on all different sources for that person (self-reports, collaborative sources-e.g. family and evaluative collaborative sources-e.g. neuropsychological test data, medical and neurological examination and neuroimaging) (Denney & Wynkoop, 2000). The information obtained by the neuropsychological assessment will also be important for the future treatment of the individual by the judge, the jurors, and other people who work for the judicial system in prisons, in psychiatric hospitals or even when these individuals with ID return back to the community. Although the main focus of using these information in the legal system is unfortunately the management of prisoners with ID, rather than the rehabilitation planning, there is evidence for example that cognitive deficits may largely contribute to the lower completion rate of alcohol and drug treatment programmes for individuals with ID (McGillivray et al., 2016), a clue that could be used in order to improve the goals and structure of rehabilitation programmes and in order to overcome possible obstacles that relate to the different cognitive profiles (Lindsay, Taylor & Sturney, 2004). In addition to that, there is a need to educate people with ID about the civil and criminal laws, and here comes the importance not only of classic cognitive-behavioral treatments, but also of the attitudes-public opinion regarding ID and law. These attitudes can shape the role that families, caregivers and society as a whole can play for the future therapeutic treatments and interventions (Lindsay, 2002).

ATTITUDES TOWARD ID AND LAW: AN EMPIRICAL STUDY

Research Rationale

ID is related to major obstacles toward social, educational, and vocational integration (Goodley, 2016). Attitudes have evolved over time, acknowledging the equality of all persons (McDonagh et al., 2018). The law today recognizes individuals with ID as citizens, who possess an equal right to education, health care, and employment. However, 'this progression was not a linear development but rather a product of periods of growth and decline, backsliding, and hard-won battles across political, cultural, and legal domains' (Conrad, 2018). Given that the conceptualization of ID has historically changed, see for example medieval English law to our days (Turner, 2018) and a relevant historical perspective regarding the USA (Conrad, 2018), in modern western societies, although many things have changed from the past toward a more positive approach of the public for individuals with ID (Morin et al., 2013; Yazbeck, McVilly & Parmenter, 2004) with the de-institutionalisation movement in the direction of the 'normalisation principle', that is by trying to make the living environment of the individuals with ID to resemble as much as possible to the independent living conditions of the 'normals' (Louhiala, 2004), still the implicit and explicit negative perceptions and attitudes lead to discrimination and stigma not only in everyday life, but also in all areas of law (Murch et al., 2018; Scully 2018; Wilson & Scior, 2015). This is supported by a cross-cultural study which reveals that the general population in ten examined countries lack an appreciation of the range of capabilities of individuals with ID and report low expectations of how much people with ID can achieve in their lives. This large-scale study also revealed that the public still believes that individuals with ID should work and learn in separate settings, apart from people without disabilities (Siperstein, 2003).

Objective

The aim of this study is to present data for the general population's attitudes toward individuals with ID, and more specifically toward a neglected topic: ID and the Greek law (Giannouli, 2016).

Participants and Procedure

Following the protocol of another study on attitudes (Giannouli & Syrmos, 2017), one hundred twenty-three healthy adults were examined. The sample came from Northern Greece. All participants were native Greek speakers and participated in the research voluntarily. The males were 45 and the females were 78. Their age varied between 22 and 62 years old. The mean age was 38 years old (SD = 8). They were divided into three age groups: from 21 to 35 years old (N = 48), from 36 to 50 years old (N = 61), and above 50 years old (N = 14). The participants had different family statuses: 32 were married, 42 were single, 13 were divorced, 12 were widowed, and 24 cohabitated. Most of them graduated from university (N = 64). A big part had secondary education (N = 44), and only a minority had a basic education (N = 15). No participant had a relative with ID or a close friend with ID. They were all given a short questionnaire to complete by themselves, which included the following questions:

Question 1: Are individuals with ID more frequently engaged with the Greek law than individuals without ID?

Question 2: Do you believe that individuals with ID have problems in Greek courts more frequently regarding civil cases or criminal cases?
Question 3: Why do you believe that individuals with ID get involved with the law?
Question 4: What kind of crimes do you expect an individual with ID to commit in Greece?
Question 5: What can we do in order to avoid possible future involvement with the criminal-civil law for individuals with ID?
Question 6: Is the Greek legal system protecting or treating individuals with ID in a special way? Is this positive or negative?
Question 7: Is this treatment characterized by you as fair? Why? Why not?

Results

The results of this study revealed for Question 1 that Greeks believe that individuals with ID engage more frequently with the law (89 participants responded that they believe this to be true). For Question 2, 56 participants responded that they believe that the civil law cases to be more frequent and 67 that criminal cases as more frequent in Greece. For Question 3, there were a variety of recorded reasons for the involvement of individuals with ID with the law: the most common reason is the fact that they do not understand what they are doing and what others are doing (70), the second reason is that they do not know what the law says (22), and the third was that they come from or end up in environments were illegal behavior is the norm (31). For Question 4, three were the most reported crimes that respondents believe that individuals with ID commit in Greece: theft (78), sexual assault (30), and homicide (15). For Question 5, there was a clear pattern in the responses of the participants of what we can do in order to change the current situation: the state must create treatment programs or institutions for this group of people to attend, where they can be controlled and educated on these issues of legal matters, but also on social behavior (101), the remaining respondents (22) did not have a clear view and did not propose anything, either because they do not believe that there is a problem, or because they could not think of anything to propose. For Question 6, respondents believe that the Greek Civil Code is giving to incapable adults and minors a different positive and protective treatment (110). For Question 7, the respondents believe that this treatment is fair (95), because according to their opinion when you have to deal with incapacitated individuals you have to change the way you are approaching him/her (94). The rest of the respondents (28) who believe that the treatment to be unfair, explain their view mainly on the basis of the fact that everyone knows what is good and what is bad in general, something that constitutes the foundation of any legal system (26). Finally, there were no statistically significant differences in the responses that the participants gave when categorized according to their age, sex, educational and family status groups in the this sample (Giannouli, 2016).

DISCUSSION AND CONCLUSIONS

The above results yield useful information to target public awareness on law and ID. Unfortunately, there are no systematic studies on the socio-demographic characteristics of individuals with ID in Greece, which could give as more information in order to compare the opinions of the participants in this sample with the documented legal reality. Greeks according to this research, do have a clear view on this unique population and it seems that a change of attitudes is necessary, with future initiatives aiming at collecting data on this topic not only locally, but also worldwide (Giannouli, 2016).

It is of interest to report here what is the reality in other Western countries during the last few years. For example, in the Nertherlands, restrictive measures, that is all measures that limit the freedom of a person, such as seclusion and mechanical and physical restraints, are generally considered most intrusive in mild ID, but Dutch staff members working in settings providing care for people with ID are aware that social restrictions could also be instrusive (Dörenberg et al., 2018). In Quebec, a recent research shows that at least half of health care providers display positive attitudes towards individuals with ID that are compatible with notions of social inclusion and equal rights (Morin et al., 2018). In a recent Greek study (southern Greece), health and social care students showed poor attitudes towards people not only with physical and intellectual disability as scored by the standardized scale CLAS-ID (Kritsotakis et al., 2017). More specifically, nursing students had slightly less positive attitudes in the "Similarity" subscale, but more positive attitudes in the "Sheltering" subscale. Previous experience, including work and contact were related to more favourable attitudes as measured by "Similarity" and "Sheltering" attitudes, and higher age to less favourable "Similarity" and "Sheltering" attitudes. Male participants had higher "Exclusion" scores regarding individuals with ID. In addition to that, participants who knew individuals with ID had less favourable "Empowerment" attitudes. Knowledge was related to more positive attitudes in all four CLAS-ID subscales (Kritsotakis et al., 2017). Of course, attitudes may change through various ways, one of which could be brief film-based digital interventions, which were found to have small positive effects on attitudes of laypeople in UK towards individuals with ID (Lindau et al., 2018). Although there is a focus on the revision and further development of scales measuring attitudes in the general and healthcare professionals population toward ID (Boo & Nie, 2018), another approach supported by some researchers state that we need to reframe the academic discussion away from attitudes and toward stigma in ID, as the latter concept makes visible possible issues of power and inequality (Cureton, 2018; Simplican, 2019).

ID, Attitudes and Legal Issues in non-Western Cultures

The relationship between intellectual disability and criminality is complex, especially if the cultural factor is taken into consideration. The cultural factor is considered to be very important, because it plays a significant role in stigma for mental illness (Scior & Werner, 2016), which seems to be less evident for example in Asian and African countries (Fabrega, 1991). In addition to that, while attitudes toward mental illness vary among non-Western cultures, the stigma of mental illness may be less severe than in Western cultures, because of the lack of differentiation between psychiatric and non-psychiatric illness in the three great non-Western medical traditions (Dols, 1987; Ng, 1997). Unfortunately, the cross-cultural studies in the western world concerning different aspects of ID and law are scarce (McAfee et al., 2001), and the existing replication studies come all from western societies (Hayes, 1996), where in general an individual's age, educational attainment and prior contact with someone with an ID may predict attitudes (Scior, 2011), while in other studies again conducted in western societies (e.g. Canada) only gender and age categories serve as predictive factors for the attitudes toward ID (Morin et al., 2014). We must keep in mind that there is always an additional influence of the culture where the individual comes from as a study with North Indian Hindu immigrants living in the mid-Western United States demonstrate on the ways in which immigrants think and talk about mental retardation even in another cultural context (Gabel, 2004). Although crime and legal issues among ID individuals in other countries besides western societies is recognized to be a little investigated topic (Kuo, 1983), there is still no adequate scientific literature on that. The main problem for this lack of information is not the existence of different legal systems, but the lack of research initiatives on this field.

There are some cross-cultural studies, such as the Scior et al. (2010), which examine and compare the attitudes among the Hong Kong Chinese public and the British public toward ID. This study found that the Chinese were less favorable than the British sample, who were less opposed to the exclusion of people with intellectual disabilities, less likely to view them as similar to themselves, and more in favor of sheltering such individuals. In Taiwan, the general attitudes of employees toward individuals with ID and their affective reactions toward their coworkers with ID are reported to be positive (Hsu et al., 2015). In India, a relevant research revealed that cultural and religious beliefs perpetuate negative attitudes towards disability (Edwardraj et al., 2010). Raw data from India indicate that ID is mainly associated with male gender, poor socio-economic status, pre-natal, peri-natal and post-natal complications, family history of ID, mental illness, and increased maternal age (Gopalan et al., 2014). High rates of comorbidity with psychiatric disorders, especially with externalizing disorders and psychosis followed by bipolar affective disorders are found in India, and ID is claimed to be associated with psychosocial adversities and psychiatric comorbidities (Gopalan et al., 2014; Kishore et al., 2004), a finding that is in line with the general trend in the western studies that offenders regardless of their IQ have in large part psychiatric comorbidities. This is supported by a recent study in Australia, where the "dual disability" group (individuals with ID and comorbid mental illness) was between 2.97 and 3.22 times more likely than those with intellectual disability alone to have a history of criminal charges, and between 2.76 and 2.97 times more likely to have been a victim of crime (Thomas et al., 2019).

Another non-western study from China revealed that the majority of mentally retarded offenders were men, with an IQ which characterized them as mildly mentally retarded, with an additional psychiatric comorbidity for nearly half of the sample and a repeated history of offenses. The offenders had committed crimes against property, while the property offenses, especially petty theft and arson were frequently seen, but there was no noteworthy above average reported frequency of sexual offenses (Su et al., 2000). Another study from China found a high percentage of individuals diagnosed with ID who are convicted of murder (Wenhua, 2005). Finally, research from Africa revealed the high vulnerability of women with learning disabilities in the mild or moderate categories for sexual abuse (Calitz, 2011; Dickman & Roux, 2005) and a similar finding is supported for a sample of women from India (Mohaparta & Mohanty, 2004).

The above findings may change as developing countries adopt western style consumer-driven economies, and in the future there might be an imitative tendency for the general public of these countries that will follow the same western trajectory of exclusion, which will impose the culture of "otherness" for the individuals with ID whose contribution to the society will be subsequently further devalued (Parmenter, 2008).

Based on the lack of information on the way that the general public form different cultural environments, perceive ID and legal issues, and on how ID individuals react in their cultural environment, it is almost impossible to propose certain steps taken in different countries towards negating stigma and discriminatory treatment of people with ID. At the same time, no recipe can be proposed concerning strategies that must be followed in every country in order to improve the way(s) the society(ies) view(s) people with ID and reduce the disadvantages faced by the people with ID and their family members in the way the legal systems conduct trial and conviction. We must keep in mind that the socially constructed phenomenon of mental retardation varies cross-culturally in important respects (Manion & Bersani,

1987), which have to be further investigated by collecting data following identical research protocols not only on what the public believes, but also on what is the 'reality' of the legal reality in terms of descriptive statistics for each country in an effort to overcome relativism (Jenkins & Angrosino, 1998).

QUO VADIS? FUTURE RESEARCH DIRECTIONS

There are more questions on issues regarding ID and law, than there are answers. Future research should move from simple prevalence and descriptive studies of the excluded individuals with ID, to attempts of investigating identification of ID and the psychological and social processes, which determine how an individual with ID gets in and out of the justice system. Of course, research until now has given little attention to the fact that there are different societies-cultures and as a consequence different attitudes toward ID and that there is no clear answer to autonomy questions (Wilker, 1979). Methodological issues from previous research should be taken into consideration since there is not one single population with ID, but numerous with different forms of ID, different levels of severity of ID, concerning the two different sexes, and different social environments. So, it will be necessary to have research from the field of civil and criminal law focusing on the different demographics of ID, the different countries and these data should have only one aim, to be used for the improvement of the assessment and treatment approaches for clinicians and for the improvement of the legal process for legal experts (Lambrick & Glaser, 2004). In addition to large-scale research, cross-cultural projects should be conducted on public protection. Based on these empirical evidence, proposals should be made to governments for mental health legislation. In addition to that, new models of care giving emphasis not only on the individuals, but also on their families (Giannouli, 2018b), should be examined for these different groups of individuals who fall under the umbrella of ID.

REFERENCES

Alexander, R. T., Chester, V., Green, F. N., Gunaratna, I., & Hoare, S. (2015). Arson or fire setting in offenders with intellectual disability: Clinical characteristics, forensic histories, and treatment outcomes. *Journal of Intellectual & Developmental Disability*, *40*(2), 1–9. doi:10.3109/13668250.2014.998182

American Psychological Association. (2005). *Assessment of older adults with diminished capacity. A handbook for lawyers.* American Bar Association Commission on Law and Aging – American Psychological Association.

American Psychological Association. (2006). *Assessment of older adults with diminished capacity. A handbook for psychologists.* American Bar Association Commission on Law and Aging – American Psychological Association.

Appelbaum, K. L., & Appelbaum, P. S. (1994). Criminal-justice-related competencies in defendants with mental retardation. *The Journal of Psychiatry & Law*, *22*(4), 483–503. doi:10.1177/009318539402200402

Baroff, G. S., Gunn, M., & Hayes, S. (2004). Legal issues. In W. Lindsay, J. Taylor, & P. Sturmey (Eds.), *Offenders with developmental disabilities* (pp. 37–65). West Sussex, UK: Wiley. doi:10.1002/9780470713440.ch3

Barron, P., Hassiotis, A., & Banes, J. (2002). Offenders with intellectual disability: The size of the problem and therapeutic outcomes. *Journal of Intellectual Disability Research, 46*(6), 454–463. doi:10.1046/j.1365-2788.2002.00432.x PMID:12354316

Beail, N. (2002). Interrogative suggestibility, memory and intellectual disability. *Journal of Applied Research in Intellectual Disabilities, 15*(2), 129–137. doi:10.1046/j.1468-3148.2002.00108.x

Benson, B. A., & Brooks, W. T. (2008). Aggressive challenging behaviour and intellectual disability. *Current Opinion in Psychiatry, 21*(5), 454–458. doi:10.1097/YCO.0b013e328306a090 PMID:18650686

Benson, B. A., & Ivins, J. (1992). Anger, depression and self-concept in adults with mental retardation. *Journal of Intellectual Disability Research, 36*(2), 169–175. doi:10.1111/j.1365-2788.1992.tb00492.x PMID:1591500

Boer, D. P., McKnight, J. M., Kinlyside, A. M., & Chan, J. P. (2018). Assessing and treating offenders with Intellectual Disabilities. In M. Ternes, P. R. Magaletta, & M. W. Patry (Eds.), *The Practice of Correctional Psychology* (pp. 71–101). Springer. doi:10.1007/978-3-030-00452-1_4

Bonnie, R. J. (1990). The competence of criminal defendants with mental retardation to participate in their own defense. *The Journal of Criminal Law & Criminology, 81*(3), 419–446. doi:10.2307/1143845

Boo, L. S. H., & Nie, Y. (2018). Attitude towards persons with intellectual disability scale: Further development. *Current Psychology (New Brunswick, N.J.), 37*(4), 760–768. doi:10.100712144-017-9560-5

Boone, K. B. (Ed.). (2007). *Assessment of feigned cognitive impairment: A neuropsychological perspective*. New York: Guilford Press.

Borromeo, A. D. (2001). Mental retardation and the death penalty. *Loyola Journal of Public Interest Law, 3*, 175.

Bush, S. S.Planning Committee. (2005). Independent and court-ordered forensic neuropsychological examinations: Official statement of the National Academy of Neuropsychology. *Archives of Clinical Neuropsychology, 20*(8), 997–1007. doi:10.1016/j.acn.2005.06.003 PMID:16076547

Calitz, F. J. (2011). Psycho-legal challenges facing the mentally retarded rape victim. *South African Journal of Psychiatry, 17*(3), 66–72. doi:10.4102ajpsychiatry.v17i3.280

Carey, A. C. (2010). *On the margins of citizenship: Intellectual disability and civil rights in twentieth-century America*. Philadelphia, PA: Temple University Press.

Carr, A., Linehan, C., O'Reilly, G., Walsh, P. N., & McEvoy, J. (Eds.). (2016). *The handbook of intellectual disability and clinical psychology practice*. Routledge. doi:10.4324/9781315739229

Cea, C. D., & Fisher, C. B. (2003). Health care decision-making by adults with mental retardation. *Journal Information, 41*(2). PMID:12622524

Clare, I. C. H., & Gudjonsson, G. H. (1993). Interrogative suggestibility, confabulation, and acquiescence in people with mild learning disabilities (mental handicap): Implications for reliability during police interview. *British Journal of Clinical Psychology, 32*(3), 295–301. doi:10.1111/j.2044-8260.1993.tb01059.x PMID:8251959

Clare, I. C. H., & Gudjonsson, G. H. (1995). The vulnerability of suspects with intellectual disabilities during police interviews: A review and experimental study of decision-making. *Mental Handicap Research*, *8*(2), 110–128. doi:10.1111/j.1468-3148.1995.tb00149.x

Cockram, J., Jackson, R., & Underwood, R. (1998). People with an intellectual disability and the criminal justice system: The family perspective. *Journal of Intellectual & Developmental Disability*, *23*(1), 41–56. doi:10.1080/13668259800033571

Conrad, J. A. (2018). On intellectual and developmental disabilities in the United States: A historical perspective. *Journal of Intellectual Disabilities*. PMID:29621909

Crocker, A. G., Mercier, C., Lachapelle, Y., Brunet, A., Morin, D., & Roy, M. E. (2006). Prevalence and types of aggressive behaviour among adults with intellectual disabilities. *Journal of Intellectual Disability Research*, *50*(9), 652–661. doi:10.1111/j.1365-2788.2006.00815.x PMID:16901292

Cureton, A. (Ed.). (2018). *Disability in practice: Attitudes, policies, and relationships*. Oxford, UK: Oxford University Press. doi:10.1093/oso/9780198812876.001.0001

Curtis, A., McVilly, K., & Day, A. (2014). Sentencing offenders with mental impairment: The case of arsonists with intellectual disability. *Journal of Intellectual Disabilities and Offending Behaviour*, *5*(2), 78–87. doi:10.1108/JIDOB-05-2014-0005

Cuskelly, M., & Bryde, R. (2004). Attitudes towards the sexuality of adults with an intellectual disability: Parents, support staff, and a community sample. *Journal of Intellectual & Developmental Disability*, *29*(3), 255–264. doi:10.1080/13668250412331285136

Daily, D. K., Ardinger, H. H., & Holmes, G. E. (2000). Identification and evaluation of mental retardation. *American Family Physician*, *61*(4), 1059–1067. PMID:10706158

Davidson, P. W., Cain, N. N., Sloane-Reeves, J. E., & Van Speybroech, A. (1994). Characteristics of community-based individuals with mental retardation and aggressive behavioral disorders. *American Journal of Mental Retardation*, *98*(6), 704–716. PMID:8054199

Day, K. (1993). Crime and mental retardation: A review. *Clinical Approaches to the Mentally Disordered Offender*, 111-44.

Day, K. (1994). Male mentally handicapped sex offenders. *The British Journal of Psychiatry*, *165*(5), 630–639. doi:10.1192/bjp.165.5.630 PMID:7866678

Demakis, G. J. (Ed.). (2011). *Civil capacities in clinical neuropsychology: Research findings and practical applications*. New York: Oxford University Press.

Denney, R. L., & Wynkoop, T. F. (2000). Clinical neuropsychology in the criminal forensic setting. *The Journal of Head Trauma Rehabilitation*, *15*(2), 804–828. doi:10.1097/00001199-200004000-00005 PMID:10739969

Devapriam, J., Raju, L., Singh, N., Collacott, R., & Bhaumik, S. (2007). Arson: Characteristics and predisposing factors in offenders with intellectual disabilities. *British Journal of Forensic Practice*, *9*(4), 23–27. doi:10.1108/14636646200700023

Dickman, B. J., & Roux, A. J. (2005). Complainants with learning disabilities in sexual abuse cases: A 10-year review of a psycho-legal project in Cape Town, South Africa. *British Journal of Learning Disabilities, 33*(3), 138–144. doi:10.1111/j.1468-3156.2005.00355.x

Dickson, K., Emerson, E., & Hatton, C. (2005). Self-reported anti-social behaviour: Prevalence and risk factors amongst adolescents with and without intellectual disability. *Journal of Intellectual Disability Research, 49*(11), 820–826. doi:10.1111/j.1365-2788.2005.00727.x PMID:16207279

Dols, M. W. (1987). Insanity and its treatment in Islamic society. *Medical History, 31*(1), 1–14. doi:10.1017/S0025727300046287 PMID:3543559

Dörenberg, V. E., de Veer, A. J., Francke, A. L., Embregts, P. J., van Nieuwenhuijzen, M., & Frederiks, B. J. (2018). Applying restrictive measures in the care of adolescents with mild intellectual disabilities: Attitudes of support staff and policy implications. *Journal of Policy and Practice in Intellectual Disabilities, 15*(1), 26–35. doi:10.1111/jppi.12223

Dwyer, R. G., & Frierson, R. L. (2006). The presence of low IQ and mental retardation among murder defendants referred for pretrial evaluation. *Journal of Forensic Sciences, 51*(3), 678–682. doi:10.1111/j.1556-4029.2006.00115.x PMID:16696721

Edwardraj, S., Mumtaj, K., Prasad, J. H., Kuruvilla, A., & Jacob, K. S. (2010). Perceptions about intellectual disability: A qualitative study from Vellore, South India. *Journal of Intellectual Disability Research, 54*(8), 736–748. doi:10.1111/j.1365-2788.2010.01301.x PMID:20633202

Everington, C., & Fulero, S. M. (1999). Competence to confess: Measuring understanding and suggestibility of defendants with mental retardation. *Mental Retardation, 37*(3), 212–220. doi:10.1352/0047-6765(1999)037<0212:CTCMUA>2.0.CO;2 PMID:10473340

Fabrega, H. Jr. (1991). Psychiatric stigma in non-Western societies. *Comprehensive Psychiatry, 32*(6), 534–551. doi:10.1016/0010-440X(91)90033-9 PMID:1778081

Fazel, S., Xenitidis, K., & Powell, J. (2008). The prevalence of intellectual disabilities among 12000 prisoners - A systematic review. *International Journal of Law and Psychiatry, 31*(4), 369–373. doi:10.1016/j.ijlp.2008.06.001 PMID:18644624

Fisher, C., Cea, C., Davidson, P., & Fried, A. (2006). Capacity of persons with mental retardation to consent to participate in randomized clinical trials. *The American Journal of Psychiatry, 163*(10), 1813–1820. doi:10.1176/ajp.2006.163.10.1813 PMID:17012694

Fogden, B. C., Thomas, S. D., Daffern, M., & Ogloff, J. R. (2016). Crime and victimisation in people with intellectual disability: A case linkage study. *BMC Psychiatry, 16*(1), 170. doi:10.118612888-016-0869-7 PMID:27234810

Fulero, S. M., & Everington, C. (1995). Assessing competency to waive Miranda rights in defendants with mental retardation. *Law and Human Behavior, 19*(5), 533–543. doi:10.1007/BF01499342

Gabel, S. (2004). South Asian Indian cultural orientations toward mental retardation. *Journal Information, 42*(1), 12–25. PMID:14720098

Giannouli, V. (2014). What do Greeks believe about elders and mental? *Agora International Journal of Juridical Sciences*, *8*(3), 1–5.

Giannouli, V. (2016). Crime and legal issues among intellectually disabled individuals. In R. T. Gopalan (Ed.), *Handbook of research on diagnosing, treating, and managing intellectual disabilities* (pp. 346–369). IGI Global. doi:10.4018/978-1-5225-0089-6.ch018

Giannouli, V. (2018a). Elder abuse and consent capacity: Our collective nemesis? In R. T. Gopalan (Ed.), *Social, psychological, and forensic perspectives on sexual abuse* (pp. 207–221). IGI Global. doi:10.4018/978-1-5225-3958-2.ch015

Giannouli, V. (2018b). On the importance of focusing on family and parent factors in multilevel analyses regarding psychopathology of adolescents with an intellectual disability who present to general hospital services. *Australasian Psychiatry*, *26*(3), 325–326. doi:10.1177/1039856217749055 PMID:29873561

Giannouli, V., Stamovlasis, D., & Tsolaki, M. (2018). Exploring the role of cognitive factors in a new instrument for elders' financial capacity assessment. *Journal of Alzheimer's Disease*, *62*(4), 1579–1594. doi:10.3233/JAD-170812 PMID:29504530

Giannouli, V., & Syrmos, N. (2017). Exploring attitudes towards endocrine diseases in Greece. *Endocrine*, *55*(2), 655–657. doi:10.100712020-016-1164-6 PMID:27822671

Giannouli, V., & Tsolaki, M. (2011). Competency and dementia: A challenge of today. [in Greek]. *Neurology*, *20*(6), 12–19.

Giannouli, V., & Tsolaki, M. (2014). Legal capacity of the elderly in Greece. *Hellenic Journal of Nuclear Medicine*, *17*, 2–6. PMID:24392459

Giannouli, V., & Tsolaki, M. (2015). A neglected drama for elders: Discrepancy between self-perception and objective performance regarding financial capacity in patients with cognitive deficits. *Psychological Thought*, *8*(2), 142–147. doi:10.5964/psyct.v8i2.130

Giannouli, V., & Tsolaki, M. (2016). Questions about Dementia with Lewy Bodies, personal beliefs and real performance for financial capacity tasks. *European Psychiatry Medicine*, *33*, 582.

Giannouli, V., & Tsolaki, M. (2019). Are left angular gyrus and amygdala volumes important for financial capacity in mild cognitive impairment? *Hellenic Journal of Nuclear Medicine*, *22*, 160–164. PMID:30877733

Glaser, W., & Deane, K. (1999). Normalisation in an abnormal world: A study of prisoners with an intellectual disability. *International Journal of Offender Therapy and Comparative Criminology*, *43*(3), 338–356. doi:10.1177/0306624X99433007

Goodley, D. (2016). *Disability studies: An interdisciplinary introduction*. London: Sage.

Gopalan, R. T., Sharma, R., & Unnikrishnan, M. P. (2014). Socio-demographic and clinical features of children with intellectual disability and their parents - An Indian study. *International Neuropsychiatric Disease Journal*, *2*(6), 2321–7235. doi:10.9734/INDJ/2014/10610

Gray, E., Beech, A., & Rose, J. (2019). Using biofeedback to improve emotion regulation in sexual offenders with intellectual disability: A feasibility study. *International Journal of Developmental Disabilities*, 1–10.

Gudjonsson, G. H., & Henry, L. (2003). Child and adult witnesses with intellectual disability: The importance of suggestibility. *Legal and Criminological Psychology*, *8*(2), 241–252. doi:10.1348/135532503322363013

Gudjonsson, G. H., Murphy, G. H., & Clare, I. C. H. (2000). Assessing the capacity of people with intellectual disabilities to be witnesses in court. *Psychological Medicine*, *30*(2), 307–314. doi:10.1017/S003329179900149X PMID:10824651

Gulati, G., Murphy, V., Clarke, A., Delcellier, K., Meagher, D., Kennedy, H., ... Dunne, C. P. (2018). Intellectual disability in Irish prisoners: Systematic review of prevalence. *International Journal of Prisoner Health*, *14*(3), 188–196. doi:10.1108/IJPH-01-2017-0003 PMID:30274556

Harris, J. E. (2019). Legal capacity at a crossroad: Mental disability and family law. *Family Court Review*, *57*(1), 14–20. doi:10.1111/fcre.12394

Hayes, S. (1996). Recent research on offenders with learning disabilities. *Tizard Learning Disability Review*, *1*(3), 7–15. doi:10.1108/13595474199600003

Heilbronner, R. (2004). A status report on the practice of forensic neuropsychology. *The Clinical Neuropsychologist*, *18*(2), 312–326. doi:10.1080/13854040490501574 PMID:15587677

Ho, P., Downs, J., Bulsara, C., Patman, S., & Hill, A. M. (2018). Addressing challenges in gaining informed consent for a research study investigating falls in people with intellectual disability. *British Journal of Learning Disabilities*, *46*(2), 92–100. doi:10.1111/bld.12217

Hockley, O. J., & Langdon, P. E. (2015). Men with intellectual disabilities with a history of sexual offending: Empathy for victims of sexual and non-sexual crimes. *Journal of Intellectual Disability Research*, *59*(4), 332–341. doi:10.1111/jir.12137 PMID:24761788

Hodgins, S. (1992). Mental disorder, intellectual deficiency, and crime: Evidence from a birth cohort. *Archives of General Psychiatry*, *49*(6), 476–483. doi:10.1001/archpsyc.1992.01820060056009 PMID:1599373

Hodgins, S., Mednick, S. A., Brennan, P. A., Schulsinger, F., & Engberg, M. (1996). Mental disorder and crime: Evidence from a Danish birth cohort. *Archives of General Psychiatry*, *53*(6), 489–496. doi:10.1001/archpsyc.1996.01830060031004 PMID:8639031

Holland, T., Clare, I. C. H., & Mukhopadhyay, T. (2002). Prevalence of 'criminal offending' by men and women with intellectual disability and the characteristics of 'offenders': Implications for research and service development. *Journal of Intellectual Disability Research*, *46*(s1), 6–20. doi:10.1046/j.1365-2788.2002.00001.x PMID:12061335

Hounsome, J., Whittington, R., Brown, A., Greenhill, B., & McGuire, J. (2018). The structured assessment of violence risk in adults with intellectual disability: A systematic review. *Journal of Applied Research in Intellectual Disabilities*, *31*(1), e1–e17. doi:10.1111/jar.12295 PMID:27891723

Hsu, T. H., Huang, Y. T., Liu, Y. H., Ososkic, J., Fried, J., & Bezyak, J. (2015). Taiwanese attitudes and affective reactions toward individuals and coworkers who have intellectual disabilities. *American Journal on Intellectual and Developmental Disabilities, 120*(2), 110–124. doi:10.1352/1944-7558-120.2.110 PMID:25715181

Huxley, A., Dalton, M., Tsui, Y. Y., & Hayhurst, K. P. (2018). Prevalence of alcohol, smoking, and illicit drug use amongst people with intellectual disabilities. *Drugs Education Prevention & Policy*, 1–20. doi:10.1080/09687637.2018.1488949

Ivanova, D., & Giannouli, V. (2017). Lesch type III alcoholism in Bulgarian women: Implications and recommendations for psychotherapy. *International Journal of Caring Sciences, 10*(3), 1569–1576.

Jahoda, A., Pert, C., Squire, J., & Trower, P. (1998). Facing stress and conflict: A comparison of the predicted responses and self-concepts of aggressive and non-aggressive people with intellectual disability. *Journal of Intellectual Disability Research, 42*(5), 360–369. doi:10.1046/j.1365-2788.1998.00143.x PMID:9828067

Jakab, I. (1990). Neuropsychological evaluation and rehabilitation in mental retardation. *Neuropsychology Review, 1*(2), 137–164. doi:10.1007/BF01108715 PMID:2152529

Jenkins, R., & Angrosino, M. V. (1998). *Questions of competence: Culture, classification and intellectual disability*. Cambridge, UK: Cambridge University Press.

Jones, J. (2007). Persons with intellectual disabilities in the criminal justice system: Review of issues. *International Journal of Offender Therapy and Comparative Criminology, 51*(6), 723–733. doi:10.1177/0306624X07299343 PMID:17636203

Kebbell, M. R., & Hatton, C. (1999). People with mental retardation as witnesses in court: A review. *Mental Retardation, 37*(3), 179–187. doi:10.1352/0047-6765(1999)037<0179:PWMRAW>2.0.CO;2 PMID:10473337

Kebbell, M. R., Hatton, C., & Johnson, S. D. (2004). Witnesses with intellectual disabilities in court: What questions are asked and what influence do they have? *Legal and Criminological Psychology, 9*(1), 23–35. doi:10.1348/135532504322776834

Kishore, M. T., Nizamie, A., Nizamie, S. H., & Jahan, M. (2004). Psychiatric diagnosis in persons with intellectual disability in India. *Journal of Intellectual Disability Research, 48*(1), 19–24. doi:10.1111/j.1365-2788.2004.00579.x PMID:14675227

Klimecki, M. R., Jenkinson, J., & Wilson, L. (1994). A study of recidivism among offenders with an intellectual disability. *Journal of Intellectual & Developmental Disability, 19*(3), 209–219.

Kritsotakis, G., Galanis, P., Papastefanakis, E., Meidani, F., Philalithis, A. E., Kalokairinou, A., & Sourtzi, P. (2017). Attitudes towards people with physical or intellectual disabilities among nursing, social work and medical students. *Journal of Clinical Nursing, 26*(23-24), 4951–4963. doi:10.1111/jocn.13988 PMID:28771877

Kuo, S. H. (1993). Forensic psychiatry in Taiwan. *International Journal of Law and Psychiatry, 6*(3-4), 457–472. doi:10.1016/0160-2527(83)90032-8 PMID:6679535

Lambrick, F., & Glaser, W. (2004). Sex offenders with an intellectual disability. *Sexual Abuse*, *16*(4), 381–392. doi:10.1177/107906320401600409 PMID:15560418

Langdon, P. E., Clare, I. C., & Murphy, G. H. (2011). Moral reasoning theory and illegal behaviour by adults with intellectual disabilities. *Psychology, Crime & Law*, *17*(2), 101–115. doi:10.1080/10683160903392384

Larrabee, G. J. (2005). *Forensic neuropsychology: A scientific approach.* New York: Oxford University Press.

Levine, K. A., Proulx, J., & Schwartz, K. (2018). Disconnected lives: Women with intellectual disabilities in conflict with the law. *Journal of Applied Research in Intellectual Disabilities*, *31*(2), 249–258. doi:10.1111/jar.12387 PMID:28718998

Lindau, N., Amin, T., Zambon, A., & Scior, K. (2018). The effect of brief digital interventions on attitudes to intellectual disability: Results from a pilot study. *Journal of Applied Research in Intellectual Disabilities*, *31*(1), 106–113. doi:10.1111/jar.12366 PMID:28503872

Lindsay, W. R. (2002). Integration of recent reviews on offenders with intellectual disabilities. *Journal of Applied Research in Intellectual Disabilities*, *15*(2), 111–119. doi:10.1046/j.1468-3148.2002.00112.x

Lindsay, W. R., Carson, D., Holland, A. J., Taylor, J. L., O'Brien, G., Wheeler, J. R., & Steptoe, L. (2013). Alcohol and its relationship to offence variables in a cohort of offenders with intellectual disability. *Journal of Intellectual & Developmental Disability*, *38*(4), 325–331. doi:10.3109/13668250.2013.837154 PMID:24279785

Lindsay, W. R., Law, J., Quinn, K., Smart, N., & Smith, A. H. (2001). A comparison of physical and sexual abuse: Histories of sexual and non-sexual offenders with intellectual disability. *Child Abuse & Neglect*, *25*(7), 989–995. doi:10.1016/S0145-2134(01)00251-4 PMID:11523873

Lindsay, W. R., Smith, A. H., Quinn, K., Anderson, A., Smith, A., Allan, R., & Law, J. (2004). Women with intellectual disability who have offended: Characteristics and outcome. *Journal of Intellectual Disability Research*, *48*(6), 580–590. doi:10.1111/j.1365-2788.2004.00627.x PMID:15312059

Lindsay, W. R., Taylor, J. L., & Sturmey, P. (Eds.). (2004). *Offenders with developmental disabilities.* Chichester, UK: John Wiley & Sons. doi:10.1002/9780470713440

Lindsay, W. R., Tinsley, S., & Emara, M. (2012). Alcohol use and offending in people with intellectual disability. *Alcohol-Related Violence. Prevention & Treatment*, 285–302.

Lorenzo, L. A. (1991). Societal prejudice reflected in our courts: The unfavorable treatment of the mentally retarded. *Seton Hall Const. LJ*, *2*, 771.

Louhiala. (2004). *Preventing intellectual disability. Ethical and clinical issues.* Cambridge, UK: Cambridge University Press.

Lund, J. (1990). Mentally retarded criminal offenders in Denmark. *The British Journal of Psychiatry*, *156*(5), 726–731. doi:10.1192/bjp.156.5.726 PMID:2095951

Lunsky, Y., Bradley, E. A., Gracey, C. D., Durbin, J., & Koegl, C. (2009). Gender differences in psychiatric diagnoses among inpatients with and without intellectual disabilities. *Journal Information*, *114*(1). PMID:19143463

Lyall, I., Holland, A. J., & Collins, S. (1995). Offending by adults with learning disabilities and the attitudes of staff to offending behaviour: Implications for service development. *Journal of Intellectual Disability Research*, *39*(6), 501–508. doi:10.1111/j.1365-2788.1995.tb00570.x PMID:8746737

Maclean, M. J., Sims, S., Bower, C., Leonard, H., Stanley, F. J., & O'Donnell, M. (2017). Maltreatment risk among children with disabilities. *Pediatrics*, *139*(4), e20161817. doi:10.1542/peds.2016-1817 PMID:28264988

Manion, M. L., & Bersani, H. A. (1987). Mental retardation as a Western sociological construct: A cross-cultural analysis. *Disability, Handicap & Society*, *2*(3), 231–245. doi:10.1080/02674648766780301

Martell, D. A. (1992). Forensic neuropsychology and the criminal law. *Law and Human Behavior*, *16*(3), 313–336. doi:10.1007/BF01044772

McAfee, J. K., Cockram, J., & Wolfe, P. S. (2001). Police reactions to crimes involving people with mental retardation: A cross-cultural experimental study. *Education and Training in Mental Retardation and Developmental Disabilities*, 160–171.

McCarthy, M., Bates, C., Triantafyllopoulou, P., Hunt, S., & Milne Skillman, K. (2019). "Put bluntly, they are targeted by the worst creeps society has to offer": Police and professionals' views and actions relating to domestic violence and women with intellectual disabilities. *Journal of Applied Research in Intellectual Disabilities*, *32*(1), 71–81. doi:10.1111/jar.12503 PMID:29992718

McDonagh, P., Goodey, C. F., & Stainton, T. (Eds.). (2018). *Intellectual disability: A conceptual history, 1200-1900*. Oxford, UK: Oxford University Press.

McGillivray, J. A., Gaskin, C. J., Newton, D. C., & Richardson, B. A. (2016). Substance use, offending, and participation in alcohol and drug treatment programmes: A comparison of prisoners with and without Intellectual Disabilities. *Journal of Applied Research in Intellectual Disabilities*, *29*(3), 289–294. doi:10.1111/jar.12175 PMID:25754684

McGillivray, J. A., & Moore, M. R. (2001). Substance use by offenders with mild intellectual disability. *Journal of Intellectual & Developmental Disability*, *26*(4), 297–310. doi:10.1080/13668250120087317

McKinlay & McGowan. (2003). Forensic issues in neuropsychology. In P. W. Halligan, U. Kischka, & J. C. Marshall (Eds.), *Handbook of clinical neuropsychology* (pp. 676–693). New York: Oxford University Press.

McNulty, C., Kissi-Deborah, R., & Newsom-Davies, I. (1995). Police involvement with clients having intellectual disabilities: A pilot study in South London. *Mental Handicap Research*, *8*(2), 129–136. doi:10.1111/j.1468-3148.1995.tb00150.x

Mohapatra, S., & Mohanty, M. (2004). *Abuse and activity limitation: A study on domestic violence against disabled women in Orissa, India*. Bhubaneswar, Orissa: Swabhiman.

Morin, D., Rivard, M., Boursier, C. P., Crocker, A. G., & Caron, J. (2015). Norms of the Attitudes Toward Intellectual Disability Questionnaire. *Journal of Intellectual Disability Research*, *59*(5), 462–467. doi:10.1111/jir.12146 PMID:25041088

Morin, D., Rivard, M., Crocker, A. G., Boursier, C. P., & Caron, J. (2013). Public attitudes towards intellectual disability: A multidimensional perspective. *Journal of Intellectual Disability Research*, *57*(3), 279–292. doi:10.1111/jir.12008 PMID:23279318

Morin, D., Valois, P., Crocker, A. G., Robitaille, C., & Lopes, T. (2018). Attitudes of health care professionals toward people with intellectual disability: A comparison with the general population. *Journal of Intellectual Disability Research*, *62*(9), 746–758. doi:10.1111/jir.12510 PMID:29968307

Morris, C. D., Niederbuhl, J. M., & Mahr, J. M. (1993). Determining the capability of individuals with mental retardation to give informed consent. *American Journal of Mental Retardation*, *98*(2), 263–272. PMID:8398085

Murch, A. J., Choudhury, T., Wilson, M., Collerton, E., Patel, M., & Scior, K. (2018). Explicit and implicit attitudes towards people with intellectual disabilities: The role of contact and participant demographics. *Journal of Applied Research in Intellectual Disabilities*, *31*(5), 778–784. doi:10.1111/jar.12429 PMID:29168267

Murphy, G., & Mason, J. (2014). Forensic and offending behaviours. In E. Tsakanikos & J. McCarthy (Eds.), Handbook of psychopathology in intellectual disability (pp. 281-303). New York: Springer. doi:10.1007/978-1-4614-8250-5_18

Neuwirth, G. S., Heisler, P. A., & Goldrich, K. S. (1974). Capacity, competence, consent: Voluntary sterilization of the mentally retarded. *Columbia Human Rights Law Review*, *6*, 447. PMID:11663600

New South Wales. Law Reform Commission. (1994). *People with an intellectual disability and the criminal justice system: Courts and sentencing issues* (Vol. 35). The Commission.

Ng, C. H. (1997). The stigma of mental illness in Asian cultures. *The Australian and New Zealand Journal of Psychiatry*, *31*(3), 382–390. doi:10.3109/00048679709073848 PMID:9226084

O'Callaghan, A. C., & Murphy, G. H. (2007). Sexual relationships in adults with intellectual disabilities: Understanding the law. *Journal of Intellectual Disability Research*, *51*(3), 197–206. doi:10.1111/j.1365-2788.2006.00857.x PMID:17300415

Olvera, D. R., Dever, R. B., & Earnest, M. A. (2000). Mental retardation and sentences for murder: Comparison of two recent court cases. *Mental Retardation*, *38*(3), 228–233. doi:10.1352/0047-6765(2000)038<0228:MRASFM>2.0.CO;2 PMID:10900930

Orchard, A. (2013). *The burning issue: Why do people with intellectual disability commit arson?* (MSc dissertation). University of Portsmouth.

Parmenter, T. R. (2008). The present, past and future of the study of intellectual disability: Challenges in developing countries. *Salud Pública de México*, *50*, s124–s131. doi:10.1590/S0036-36342008000800004 PMID:18470339

Parry, J., & Drogin, E. Y. (2007). *Mental disability law, evidence, and testimony: A comprehensive reference manual for lawyers, judges, and mental disability professionals*. American Bar Association.

Perske, R. (1991). *Unequal justice? What can happen when persons with retardation or other developmental disabilities encounter the criminal justice system*. Nashville, TN: Abingdon Press.

Perske, R. (2005). Search for persons with intellectual disabilities who confessed to serious crimes they did not commit. *Journal Information*, *43*(1), 58–65. PMID:15628935

Perske, R. (2008). False confessions from 53 persons with intellectual disabilities: The list keeps growing. *Intellectual and Developmental Disabilities*, *46*(6), 468–479. doi:10.1352/2008.46:468-479 PMID:19006433

Perske, R. (2011). Perske's list: False confessions from 75 persons with intellectual disability. *Intellectual and Developmental Disabilities*, *49*(5), 365–373. doi:10.1352/1934-9556-49.5.365 PMID:21905830

Plant, A., McDermott, E., Chester, V., & Alexander, R. T. (2011). Substance misuse among offenders in a forensic intellectual disability service. *Journal of Learning Disabilities and Offending Behaviour*, *2*(3), 127–135. doi:10.1108/20420921111186589

Polloway, E. A. (2015). *The death penalty and intellectual disability*. Washington, DC: American Association on Intellectual and Developmental Disabilities.

Raina, P., & Lunsky, Y. (2010). A comparison study of adults with intellectual disability and psychiatric disorder with and without forensic involvement. *Research in Developmental Disabilities*, *31*(1), 218–223. doi:10.1016/j.ridd.2009.09.008 PMID:19854026

Reed, E. J. (1997). Criminal law and the capacity of mentally retarded persons to consent to sexual activity. *Virginia Law Review*, *83*(4), 799–827. doi:10.2307/1073749

Ricciardelli, L. A., & Jaskyte, K. (2019). A value-critical policy analysis of Georgia's beyond a reasonable doubt standard of proof of Intellectual Disability. *Journal of Disability Policy Studies*.

Ridley, A. M., Gabbert, F., & La Rooy, D. J. (2012). *Suggestibility in legal contexts: psychological research and forensic implications*. Chichester, UK: John Wiley & Sons.

Robertson, J., Emerson, E., Baines, S., & Hatton, C. (2018). Self-reported smoking, alcohol and drug use among adolescents and young adults with and without mild to moderate intellectual disability. *Journal of Intellectual & Developmental Disability*, 1–11. doi:10.3109/13668250.2018.1440773

Ruff, C. F., Templer, D. I., & Ayers, J. L. (1976). The intelligence of rapists. *Archives of Sexual Behavior*, *5*(4), 327–329. doi:10.1007/BF01542085 PMID:952615

Salavert, J., Clarabuch, A., Fernández-Gómez, M. J., Barrau, V., Giráldez, M. P., & Borràs, J. (2018). Substance use disorders in patients with intellectual disability admitted to psychiatric hospitalisation. *Journal of Intellectual Disability Research*, *62*(11), 923–930. doi:10.1111/jir.12514 PMID:29961996

Salekin, K. L., Olley, J. G., & Hedge, K. A. (2010). Offenders with intellectual disability: Characteristics, prevalence, and issues in forensic assessment. *Journal of Mental Health Research in Intellectual Disabilities*, *3*(2), 97–116. doi:10.1080/19315861003695769

Salkind, N. J. (2002). *Child development.* New York: Macmillan Reference USA.

Schalock, R. L., Luckasson, R. A., & Shogren, K. A. (2007). The renaming of mental retardation: Understanding the change to the term intellectual disability. *Journal Information, 45*(2). PMID:17428134

Schatz, S. J. (2018). Interrogated with Intellectual Disabilities: The risks of false confession. *Stanford Law Review, 70*, 643. PMID:29486553

Schoenberg, M. R., & Scott, J. G. (2011). *The little black book of neuropsychology: a syndrome-based approach.* New York: Springer Science & Business Media. doi:10.1007/978-0-387-76978-3

Scior, K. (2011). Public awareness, attitudes and beliefs regarding intellectual disability: A systematic review. *Research in Developmental Disabilities, 32*(6), 2164–2182. doi:10.1016/j.ridd.2011.07.005 PMID:21798712

Scior, K., Kan, K. Y., McLoughlin, A., & Sheridan, J. (2010). Public attitudes toward people with intellectual disabilities: A cross-cultural study. *Intellectual and Developmental Disabilities, 48*(4), 278–289. doi:10.1352/1934-9556-48.4.278 PMID:20722478

Scior, K., & Werner, S. (Eds.). (2016). *Intellectual disability and stigma: Stepping out from the margins.* London: Palgrave McMillan. doi:10.1057/978-1-137-52499-7

Scully, J. L. (2018). Epistemic Exclusion, Injustice, and Disability. In D. T. Wasserman & A. Cureton (Eds.), *The Oxford Handbook of Philosophy and Disability*. Oxford, UK: Oxford University Press.

Segeren, M. W., Fassaert, T. J., Kea, R., de Wit, M. A., & Popma, A. (2018). Exploring differences in criminogenic risk factors and criminal behavior between young adult violent offenders with and without mild to borderline intellectual disability. *International Journal of Offender Therapy and Comparative Criminology, 62*(4), 978–999. doi:10.1177/0306624X16674009 PMID:29409403

Simplican, S. C. (2019). Intellectual disability and stigma: Stepping out from the margins. *Disability & Society, 34*(2), 335-337.

Simpson, M. K., & Hogg, J. (2001). Patterns of offending among people with intellectual disability: A systematic review. Part I: Methodology and prevalence data. *Journal of Intellectual Disability Research, 45*(5), 384–396. doi:10.1046/j.1365-2788.2001.00345.x PMID:11679044

Siperstein, G. N. (2003). *Multinational study of attitudes towards individuals with intellectual disabilities: General findings and calls to action.* Special Olympics.

Sjgafoos, J., Elkins, J., Kerr, M., & Attwood, T. (1994). A survey of aggressive behaviour among a population of persons with intellectual disability in Queensland. *Journal of Intellectual Disability Research, 38*(4), 369–381. doi:10.1111/j.1365-2788.1994.tb00417.x PMID:7949789

Søndenaa, E., Rasmussen, K., & Nøttestad, J. A. (2008). Forensic issues in intellectual disability. *Current Opinion in Psychiatry, 21*(5), 449–453. doi:10.1097/YCO.0b013e328305e5e9 PMID:18650685

Søndenaa, E., Rasmussen, K., Palmstierna, T., & Nøttestad, J. A. (2008). The prevalence and nature of intellectual disability in Norwegian prisons. *Journal of Intellectual Disability Research, 52*(12), 1129–1137. doi:10.1111/j.1365-2788.2008.01072.x PMID:18498332

Stavrakantonaki, M., & Johnson, T. P. (2018). Effects of Rosa's Law on Intellectual-Disability reporting. *Public Opinion Quarterly*, *82*(3), 593–604. doi:10.1093/poq/nfy024

Stoyanova, S., & Giannouli, V. (2018). Bulgarian students' impulsivity differentiated by gender, age, and some scientific areas. *Psychological Thought*, *11*(2), 138–147. doi:10.5964/psyct.v11i2.250

Strømme, P., & Magnus, P. (2000). Correlations between socioeconomic status, IQ and aetiology in mental retardation: A population-based study of Norwegian children. *Social Psychiatry and Psychiatric Epidemiology*, *35*(1), 12–18. doi:10.1007001270050003 PMID:10741531

Su, K. P., Yu, J. M., Yang, T. W., Tsai, S. Y., & Chen, C. C. (2000). Characteristics of mentally retarded criminal offenders in Northern Taiwan. *Journal of Forensic Sciences*, *45*(6), 1207–1209. doi:10.1520/JFS14869J PMID:11110172

Sullivan, P. M., & Knutson, J. F. (2000). Maltreatment and disabilities: A population-based epidemiological study. *Child Abuse & Neglect*, *24*(10), 1257–1273. doi:10.1016/S0145-2134(00)00190-3 PMID:11075694

Suto, W. M. I., Clare, I. C. H., Holland, A. J., & Watson, P. C. (2005). Capacity to make financial decisions among people with mild intellectual disabilities. *Journal of Intellectual Disability Research*, *49*(3), 199–209. doi:10.1111/j.1365-2788.2005.00635.x PMID:15713195

Sweet, J. J., King, J. H., Malina, A. C., Bergman, M. A., & Simmons, A. (2002). Documenting the prominence of forensic neuropsychology at national meetings and in relevant professional journals from 1990 to 2000. *The Clinical Neuropsychologist*, *16*(4), 481–494. doi:10.1076/clin.16.4.481.13914 PMID:12822057

Thomas, S. D., Nixon, M., Ogloff, J. R., & Daffern, M. (2019). Crime and victimization among people with intellectual disability with and without comorbid mental illness. *Journal of Applied Research in Intellectual Disabilities*, jar.12598. doi:10.1111/jar.12598 PMID:30990251

Timms, S., & Goreczny, A. J. (2002). Adolescent sex offenders with mental retardation: Literature review and assessment considerations. *Aggression and Violent Behavior*, *7*(1), 1–19. doi:10.1016/S1359-1789(00)00031-8

Turner, W. J. (2018). Conceptualization of intellectual disability in medieval English law. In *Intellectual disability*. Manchester University Press.

Vandevelde, S., Broekaert, E., Schuyten, G., & Van Hove, G. (2005). Intellectual abilities and motivation toward substance abuse treatment in drug-involved offenders: A pilot study in the Belgian criminal justice system. *International Journal of Offender Therapy and Comparative Criminology*, *49*(3), 277–297. doi:10.1177/0306624X04270779 PMID:15851508

Vaughan, P. J., Pullen, N., & Kelly, M. (2000). Services for mentally disordered offenders in community psychiatry teams. *Journal of Forensic Psychiatry*, *11*(3), 571–586. doi:10.1080/09585180010004829

Vera, H., Barnard, G. W., & Holzer, C. (1979). The intelligence of rapists: New data. *Archives of Sexual Behavior*, *8*(4), 375–377. doi:10.1007/BF01541880 PMID:475583

Wallinius, M., Nordholm, J., Wagnström, F., & Billstedt, E. (2019). Cognitive functioning and aggressive antisocial behaviors in young violent offenders. *Psychiatry Research, 272*, 572–580. doi:10.1016/j.psychres.2018.12.140 PMID:30616126

Wenhua, L. (2005). Analysis of 294 cases of murder in forensic psychiatric expertise. *Journal of Clinical Psychosomatic Diseases, 4*, 25.

Wikler, D. (1979). Paternalism and the mildly retarded. *Philosophy & Public Affairs*, 377–392.

Williams, F., Kouimtsidis, C., & Baldacchino, A. (2018). Alcohol use disorders in people with intellectual disability. *BJPsych Advances, 24*(4), 264–272. doi:10.1192/bja.2017.37

Wilson, M. C., & Scior, K. (2015). Implicit attitudes towards people with intellectual disabilities: Their relationship with explicit attitudes, social distance, emotions and contact. *PLoS One, 10*(9), e0137902. doi:10.1371/journal.pone.0137902 PMID:26366575

Yazbeck, M., McVilly, K., & Parmenter, T. R. (2004). Attitudes toward people with intellectual disabilities an Australian perspective. *Journal of Disability Policy Studies, 15*(2), 97–111. doi:10.1177/10442073040150020401

ADDITIONAL READING

Boone, K. B. (2012). *Clinical practice of forensic neuropsychology: An evidence-based approach*. New York: Guilford Press.

Demakis, G. J. (Ed.). (2011). *Civil capacities in clinical neuropsychology: Research findings and practical applications*. New York: Oxford University Press.

Denney, R. L., & Sullivan, J. P. (Eds.). (2008). *Clinical neuropsychology in the criminal forensic setting*. New York: Guilford Press.

Horton, A. M., & Hartlage, L. C. (Eds.). (2010). *Handbook of forensic neuropsychology*. New York: Springer Publishing Company.

Larrabee, G. J. (Ed.). (2011). *Forensic neuropsychology: A scientific approach*. New York: Oxford University Press.

Lindsay, W. R., & Taylor, J. L. (Eds.). (2018). *The Wiley handbook on offenders with intellectual and developmental disabilities: Research, training, and practice*. UK: John Wiley & Sons. doi:10.1002/9781118752982

Morgan, J. E., & Sweet, J. J. (Eds.). (2010). *Neuropsychology of malingering casebook*. New York: Psychology Press.

Parckard, W. B. (2013). *Intellectual disability and the criminal justice system: Solutions through collaboration*. Create Space Independent Publishing Platform.

Søndenaa, E. (2009). *Intellectual disabilities in the criminal justice system*. Norwegian University of Science and Technology.

Towl, G. J., & Crighton, D. A. (2010). *Forensic psychology*. London: BPS Blackwell.

Wehmeyer, M. L. (2013). *The story of intellectual disability: An evolution of meaning, understanding, and public perception*. Baltimore: Paul H. Brookes Publishing.

Young, S., Kopelman, M., & Gudjonsson, G. (Eds.). (2009). *Forensic neuropsychology in practice: A guide to assessment and legal processes*. New York: Oxford University Press. doi:10.1093/med/9780198566830.001.0001

KEY TERMS AND DEFINITIONS

Civil Law: Civil law is a branch of law that consists of non-criminal law.

Crime: This general term denotes an unlawful act punishable by the state.

Criminal Law: Criminal law is a branch of law that relates to crime.

Financial Capacity: The capacity of an individual to manage his/her own money-financial affairs and make relevant decisions while keeping in mind all possible financial-legal consequences of his/her acts.

Forensic Neuropsychological Assessment: The evaluation of performance on various areas of functioning, which is based on the use of standardized testing methods focusing on cognitive, behavioral and emotional functioning which aim at clarifying issues for legal decision making.

Intellectual Disability: A new term used for disability characterized by significant limitations in both intellectual functioning and non-adaptive behavior, which covers many everyday social and practical skills and refers to individuals who are under 18 years of age. Intellectual disability has replaced the term mental retardation.

Miranda Rights or Miranda Warning: Warning given by the police in the USA to criminal suspects in police custody or in a custodial interrogation stating that: You have the right to remain silent. Anything you say or do can or will be used against you in a court of law. You have the right to an attorney. If you cannot afford an attorney, one will be appointed to you. Do you understand these rights as they have been read to you?

Sexual Abuse: Any form of forced-undesired sexual behavior by one person upon another.

Chapter 15

Sexuality, Sexual Abuse, Marriage, Partner Violence, and Parenting Skills Among Persons With Intellectual Disability

Rejani Thudalikunnil Gopalan
https://orcid.org/0000-0002-5957-8144
Mahatma Gandhi Medical College and Hospital, India

Prathibha Augustus Kurishinkal
Gujarat Forensic Sciences University, India

ABSTRACT

Sexuality begins from the moment of birth and has an active role in the development, evolution, emotional balance, and affective stability of the individual. It has a significant role in interpersonal and couple's relationships. The sexuality of people with intellectual disability is important from the view of medical, pedagogical, psychological, and ethical aspects. As intellectually disabled person approach puberty their control of behavior and expression of sexuality may manifest in unacceptable ways. They are also at increased risk for physical, sexual, and emotional abuse. The chapter focused on the sexuality, the risk of sexual abuse, marriage, partner violence among people with intellectual disability. The requirement of sex education and components of sex education for various age ranges were also explained and effectiveness of such programs were also discussed. The chapter also discussed the parenting and challenges involved in parenting among intellectually disabled individuals.

OVERVIEW

Sexuality is one of the most important aspects of human life that relates to sex, one's identification, sexual role, sexual preferences, eroticism, pleasure and intimacy. It fulfils such functions as procreative, hedonistic and relationship-building as well as constitutes an integral part of human's personality. Sexu-

DOI: 10.4018/978-1-7998-1223-4.ch015

ality begins from the moment of birth and has an active role in the development, evolution, emotional balance and affective stability of the individual. The primary objective of sexuality is pleasure hence human beings tend to focus their minds on obtaining and giving pleasure and relate to one another. This could be found in persons with intellectual disability also. The sexuality of people with intellectual disability is a special case - both from medical, pedagogical, psychological and ethical point of view. Little available research shows that it may become a significant factor that modifies their psychological and sexual functioning (Kijak, 2013; Clarke &O'toole, 2007).

Individuals with disabilities are commonly viewed as asexual due to a predominant heteronormative idea of sex and what is considered natural. A lack of information and education on sexuality and disability was felt to be a major contributing factors towards the stigma attached to disability and sexuality. Stigma can lead individuals to internalise concepts of asexuality and may negatively impact confidence, desire and ability to find a partner while distorting one's overall sexual self-concept. Societal attitudes and perceptions are driven by education and knowledge, if there is no exposure to sexuality and disability, it follows suit that society would have a narrow understanding of these issues (Esmail, Darry, Walter & Knupp, 2010).

People with intellectual disability have the same sexual needs as those without any disability, yet their sexuality is often restricted by reluctant attitudes and/or fears based on irrational beliefs. In a study on sexuality among adults with mild or moderate intellectual disability, Gil-Llario, Morell-Mengual, Ballester-Arnal & Díaz-Rodríguez (2018) reported that 84.2% have had sexual relationships with another person, this percentage being higher in females and in people aged between 38 and 55 years old. A study in England reported that most young people with mild/moderate intellectual disabilities have had sexual intercourse by age 19/20, although young women were less likely to have sex prior to 16 than their peers and both men and women with intellectual disabilities were more likely to have unsafe sex 50% or more of the time than their peers. Women with intellectual disabilities were likely to have been pregnant and more likely to be a mother. (Baines, Emerson, Robertson,& Hatton, 2018).

Examining literature that tells us what people with intellectual disability (PWID) think and feel about their sexual lives may enable families and professionals to offer a more person-centered approach to education and support. In a metasynthesis of people with intellectual disability speaking about sex and relationships, participants across studies desired friendships and close interpersonal relationships, yet were restricted from developing these relationships by policies, program staff, and family members (Black & Kammes, 2019). It is s been reported that mothers of young people with intellectual disability held more cautious attitudes about contraception, readiness to learn about sex, and decisions about intimate relationships. Mothers expressed concerns about their children with intellectual disability and sexual vulnerability and speak about fewer sexual topics with their children and began these discussions when their children were older (Pownall, Jahoda, & Hastings, 2012). Given the complexity of intellectual disability, the development of socially appropriate sexual attitudes and behaviours in intellectually disabled persons is challenging and depends on the participation of parents, teachers and society as a whole. This is important to get adequately integrated into society as it would help them to interact appropriately in social, work and family domains (Rademakers, Mouthaan&deNeef, 2005).

As intellectually disabled person approach puberty their control of behaviour and expression of sexuality may manifest in unacceptable ways. Aberrant or delinquent behaviour can be seen in adolescence and adult age (McDonald, Keys &Balcazar, 2007). Adults with a higher degree of ID have certain sexual experience but not enough knowledge on human sexual life and the sexual development is delayed by an average period of 3 years. Masturbation and petting were found to be the most frequent ways of expressing one's sexual needs, with masturbation playing the major role, whereas touching and sexual intercourse proved less popular. The masturbation activities were found to occur in various circumstances, most frequently in intimate situations (Kijak, 2013).

On sexual lives of people with disabilities within low- and middle-income countries **(LMICs),** Carew, Braathen, Swartz, Hunt, & rohleder (2017) reported the major topics researched so far and the topics were focused on themes of Self-attitudes, knowledge, and experiences, Community, parental, and professional attitudes, Access to sexual and reproductive healthcare, access to sexual education, sexual abuse/violence and Intersectionality. Researches on these themes highlighted the fact that People with disabilities may engage in risky sexual behaviors and possess low levels of knowledge about safe sexual practices. Although many face challenges to leading sexual lives, such as low sexual self-esteem, people with disabilities are sexual beings and have the same needs as people without disabilities. While the attitudes of people with disabilities are not uniformly negative, people with disabilities are not seen as fully sexual by community members. Parents of children with disabilities may be reluctant to accept the sexual desires of their offspring, especially if they have intellectual disabilities. Professionals may not know how best to address or teach common sexual topics when working with people with disabilities. While the attitudes of people with disabilities are not uniformly negative, people with disabilities are not seen as fully sexual by community members. Parents of children with disabilities may be reluctant to accept the sexual desires of their offspring, especially if they have intellectual disabilities. Professionals may not know how best to address or teach common sexual topics when working with people with disabilities. There are many barriers to accessing sexual and reproductive healthcare among people with disabilities, several of which are exacerbated by poor infrastructure and greater levels of poverty in LMICs. Examples include inaccessible healthcare facilities, poor provision of adequate transportation, and negative attitudes of healthcare providers. There are also several barriers to accessing sexual education, for example, lack of provision of accessible information and lack of knowledge among teachers and parents. People with disabilities, particularly women, children, or individuals with intellectual disabilities, may be vulnerable to sexual abuse, exploitation, and violence. Disability and sexuality may intersect with other factors, such as gender and culture, to disadvantage certain people with disabilities in terms of their access to sexual healthcare or ability to live a fulfilling sexual life.

It is also important address the issues of sexual orientation among intellectually disabled individuals. Empirical research that addresses sexual orientation in people with an intellectual disability (ID) is limited and very little is known regarding the personal experiences of lesbian and bisexual women with ID. Stoffelen, Schaafsma, Kok, & Curfs (2018) have studied ten lesbian and bisexual women (average age of 33 years) with a mild intellectual disability. Participants reported that they had found it hard to talk to others about sensitive subjects such as their sexuality, and had been left to figure out information regarding their sexual orientation without support or guidance. It point to a lack of information, sexual education and role models when it comes to lesbian sex and women with an intellectual disability. Social contact was often limited, and participants experienced difficulties finding a partner. Furthermore, participants often had to cope with mental health problems and had struggled with loneliness, depression and addiction and they had been discriminated against. Coming out (revealing your sexual orientation) is not easy when you have an intellectual disability. To enable women with ID who have lesbian or bisexual feelings to understand and secure their sexual rights in their daily lives is important. Therefore, it is necessary to provide support in sexual education and training, social contact and assertiveness.

Intellectual disability may not interfere with healthy display of sexuality in all cases. Their needs are often stigmatized when identified with inability to express age appropriate sexual development. With training such people can be helped to express their sexuality with respect and in accordance with the norms (Carrier, 2007). Presence of weak self esteem due to continuous reflection from society or inability to control impulses due to cerebral damage which accompanies intellectual disability are some of the factors that should be considered while looking into sexuality issues in persons with intellectual disability (Katz &Lazcano- Ponce, 2008).

Though not many studies are addressing the sexuality and sexual orientation among people with intellectual disabilities, clinicians and other mental health professionals always need to address these issues in their daily practice. Parents often feel helpless when adolescence or adult with disabilities express sexual desires and many parents become perplexed or deny the issues, at time become over involved with the son or the daughter that they assist him/her or become a partner in sexual activities, more frequently in masturbation. Some parents undergo feelings of shame or guilt while engaging in such activities. Some may do such activities while thinking that their children never get an opportunity to marry or engage in sexual activities. Adolescents or adults with mild intellectual disability often express the desire to get marry though they don't fully understand the responsibilities involved in marriage. It is very important to deal with such issues much more empathetic way and teach healthy way of expressing sexual desires and sexual gratification. Awareness program to parents and teaching parents, teachers and other caregivers how to deal with sexual expressions and desires are to be focused in future. It is also necessary to encourage individuals with disability to talk about their sexual desires and doubts, healthy way of expressing sexual desires and gratification, and to teach how to prevent sexual abuse.

Sexual Abuse in Persons with Intellectual Disability

Persons with intellectual disabilities are at increased risk for physical, sexual and emotional abuse. With regard to sexual abuse an incidence rate of 50% is seen among such individuals (Van Dyke, McBrien&Sherbondy, 1995). Gil-Llario et al, (2018) reported 9.4% of the women and 2.8% of the men has experienced sexual abuse among adults with mild or moderate intellectual disability. It has been found that about 90 percent of people with developmental disabilities will experience sexual abuse at some point in their lives. Mostly, females are victims of sexual abuse and those with borderline to mild mental retardation. The incidence of abuse tend to decrease as the level of disability become severe (Schor, 1987).

In a study conducted in Australia it was found that persons with developmental disabilities (intellectual disability, autism, cerebral palsy, epilepsy and learning disabilities) were sexually assaulted 10.7 times more than the rate of nondisabled persons. Though studies consistently report high prevalence of sexual abuse in intellectually disabled individuals, only 3% of such cases involving people with developmental disabilities get reported (Valenti-Hein & Schwartz, 1995). There are a multitude of factors which predispose these individuals to sexual abuse. Social isolation, communication skill deficits, cognitive problems like diminished ability to protect oneself due to lack of instruction and/or resources and impaired judgment (the inability to detect who is safe to be around). Some researchers have suggested that people with mental retardation are more likely to give and receive affection (Kempton &Gochros, 1986; Schor, 1987). Since intellectually disabled individuals feel lonely, they would be grateful for any form of attention. Their desire to be normal and the anxiety to please others predispose the individual to abuse (Heaton, 1995) The living arrangements like institutional setting, such as residential and group homes where there are multiple and transient care takers also increases the risk for abuse (Sobsey&Mansell, 1990). Mostly abusers (97%) are known and trusted by the victim who has developmental disability. This includes family members and acquaintances which could be residential care staff, transportation providers and personal care attendants (Baladerian, 1991).

Gender is significant in explaining the type of violence experienced and the experience of discrimination. Dammeyer &, Chapman(2018) analyzed data on self-reported violence and discrimination from a Danish national survey of 18,019 citizens, of whom 4519 reported a physical disability and 1398 reported a mental disability. Individuals with disabilities reported significantly higher levels of violence than those without. Specifically, individuals reporting a mental disability reported higher levels of violence and discrimination. Significant gender differences were found with regard to type of violence: while men with disabilities were more likely to report physical violence, women with disabilities were more likely to report major sexual violence, humiliation and discrimination. Neither severity nor visibility of disability was found to be a significant factor for risk of violence. This large-scale study lends support to existing research showing that people with disabilities are at greater risk of violence than people without disabilities. Further, the study found that people with mental disabilities were significantly more likely to report all types of violence and discrimination than those with physical disabilities.

The effects of sexual abuse are manifold. Pregnancy, sexually transmitted diseases, bruises, lacerations and other physical abuse are issues which often follow sexual abuse. Psychosomatic symptoms such as stomach aches, headaches, seizures and problems with sleep manifest. Low self-esteem, shame and guilt, irrational fear, depression and loss of trust are the psychological symptoms that follow sexual abuse. Behavioural symptoms include withdrawal, as well as noncompliant, aggressive, self-injurious and sexually inappropriate behaviour (Sobsey, 1994).

Reporting abuse may be difficult for a person with limited verbal skills, and may lack the capacity to give valid consent to medical treatment. Their reproductive choices may be limited by their support needs, by social pressures or by sterilisation at a young age. (Eastgate,G.,201; Eastgate,2005). This scenario calls for comprehensive training programs which include sex education, training in personal and emotional safety as well as relationship issues that should be part any educational or rehabilitative work with population of intellectual disability .

Affective dimensions along with intellectual disability increases the likelihood of being sexually abused (Steptoe, Lindsay, Forrest & Power, 2006). This point out the need for sex education and counselling from an early age. From infancy onwards persons with intellectual disability should receive continuous sexual guidance in such concepts as intellectual deficiency limits their capacity to learn from role models or experiences in life which in turns affects generalization processes (Piaget, 1977).

Teaching the skills to protect themselves from sexual abuse is found to be effective among persons with intellectual disability. Kucuk, Platin & Erdem (2017) conducted a study to raise awareness about sexual abuse in children with intellectual disabilities with 15 children who had mild intellectual disabilities as a pre-posttest experimental design. Informative pictures, designed according to age and intellectual level, suitable stories linked with these pictures and homework, were used in an educational setting. It was determined that there was a significant difference relating to the scores for all the subjects before and after the assignment. After education, awareness of them in protecting from a possible sexual abuse increased with protection educations for intellectual disabilities children, as desired.

Research repeatedly shown that children and adults with an intellectual disability are at a higher risk of sexual abuse than nondisabled peers and there is no single diagnostic trajectory when dealing with the sequelae of sexual abuse among those with an intellectual disability. The impact of sexual abuse among those with an intellectual disability is an area in need of further research (Byrne, 2018). People with intellectual disability require education to help them resist abuse, and advocacy to ensure that their environment protects them. They require support and education when making reproductive choices and health care decisions. In cases where they do not have the capacity for informed consent, a substitute decision maker is required (Eastgate,2005). ID children should be educated more regarding sexuality and 'empowered' by programs. Perpetrators of sexual abuse of ID children are often ID peers who have been abused. Care providers should be trained in open communication and recognition of signals of abuse (Wissink, Vugt, Moonen, Stams & Hendriks,2015).

Sexual Assault by Individuals with Intellectual Disability

Though the exact prevalence is not available, Day (1997) reported sex offenses to be the second most common crime among people with intellectual disability and that sex offenses are crimes for which most offenders with intellectual disability are incarcerated. According to Murphy et al. (1983) approximately 10% to 15% of all sexual offenses are committed by people with intellectual disability and Gross (1985) reported almost 50% of incarcerated offenders with intellectual disability and 34% of those living in the community had been convicted of sex offenses.

Brown and Stein (1997) compared cases of sexual abuse of adults with intellectual disabilities, reported across the South East of England, which were perpetrated by men with intellectual disabilities, with those committed by other male perpetrators. The comparison provides some support for the findings of other studies, which have suggested that men with intellectual disabilities offend against more male victims than non-disabled sex offenders and that their offences are somewhat less serious, but otherwise indicates common patterns of abusive behaviour across this divide but differential service responses and support for victims. So called 'peer abuse' is a widespread problem which service agencies have failed to address: repeated offences are frequent and lack of appropriate intervention is the norm. Other studies noted the most frequent sexual offenses by individuals with intellectual disability were indecent exposure, other minor offenses, and sexual assault of young girls, inappropriate sexual behavior in public, sexual behaviors and stimulation that inappropriately involved others, sexual activity involving minors and assaultive/nonconsensual sexual activity not involving minors (Day, 1997; Ward et al, 2001).

Although the cognitively impaired are frequently included in heterogeneous studies of problematic sexual behavior, the epidemiology, etiology, and approach to assessment and treatment of persons with intellectual disability are distinct from those of the general population. The incidence of inappropriate sexual behavior among the intellectually disabled is 15-33%; however, the nature tends to be more socially inappropriate than with violative intent. Limited sociosexual education is a large contributor, and better addressing this area offers a target for prevention and treatment. A thorough clinical assessment of problematic sexual behaviors in the cognitively impaired requires understanding the patient's internal experience, which can be challenging. Assessment tools validated for the general population have not been validated for this population. Very few studies have assessed treatment approaches specifically among the cognitively impaired; however, research does suggest utility in habilitative, psychotherapeutic, and pharmacologic approaches which have been validated among the general population(Thom, Grudzinskas &Saleh, 2017).

People with intellectual disabilities (ID) are at greater risk of being a victim of sexual abuse and may also be more predisposed to perpetrating sexual abuse. Although the prevalence of sexual abuse among people with ID is difficult to determine, it is clear that there are serious consequences for both victims and perpetrators, and professional support is needed. Psychologists play an important role in the assessment of sexual abuse in both victims and perpetrators and require specific knowledge and skills to execute the assessments (Embregts, Heestermans & Van den Bogaard, 2017). Clay, Bloom & Joseph Lambert (2018) reported insufficient evidence exists to consider any specific response-suppression technique an overarching treatment for decreasing Inappropriate sexual behavior (ISB). However, broadly speaking, behavior analytic approaches have been highly effective. Practitioners should consider function-based intervention and draw from studies identified as having strong supporting evidence.

SEX EDUCATION IN CHILDHOOD, ADOLESCENCE AND ADULTHOOD IN PERSONS WITH INTELLECTUAL DISABILITY

Sex Education in Childhood

In their early years children show their feelings through behaviour and which depends on the emotional development level of each person. They notice that their behaviour elicit certain reactions in parents and others. Gradually, as they mature they realize that their behaviour affects people and society as a whole. This leads to the formation of behaviour in children and the incorporation of norms and rules of the society. In children with intellectual disability emotional development does not follow the same way and they lack the ability to generalize or assimilate norms and rules. Therefore, they require a specific way for handling such behaviour.

Children with intellectual disability tend to search for gratification through pleasant sensations because of poor impulse control, low tolerance of frustration and limited comprehension. As a response to such behaviour authority figures try to exercise control these sensations which in turn the child interprets as the person`s effort to impede their experiencing pleasure. They require more time to understand this exercise of control is to prevent them from injury or abuse. Authority figures in collaboration with a counselor should therefore create a system of cause and effect marked by consistency, firmness, clarity and should not impart double messages and not use physical or verbal aggression. Intellectually disabled children should be made aware of public and private conducts. Public conducts are those that do not offend or hurt anyone and are accepted by the society. Examples are greeting someone, sitting with legs together when wearing a dress, being quiet, not lowering pants except in bathroom, not yelling among others. Private conducts, though easy for normal children, are abstractions for children with intellectual disability. They should be counselled not to burp in public, pass gases, pick the nose, touch their genitals, masturbate or take off clothes in public. When children assimilate the concept of public and private, they are able to differentiate from sexual behaviour from predominant social behaviour. When improvement is evident and new behaviour appear the repertoire of behaviours can be broadened. It is important to deal with behaviours that are related to how and when behaviour occurs rather than why behaviour occurs. Children should be trained to develop responsibility for impulse control. The formation of moral judgement should be facilitated which would help them to respect their body and that of others. It is important for the counsellor to work together with parents and other family members as they spend more time with the child and majority of inappropriate behaviour occurs at home. Guidance imparted to parents is equally important. They should be counselled about the general ways of dealing with behaviour and breaking the generalised taboos of the society Parents should also be helped to overcome the feelings of denial, rejection and grief(Walter, 2002).

Sex Education in Adolescence

The arrival of puberty is marked by changes in physical and mental aspects of a normal adolescent. The development of secondary sexual traits transforms the body of the child which provoke a state of anxiety about how their body will look in the end. At the cognitive level, stage of formal operations begins, which help them to understand the experiences they face. However, the emerging sexuality overwhelms them and the adolescent is preoccupied with doubt, uncertainty and insecurity. This does not seem to be the process in an adolescent with intellectual disability. Their sexual development is late when compared to that of adolescents with normal development. The average age at which disabled females attain menarche is 14 and the first wet dream experience among men with intellectual disability occurs at the age of 15. It is rarely that a premature sexual development is observed among such people (Kijak, 2011).

Adolescents with intellectual disability unaware about the development of secondary sexual characteristics and they conceptualize gender through their external experience (image). At the cognitive level, they never reach the stage of formal operations and sexual impulses are not questioned in conceptual terms. They do not acquire self-control and therefore impulses are acted upon without repression or guilt. This scenario calls for sex education starting from early childhood (Berman et al., 1999). If sexual education is imparted during childhoodwithout affecting the child's need to display sexual curiosity and expression of sexual tension, then the individual is equipped to deal with the sexual processes that appear in adolescence. If this has not been imparted or achieved then the process becomes more complicated and requires greater effort. In this context before beginning the sexual counselling that is appropriate for this (adolescence) stage of development, it is necessary for the individual to be trained to control sexual impulses ideally through a humanistic-behavioural therapeutic program. Incorporation of the social concept of public and private conduct with regard to control of sexual impulses is the primary aim of this program. Once this is achieved, the adolescent is ready to receive sexual education. The main components of sexual education include the following:

1. Anatomy and physiology
2. Maturation and changes in physical appearance
3. Public and private conducts
4. Masturbation
5. Responsibility for sexual conduct

1. **Anatomy and Physiology of the Reproductive Apparatus:** Adolescents with intellectual disability often believe that there is no difference between both genders. Therefore, it is necessary to provide them the basic information about sexual organs and their functions. Different methods are to be used to allow these individuals to explore the difference between men and women. The concepts that have to be emphasized include: 1.The same sex organs always exist for each gender and 2. They vary in terms of shape, size and certain characteristics. Adolescents should be explained that genitals are intimate parts and has to be dealt privately. They should be also helped to broaden their vocabulary and use appropriate terms (Angelopoulou et al., 1999).
2. **Maturation and Changes in Physical Appearance:** This includes the use of coloured drawings or anatomically suitable dolls to explain the process of maturation of body. Adolescent should be helped to identify his or her gender, recognize what his or her body is like at that moment, what it was like during childhood, and how it will transform in future. Questions from adolescents should

be encouraged and clarified. Self-care methods can be taught using this method. For girls menstrual hygiene, use of deodorants, genital cleanliness, what to do with vaginal secretions removal of axillary and leg hair are described. Boys are taught skills such as shaving, combing their hair, use of deodorants, genital cleanliness and information about erections and night ejaculations are provided.

3. **Public and Private Conduct:** This include situations typically found in adolescence. The areas addressed in public conduct include development of skills with regard to social adaptation, maturation of friendship relationships within groups of belonging and identification of all non-sexual behaviour. This is a complex task due to its abstract nature as the individuals have to develop attitudes with regard to respect for other people in general and create a place in the world for belonging. The counsellor can develop a moral code of public and private conduct which incorporates the norms of the society and culture. At this point it is necessary to take care not to neglect the difficulty in carrying out any kind of behavioural control in adolescence. Adolescents are taught about normal behaviour in social situations such as going to the movies, gatherings etc so as to differentiate what behaviours are acceptable at particular places. The purpose of this is to help the person generalize appropriate behaviours regardless of the place involved and to identify places suitable for carrying out public or private conduct.
4. **Masturbation:** It is a resource that an adolescent with intellectual disability frequently use for sexual gratification. Individuals should be helped to recognize that manipulation of genitals is a private conduct and doing it appropriately is a normal process in adolescence and should not cause guilt. They should be made aware about how prevent from hurting themselves, especially when using sharp objects. Individuals should be encouraged to express the feelings associated with masturbation and control the negative sensations that accompany this practice. With those who engage in masturbation excessively, help should be offered to deal with anxiety constructively. For individuals who do not engage in this practice or do not want to talk about it or causes conflict, it need to be respected (Scott, 1998).
5. **Taking Responsibility for Sexual Behaviour:** This area should be considered with utmost care as it involves ethical and moral issues surrounding intellectual disability. The counsellor works with the individual on the consequences of sexual behaviour. At first the individuals are provided information to fill in gaps in their knowledge so that they form a functional pattern of appropriate sexual behaviour. Parents, teachers, family members and others are counselled so that they reinforce appropriate social behaviour when they occur. This would help the person to build self-esteem. It is also important to notify the counselor about any inappropriate behaviour. Secondly, role playing is employed to correct inappropriate behaviour and their consequences. The counselor recreates the scene where the behaviour occurred and through discussion offer alternative possibilities. Consistent display of appropriate sexual behaviour by an adolescent who is intellectually disabled depends on sexual education and counselling. Only by this they can be prepared to begin a sexual life appropriate to their ageand establish relationships for a successful marriage .

Sex Education During Adulthood

Adults with intellectual disability display appropriate sexual behaviour if sexual education and counselling is imparted in childhood or adolescence. If an individual is untrained with regard to what is socially appropriate sexual behaviour for that age, training programs could include the following components:

1. Taking responsibility for sexual behaviour
2. Sexual activity with same gender and opposite gender
3. Birth control
4. Marriage and parenthood
5. Sexual transmission of infections and their prevention
6. Unacceptable and criminal sexual conduct

1. **Taking Responsibility for Sexual Behaviour:** It involves efforts to make the behaviour of all intellectually disabled persons to be similar to adults without intellectual disability. The counselor should always remember that the maximum mental age that persons with intellectual disability attain is 12 years which means that they lack the ability to evaluate the risk associated with relationships motivated by sexual gratification. Hence, they should be assisted to make decisions and delineate behaviours determined by conventional societal values.
2. **Sexual Activity with Same and Opposite Gender:** Due to affective deficiency in persons with intellectual disability they constantly seek sexual pleasure. Parents often deny the sexuality aspect of such persons which leads the individual to engage in sexual activity with same gender. In such cases it is difficult to discuss about homosexual tendencies as it may be due to the inability to relate with persons of opposite gender or a comparative choice over past unsatisfactory sexual relationships.
3. **Birth Control:** Programs should teach about different contraceptive methods to avoid unwanted pregnancy. It is also important to evaluate the use of sterilization techniques for men and women as permanent birth control alternative.
4. **Marriage and Parenthood:** Individuals with mild intellectual disability has the ability to fully experience sexuality and have stable relationship with a partner through marriage. Some of the difficulties faced by such persons include lack of economic support from families and presence of children. Due to high social vulnerability and low frustration tolerance individuals tend to regress in stressful conditions and act impulsively. The decision to have children would be due to lack of knowledge regarding what it means to have a child. Sexual counselling programs should assist the individual to understand their limitations to assume the role of a parent and take responsibility for choosing a birth control method which ensures marriage without children.
5. **Sexually Transmitted Infections and their Prevention:** Individuals should be provided adequate information regarding risks of sexually transmitted diseases and how to protect themselves. They should be helped to identify the symptoms of diseases, use of condoms or abstinence in view of possible infection. The counselor should make sure that the subjects have comprehended the information and they are equipped to prevent any type of infection.
6. **Unacceptable or Criminal Conducts:** This comes under the purview of private conducts and the norms of society regarding conventionally acceptable sexual behaviour. Intellectually disabled adults should be made aware about unacceptable behaviours like incest, sexual abuse or violation. The incorporation of norms is carried out through cause and effect relationships and identification of behaviours with their consequences. Moral and legal implications of unacceptable behaviours are looked into to behave as per the norms of the society (Katz &Lazcano-Ponce, 2008).

As a relevant evidence base remains largely unavailable, program developers intending to prevent sexual violence against women with intellectual disabilities should draw on the prevention science literature and what is known about effective prevention programs in general. Morrissey et al. (1997) have developed a set of evidence-based criteria for effective programs, all of which should be applied to the prevention of sexual violence against women with intellectual disabilities. They suggested that program should be *comprehensive* (The program should involve all the systems that have a direct impact on the participants. For a woman with intellectual disabilities, this may include family, friends, partners, caretakers, case workers, therapists, or employment support professionals), *theoretically based* (The program should be based on a clear theoretical model that explains the problem of sexual violence against women with intellectual disabilities. Applying a theoretical foundation encourages consistency throughout all aspects of the program), *intensive* (The program should offer sufficient contact between the trainer and participants. For participants with intellectual disabilities, short and frequent sessions that use a variety of teaching methods may prove most effective), *tailored to the needs of the participants* (The program should account for participants' age, communication abilities, care needs, cognitive functioning, and developmental level. The material should be intellectually appropriate and flexible enough to accommodate the varying communication and learning needs of the participants), *focused on skill development* (The program's curriculum should be active and provide hands-on experiences to increase participants' skill level. The program should offer practical and feasible tools that are relevant to real life for women with intellectual disabilities), *sufficient follow up* (In general, the positive effects of prevention programs wane over time without appropriate follow up. Participants with intellectual disabilities may need to attend supplemental sessions (i.e., "booster" sessions) while the program is continuously evaluated), and to have *consumer ownership* (The people for whom the program is intended (women with intellectual disabilities) should be involved in all levels of the program development, including planning, implementation, evaluation, and advisory boards).

Embregts, Heestermans, and Van den Bogaard (2017) developed a five-day training course, sessions focusing on theories about diagnostic models were combined with sessions focusing on the assessment of sexual abuse of victims and perpetrators and its effectives was evaluated. The effectiveness of the training course was determined in terms of (applied) knowledge via the administration of a study-specific questionnaire including a hypothetical case vignette before, immediately after, and six months after completion of the course. The results show that the knowledge of the psychologists related to sexual abuse and the assessment process for sexual abuse increased significantly, and remained above pre-test level at six-month follow-up. These results are promising, but more research is needed to see if the increased (applied) knowledge in turn leads to application in practice and better care for both victims and perpetrators. Despite limitations of the current study regarding the transfer of knowledge, it seems likely that enhanced knowledge of sexual abuse and the assessment process will lead to greater sensitivity to potential cases of sexual abuse in practice and to a more efficient assessment process following a disclosure. Assessment is an important step in the treatment of the consequences of sexual abuse as well as the prevention of sexual abuse by potential perpetrators. Trained psychologists will be better equipped to confirm/disconfirm their suspicions of sexual abuse and to deal with cases of (alleged) sexual abuse, which will ultimately benefit wellbeing of people with ID.

Chou, Lu, Chen, & Lin (2019) evaluated the impact of the sexual health programs that involved the parents and service workers intended to promote sexual health in adults with an intellectual disability (ID) in Taiwan. The findings revealed that after the programs were implemented, attitudes towards the sexual rights of people with ID were significantly more positive among both the parents and service workers. Participation in the sexual health programs facilitated constructive dialogue by revealing hidden concerns and by transforming the perspectives of the parents and service workers from viewing sexuality as a social problem to understanding the sexual rights of adults with ID. Both the quantitative and qualitative results demonstrate that the programs had a positive impact on the parents and service workers in terms of their attitudes towards the sexual rights of people with ID. Open dialogue and reciprocal interaction strategies caused transformations in the perspectives of parents and service workers on sexual health.

The interventions tried to deal with sexual issues among people with intellectual disabilities through caregivers and midwives too. According to Whittle & Butler (2018) application of the hierarchical Coordinated Management of Meaning model suggested caregivers contextual beliefs about people with intellectual disabilities' sexuality inhibited or facilitated positive expressions of sexuality over and above individual needs and desires. Rights-based cultural messages provided the only context that led to positive sexuality outcomes and research that explores sexuality within this context is much needed. The Coordinated Management of Meaning model may act as a framework to support the reflective-practice of caregivers.

Family planning counselling is an essential part of sexual and reproductive health care; however, health care professionals often fail to offer sexual and reproductive health services to women with intellectual disability (ID), based on a misconception of inactive sexuality. Few women with ID request contraceptive counselling, which limits midwives' knowledge, experience and competence. Midwives, therefore, plan consultations carefully and strive to enable women with ID to make informed contraceptive choices. Increased teamwork could be a way to strengthen the role of midwives and thereby improve counselling (Höglund & Larsson, 2019).

Attempt were also done to provide sex education through genetic counselling as an additional component or as a part of genetic counselling and sessions may include discussions of reproductive implications and other issues related to sex education. Patients with ID regularly meet barriers when trying to obtain sex education due to the misperceptions of others as being either asexual or that such education would promote inappropriate sexual behavior. Caregivers and patients most frequently requested information on puberty, sex abuse prevention, and reproductive health. Genetic counselors were most comfortable when they could provide sex education counseling within the context of a particular condition or constellation of features. They were least comfortable when they lacked familiarity with the patient, caregiver, or the family's culture. The most frequently cited barriers that prevented genetic counselors from providing sex education counseling were lack of time, lack of training, the patient's ID being too profound, and a belief that genetic counselors should not be responsible for providing sex education counseling. While many respondents reported that providing sex education counseling is not considered within the scope of a genetic counselor's practice, they also noted that patients' families initiate discussions for which counselors should be prepared. Respondents indicated that resource guides specifically designed for use by genetic counselors would be beneficial to their practice. Genetic counselors have the opportunity to embrace the role of advocate and broach the issue of sexual health with caregivers and patients by directing them toward educational resources, if not providing sex education directly to effectively serve the needs of patients and caregivers (Murphy, Lincoln, Meredith, Cross & Rintell, 2016).

Sex education should include social skills, such as those that allow individuals to relate, socialize, and communicate with others, to assist people with intellectual disability (ID) to live life fully in the community and sex education program involving social skills training for people with ID found to have significant effects (Hayashi, Arakida, & Ohashi, 2011).

Schaafsma, Kok, Stoffelen, & Curfs (2015) reported the results of a systematic review identifying methods for sex education programs aimed at individuals with intellectual disabilities. They reported that there are some indications that skills and knowledge can be increased, and attitudes can indeed be improved. It also became apparent that some studies used similar methods. Furthermore, it became clear that there is room for improvement. What exactly was taught to individuals with intellectual disabilities and how it was taught was rarely reported in sufficient detail. It seems as if the underlying assumption is that the sex education materials and programs used in the studies are effective in positively changing the determinants (e.g., knowledge, skills, and attitudes) they focus on, yet most studies do not provide any evidence of the quality of the program that was used or information on how these programs or training sessions were developed. It has been shown that sex education programs for individuals with intellectual disabilities often have an insufficient theory or evidence base and have not been properly evaluated. It is likely that any references to theory and evidence in terms of the development of such programs are omitted because the research lacks this theory and evidence base. Many studies are required to find effectiveness of sex education programs especially to focus on the components to be included and to have success in real life situation.

FUTURE DIRECTIONS

In order for persons with intellectual disability to express their sexuality in accordance with their developmental stage and societal norms and also to safeguard them from any form of sexual abuse the following factors could be considered:

- Primary prevention involving prevention programs to identify high risk factors, personal factors, and cultural factors associated with sexual abuse.
- Secondary prevention involving identification of vulnerable sub groups in this population and deliver services promptly.
- Tertiary care which includes well structured, personalised, well responsive sytems to act effectively when intellectually disabled individuals are harmed through sexual abuse.
- Education and training programs to provide information about sexuality and sexual health to enhance personal and emotional safety.
- Training programmes for multitude of professionals who are associated with service delivery to this population in preventing as well as handling sexuality related issues.
- Meaningful and well-articulated government policies to safeguard the rights of persons with intellectual disability.
- Research work intended to study sexuality related issues in people with intellectual disability across cultural, familial, institutional,legal and personal paradigms.

PARENTHOOD AND INTELLECTUAL DISABILITY

The ability of persons with intellectual disability to take the role of parent is a matter of great concern as it involves moral, financial, technical, medical and legal implications. These individuals, like others, have feelings and want relationships and are able to have children.

The attitude of society has changed through time from the early eugenic concern with heredity and fertility, to a focus on the risk to the children due to parental neglect or abuse, to acceptance and a search for solutions to parental training and support. This change can be seen as a result of a shift from institutional care to community care and normalization. It is reported that, in the case of such a union resulting in children, although they require some supervision, family, friends, and social welfare agencies have scrutinized these families so much they are in constant fear of their child being taken away. (Kandel, Morad, Vardi& Merrick, 2005). Most people with intellectual disability have normal fertility, and many desire children. They may encounter opposition to their intention to have children, making it difficult to plan for pregnancy and parenting and to access the social support they and their children are likely to need. While parents with intellectual disability usually need support, so do many other groups such as very young parents and those with substance use or mental health issues. Parents with intellectual disability may have difficulty understanding and responding to their children's needs. Most have low incomes, limiting their children's access to important developmental activities. Depending on the cause of the parents' disability, their children may be at increased risk of having an intellectual disability. Children who do not have intellectual disability may surpass their parents' cognitive ability at a young age. However, such children are generally positive about their parents and good outcomes are possible with appropriate support (Eastgate, 2011).

The prevalence rate of parents with intellectual disability is not known fully. Literature suggest a possible prevalence rate of less than 1 per cent in Australia i. e 0.99 per cent of the general population has intellectual disability (stereo). Another study conducted in New Zealand ascertained a prevalence figure of 0.25 per cent. Though information regarding the prevalence rates lacks clarity, there is general consensus in the literature that more people with intellectual disability become parents as opportunities for community living expand (McConnel& Llewellyn, 2002). As there is no clear definitions regarding adequate parenting and parental competence, assessing minimal parental competence remains significant issue in this area. This become even more complex when intellectually disabled parents are concerned (Lamont & Bromfield, 2009).

Individuals with intellectual disability are considered to be unable to provide adequate care for their children. It is likely that parents with intellectual disability may neglect their child, subject them to physical and sexual abuse or witness violence (James, 2004; Booth & Booth, 1998). There are certain factors which are identified to be associated with maltreatment of children by parents who are intellectually disabled. They include the following: social isolation, parental stress, parents with past histories of being abused or neglected as children, „ demographic characteristics such as parental income, education, and employment status, parental physical and mental health problems, children with physical or mental health problems, behavioural problems or disability, parental substance abuse; and domestic/family violence (Cleaver, Unell, &Aldgate, 1999; Feldman et al., 2002).

Records of data from the U. S, U. K and Australia reveals that parents with intellectual disability is less likely to have received support in their parenting. They are over-represented in child care proceedings and are at greater risk to have their parental responsibility terminated. They are likely to be judged against stricter criteria and are more likely to have their children removed. They are also less likely to receive support in correcting the condition (Kandel, Morad, Verdi &Merrick, 2005).

Mothers with intellectual and developmental disabilities (IDD) frequently experience mental health problems. Yet, they are excluded from broader women's mental health efforts, and few services exist to support their unique mental health needs. Heifetz, Brown, Chacra, Tint,Vigod, Bluestein, & Lunsky (2019) have identified nine thematic categories which were organized into risks, protective factors, and resilience factors. Risks were parenting stress, life stressors, feelings of powerlessness with the child welfare system, and feeling judged. Protective factors were formal and informal supports. Resilience factors were motherhood enjoyment, having a good family life, and wishing to be independent. Efforts to improve mental health among mothers with IDD should minimize risks that undermine adaptive capabilities and promote resilience to restore efficacy of protective systems. Better training of service-providers working with individuals with IDD, using strength-based approaches and developing alternative, autonomy-building sources of support in the form of peer support groups is recommended

Parents with intellectual disabilities face particular challenges, such as lack of sufficient support with their parenting. Peers can be an important source of support for parents in the general population; however, there is a limited knowledge about peer support for parents with intellectual disabilities. The source of support was less important than the way support was offered. Parents valued support offered by someone who respected them as a person and parent, and was interested in what they wanted and needed (Strnadová , Collings, Loblinzk, & Danker, 2019).

Parents with intellectual disabilities (ID) are at risk for high levels of parenting stress. The study evaluated resources, including parental adaptive functioning, financial resources and access to a support network, as moderators of the association between child behaviour problems and parenting stress. A total of 134 parents with ID and their children (ages 1-7 years) were recruited from 10 Dutch care organisations. Parents experienced more stress with regard to their children than towards their own functioning and situation. Parenting stress was less in parents who were not experiencing financial hardship. Child behaviour problems were associated with high child-related parenting stress, not parent-related parenting stress. Large support networks decreased the association between child behaviour problems and child-related parenting stress. Financial resources did not significantly moderate the association. Parenting stress among parents with ID is focused on problems with the child, especially when little social support is available (Meppelder, Hodes, Kef & Schuengel, 2015).

United Nations human rights treaties and domestic law require social workers to support the parenting rights of persons with intellectual disabilities. Social workers are also required to protect the health and well-being of those clients' children. Gur & Stein (2019) explored the experiences, challenges, and complex attitudes of Israeli social workers regarding parenthood by their clients with intellectual disabilities. A qualitative method employed semi-structured interviews with twenty-one social workers. A thematic analysis identified major themes. Social workers recognized the parental desires of clients with intellectual disabilities and acknowledged their role in supporting those individuals. Nevertheless, most of the social workers expressed negative perceptions regarding the right or capability of clients with intellectual disabilities to parent. Social workers thus felt the tension between their personal reservations and their professional duty to support these clients. Regardless of individual attitudes, social workers uniformly asserted that greater state and community support was needed to enable the parental capacity of their clients.In addition to increasing state and community support for parents with intellectual disabilities, additional training is needed for empowering social workers to act on behalf of these clients in Israel. Implications for Rehabilitation Social workers hold critical roles for parents with intellectual disabilities and are required to support their clients' parenting while ensuring the health and well-being of their children. Israeli social workers balance negative or ambivalent attitudes regarding the capability of parents with intellectual disabilities against a desire to honor their duty to support these clients. State and community support for parents with intellectual disabilities must be increased. Additional training is needed for empowering social workers to act on behalf of these clients in Israel.

Partner Violence

It is also important to mention that individuals with intellectual disabilities (IDs) are at increased risk of violence perpetration and victimization. Bowen & Swift (2017) did a systematic review to identify and critically evaluate the existing empirical research concerning the use and experience of partner violence by adults with IDs. A partner violence victimization rate of 60% was identified in one nonrepresentative sample. Two superordinate themes emerged from the qualitative data: nature of partner violence experience and help seeking. Children were the cross-cutting theme within the two superordinate themes. Participants reported experiencing a range of physical, emotional, and sexual violence leading to serious injury and psychological consequences. Participants reported experiences of positive and negative help-seeking reactions from professionals and specific requirements of services for victims with IDs. Children were identified as involved in the experience of abuse, the impact of abuse, and decisions to seek help. The findings indicate that training of clinical staff to detect partner violence is needed. In addition, adults with IDs need education concerning healthy relationships. Research is needed to better understand the difference between "challenging behavior" that is behavior displayed by an individual which challenges services, family members, and carers. Such behavior is more common in individuals with a severe ID for whom it would not be appropriate to be dealt with through the criminal justice system, and partner violence, in order to develop appropriate interventions for victims and perpetrators with ID.

Providing Support Services

Early provision of support services should be ensured where intellectual disability of the parent is affecting the welfare of the child. Research in this area suggests that support programs are effective if they are family-centred,provided over the long-term, focused on strengths rather than deficits, home based, feature participatory rather than relational elements of practice and performance rather than knowledge based (Lamont & Bromfield, 2009).

Contraception

The need for contraception in adolescents with ID is a frequent reason for gynaecological consultation, despite their younger age and lower number who are sexually active. Combined oral contraception is the most prescribed method in adolescents with ID; however, the transdermal patch also plays an important role in this group (Nunes, Neves, Geraldes, & Lopes,2017). The most frequently used contraceptive methods are condoms (41.4%), the pill (39.6%), transdermal patch (30.2%) and intrauterine device (6.7%) (Gil-Llario, Morell-Mengual, Ballester-Arnal & Díaz-Rodríguez (2018). Currently there is limited knowledge on the use of contraception among intellectually disabled individuals hence future studies need to focus on this aspect.

CONCLUSION

There is a growing and evolving research evidence base regarding sexuality issues and adults with intellectual disabilities. However, the experiences and views of families and direct care support workers and their support and development needs in the topic area are unclear. Families and direct care support workers have specific support and education needs. Future healthcare initiatives need to be developed that are fully responsive to the identified concerns and requirements of families and direct care support workers (Brown & McCann, 2019). There is a need to draw up educational programmes, differentiated according to gender and adapted to their reality, which include contents related with sexual health, sexual abuse and condom use (Gil-Llario., Morell-Mengual., Ballester-Arnal., & Díaz-Rodríguez, 2018). There is a large unmet need for well designed, properly evaluated sex education for people with intellectual disability, families and support workers. There is also a need for clarification of legal and ethical issues. Family members and professionals alike need to remain aware of the risk of abuse and its effect on the health and lives of people with intellectual disability (Eastgate, Scheermeyer, van Driel, &Lennox, 2012).

As sexual violence against women with intellectual disabilities continues to pose a pervasive and largely overlooked problem, disability and sexual assault prevention advocates must coordinate their resources and efforts to develop an evidence-based program that will limit such violence. Interventions must be as multifaceted as the lives of women with intellectual disabilities, incorporating the many service systems and individuals involved to meet their complex needs. Similarly, sexual violence practitioners must feel necessarily concerned with the needs of women with disabilities, as no woman is truly safe if she is not assured that her most vulnerable peers enjoy the same protection (Barger, Wacker, Macy, & Parish (2009).

There is limited consideration of the importance of pleasure in published discussions of sexuality and intellectual disability. The literature is dominated by conversations about the need for sex education, vulnerability to sexual exploitation, capacity to consent, and protection/safeguarding. Of course, this is essential and necessary, but there is plenty of room for more discourse about pleasure, sensuality, and feeling good. These conversations can be hard for professionals to have within public services. Parents and carers may feel uncomfortable about raising these issues with other people within the support system. For disability organisations, there are many obstacles to supporting safe sexual expression in their customers with disabilities, such as facing family opposition, feeling confusion over the legality of their support, personal prejudices may take precedence over their professional obligations, and lack of organisational consideration for support workers at the frontline of the privacy issues for people for whom they provide care. People with intellectual disability, in particular, are not often given support to understand their sexual rights, nor the opportunity or indeed the education, to explore their sexuality and sexual expression. We teach people many life skills; everything from cleaning their teeth to understanding public and private spaces. Why do we not routinely teach people to have healthy and intimate relationships? Why are the values and beliefs of staff paramount for this particular issue, when we are supposed to be person-centred regarding everything else? (Turner, 2016; Turne, & Crane,2016; Alexander & Gomez, 2016).

Like any other individual a person with intellectual disability possess the biological ability to conceive and bear offspring. They enjoy the legal right to raise a family. But these individuals are faced with multitude of issues related to personal and societal factors. If support services are organised, delivered promptly and systematically to handle such issues they will be able to ensure the welfare of their children. Collaborative services by governmental, medical, legal, familial, educational and community level agencies can provide these individuals with the necessary support and prevent from compromising the welfare of the child.

REFERENCES

Alexander, N., & Gomez, M.T. (2017). Pleasure, sex, prohibition, intellectual disability, and dangerous ideas. *An International Journal on Sexual and Reproductive Health And rights, 25*(50), 114-120. doi: 10.1080/09688080.2017.1331690

Angelopoulou, N., Souftas, V., Sakadamis, A., Matziari, C., Papameletiou, V., & Mandroukas, K. (1999). Gonadal function in young women with Down syndrome. *International Journal of Gynaecology and Obstetrics: the Official Organ of the International Federation of Gynaecology and Obstetrics, 67*(1), 15–21. doi:10.1016/S0020-7292(99)00123-X PMID:10576235

Baines, S., Emerson, E., Robertson, J., & Hatton, C. (2018). Sexual activity and sexual health among young adults with and without mild/moderate intellectual disability. *BMC Public Health, 18*(1), 667. doi:10.118612889-018-5572-9

Balderian, N. (1991). Sexual abuse of people with developmental disabilities. *Sexuality and Disability, 9*(4), 323–335. doi:10.1007/BF01102020

Barger, E., Wacker, J., Macy, R., & Parish, S. (2009). Sexual Assault Prevention for Women With Intellectual Disabilities: A Critical Review of the Evidence. *Intellectual and Developmental Disabilities, 47*(4), 249–262. doi:10.1352/1934-9556-47.4.249 PMID:19650680

Berman, H., Harris, D., Enright, R., Gilpin, M., Cathers, T., & Bukovy, G. (1999). Sexuality and the adolescent with a physical disability: Understandings and misunderstandings. *Issues in Comprehensive Pediatric Nursing, 22*(4), 183–196. doi:10.1080/014608699265275 PMID:10827606

Black, R. S., & Kammes, R. R. (2019). Restrictions, Power, Companionship, and Intimacy: A Metasynthesis of People With Intellectual Disability Speaking About Sex and Relationships. *Intellectual and Developmental Disabilities, 57*(3), 212–233. doi:10.1352/1934-9556-57.3.212 PMID:31120408

Booth, T., & Booth, W. (1998). *Growing up with parents who have learning difficulties*. London: Routledge.

Bowen, E., & Swift, C. (2017). The Prevalence and Correlates of Partner Violence Used and Experienced by Adults With Intellectual Disabilities: A Systematic Review and Call to Action. *Trauma, Violence & Abuse, 1*. doi:10.1177/1524838017728707 PMID:29333986

Brown, H., & Stein, J. (1997). Sexual abuse perpetrated by men with intellectual disabilities: A comparative study. *Journal of Intellectual Disability Research, 41*(3), 215–224. doi:10.1111/j.1365-2788.1997.tb00700.x PMID:9219070

Brown, M., & McCann, E. (2019). The views and experiences of families and direct care support workers regarding the expression of sexuality by adults with intellectual disabilities: A narrative review of the international research evidence. *Research in Developmental Disabilities, 90*, 80–91. doi:10.1016/j.ridd.2019.04.012 PMID:31082682

Byrne, G. (2018). Prevalence and psychological sequelae of sexual abuse among individuals with an intellectual disability: A review of the recent literature. *Journal of Intellectual & Developmental Disability, 22*(3), 294–310. doi:10.1177/1744629517698844 PMID:30134783

Carew, M. T., Braathen, S. H., Swartz, L., Hunt, X., & Rohleder, P. (2017). The sexual lives of people with disabilities within low- and middle-income countries: A scoping study of studies published in English. *Global Health Action, 10*(1), 1337342. doi:10.1080/16549716.2017.1337342 PMID:28678682

Carrier, S. (2007). Understanding social and professional integration as an adjustment process: Contribution to a theory of coadaptation. *Intellectual and Developmental Disabilities, 45*(1), 10–22. doi:10.1352/1934-9556(2007)45[10:USAPIA]2.0.CO;2 PMID:17428122

Chou, Y. C., Lu, Z. J., Chen, B. W., & Lin, C. J. (2019). Transformed rights' sexual health programme evaluation for the parents and service workers of adults with an intellectual disability. *Journal of Intellectual Disability Research, 23*. doi:10.1111/jir.12624 PMID:31016807

Clark, L. I., & O'toole, M. S. (2007). Intellectual impairment and sexual health: Information needs. *British Journal of Nursing (Mark Allen Publishing), 16*(3), 154–156. doi:10.12968/bjon.2007.16.3.22968 PMID:17363881

Clay, C. J., Bloom, S. E., & Lambert, J. M. (2018). Behavioral Interventions for inappropriate sexual behavior in individuals with developmental disabilities and acquired brain injury: A review. *American Journal on Intellectual and Developmental Disabilities, 123*(3), 254–282. doi:10.1352/1944-7558-123.3.254 PMID:29671636

Cleaver, H., Unell, I., & Aldgate, J. (1999). *Children's needs, parenting capacity: The impact of parental mental illness, problem alcohol and drug use and domestic violence on children's development*. London: Department of Health, Stationary Office.

Dammeyer, J., & Chapman, M. (2018). A national survey on violence and discrimination among people with disabilities. *BMC Public Health, 18*(1), 355. doi:10.118612889-018-5277-0

Day, K. (1997). Clinical features and offense behavior of mentally retarded sex offenders: A review of research. *The NADD Newsletter, 14*, 86–89.

Eastgate, G. (2005). Sex, consent and intellectual disability. *Australian Family Physician, 34*(3), 163–166. PMID:15799666

Eastgate, G. (2011). Sex and intellectual disability: Dealing with sexual health issues. *Disability, 40*, 188–191. PMID:21597526

Eastgate, G., Scheermeyer, E., van Driel, M., & Lennox, N. G. (2012). Intellectual disability, sexuality and sexual abuse prevention: A study of family members and support workers. *Disability, 41*(3), 135-139. Retrieved from https://www.racgp.org.au/afp/2012/march/intellectual-disability,-sexuality-and-sexual-abuse-prevention/

Embregts, P. J. C. M., Heestermans, M., & Van den Bogaard, K. J. H. M. (2017). A Training Course for Psychologists: Learning to Assess (Alleged) Sexual Abuse Among Victims and Perpetrators Who Have Intellectual Disabilities. *Sexuality and Disability, 35*(1), 39–44. doi:10.100711195-017-9476-x PMID:28250542

Esmail, S., Darry, K., Walter, A., & Knupp, H. (2010). Attitudes and perceptions towards disability and sexuality. *Journal Disability and Rehabilitation*, *32*(14), 1148–1155. doi:10.3109/09638280903419277 PMID:20131952

Feldman, M., Varhese, J., Ramsay, J., & Rajska, D. (2002). Relationships between social support, stress and mother–child interactions in mothers with intellectual disabilities. *Journal of Applied Research in Intellectual Disabilities*, *15*(4), 314–323. doi:10.1046/j.1468-3148.2002.00132.x

Gil-Llario, M. D., Morell-Mengual, V., Ballester-Arnal, R., & Díaz-Rodríguez, I. (2018). The experience of sexuality in adults with intellectual disability. *Journal of Intellectual Disability Research*, *62*(1), 72–80. doi:10.1111/jir.12455 PMID:29159891

Gross, G. (1985). *Activities of the developmental disabilities adult offender project*. Olympia, WA: Washington State Developmental Disability Planning Council.

Gur, A., & Stein, M. A. (2019). Social worker attitudes toward parents with intellectual disabilities in Israel. *Disability and Rehabilitation*, *7*, 1–11. doi:10.1080/09638288.2018.1537382 PMID:30616429

Hayashi, M., Arakida, M., & Ohashi, K. (2011). The effectiveness of a sex education program facilitating social skills for people with intellectual disability in Japan. *Journal of Intellectual & Developmental Disability*, *36*(1), 11–19. doi:10.3109/13668250.2010.549463 PMID:21284415

Heifetz, M., Brown, H. K., Chacra, M. A., Tint, A., Vigod, S., Bluestein, D., & Lunsky, Y. (2019). Mental health challenges and resilience among mothers with intellectual and developmental disabilities. *Disability and Health Journal*, *19*, 30107–4. doi:10.1016/j.dhjo.2019.06.006 PMID:31235446

Höglund, B., & Larsson, M. (2019). Midwives' work and attitudes towards contraceptive counselling and contraception among women with intellectual disability: Focus group interviews in Sweden. *The European Journal of Contraception & Reproductive Health Care*, *24*(1), 39–44. doi:10.1080/13625187.2018.1555640 PMID:30633574

James, H. (2004). Promoting effective working with parents with learning disabilities. *Child Abuse Review*, *13*(1), 31–41. doi:10.1002/car.823

Kandel, I., Morad, M., Vardi, G., & Merrick, J. (2005). Intellectual disability and parenthood. *The Scientific World Journal*, *5*, 50–57. doi:10.1100/tsw.2005.12 PMID:15674450

Katz, G., & Lazcano-Ponce, E. (2008). Sexuality in subjects with intellectual disability: An educational intervention proposal for parents and counsellors in developing countries. *Salud Pública de México*, *2*, 239–254. doi:10.1590/S0036-36342008000800018

Kempton, W., & Gochros, J. (1986). The developmentally disabled. In H. L. Gochros, J. S. Gochros, & J. Fisher (Eds.), *Helping the sexually oppressed* (pp. 224–237). Englewood Cliffs, NJ: Prentice-Hall.

Kijak, R. (2013). The Sexuality of Adults with Intellectual Disability in Poland. *Sexuality and Disability*, *31*(2), 109–123. doi:10.100711195-013-9294-8 PMID:23704799

Kijak, R. J. (2011). Desire for love: Considerations on sexuality and sex education of people with intellectual disability in Poland. *Sexuality and Disability*, *29*(1), 65–74. doi:10.100711195-010-9184-2 PMID:21423325

Kucuk, S., Platin, N., & Erdem, E. (2017). Increasing awareness of protection from sexual abuse in children with mild intellectualdisabilities: An education study. *Applied Nursing Research*, *38*, 153–158. doi:10.1016/j.apnr.2017.10.016 PMID:29241509

Lamont, A., & Bromfield, L. (2009). Parental intellectual disability and child protection: Key issues. National Child Protection Clearing house. *Issues (Chicago, Ill.)*, *31*. Retrieved from http://www.aifs. gov

McConnel, D., & Llewllyn, G. (2002). Stereotypes, parents with intellectual disability and child protection. *Journal of Social Welfare and Family*, *24*(3), 297–317. doi:10.1080/09649060210161294

McDonald, K. E., Keys, C. B., & Balcazar, F. E. (2007). Disability, race/ethnicity and gender: Themes of cultural oppression, acts of individual resistance. *American Journal of Community Psychology*, *39*(1-2), 145–161. doi:10.100710464-007-9094-3 PMID:17294120

Meppelder, M., Hodes, M., Kef, S., & Schuengel, C. (2015). Parenting stress and child behaviour problems among parents with intellectual disabilities: The buffering role of resources. *Journal of Intellectual Disability Research*, *59*(7), 664–677. doi:10.1111/jir.12170 PMID:25472805

Morrissey, E., Wandersman, A., Seybolt, D., Nation, M., Crusto, C., & Davino, K. (1997). Toward a framework for bridging the gap between science and practice in prevention: A focus on evaluator and practitioner perspectives. *Evaluation and Program Planning*, *20*(3), 367–377. doi:10.1016/S0149-7189(97)00016-5

Murphy, C., Lincoln, S., Meredith, S., Cross, E. M., & Rintell, D. (2016). Sex Education and Intellectual Disability: Practices and Insight from Pediatric Genetic Counselors. *Journal of Genetic Counseling*, *25*(3), 552–560. doi:10.100710897-015-9909-6 PMID:26581379

Murphy, W., Coleman, E., & Haynes, M. (1983). Treatment and evaluation issues with the mentally retarded sex offender. In J. G. Greer & I. R. Stuart (Eds.), *The sexual aggressor: Current perspectives on treatment* (pp. 22–41). New York: Van Nostrand Reinhold.

Nunes, F. R. P., Neves, F. A. D., Geraldes, F. D. P. B., & Lopes, A. M. F. R. (2017). Contraception in adolescents with intellectual disability. *The European Journal of Contraception & Reproductive Health Care*, *22*(6), 401–406. doi:10.1080/13625187.2017.1402875 PMID:29188744

Piaget, J. (1997). The essential Piaget. In R. E. Gruber & J. J. Voneche (Eds.), *The language and thought of the child* (p. 85). New York: Basic Books, Inc. Publishers.

Pownall, J. D., Jahoda, A., & Hastings, R. P. (2012). Sexuality and sex education of adolescents with intellectual disability: Mothers' attitudes, experiences, and support needs. *Journal of Intellectual & Developmental Disability*, *50*(2), 140–154. doi:10.1352/1934-9556-50.2.140 PMID:22642968

Rademakers, J., Mouthaan, I., & de Neef, M. (2005). Diversity in sexual health: Problems and dilemmas. *The European Journal of Contraception & Reproductive Health Care*, *10*(4), 207–211. doi:10.1080/13625180500279847 PMID:16448946

Schaafsma, D., Kok, G., Stoffelen, J.M.T., & Curfs, L.M.G. (2015). Identifying Effective Methods for Teaching Sex Education to Individuals With Intellectual Disabilities: A Systematic Review. *The Journal of Sex Research*, *52*(4), 412–432. doi:10.1080/00224499.2014.919373

Schor, D. P. (1987). Sex and sexual abuse in developmentally disabled adolescents. *Seminars in Adolescent Medicine*, *3*, 1–7. PMID:2955493

Scott, H. (1998). Helping clients in their sexual expression. *British Journal of Nursing (Mark Allen Publishing)*, *7*(10), 568. doi:10.12968/bjon.1998.7.10.5678 PMID:9775763

Sobsey, D. (1994). *Violence and abuse in the lives of people with disabilities: The end of silent acceptance?* Baltimore, MD: Paul H. Brookes Publishing Co.

Sobsey, D., & Mansell, S. (1990). The prevention of sexual abuse and assault: Sexual exploitation of people with disabilities. *Sexuality and Disability*, *9*, 243–259. doi:10.1007/BF01102395

Steptoe, L., Lindsay, W. R., Forrest, D., & Power, M. (2006). Quality of life and relationships in sex offenders with intellectual disability. *Journal of Intellectual and Developmental Disabilities*, *31*(1), 13-19.

Stoffelen, J. M. T., Schaafsma, D., Kok, G., & Curfs, L. M. G. (2018, September). Women Who Love: An Explorative Study on Experiences of Lesbian and Bisexual Women with a Mild Intellectual Disability in The Netherlands. *Sexuality and Disability*, *36*(3), 249–264. doi:10.100711195-018-9519-y PMID:30220750

Strnadová, I., Collings, S., Loblinzk, J., & Danker, J. (2019). Parents with intellectual disabilities and their perspective of peer support: "It depends on how they give it. *Journal of Applied Research in Intellectual Disabilities*, *32*(4), 879–889. doi:10.1111/jar.12579 PMID:30790398

Thom, R. P., Grudzinskas, A. J. Jr, & Saleh, F. M. (2017). Sexual Behavior Among Persons With Cognitive Impairments. *Current Psychiatry Reports*, *19*(5), 25. doi:10.100711920-017-0777-7 PMID:28417268

Tower, C. (1989). *Understanding child abuse and neglect*. Boston: Allyn and Bacon.

Turner, G. W., & Crane, B. (2016). Pleasure is paramount: Adults with intellectual disabilities discuss sensuality and intimacy. *Sexualities*, *19*(5–6), 677–697. doi:10.1177/1363460715620573

Turner, G. W., & Crane, B. (2016). Sexually silenced no more, adults with learning disabilities speak up: A call to action for social work to frame sexual voice as a social justice issue. *British Journal of Social Work*, *46*(8), 2300–2317. doi:10.1093/bjsw/bcw133

Van Dyke, D. E., Mc Brien, D. M., & Sherbondy, A. (1995). Issues of sexuality in Down Syndrome. *Down's Syndrome: Research and Practice*, *3*(2), 65–69. doi:10.3104/reviews.53

Walter, J. (n.d.). From taboo to self-actualization–acceptance problems and learning processes in working with mentally handicapped patients. *Praxis der Kinderpsychologie und Kinderpsy*chiatrie, *51*(8), 587-597.

Ward, K., Trigler, J., & Pfeiffer, K. (2001). Community services, issues, and service gaps for individuals with developmental disabilities who exhibit inappropriate sexual behaviors. *Mental Retardation*, *39*(1), 11–19. doi:10.1352/0047-6765(2001)039<0011:CSIASG>2.0.CO;2 PMID:11270210

Whittle, C., & Butler, C. (2018). Sexuality in the lives of people with intellectual disabilities: A meta-ethnographic synthesis of qualitative studies. *Research in Developmental Disabilities*, *75*, 68–81. doi:10.1016/j.ridd.2018.02.008 PMID:29486384

Wissink, I. B., Vugt, V. E., Moonen, X., Stams, G. J., & Hendriks, J. (2015). Sexual abuse involving children with an intellectual disability (ID): A narrative review. *Research in Developmental Disabilities*, *36*, 20–35. doi:10.1016/j.ridd.2014.09.007 PMID:25310832

Compilation of References

<unknown>Derigne, L., & Porterfield, S. L. (2017). Employment change among married parents of children with special health care needs. Journal of Family Issues, 38(5), 579-606.</unknown>

<unknown>Leonard, H., Petterson, B., Bower, C., & Sanders, R. (2003). Prevalence of intellectual disability in western australia. Paediatric and Perinatal Epidemiology, 17(1), 58-67.</unknown>

<unknown>No child left behind act of 2001, 20 u.s.c., pub. L. No. 107-110 (2002).</unknown>

<unknown>Nota, L., Ferrari, L., Soresi, S., & Wehmeyer, M. (2007). Self-determination, social abilities and the quality of life of people with intellectual disability. Journal of Intellectual Disability Research, 51(11), 850-865.</unknown>

<unknown>Richardson, S. A., & Koller, H. (1996). Twenty-two years: Causes and consequences of mental retardation. Harvard University Press.</unknown>

<unknown>Roeleveld, N., & Zielhuis, G. A. (1997). The prevalence of mental retardation: a critical review of recent literature. Developmental Medicine & Child Neurology, 39(2), 125-132.</unknown>

Abbeduto, L., Seltzer, M. M., Shattuck, P., Krauss, M. W., Orsmond, G., & Murphy, M. M. (2004). Psychological well-being and coping in mothers of youths with autism, down syndrome, or fragile x syndrome. *Journal Information, 109*(3).

Abbeduto, L., Furman, L., & Davies, B. (1989). Relation between the receptive language and mental age of persons with mental retardation. *American Journal of Mental Retardation, 93*, 535–543. PMID:2706121

Abbeduto, L., Krauss, M. W., Murphy, M. M., Orsmond, G., Seltzer, M. M., & Shattuck, P. (2004). Psychological well-being and coping in mothers of youths with autism, down syndrome, or fragile x syndrome. *American Journal of Mental Retardation, 109*(3), 237–254. doi:10.1352/0895-8017(2004)109<237:PWACIM>2.0.CO;2 PMID:15072518

Abberley, P. (1987). The concept of oppression and the development of a social theory of disability. *Disability, Handicap & Society, 2*(1), 5–19. doi:10.1080/02674648766780021

Abbey, A., & Andrews, F. M. (1986). Modeling the psychological determinants of life quality. In F. M. Andrews (Ed.), *Research on the quality of life*. Ann Arbor, MI: Institute for Social Research, University of Michigan.

Abbott, D. A., & Meredith, W. H. (1986). Strengths of parents with retarded children. *Family Relations, 35*(3), 371–375. doi:10.2307/584363

Abidi, J. (1999). Current status of employment of disabled people in Indian industries. *Asia Pacific Disability Rehabilitation Journal, 10*(2).

Achenbach, T. M., & Rescorla, L. A. (2000). *Manual for the ASEBA Preschool Forms & Profiles*. Burlington, VT: University of Vermont, Research Center for Children, Youth, & Families.

Adolphs, R., Russell, J. A., & Tranel, D. (1999). A role for the human amygdala in recognizing emotional arousal from unpleasant stimuli. *Psychological Science, 10*(2), 167–171. doi:10.1111/1467-9280.00126

Ageranioti-Bélanger, S., Brunet, S., D'Anjou, G., Tellier, G., Boivin, J., & Gauthier, M. (2012). Behaviour disorders in children with an intellectual disability. *Paediatrics & Child Health, 17*(2), 84–88. doi:10.1093/pch/17.2.84 PMID:23372399

Agnoli, S., Mancini, G., Pozzoli, T., Russo, P. M., Baldaro, B., & Surcinelli, P. (2012). The Interaction Between Emotional Intelligence and Cognitive Abilities in Predicting Scholastic Performance in School Aged Children. *Journal of Personality and Individual Differences, 53*(5), 660–665. doi:10.1016/j.paid.2012.05.020

Ahmedani, B. K., & Hock, R. (2012). Parent perceptions of autism severity: Exploring social-ecological context. *Disability and Health Journal, 5*(4), 298–304. doi:10.1016/j.dhjo.2012.06.002 PMID:23021742

Ahuja, N. (2007). *Short Text Book of Psychiatry*. Academic Press.

Ahuja, N. (2011). *A Short Textbook of Psychiatry. VII 01*. JP Brothers. doi:10.5005/jp/books/11464

Aicardi, J. (1998). The etiology of developmental delay. *Seminars in Pediatric Neurology, 5*(1), 15–20. doi:10.1016/S1071-9091(98)80013-2 PMID:9548636

Ainsworth, M. D. (1985). Attachments across the life span. *Bulletin of the New York Academy of Medicine, 61*, 792–812. PMID:3864511

Ainsworth, M. S., Blehar, M. C., & Everett Waters, E. (1978). *Patterns of attachment: A psychological study of the strange situation*. New York: Lawrence Erlbaum.

Ainsworth, M. S., & Bowlby, J. (1991). An ethological approach to personality development. *The American Psychologist, 46*(4), 333–341. doi:10.1037/0003-066X.46.4.333

Alaghband, M., Tavakoli, S., & Alaghband, L. (2002). The relationship between communication skills and emotional intelligence of female high school students. *Research in Social Psychology, 2*(6).

Alderson, E. (2013). *Supporting People with Intellectual Disability to Express Appropriate Sexual Behaviors*. Retrieved from http://www.ndis.gov.au/sites/default/files/documents/5_Supporting_People_with_Intellectual_Disability_to_Express_Appropriate.docx

Alexander, N., & Gomez, M.T. (2017). Pleasure, sex, prohibition, intellectual disability, and dangerous ideas. *An International Journal on Sexual and Reproductive Health And rights, 25*(50), 114-120. doi:10.1080/09688080.2017.1331690

Alexander, R. T., Chester, V., Green, F. N., Gunaratna, I., & Hoare, S. (2015). Arson or fire setting in offenders with intellectual disability: Clinical characteristics, forensic histories, and treatment outcomes. *Journal of Intellectual & Developmental Disability, 40*(2), 1–9. doi:10.3109/13668250.2014.998182

Ali, A., Hassiotis, A., Strydom, A., & King, M. (2012). Self stigma in people with intellectual disabilities and courtesy stigma in family carers: A systematic review. *Research in Developmental Disabilities, 33*(6), 2122–2140. doi:10.1016/j.ridd.2012.06.013 PMID:22784823

Alimovic, S. (2013). Emotional and behavioural problems in children with visual impairment, intellectual and multiple disabilities. *Journal of Intellectual Disability Research, 57*(2), 153–160. doi:10.1111/j.1365-2788.2012.01562.x PMID:22563696

Al-Krenawi, A., Graham, J. R., & Al Gharaibeh, F. (2011). The impact of intellectual disability, caregiver burden, family functioning, marital quality, and sense of coherence. *Disability & Society, 26*(2), 139–150. doi:10.1080/09687599.2011.543861

Allen, D. (2008). The relationship between challenging behaviour and mental ill-health in people with intellectual disabilities: A review of current theories and evidence. *Journal of Intellectual Disabilities*, *12*(4), 267–294. doi:10.1177/1744629508100494 PMID:19074934

Allen, K. D., Wallace, D. P., Renes, D., Bowen, S. L., & Burke, R. V. (2010). Use of video modeling to teach vocational skills to adolescents and young adults with autism spectrum disorders. *Education & Treatment of Children*, *33*(3), 339–349. doi:10.1353/etc.0.0101

Allen, L. B., McHugh, R. K., & Barlow, D. H. (2008). Emotional disorders: A unified protocol. In D. H. Barlow (Ed.), *Clinical handbook of psychological disorders: A step-bystep treatment manual* (4th ed.; pp. 216–249). New York, NY: Guilford Press.

Alnahdi, G. H. (2019). The positive impact of including students with intellectual disabilities in schools: Children's attitudes towards peers with disabilities in Saudi Arabia. *Research in Developmental Disabilities*, 1–7. doi:10.1016/j.ridd.2018.10.004 PMID:30388506

American Association on Intellectual & Developmental Disabilities. (2012) *Definition of Intellectual Disability*. Author.

American Association on Intellectual and Developmental Disabilities. (2011). *What is the AAIDD definition of intellectual disability?* Retrieved from http://www.aaidd.org/IntellectualDisabilityBook/content_7473.cfm?navID=366

American Association on Intellectual and Developmental Disabilities. (2013). *Definition of intellectual disability*. Retrieved from www.aaidd.org

American Association on Intellectual Developmental Disabilities. (2010). *Intellectual disability: Definition, classification, and systems of supports*. Washington, DC: AAIDD.

American Psychiatric Association. (1994). *Diagnostic and Statistical Manual of mental disorders: DSM-IV*. Washington, DC: Author.

American Psychiatric Association. (2012). *Diagnostic and statistical manual of mental disorders (5th. text revision)*. Arlington, VA: Author.

American Psychiatric Association. (2013). *Diagnostic and Statistical Manual of Mental Disorders* (5th ed.). American Psychiatric Publishing, Incorporated.

American Psychiatric Association. (2013). *Diagnostic and statistical manual of mental disorders* (5th ed.). Retrieved from: http://www.dsm5.org/Pages/Default.aspx

American Psychiatric Association. (2013). *Diagnostic and statistical manual of mental disorders* (5th ed.). Washington, DC: Author.

American Psychological Association. (2005). *Assessment of older adults with diminished capacity. A handbook for lawyers*. American Bar Association Commission on Law and Aging – American Psychological Association.

American Psychological Association. (2006). *Assessment of older adults with diminished capacity. A handbook for psychologists*. American Bar Association Commission on Law and Aging – American Psychological Association.

American Psychological Association. (2015). Diagnostic and Statistical Manual of Mental Disorder: Publication manual of the American Psychological Association (5th ed.). Washington, DC: Author.

Anderson, D. J., Lakin, K. C., Hill, B. K., & Chen, T. (1992). Social integration of older persons with mental retardation in residential facilities. *American Journal of Mental Retardation*. PMID:1562307

Andreou, E., Didaskalou, E., & Vlachou, A. (2013). Bully/victim problems among Greek pupils with special educational needs: Associations with loneliness and self-efficacy for peer interactions. *Journal of Research in Special Educational Needs.*

Andrews, G., Henderson, S., & Hall, W. (2001). *Prevalence, comorbidity, disability and service utilisation* (vol. 178). Academic Press.

Andrews, F. M. (1974). Social indicators of perceived life quality. *Social Indicators Research, 1*(3), 279–299. doi:10.1007/BF00303860

Angelopoulou, N., Souftas, V., Sakadamis, A., Matziari, C., Papameletiou, V., & Mandroukas, K. (1999). Gonadal function in young women with Down syndrome. *International Journal of Gynaecology and Obstetrics: the Official Organ of the International Federation of Gynaecology and Obstetrics, 67*(1), 15–21. doi:10.1016/S0020-7292(99)00123-X PMID:10576235

Annalakshmi, N. (2009). Bharathiar University Resilience Scale. In Research Methodology Tools and Techniques, (pp. 105-121). Retrieved from Google Scholar.

APA. (2013). *Diagnostic and statistical manual of mental disorders - fifth edition (dsm-5).* Washington, DC: American Psychiatric Publishing.

Appelbaum, K. L., & Appelbaum, P. S. (1994). Criminal-justice-related competencies in defendants with mental retardation. *The Journal of Psychiatry & Law, 22*(4), 483–503. doi:10.1177/009318539402200402

Aqil, Z., & Ahmed, E. (2014). A comparative study of IQ and EQ in physically disabled and abled adults. *International Journal of Scientific Engineering and Research,* 2347-3878.

Arendt, S. W., & Paez, P. (2014). Managers' Attitudes Towards Employees with Disabilities in the Hospitality Industry. *International Journal of Hospitality & Tourism Administration, 15*(2), 172–190. doi:10.1080/15256480.2014.901065

Arim, R. G., Garner, R. E., Brehaut, J. C., Lach, L. M., MacKenzie, M. J., Rosenbaum, P. L., & Kohen, D. E. (2012). Contextual influences of parenting behaviors for children with neurodevelopmental disorders: Results from a Canadian national survey. *Disability and Rehabilitation, 34*(26), 2222–2233. doi:10.3109/09638288.2012.680650 PMID:22663074

Armatas, V. (2009). Mental retardation: Definitions, etiology, epidemiology and diagnosis. *Journal of Sport and Health Research, 1*(2), 112–122.

Armstrong, K., DeLoatche, K. J., Preece, K. K., & Agazzi, H. (2015). Combining Parent–Child Interaction Therapy and Visual Supports for the Treatment of Challenging Behavior in a Child With Autism and Intellectual Disabilities and Comorbid Epilepsy. *Clinical Case Studies, 14*(1), 3–14. doi:10.1177/1534650114531451

Arthur, M. (1998). *Socio-communicative variables and behaviour states in students with the most severe and multiple disabilities: An observational study* (Unpublished PhD dissertation). Macquarie University, Sydney, Australia.

Atik, G., & Guneri, O. Y. (2013). Bullying and victimization: Predictive role of individual, parental, and academic factors. *School Psychology International, 34*(6), 658–673. doi:10.1177/0143034313479699

Axmon, A., Sandberg, M., & Ahlström, G. (2017). Gender differences in psychiatric diagnoses in older people with intellectual disability: A register study. *BMC Psychiatry, 17*(1), 192.

Azad, G., Blacher, J., & Marcoulides, G. A. (2013). Mothers of children with developmental disabilities: Stress in early and middle childhood. *Research in Developmental Disabilities, 34*(10), 3449–3459. doi:10.1016/j.ridd.2013.07.009 PMID:23920028

Azar, M., & Badr, L. K. (2010). Predictors of coping in parents of children with an intellectual disability: Comparison between Lebanese mothers and fathers. *Journal of Pediatric Nursing*, *25*(1), 46–56. doi:10.1016/j.pedn.2008.11.001 PMID:20117676

Azeem, M.W., Dogar, I.A., & Shah, S. (2013). Anxiety and Depression among Parents of Children with Intellectual Disability in Pakistan. *Journal of the Canadian Academy of Child and Adolescent Psychiatry*, *22*(4), 290-296.

Azrin, N. H., & Foxx, R. M. (1971). A rapid method of toilet training the institutionalized retarded. *Journal of Applied Behavior Analysis*, *4*(2), 89–99. doi:10.1901/jaba.1971.4-89 PMID:16795291

Bachrach, S. (2004). In the name of public health – Nazi racial hygiene. *The New England Journal of Medicine*, *351*(5), 417–420. doi:10.1056/NEJMp048136 PMID:15282346

Baer, D. M., Wolf, M. M., & Risley, T. R. (1968). Some current dimensions of applied behavior analysis. *Journal of Applied Behavior Analysis*, *1*(1), 91–97. doi:10.1901/jaba.1968.1-91 PMID:16795165

Bagner, D. M., & Eyberg, S. M. (2007). Parent–child interaction therapy for disruptive behavior in children with mental retardation: A randomized controlled trial. *Journal of Clinical Child and Adolescent Psychology*, *36*(3), 418–429. doi:10.1080/15374410701448448 PMID:17658985

Bailey, D. B. Jr, Golden, R. N., Roberts, J., & Ford, A. (2007). Maternal depression and developmental disability: Research critique. *Mental Retardation and Developmental Disabilities Research Reviews*, *13*(4), 321–329. doi:10.1002/mrdd.20172 PMID:17979207

Baines, S., Emerson, E., Robertson, J., & Hatton, C. (2018). Sexual activity and sexual health among young adults with and without mild/moderate intellectual disability. *BMC Public Health*, *18*(1), 667. doi:10.118612889-018-5572-9

Baker, B. L., Landen, S. J., & Kashima, K. J. (1991). Effects of parent training on families of children with mental retardation: Increased burden or generalized benefit? *American Journal of Mental Retardation*. PMID:1930946

Baker, B. L., Blacher, J., Crnic, K. A., & Edelbrock, C. (2002). Behavior problems and parenting stress in families of three-year-old children with and without developmental delays. *American Journal of Mental Retardation*, *107*(6), 433–444. doi:10.1352/0895-8017(2002)107<0433:BPAPSI>2.0.CO;2 PMID:12323068

Baker, B. L., Blacher, J., & Olsson, M. B. (2005). Preschool children with and without developmental delay: Behaviour problems, parents' optimism and well-being. *Journal of Intellectual Disability Research*, *49*(8), 575–590. doi:10.1111/j.1365-2788.2005.00691.x PMID:16011551

Baker, B. L., McIntyre, L. L., Blacher, J., Crnic, K., Edelbrock, C., & Low, C. (2003). Pre-school children with and without developmental delay: Behaviour problems and parenting stress over time. *Journal of Intellectual Disability Research*, *47*(4-5), 217–230. doi:10.1046/j.1365-2788.2003.00484.x PMID:12787154

Baker, B. L., Neece, C. L., Fenning, R. M., Crnic, K. A., & Blacher, J. (2010). Mental disorders in five-year-old children with or without developmental delay: Focus on ADHD. *Journal of Clinical Child and Adolescent Psychology*, *39*(4), 492–505. doi:10.1080/15374416.2010.486321 PMID:20589561

Baker, B., & Brightman, A. (2004). *Steps to independence: Teaching everyday skills to children with special needs* (4th ed.). Baltimore, MD: Paul H. Brookes.

Bakken, T. L., Helverschou, S. B., Eilertsen, D. E., Heggelund, T., Myrbakk, E., & Martinsen, H. (2010). Psychiatric disorders in adolescents and adults with autism and intellectual disability: A representative study in one county in Norway. *Research in Developmental Disabilities*, *31*(6), 1669–1677. doi:10.1016/j.ridd.2010.04.009 PMID:20493660

Balderian, N. (1991). Sexual abuse of people with developmental disabilities. *Sexuality and Disability*, *9*(4), 323–335. doi:10.1007/BF01102020

Baldry, A. C., & Farrington, D. (2000). Bullies and delinquents: Personal characteristics and parental styles. *Journal of Community & Applied Social Psychology*, *10*(1), 17–31. doi:10.1002/(SICI)1099-1298(200001/02)10:1<17::AID-CASP526>3.0.CO;2-M

Bandura, A. (1969). *Principles of Behavior Modification*. New York: Holt, Rinehart and Winston.

Bandura, A. (1991). Social cognitive theory of self-regulation. *Theories of Cognitive Self-Regulation*, *50*, 248–287.

Banks, R. (1997). *Bullying in Schools*. Washington, DC: U.S. Government Printing Office.

Barak-Levy, Y., & Atzaba-Poria, N. (2013). Paternal versus maternal coping styles with child diagnosis of developmental delay. *Research in Developmental Disabilities*, *34*(6), 2040–2046. doi:10.1016/j.ridd.2013.02.026 PMID:23584184

Barger, E., Wacker, J., Macy, R., & Parish, S. (2009). Sexual Assault Prevention for Women With Intellectual Disabilities: A Critical Review of the Evidence. *Intellectual and Developmental Disabilities*, *47*(4), 249–262. doi:10.1352/1934-9556-47.4.249 PMID:19650680

Barker, E. T., Greenberg, J. S., Seltzer, M. M., & Almeida, D. M. (2012). Daily Stress and Cortisol Patterns in Parents of Adult Children with a Serious Mental Illness. *Journal of Health Psychology*, *31*(1), 130–134. doi:10.1037/a0025325 PMID:21895369

Baroff, G. S., Gunn, M., & Hayes, S. (2004). Legal issues. In W. Lindsay, J. Taylor, & P. Sturmey (Eds.), *Offenders with developmental disabilities* (pp. 37–65). West Sussex, UK: Wiley. doi:10.1002/9780470713440.ch3

Barron, P., Hassiotis, A., & Banes, J. (2002). Offenders with intellectual disability: The size of the problem and therapeutic outcomes. *Journal of Intellectual Disability Research*, *46*(6), 454–463. doi:10.1046/j.1365-2788.2002.00432.x PMID:12354316

Basser, L. A., & Jones, M. (2002). The Disability Discrimination Act 1992 (Cth): A three-dimensional approach to operationalising human rights. *Melb. UL Rev.*, *26*, 254.

Bauman, S. (2004). *Parents of children with mental retardation, coping mechanisms and support needs*. College Park: Dissertation, Faculty of the Graduate School of University of Maryland.

Bauminger, N., Solomon, M., & Rogers, S. J. (2010). Externalizing and internalizing behaviors in ASD. *Autism Research*, *3*(3), 101–112. doi:10.1002/aur.131 PMID:20575109

Bazzano, A., Wolfe, C., Zylowska, L., Wang, S., Schuster, E., Barrett, C., & Lehrer, D. (2015). Mindfulness Based Stress Reduction (MBSR) for parents and caregivers of individuals with developmental disabilities: A community-based approach. *Journal of Child and Family Studies*, *24*(2), 298–308. doi:10.100710826-013-9836-9

Beail, N. (2002). Interrogative suggestibility, memory and intellectual disability. *Journal of Applied Research in Intellectual Disabilities*, *15*(2), 129–137. doi:10.1046/j.1468-3148.2002.00108.x

Bear, G. G., Mantz, L. S., Glutting, J. J., Yang, C., & Boyer, D. E. (2015). Differences in bullying victimization between students with and without disabilities. *School Psychology Review*, *44*(1), 98–116. doi:10.17105/SPR44-1.98-116

Beavers, G. A., Iwata, B. A., & Lerman, D. C. (2013). Thirty years of research on the functional analysis of problem behavior. *Journal of Applied Behavior Analysis*, *46*(1), 1. doi:10.1111/j.1365-2788.2006.00948.x

Begg, S., Vos, T., Barker, B., Stevenson, C., Stanley, L., & Lopez, A. (2007). *Burden of disease and injury in Australia, 2003*. Australian Institute of Health and Welfare.

Beirne, S. M., Patton, J. R., & Kim, S. H. (2006). *Mental retardation: An introduction to intellectual disabilities*. Upper Saddle River, NJ: Pearson Merrill Prentice Hall.

Bellini, S., & Akullian, J. (2007). A meta-analysis of video modeling and video self-modeling interventions for children and adolescents with autism spectrum disorders. *Exceptional Children*, *73*(3), 264–287. doi:10.1177/001440290707300301

Belva, B. C., Matson, J. L., Sipes, M., & Bamburg, J. W. (2012). An examination of specific communication deficits in adults with profound intellectual disabilities. *Research in Developmental Disabilities*, *33*(2), 525–529. doi:10.1016/j.ridd.2011.10.019 PMID:22119701

Benderix, Y., & Sivberg, B. (2007). Siblings' experiences of having a brother or sister with autism and mental retardation: A case study of 14 siblings from five families. *Journal of Pediatric Nursing*, *22*(5), 410–418. doi:10.1016/j.pedn.2007.08.013 PMID:17889735

Benomir, A. M., Nicolson, R. I., & Beail, N. (2016). Attitudes towards people with intellectual disability in the UK and Libya: A cross-cultural comparison. *Research in Developmental Disabilities*, *51-52*, 1–9. doi:10.1016/j.ridd.2015.12.009 PMID:26773692

Bensberg, G. J., Colwell, C. N., & Cassel, R. (1965). Teaching the profoundly retarded self-help activities by behavior shaping techniques. *American Journal of Mental Deficiency*, *69*, 674–679. PMID:14286827

Benson, B. A., & Brooks, W. T. (2008). Aggressive challenging behaviour and intellectual disability. *Current Opinion in Psychiatry*, *21*(5), 454–458. doi:10.1097/YCO.0b013e328306a090 PMID:18650686

Benson, B. A., & Fuchs, C. (1999). Anger arousing situations and coping responses of aggressive adults with intellectual disability. *Journal of Intellectual & Developmental Disability*, *24*(3), 207–214. doi:10.1080/13668259900033991

Benson, B. A., & Ivins, J. (1992). Anger, depression and self-concept in adults with mental retardation. *Journal of Intellectual Disability Research*, *36*(2), 169–175. doi:10.1111/j.1365-2788.1992.tb00492.x PMID:1591500

Bergen, D. C. (2008). Effects of poverty on cognitive function: A hidden neurologic epidemic. *Neurology*, *71*(6), 447–451. doi:10.1212/01.wnl.0000324420.03960.36 PMID:18678828

Berkson, G., Tupa, M., & Sherman, L. (2001). Early development of stereotyped and self-injurious behaviors: Incidence. *American Journal of Mental Retardation*, *106*(6), 539–547. doi:10.1352/0895-8017(2001)106<0539:EDOSAS>2.0.CO;2 PMID:11708939

Berman, H., Harris, D., Enright, R., Gilpin, M., Cathers, T., & Bukovy, G. (1999). Sexuality and the adolescent with a physical disability: Understandings and misunderstandings. *Issues in Comprehensive Pediatric Nursing*, *22*(4), 183–196. doi:10.1080/014608699265275 PMID:10827606

Bernard-Opitz, V., Sriram, N., & Nakhoda-Sapuan, S. (2001). Enhancing social problem solving in children with autism and normal children through computer-assisted instruction. *Journal of Autism and Developmental Disorders*, *31*(4), 377–384. doi:10.1023/A:1010660502130 PMID:11569584

Bernard, S. H. (2009). Mental health and behavioural problems in children and adolescents with learning disabilities. *Psychiatry*, *8*(10), 387–390. doi:10.1016/j.mppsy.2009.06.017

Berry, B. S., & Kymar, K. R. (2012). Human resource professionals' perception on disability related barriers to employment of individuals with intellectual disability. *The Indian Journal of Occupational Therapy*, *44*(2).

Berry, P. B. (1972). Comprehension of possessive and present continuous sentences by nonretarded, mildly retarded, and severely retarded children. *American Journal of Mental Deficiency*, *76*, 540–544. PMID:5012135

Berthold, K., & Hoover, J. (2000). Correlates of bullying and victimization among intermediate students in Midwestern USA. *School Psychology International, 21*(1), 65–79. doi:10.1177/0143034300211005

Bharath Raj, J. (1971). AHSH Norms on seguin form board with Indian Children. *J. of AHSH, II*, 34–39.

Bharath Raj, J. (2004). *The developmental screening test manual.4th rd.* Mysore: SwayamsiddhaPrakashana.

Bhat, A.M., Sharma, V. & Jena, S.P. (2013). Managing stress in parents of children with intellectual disability. *Indian Journal of Health and Well-Being, 4*(9), 1790-1793.

Bickenbach, J. E. (1993). *Physical disability and social policy*. Toronto, ON: University of Toronto Press.

Bigby, C. (1997). Parental substitutes? The role of siblings in the lives of older people with intellectual disability. *Journal of Gerontological Social Work, 29*(1), 3–21. doi:10.1300/J083v29n01_02

Bigby, C. (2004). *Ageing with a Lifelong Disability: A Guide to Practice, Program and Policy Issues for Human Services Professionals*. London: Jessica Kingsley.

Bigby, C., & Balandin, S. (2004). Issues in researching the ageing of people with intellectual disability. In E. Emerson, C. Hatton, T. Thompson, & T. R. Parmenter (Eds.), *The International Handbook of Applied Research in Intellectual Disabilities* (pp. 221–236). West Sussex, UK: Wiley. doi:10.1002/9780470713198.ch10

Bijou, S. W., Peterson, R. F., & Ault, M. H. (1968). A method to integrate descriptive and experimental field studies at the level of data and empirical concepts. *Journal of Applied Behavior Analysis, 1*(2), 175–191. doi:10.1901/jaba.1968.1-175 PMID:16795175

Blacher, J. (1984). Sequential stages of parental adjustment to the birth of a child with handicaps: Fact or artifact? *Mental Retardation, 22*, 55–68. PMID:6234448

Blacher, J., Baker, B. L., & Eisenhower, A. S. (2009). Student–teacher relationship stability across early school years for children with intellectual disability or typical development. *American Journal on Intellectual and Developmental Disabilities, 114*(5), 322–339. doi:10.1352/1944-7558-114.5.322 PMID:19928015

Blacher, J., & Bromley, B. E. (1990). Correlates of out-of-home placement of handicapped children: Who places and why? *Journal of Children in Contemporary Society, 21*, 3–41. doi:10.1300/J274v21n03_02

Blacher, J., Neece, C. L., & Paczkowski, E. (2005). Families and intellectual disability. *Current Opinion in Psychiatry, 18*(5), 507–513. doi:10.1097/01.yco.0000179488.92885.e8 PMID:16639109

Black, L., Cullen, C., & Novaco, R. W. (1997). Anger assessment for people with mild learning disabilities in secure settings. In B. S. Kroese, D. Dagnan, & K. Loumidis (Eds.), *Cognitive-behaviour therapy for people with learning disabilities*. London: Routledge.

Black, R. S., & Kammes, R. R. (2019). Restrictions, Power, Companionship, and Intimacy: A Metasynthesis of People With Intellectual Disability Speaking About Sex and Relationships. *Intellectual and Developmental Disabilities, 57*(3), 212–233. doi:10.1352/1934-9556-57.3.212 PMID:31120408

Blake, J. J., Lund, E. M., Zhou, Q., Kwok, O., & Benz, M. (2012). National prevalence rates of bully victimization among students with disabilities in the United States. *School Psychology Quarterly, 27*(4), 2100–2222. doi:10.1037pq0000008 PMID:23294235

Block, P. (2000). Sexuality, fertility and danger: Twentieth-century images of women with cognitive disabilities. *Sexuality and Disability, 18*(4), 239–254. doi:10.1023/A:1005642226413

Blumberg, E. R., Horner, R. H., Irvin, L. K., Laverty, R., Lucyshyn, J. M., & Sprague, J. R. (2004). Validating the construct of coercion in family routines: Expanding the unit of analysis in behavioral assessment with families of children with developmental disabilities. *Research and Practice for Persons with Severe Disabilities*, *29*(2), 104–121. doi:10.2511/rpsd.29.2.104 PMID:26321883

Boer, D. P., McKnight, J. M., Kinlyside, A. M., & Chan, J. P. (2018). Assessing and treating offenders with Intellectual Disabilities. In M. Ternes, P. R. Magaletta, & M. W. Patry (Eds.), *The Practice of Correctional Psychology* (pp. 71–101). Springer. doi:10.1007/978-3-030-00452-1_4

Bonham, G. S., Basehart, S., Schalock, R. L., Marchand, C. B., Kirchner, N., & Rumenap, J. M. (2004). Consumer-based quality of life assessment: The Maryland Ask Me! Project. *Mental Retardation*, *42*(5), 338–355. doi:10.1352/0047-6765(2004)42<338:CQOLAT>2.0.CO;2 PMID:15335259

Bonnie, R. J. (1990). The competence of criminal defendants with mental retardation to participate in their own defense. *The Journal of Criminal Law & Criminology*, *81*(3), 419–446. doi:10.2307/1143845

Boo, L. S. H., & Nie, Y. (2018). Attitude towards persons with intellectual disability scale: Further development. *Current Psychology (New Brunswick, N.J.)*, *37*(4), 760–768. doi:10.100712144-017-9560-5

Boone, K. B. (Ed.). (2007). *Assessment of feigned cognitive impairment: A neuropsychological perspective*. New York: Guilford Press.

Booth, T., & Booth, W. (1998). *Growing up with parents who have learning difficulties*. London: Routledge.

Borromeo, A. D. (2001). Mental retardation and the death penalty. *Loyola Journal of Public Interest Law*, *3*, 175.

Borthwick-Duffy, S. A., & Eyman, R. K. (1990). Who are the dually diagnosed? *American Journal of Mental Retardation*. PMID:2340136

Bouras, N. (2011). Mental health problems and related issues for people with developmental and intellectual disability. *Current Opinion in Psychiatry, 24*(5), 365-366.

Bouras, N., & Holt, G. (2007). *Psychiatric and behavioural disorders in developmental disabilities and mental retardation*. Cambridge, UK: Cambridge University Press.

Bourke, J., Ricciardo, B., Bebbington, A., Aiberti, K., Jacoby, P., Dyke, P., . . . Leonard, H. (2008). Physical and mental health in mothers of children with down syndrome. *The Journal of Pediatrics, 153*(3), 320-326.

Bourke-Taylor, H., Law, M., Howie, L., & Pallant, J. F. (2010). Development of the Child's Challenging Behaviour Scale (CCBS) for mothers of school-aged children with disabilities. *Child: Care, Health and Development*, *36*(4), 491–498. doi:10.1111/j.1365-2214.2009.01055.x PMID:20047597

Bourke-Taylor, H., Pallant, J. F., Law, M., & Howie, L. (2012). Predicting mental health among mothers of school-aged children with developmental disabilities: The relative contribution of child, maternal and environmental factors. *Research in Developmental Disabilities*, *32*(6), 1732–1740. doi:10.1016/j.ridd.2012.04.011 PMID:22699247

Bowe, F. (1978). *Handicapping America: Barriers to Disabled People*. New York: Harper and Row.

Bowen, E., & Swift, C. (2017). The Prevalence and Correlates of Partner Violence Used and Experienced by Adults With Intellectual Disabilities: A Systematic Review and Call to Action. *Trauma, Violence & Abuse*, *1*. doi:10.1177/1524838017728707 PMID:29333986

Bowlby, J. (1988a). *A secure base: clinical applications of attachment theory*. Hove, NY: Brunner-Routledge, Taylor & Francis Group.

Bowlby, J. (1988b). *A secure base: Parent-child attachment and healthy human development.* New York: Basic Books.

Bowlby, J. (1989). *The Making and Breaking of Affectional Bonds.* New York: Routledge, Taylor and Francis Group.

Boyes, M. E., Bowes, L., Cluver, L. C., Ward, C. L., & Badcock, N. A. (2014). Bullying victimization, internalizing symptoms, and conduct problems in South African children and adolescents: A longitudinal investigation. *Journal of Abnormal Child Psychology, 42*(8), 1313–1324. doi:10.100710802-014-9888-3 PMID:24882504

Boyle, C.A. & Lary, J.M. (1996). Prevalence of selected developmental disabilities in children 3-10 years of age: The Metropolitan Atlanta Developmental Disabilities Surveillance Program, 1991. *Morbidity and Mortality Weekly Report.*

Braddock, D., & Parish, S. L. (2002). *An institutional history of disability.* Washington, DC: American Association of Mental Retardation.

Bradley, E., Burke, L., Drummond, C., Korossy, M., Lunsky, Y., & Morris, S. (2010). *Guidelines for managing the patient with developmental disability in the emergency room.* Retrieved fromwww.camh.net/Publications/Resources_for_Professionals/guidelines_manageclient_emerg2 003.pdf

Bradley, R. H., Corwyn, R. F., Burchinal, M., McAdoo, H. P., & Garcia Coll, C. (2001). The home environments of children in the United States Part II: Relations with behavioral development through age thirteen. *Child Development, 72*(6), 1868–1886. doi:10.1111/1467-8624.t01-1-00383 PMID:11768150

Bradshaw, C. P., Stuart, E. A., & Zablotsky, B. (2013). The association between mental health, stress, and coping supports in mothers of children with autism spectrum disorders. *Journal of Autism and Developmental Disorders, 43*(6), 1380–1393. doi:10.100710803-012-1693-7 PMID:23100053

Bradshaw, C. P., Waasdorp, T. E., & Johnson, S. L. (2015). Overlapping verbal, relational, physical, and electronic forms of bullying in adolescence: Influence of school context. *Journal of Clinical Child and Adolescent Psychology, 44*(3), 494–508. doi:10.1080/15374416.2014.893516 PMID:24738548

Braithwaite, D. O., & Thompson, T. L. (1999). *Handbook of Communication and People With Disabilities: Research and Application.* Retrieved from https://books.google.co.in/books?isbn=1135675805

Brehaut, J. C., Kohen, D. E., Raina, P., Walter, S. D., Russell, D. J., Swinton, M., ... Rosenbaum, P. (2004). The health of primary caregivers of children with cerebral palsy: How does it compare with that of other Canadian caregivers? *Pediatrics, 4*(2), e182–e191. doi:10.1542/peds.114.2.e182 PMID:15286255

Breslau, N., & Prabucki, K. (1987). Siblings of disabled children: Effects of chronic stress in the family. *Archives of General Psychiatry, 44*(12), 1040–1046. doi:10.1001/archpsyc.1987.01800240014003 PMID:2961319

Breslau, N., Staruch, K. S., & Mortimer, E. A. (1982). Psychological distress in mothers of disabled children. *American Journal of Diseases of Children, 136*, 682–686. PMID:6213143

Brighi, A., Guarini, A., Melotti, G., Galli, S., & Genta, M. L. (2012). Predictors of victimization across direct bullying, indirect bullying and cyberbullying. *Emotional & Behavioural Difficulties, 17*(3-4), 375–388. doi:10.1080/13632752.2012.704684

Britton, L. N., Carr, J. E., Kellum, K. K., Dozier, C. L., & Weil, T. M. (2000). A variation of noncontingent reinforcement in the treatment of aberrant behavior. *Research in Developmental Disabilities, 21*(6), 425–435. doi:10.1016/S0891-4222(00)00056-1 PMID:11153827

Brooks, A., Todd, A. W., Tofflemoyer, S., & Horner, R. H. (2003). Use of functional assessment and a self-management system to increase academic engagement and work completion. *Journal of Positive Behavior Interventions, 5*(3), 144–152. doi:10.1177/10983007030050030301

Browder, D. M., Wood, L., Thompson, J., & Ribuffo, C. (2014). *Evidence-based practices for students with severe dis abilities* (Document No. IC-3). Retrieved from University of Florida, Collaboration for Effective Educator, Development, Accountability, and Reform Center website: http://ceedar.education.ufl.edu/tools/innovation-configurations/

Brown & Randel. (1997). *The Individual with Intellectual Disabilities and Sex Education: Perspectives of Involved Adults*. Presented at the *7th Annual Meeting of the International Society for the Study of Human Subjectivity*, Columbia.

Brown, I., & Brown, R. I. (2009). Choice as an aspect of quality of life for people with intellectual disabilities. *Journal of Policy and Practice in Intellectual Disabilities, 6*, 10 17.

Brown, J. (2011). The Skills System instructor's guide: An emotion regulation skills curriculum for all learning abilities. Bloomington, IN: IUniverse.

Brown, R. I. (1998). *Conceptualisation of quality of life: An overview*. Paper presented at the 1998 Australian Society for the Study of Intellectual Disability (ASSID) Conference: Conceptualisation of quality of life workshop, Flinders University of South Australia, Adelaide, Australia.

Brown, B. J., Mansell, J., & Kozma, A. (2007). Deinstitutionalization in intellectual disabilities. *Current Opinion in Psychiatry, 20*(5), 437–442. doi:10.1097/YCO.0b013e32827b14ab PMID:17762584

Browne, G., & Bramston, P. (1998). Stress and the quality of life in the parents of young people with intellectual disabilities. *Journal of Psychiatric and Mental Health Nursing, 5*(5), 415-421.

Brown, H., & Stein, J. (1997). Sexual abuse perpetrated by men with intellectual disabilities: A comparative study. *Journal of Intellectual Disability Research, 41*(3), 215–224. doi:10.1111/j.1365-2788.1997.tb00700.x PMID:9219070

Brown, I. (2006). *Family Quality of Life Survey: Main caregivers of people with intellectual or developmental disabilities*. Toronto: Surrey Place Centre.

Brown, I., & Brown, R. I. (2003). *Quality of Life and Disability: An Approach for Community Practitioners*. London, UK: Jessica Kingsley.

Brown, M. A., McIntyre, L. L., Crnic, K. A., Baker, B. L., & Blacher, J. (2011). Preschool children with and without developmental delay: Risk, parenting, and child demandingness. *Journal of Mental Health Research in Intellectual Disabilities, 4*(3), 206–226. doi:10.1080/19315864.2011.596990 PMID:22778798

Brown, M., & McCann, E. (2019). The views and experiences of families and direct care support workers regarding the expression of sexuality by adults with intellectual disabilities: A narrative review of the international research evidence. *Research in Developmental Disabilities, 90*, 80–91. doi:10.1016/j.ridd.2019.04.012 PMID:31082682

Brown, N., McLinden, M., & Porter, J. (1998). Sensory needs. In P. Lacey & C. Ouvry (Eds.), *People with profound and multiple learning disabilities: A collaborative approach to meeting complex needs* (pp. 29–38). London: David Fulton.

Brown, R. I. (1995). Measuring new dimensions through quality of life: The personal equation. *Evaluation Journal of Australasia, 7*(1), 14–23.

Brown, R. I., Bayer, M. B., & MacFarlane, C. (1989). *Rehabilitation programs: Performance and Quality of Life of adults with developmental handicaps*. Toronto: Lugus Productions.

Brown, R. I., & Brown, I. (2005). The application of quality of life. *Journal of Intellectual Disability Research, 49*(10), 718–727. doi:10.1111/j.1365-2788.2005.00740.x PMID:16162116

Bruce, E. J., Schultz, C. L., Smyrnios, K. X., & Schultz, N. C. (1994). Grieving related to development: A preliminary comparison of three age cohorts of parents of children with intellectual disability. *The British Journal of Medical Psychology*, *67*(1), 37–52. doi:10.1111/j.2044-8341.1994.tb01769.x PMID:7515655

Bruininks, H., Hill, B. K., & Morreau, L. E. (1988). Prevalence and implications of maladaptive behaviors and dual diagnosis in residential and other service programs. In Mental Retardation and Mental Health (pp. 3-29). Springer.

Buckley, S., Bird, G., Sacks, B., & Archer, T. (2002). A comparison of mainstream and special school education for teenagers with Down syndrome: Effects of social and academic development. *Down's Syndrome: Research and Practice*, *2*(2), 46–54.

Bush, S. S.Planning Committee. (2005). Independent and court-ordered forensic neuropsychological examinations: Official statement of the National Academy of Neuropsychology. *Archives of Clinical Neuropsychology*, *20*(8), 997–1007. doi:10.1016/j.acn.2005.06.003 PMID:16076547

Butterfield, N., Arthur, M., & Linfoot, K. (1992). Meeting communication needs in communication programming for students with severe intellectual disability: The creating communicative contexts manual. *Special Education Perspectives*, *1*(1), 35–43.

Byrne, G. (2018). Prevalence and psychological sequelae of sexual abuse among individuals with an intellectual disability: A review of the recent literature. *Journal of Intellectual & Developmental Disability*, *22*(3), 294–310. doi:10.1177/1744629517698844 PMID:30134783

Cabrera, N. J., Shannon, J. D., & Tamis-LeMonda, C. (2007). Fathers' influence on their children's cognitive and emotional development: From toddlers to pre-K. *Applied Developmental Science*, *11*(4), 208–213. doi:10.1080/10888690701762100

Calitz, F. J. (2011). Psycho-legal challenges facing the mentally retarded rape victim. *South African Journal of Psychiatry*, *17*(3), 66–72. doi:10.4102ajpsychiatry.v17i3.280

Camp, B. W., Broman, S. H., Nichols, P. L., & Leff, M. (1998). Maternal and neonatal risk factors for mental retardation: Defining the "at-risk" child. *Early Human Development*, *50*(2), 159–173. doi:10.1016/S0378-3732(97)00034-9 PMID:9483389

Campbell-Sills, L., & Barlow, D. H. (2007). Incorporating emotion regulation into conceptualizations and treatments of anxiety and mood disorders. In J. J. Gross (Ed.), *Handbook of Emotion Regulation* (pp. 542–559). New York: Guilford Press.

Campos, J. J., Campos, R. G., & Barrett, K. C. (1989). Emergent themes in the study of emotional development and emotion regulation. *Developmental Psychology*, *25*(3), 394–402. doi:10.1037/0012-1649.25.3.394

Cantwell, J., Muldoon, O. T., & Gallagher, S. (2014). Social support and mastery influence the association between stress and poor physical health in parents caring for children with developmental disabilities. *Research in Developmental Disabilities*, *35*(9), 2215–2223. doi:10.1016/j.ridd.2014.05.012 PMID:24927515

Caplan, B., Neece, C. L., & Baker, B. L. (2015). Developmental level and psychopathology: Comparing children with developmental delays to chronological and mental age matched controls. *Research in Developmental Disabilities*, *37*, 143–151. doi:10.1016/j.ridd.2014.10.045 PMID:25498740

Cappadocia, M. C., Weiss, J. A., & Pepler, D. (2012). Bullying experiences among children and youth with autism spectrum disorders. *Journal of Autism and Developmental Disorders*, *42*(2), 266–277. doi:10.100710803-011-1241-x PMID:21499672

Carbone-Lopez, K., Esbensen, F. A., & Brick, B. T. (2010). Correlates and consequences of peer victimization: Gender differences in direct and indirect forms of bullying. *Youth Violence and Juvenile Justice*, *8*(4), 332–350. doi:10.1177/1541204010362954

Card, N. A., & Hodges, E. V. E. (2008). Peer victimization among schoolchildren: Correlations, causes, consequences, and considerations in assessment and intervention. *School Psychology Quarterly*, *23*(4), 451–461. doi:10.1037/a0012769

Carew, M. T., Braathen, S. H., Swartz, L., Hunt, X., & Rohleder, P. (2017). The sexual lives of people with disabilities within low- and middle-income countries: A scoping study of studies published in English. *Global Health Action*, *10*(1), 1337342. doi:10.1080/16549716.2017.1337342 PMID:28678682

Carey, A. C. (2010). *On the margins of citizenship: Intellectual disability and civil rights in twentieth-century America*. Philadelphia, PA: Temple University Press.

Carlesimo, G. A., Marotta, L., & Vicari, S. (1997). Long-term memory in mental retardation: Evidence for a specific impairment in subjects with Down's syndrome. *Neuropsychologia*, *35*(1), 71–79. doi:10.1016/S0028-3932(96)00055-3 PMID:8981379

Carlson, I. W., & Cornell, D. W. (2008). Differences between persistent and desistent middle school bullies. *School Psychology International*, *29*(4), 442–451. doi:10.1177/0143034308096433

Carney, A., & Merrell, K. (2001). Bullying in schools: Perspectives on understanding and preventing an international problem. *School Psychology International*, *21*(3), 364–382. doi:10.1177/0143034301223011

Carr, J. (2004). *Understanding intellectual disability and health*. Retrieved from http://www.intellectualdisability.info/mental-health/behaviour-management

Carr, A., Linehan, C., O'Reilly, G., Walsh, P. N., & McEvoy, J. (Eds.). (2016). *The handbook of intellectual disability and clinical psychology practice*. Routledge. doi:10.4324/9781315739229

Carr, E. G., Horner, R. H., & Turnbull, A. P. (1999). *Positive Behavior Support for People with Developmental Disabilities: A Research Synthesis*. American Association on Mental Retardation.

Carr, E., Horner, R., Turnbull, A., Marquis, J., McLaughlin, D., & McAtee, M. (1999). *Positive behavior support for people with developmental disabilities: A research synthesis*. Washington, DC: American Association on Mental Retardation.

Carr, E., Levin, L., McConnachie, G., Carlson, J., Kemp, D., & Smith, C. (1994). *Communication-based intervention for problem behavior*. Baltimore, MD: Paul H. Brookes.

Carrier, S. (2007). Understanding social and professional integration as an adjustment process: Contribution to a theory of coadaptation. *Intellectual and Developmental Disabilities*, *45*(1), 10–22. doi:10.1352/1934-9556(2007)45[10:USAPIA]2.0.CO;2 PMID:17428122

Carter, B. B., & Spencer, V. G. (2006). The Fear Factor: Bullying and Students with Disabilities. *International Journal of Special Education*, *21*(1). Retrieved from http://www.forockids.org/PDF Docs/Bullying.pdf

Carter, M., & Hook, J. (1998). Communication programming for students with high support needs: A model for deciding what to teach. *Special Education Perspectives*, *7*(1), 42–55.

Carulla, L. S., Reed, G. M., Vaezazizi, L. M., Cooper, S. N., Leal, R. M., Bertelli, M., ... Saxena, S. (2011). Intellectual developmental disorders: Towards a new name, definition and framework for "mental retardation/intellectual disability. *World Psychiatry; Official Journal of the World Psychiatric Association (WPA)*, *10*(3), 175–180. doi:10.1002/j.2051-5545.2011.tb00045.x PMID:21991267

Cascella, P. W. (2004). *Receptive communication abilities among adults with significant intellectual disability*. Taylor & Francis Ltd.

Cascella, P. W. (2006). Standardised speech-language tests and students with intellectual disability: A review of normative data. *Journal of Intellectual & Developmental Disability, 31*(2), 120–124. doi:10.1080/13668250600681503 PMID:16782597

Cassidy, S. B., & Morris, C. A. (2001). Behavioral phenotypes in genetic syndromes: Genetic clues to human behavior. *Advances in Pediatrics, 49*, 59–86. PMID:12214780

Cea, C. D., & Fisher, C. B. (2003). Health care decision-making by adults with mental retardation. *Journal Information, 41*(2). PMID:12622524

Census of India. (2011). *Central Statistics Office Ministry of Statistics & Programme Implementation Government of India*. Retrieved from: http://mospi.nic.in/Mospi_New/site/home.aspx

Cermak, S. A., & Aberson, J. R. (1998). Social skills in children with learning disabilities. *Occupational Therapy in Mental Health, 13*(4), 1–24. doi:10.1300/J004v13n04_01

Chadwick, O., Kusel, Y., Cuddy, M., & Taylor, E. (2005). Psychiatric diagnoses and behaviour problems from childhood to early adolescence in young people with severe intellectual disabilities. *Psychological Medicine, 35*(5), 751-760.

Chandravanshi, G., Sharma, K. K., Jilowa, C. S., Meena, P. S., Jain, M., & Prakash, O. (2017). Prevalence of depression in mothers of intellectually disabled children: A cross-sectional study. *Medical Journal of Dr. D.Y. Patil Vidyapeeth, 10*(2), 156–161.

Chan, J. B., & Sigafoos, J. (2001). Does respite care reduce parental stress in families with developmentally disabled children? *Child and Youth Care Forum, 30*(5), 253–263. doi:10.1023/A:1014467226528

Chapman, R. A., Shedlack, K. J., & France, J. (2006). Stop-think-relax: An adapted self control training strategy for individuals with mental retardation and coexisting psychiatric illness. *Cognitive and Behavioral Practice, 13*(3), 205–214. doi:10.1016/j.cbpra.2005.08.002

Charach, A., Pepler, D., & Ziegler, S. (1995). Bullying at school. *Education Canada, 37*, 12–18.

Chaturvedi, S. K., & Malhotra, S. (1984). A follow up study of mental retardation focussing parental attitudes. *Indian Journal of Psychiatry, 26*(4), 370–376. PMID:21966015

Chavan, B. S., & Rozatkar, A. S. (2014). Intellectual disability in India: Charity to right based. *Indian Journal of Psychiatry, 56*(2), 113–116. doi:10.4103/0019-5545.130477 PMID:24891695

Chawner, S., Owen, M., Holmans, P., Raymond, L., Skuse, D., Hall, J., . . . Consortium, I.-I. (2019). Genotype-phenotype relationships in children with copy number variants associated with high neuropsychiatric risk: findings from the intellectual disability & mental health: assessing the genomic impact on neurodevelopment (imagine-id) study. *Biorxiv*, 535708.

Cheslock, M. A., Barton-Hulsey, A., Romski, M., & Sevcik, R. A. (2008). Using a speech-generating device to enhance communicative abilities for an adult with moderate intellectual disability. *Intellectual and Developmental Disabilities, 46*(5), 376–386. doi:10.1352/2008.46:376-386 PMID:19090639

Chiner, E., & Cardona, M. C. (2012). Inclusive education in Spain: How do skills, resources, and supports affect regular education teachers' perceptions of inclusion? *International Journal of Inclusive Education, 17*(5), 526–541. doi:10.1080/13603116.2012.689864

Chou, Y. C., Lu, Z. J., Chen, B. W., & Lin, C. J. (2019). Transformed rights' sexual health programme evaluation for the parents and service workers of adults with an intellectual disability. *Journal of Intellectual Disability Research, 23*. doi:10.1111/jir.12624 PMID:31016807

Christensen, H., Calear, A., Tait, R., Gosling, J., Griffiths, K., & Murray, K. (2011). *School based intervention programs and shared care collaborative models targeting the prevention of or early intervention in child and adolescent mental health problems: an evidence check rapid review brokered by the sax institute for the nsw ministry of health*. Academic Press.

Christensen, L., Fraynt, B., Neece, C. L., & Baker, B. L. (2012). Bullying adolescents with intellectual disability. *Journal of Mental Health Research in Intellectual Disabilities*, *5*(1), 49–65. doi:10.1080/19315864.2011.637660

Cihak, D., Fahrenkrog, C., Ayres, K. M., & Smith, C. (2009). The use of video modeling via a video iPod and a system of least prompts to improve transitional behaviors for students with autism spectrum disorders in the general education classroom. *Journal of Positive Behavior Interventions*. doi:10.1177/1098300709332346

Cirrin, F. M., & Rowland, C. M. (1985). Communicative assessment of non-verbal youths with severe/profound mental retardation. *Mental Retardation*, *23*(2), 52–62. PMID:3990553

Clare, I. C. H., & Gudjonsson, G. H. (1993). Interrogative suggestibility, confabulation, and acquiescence in people with mild learning disabilities (mental handicap): Implications for reliability during police interview. *British Journal of Clinical Psychology*, *32*(3), 295–301. doi:10.1111/j.2044-8260.1993.tb01059.x PMID:8251959

Clare, I. C. H., & Gudjonsson, G. H. (1995). The vulnerability of suspects with intellectual disabilities during police interviews: A review and experimental study of decision-making. *Mental Handicap Research*, *8*(2), 110–128. doi:10.1111/j.1468-3148.1995.tb00149.x

Clarke, J., Littlejohns, C. S., Corbett, J. A., & Joseph, S. (1989). Pervasive developmental disorders and psychoses in adult life. *The British Journal of Psychiatry*, *155*(5), 692–699. doi:10.1192/bjp.155.5.692 PMID:2611600

Clark, K. E., & Ladd, G. W. (2000). Connectedness and autonomy support in parent–child relationships: Links to children's socioemotional orientation and peer relationships. *Developmental Psychology*, *36*(4), 485–498. doi:10.1037/0012-1649.36.4.485 PMID:10902700

Clark, L. I., & O'toole, M. S. (2007). Intellectual impairment and sexual health: Information needs. *British Journal of Nursing (Mark Allen Publishing)*, *16*(3), 154–156. doi:10.12968/bjon.2007.16.3.22968 PMID:17363881

Clay, C. J., Bloom, S. E., & Lambert, J. M. (2018). Behavioral Interventions for inappropriate sexual behavior in individuals with developmental disabilities and acquired brain injury: A review. *American Journal on Intellectual and Developmental Disabilities*, *123*(3), 254–282. doi:10.1352/1944-7558-123.3.254 PMID:29671636

Cleaver, H., Unell, I., & Aldgate, J. (1999). *Children's needs, parenting capacity: The impact of parental mental illness, problem alcohol and drug use and domestic violence on children's development*. London: Department of Health, Stationary Office.

Cleveland, D. S., & Miller, N. B. (1977). Attitudes and life commitments of older siblings of mentally retarded adults: An exploratory study. *Mental Retardation*, *15*, 38–41. PMID:875727

Cockram, J., Jackson, R., & Underwood, R. (1998). People with an intellectual disability and the criminal justice system: The family perspective. *Journal of Intellectual & Developmental Disability*, *23*(1), 41–56. doi:10.1080/13668259800033571

Coffee, B., Keith, K., Albizua, I., Malone, T., Jowrey, J., Sherman, L., & Warren, T. (2009). Incidence of fragile X syndrome by newborn screening for methylated FMR1 DNA. *American Journal of Human Genetics*, *85*(4), 503–514. doi:10.1016/j.ajhg.2009.09.007 PMID:19804849

Cole, P. M., Michel, M. K., & Teti, L. O. (1994). The development of emotion regulation and dysregulation: A clinical perspective. *Monographs of the Society for Research in Child Development*, *59*(2/3), 73–102. doi:10.2307/1166139 PMID:7984169

Cologon, K. (2012). Confidence in their own ability: Postgraduate early childhood students examining their attitudes towards inclusive education. *International Journal of Inclusive Education*, *16*(11), 1155–1173. doi:10.1080/13603116.2010.548106

Conrad, J. A. (2018). On intellectual and developmental disabilities in the United States: A historical perspective. *Journal of Intellectual Disabilities*. PMID:29621909

Cook, B. G., Tankersley, M., Cook, L., & Landrum, T. (2000). Abstract of Teachers' Attitudes toward their included students with disabilities. *Exceptional Children*, *67*(1), 115–135. doi:10.1177/001440290006700108

Cooper, J. O., Heron, T. E., & Heward, W. L. (2007). Applied Behavior Analysis (2nd ed.). Academic Press.

Cooper. (1997). High prevalence of dementia among people with learning disabilities not attributable to down's syndrome. *Psychological Medicine*, *27*(3), 609–616. doi:10.1017/S0033291796004655 PMID:9153681

Cooper, A. (1997). Psychiatry of elderly compared to younger adults with intellectual disabilities. *Journal of Applied Research in Intellectual Disabilities*, *10*(4), 303–311. doi:10.1111/j.1468-3148.1997.tb00025.x

Cooper, A., Smiley, E., Morrison, J., Williamson, A., & Allan, L. (2007). Mental ill-health in adults with intellectual disabilities: Prevalence and associated factors. *The British Journal of Psychiatry*, *190*(1), 27–35. doi:10.1192/bjp.bp.106.022483 PMID:17197653

Cooper, S. A., McLean, G., Guthrie, B., McConnachie, A., Mercer, S., Sullivan, F., & Morrison, J. (2015). Multiple physical and mental health comorbidity in adults with intellectual disabilities: Population-based cross-sectional analysis. *BMC Family Practice*, *16*(1), 110. doi:10.118612875-015-0329-3 PMID:26310664

Corbett, A. (1979). Psychiatric morbidity and mental retardation. In F. E. James & R. P. Snaith (Eds.), Psychiatric illness and mental handicap (pp. 11-25). London: Royal College of Psychiatry, Gaskell.

Cornelius, D. J. K. (2009). *Vocational Training and Employment for Individuals with mental retardation to meet the needs of 21st Century*. Report of the National Seminar - Planning for Comprehensive Rehabilitation of Individuals with mental retardation, Chennai, India.

Costeff, H., Cohen, B. E., Weller, L., & Kleckner, H. (1981). Pathogenic factors in idiopathic mental retardation. *Developmental Medicine and Child Neurology*, *23*(5), 484–493. doi:10.1111/j.1469-8749.1981.tb02022.x PMID:7196853

Costello, H., & Bouras, N. (2006). Assessment of mental health problems in people with intellectual disabilities. *Israel Journal of Psychiatry and Related Sciences, 43*(4), 241.

Craig, W. M., & Pepler, D. J. (1995). Peer processes in bullying and victimization: An observational study. *Exceptionality Education Canada*, *5*, 81–95.

Cramm, J. M., & Nieboer, A. P. (2011). Psychological well-being of caregivers of children with intellectual disabilities: Using parental stress as a mediating factor. *Journal of Intellectual Disabilities*, *15*(2), 101–113. doi:10.1177/1744629511410922 PMID:21750213

Crick, N. R., & Grotpeter, J. K. (1995). Relational aggression, gender, and social-psychological adjustment. *Child Development*, *66*(3), 710–722. doi:10.2307/1131945 PMID:7789197

Crnic, A., Neece, C. L., McIntyre, L. L., Blacher, J., & Baker, B. L. (2017). Intellectual disability and developmental risk: Promoting intervention to improve child and family well-being. *Child Development*, *88*(2), 436–445. doi:10.1111/cdev.12740 PMID:28138976

Crnic, K., Hoffman, C., Gaze, C., & Edelbrock, C. (2004). Understanding the emergence of behavior problems in young children with developmental delays. *Infants and Young Children*, *17*(3), 223–235. doi:10.1097/00001163-200407000-00004

Crocker, A. G., Mercier, C., Allaire, J., & Roy, M. (2007). Profiles and correlates aggressive behaviour among adults with intellectual disabilities. *Journal of Intellectual Disability Research: JIDR*, *51*(10), 786–801. doi:10.1111/j.1365-2788.2007.00953.x PMID:17803497

Croen, A., Grether, J. K., & Selvin, S. (2001). The epidemiology of mental retardation of unknown cause. *Pediatrics*, *107*(6), e86–e86. doi:10.1542/peds.107.6.e86 PMID:11389284

Crowe, T. K., Cunningham-Sabo, L. D., Helitzer, D. L., & Vanleit, B. (2002). Perceived changes in self-image and coping strategies of mothers of children with disabilities. *The Occupational Therapy Journal of Research*, *22*(1), 25–33.

Cummings, J., Pepler, D. J., Mishna, F., & Craig, W. M. (2006). Bullying and victimization among children with exceptionalities. *Exceptionality Education Canada*, *16*, 193–222.

Cummins, R.A. (1996). The domains of life satisfaction: An attempt to order chaos. *Social Indicators Research, 38*, 303-28.

Cummins, R. A. (1996). Assessing quality of life. In R. L. Schalock (Ed.), *Quality of life. Volume Conceptualization and measurement*. Washington, DC: American Association on Mental Retardation.

Cummins, R. A. (2005). Moving from the quality of life concept to a theory. *Journal of Intellectual Disability Research*, *49*(10), 699–706. doi:10.1111/j.1365-2788.2005.00738.x PMID:16162114

Cunningham, C. E., Clark, M. L., Heaven, R. K., Durrant, J., & Cunningham, L. H. (1989). The effects of coping-modelling problem solving and contingency management procedures on the positive and negative interactions of learning disabled and attention deficit disordered children with an autistic peer. *Child & Family Behavior Therapy*, *11*(3-4), 89–106. doi:10.1300/J019v11n03_06

Cureton, A. (Ed.). (2018). *Disability in practice: Attitudes, policies, and relationships*. Oxford, UK: Oxford University Press. doi:10.1093/oso/9780198812876.001.0001

Curtis, A., McVilly, K., & Day, A. (2014). Sentencing offenders with mental impairment: The case of arsonists with intellectual disability. *Journal of Intellectual Disabilities and Offending Behaviour*, *5*(2), 78–87. doi:10.1108/JIDOB-05-2014-0005

Cuskelly, M., & Bryde, R. (2004). Attitudes towards the sexuality of adults with an intellectual disability: Parents, support staff, and a community sample. *Journal of Intellectual & Developmental Disability*, *29*(3), 255–264. doi:10.1080/13668250412331285136

Dabrowska, A., & Pisula, E. (2010). Parenting stress and coping styles in mothers and fathers of pre-school children with autism and down syndrome. *Journal of Intellectual Disability Research, 54*(3), 266-280.

Dabrowska, A., & Pisula, E. (2010). Parenting stress and coping styles in mothers and fathers of pre-school children with autism and Down syndrome. *Journal of Intellectual Disability Research*, *54*(3), 266–280. doi:10.1111/j.1365-2788.2010.01258.x PMID:20146741

Dahl, A., Joseph, J., & David. (2011). Emotional action and communication in early moral development. *International Society for Research of Emotion*, *3*, 147. doi:10.1177/1754073910387948

Daily, D. K., Ardinger, H. H., & Holmes, G. E. (2000). Identification and evaluation of mental retardation. *American Family Physician, 61*(4), 1059–1067. PMID:10706158

Dalal, A. (1998). CBR in Action - Some Reflections from the Sirathu Project. *Asia Pacific Disability Rehabilitation Journal, 9*(1), 29–31.

Dammeyer, J., & Chapman, M. (2018). A national survey on violence and discrimination among people with disabilities. *BMC Public Health, 18*(1), 355. doi:10.118612889-018-5277-0

Davidson, P. W., Cain, N. N., Sloane-Reeves, J. E., & Van Speybroech, A. (1994). Characteristics of community-based individuals with mental retardation and aggressive behavioral disorders. *American Journal of Mental Retardation, 98*(6), 704–716. PMID:8054199

Davis, S., & Nixon, C. (2010). *The youth voice research project: Victimization and strategies.* Retrieved from: http://njbullying.org/documents/YVPMarch2010.pdf

Davis, C., Oliver, C., Tang, C. S., & Wu, A. (2000). Chinese children's attitudes towards mental retardation. *Journal of Developmental and Physical Disabilities, 12.*

Dawkins, J. L. (1996). Bullying, physical disability and the pediatric patient. *Developmental Medicine and Child Neurology, 38*(7), 603–612. doi:10.1111/j.1469-8749.1996.tb12125.x PMID:8674911

Day, K. (1993). Crime and mental retardation: A review. *Clinical Approaches to the Mentally Disordered Offender*, 111-44.

Day, K. (1994). Male mentally handicapped sex offenders. *The British Journal of Psychiatry, 165*(5), 630–639. doi:10.1192/bjp.165.5.630 PMID:7866678

Day, K. (1997). Clinical features and offense behavior of mentally retarded sex offenders: A review of research. *The NADD Newsletter, 14*, 86–89.

De Caroli, M. E., & Sagone, E. (2013). Siblings and disability: A study on social attitudes toward disabled brothers and sisters. *Procedia: Social and Behavioral Sciences, 93*, 1217–1223. doi:10.1016/j.sbspro.2013.10.018

De Falco, S., Esposito, G., Venuti, P., & Bornstein, M. H. (2008). Fathers' play with their Down syndrome children. *Journal of Intellectual Disability Research, 52*(6), 490–502. doi:10.1111/j.1365-2788.2008.01052.x PMID:18373561

de Falco, S., Venuti, P., Esposito, G., & Bornstein, M. H. (2009). Mother–child and father–child emotional availability in families of children with Down syndrome. *Parenting, Science and Practice, 9*(3-4), 198–215. doi:10.1080/15295190902844381

Deater-Deckard, K. (2005). Parenting stress and children's development: Introduction to the special issue. *Infant and Child Development, 13*(2), 111–115. doi:10.1002/icd.383

Deb, S., Thomas, M., & Bright, C. (2001). Mental disorder in adults with intellectual disability. 1: prevalence of functional psychiatric illness among a community-based population aged between 16 and 64 years. *Journal of Intellectual Disability Research, 45*(6), 495-505.

Deb, S., Thomas, M., & Bright, C. (2001). Mental disorder in adults with intellectual disability: Prevalence of functional psychiatric illness among a community-based population aged between 16 and 64 years. *Journal of Intellectual Disability Research, 46*(6), 495–505. doi:10.1046/j.1365-2788.2001.00374.x PMID:11737536

Deitz, D. E., & Repp, A. C. (1983). Reducing Behavior through Reinforcement. *Exceptional Education Quarterly, 3*(4), 34–46. doi:10.1177/074193258300300410

Dekker, C., & Koot, H. M. (2003a). Dsm-iv disorders in children with borderline to moderate intellectual disability. I: Prevalence and impact. *Journal of the American Academy of Child and Adolescent Psychiatry*, *42*(8), 915–922. doi:10.1097/01.CHI.0000046892.27264.1A PMID:12874493

Dekker, C., & Koot, H. M. (2003b). Dsm-iv disorders in children with borderline to moderate intellectual disability. Ii: Child and family predictors. *Journal of the American Academy of Child and Adolescent Psychiatry*, *42*(8), 923–931. doi:10.1097/01.CHI.0000046891.27264.C1 PMID:12874494

Dekker, M. C., Koot, H. M., van der Ende, J., & … . (2002). Emotional and behavioral problems in children and adolescents with and without intellectual disability. *Journal of Child Psychology and Psychiatry, and Allied Disciplines*, *43*(8), 1087–1098. doi:10.1111/1469-7610.00235 PMID:12455929

DeLambo, D., Chung, W., & Huang, W. (2011). Stress and age: A comparison of Asian American and Non-Asian American parents of children with developmental disabilities. *Journal of Developmental and Physical Disabilities*, *23*(2), 129–141. doi:10.100710882-010-9211-3

Delano, M. E. (2007). Video modeling interventions for individuals with autism. *Remedial and Special Education*, *28*(1), 33–42. doi:10.1177/07419325070280010401

DeLoache, J. S., & Burns, N. M. (1994). Symbolic functioning in preschool children. *Journal of Applied Developmental Psychology*, *15*(4), 513–527. doi:10.1016/0193-3973(94)90020-5

Demakis, G. J. (Ed.). (2011). *Civil capacities in clinical neuropsychology: Research findings and practical applications*. New York: Oxford University Press.

Dempsey, I. (2003). The impact of the Disability Discrimination Act on school students with a disability in Australia. *Austl. & NZJL & Educ.*, *8*, 35.

Denney, R. L., & Wynkoop, T. F. (2000). Clinical neuropsychology in the criminal forensic setting. *The Journal of Head Trauma Rehabilitation*, *15*(2), 804–828. doi:10.1097/00001199-200004000-00005 PMID:10739969

Dervishaliaj, E. (2013). Parental stress in families with disabilities: A literature review. *Journal of Educational and Social Research*, *3*(7), 579–584.

Devapriam, J., Raju, L., Singh, N., Collacott, R., & Bhaumik, S. (2007). Arson: Characteristics and predisposing factors in offenders with intellectual disabilities. *British Journal of Forensic Practice*, *9*(4), 23–27. doi:10.1108/14636646200700023

Dew, A., Llewellyn, G., & Balandin, S. (2004). Post-parental care: A new generation of siblingcarers. *Journal of Intellectual & Developmental Disability*, *29*(2), 176–179. doi:10.1080/13668250410001709520

DeWeaver, K. L., & Kropf, N. P. (1992). Persons with mental retardation: A forgotten minority in education. *Journal of Social Work Education*, *28*(1), 36–46. doi:10.1080/10437797.1992.10778756

Dhanesh, K. G., & Karthikeyan, S. (2012). *Gender difference in level of intelligence and social quotient among children with autism spectrum disorders*. International Journal of Scientific and Research Publications.

Di Nuovo, S. F., & Buono, S. (2007). Psychiatric syndromes comorbid with mental retardation: Differences in cognitive and adaptive skills. *Journal of Psychiatric Research*, *41*(9), 795–800. doi:10.1016/j.jpsychires.2006.02.011 PMID:16697412

Dickerson Mayes, S., Baweja, R., Calhoun, S. L., Syed, E., Mahr, F., & Siddiqui, F. (2014). Suicide ideation and attempts and bullying in children and adolescents: Psychiatric and general population samples. *Crisis*, *35*(5), 301–309. doi:10.1027/0227-5910/a000264 PMID:25115491

Dickman, B. J., & Roux, A. J. (2005). Complainants with learning disabilities in sexual abuse cases: A 10-year review of a psycho-legal project in Cape Town, South Africa. *British Journal of Learning Disabilities, 33*(3), 138–144. doi:10.1111/j.1468-3156.2005.00355.x

Dickson, K., Emerson, E., & Hatton, C. (2005). Self-reported anti-social behaviour: Prevalence and risk factors amongst adolescents with and without intellectual disability. *Journal of Intellectual Disability Research, 49*(11), 820–826. doi:10.1111/j.1365-2788.2005.00727.x PMID:16207279

Didden, R. (2007). Functional analysis methodology in developmental disabilities. In P. Strumey (Ed.), *Functional analysis in clinical treatment: Practical resources for mental health professional* (pp. 65–86). San Diego, CA: Elsevier Academic Press. doi:10.1016/B978-012372544-8/50005-7

Didden, R., Duker, P. C., & Korzilius, H. (1997). Meta-analytic study on treatment effectiveness for problem behaviors with individuals who have mental retardation. *American Journal of Mental Retardation, 101*(4), 387–399. PMID:9017085

Didden, R., Scholte, R. H. J., Korzilius, H., De Moor, J. M. H., Vermeulen, A., O'Reilly, M., & Lancioni, G. E. (2009). Cyberbullying among students with intellectual and developmental disability in special education settings. *Developmental Neurorehabilitation, 12*(3), 146–151. doi:10.1080/17518420902971356 PMID:19466622

Diekema, D. (2003). Involuntary sterilization of persons with mental retardation: Ethical analysis. *Mental Retardation and Developmental Disabilities Research Reviews, 9*(1), 21–26. doi:10.1002/mrdd.10053 PMID:12587134

Diez Roux, A. V. (2004). The study of group-level factors in epidemiology: rethinking variables, study designs, and analytical approaches. *Epidemiologic Reviews, 26*(1), 104-111. doi:10.1093/epirev/mxh006

Dinkes, R., Kemp, J., Baum, K., & Snyder, T. (2009). *Indicators of school crime and safety: 2009 (NCES 2010–012/NCJ 228478).* Washington, DC: National Center for Education Statistics, Institute of Education Sciences, U.S. Department of Education, and Bureau of Justice Statistics, Office of Justice Programs, U.S. Department of Justice.

Disability Information. (2013). *Department of communities and social inclusion.* Government of South Australia.

Disabled Individuals in India. (2002). *National sample survey 58th round.Ministry of statistics and programme implementation.* New Delhi: Govt. of India.

Dols, M. W. (1987). Insanity and its treatment in Islamic society. *Medical History, 31*(1), 1–14. doi:10.1017/S0025727300046287 PMID:3543559

Doornbos, M. M. (2002). Predicting family health in families of young adults with severe mental illness. *Journal of Family Nursing, 8*(3), 241–263. doi:10.1177/107484070200800306

Doran, C. M., Einfeld, S. L., Madden, R. H., Otim, M., Horstead, S. K., Ellis, L. A., & Emerson, E. (2012). How much does intellectual disability really cost? First estimates for australia. *Journal of Intellectual and Developmental Disability, 37*(1), 42-49.

Doren, B., Bullis, M., & Benz, M. R. (1996). Predictors of victimization: Experiences of adolescents with disabilities in transition. *Exceptional Children, 63*(1), 7–18. doi:10.1177/001440299606300101

Dörenberg, V. E., de Veer, A. J., Francke, A. L., Embregts, P. J., van Nieuwenhuijzen, M., & Frederiks, B. J. (2018). Applying restrictive measures in the care of adolescents with mild intellectual disabilities: Attitudes of support staff and policy implications. *Journal of Policy and Practice in Intellectual Disabilities, 15*(1), 26–35. doi:10.1111/jppi.12223

Dosen, A. (2007). Integrative treatment in persons with intellectual disability and mental health problems. *Journal of Intellectual Disability Research, 51*(1), 66-74. doi:10.1111/j.1365-2788.2006.00868.x

Dufrene, B. A., Doggett, R. A., Henington, C., & Watson, T. S. (2007). Functional assessment and intervention for disruptive classroom behaviors in preschool and head start classrooms. *Journal of Behavioral Education, 16*(4), 368–388. doi:10.100710864-007-9048-8

Dumont, M., & Beaulieu, C. (2007). Light exposure in the natural environment: Relevance to mood and sleep disorders. *Sleep Medicine, 8*(6), 557–565. doi:10.1016/j.sleep.2006.11.008 PMID:17383230

Duncan, N. (1999). *Sexual bullying: Gender conflict and pupil culture in secondary schools.* New York, NY: Routledge.

Durand, V. M., & Carr, E. G. (1991). Functional communication training to reduce challenging behavior: Maintenance and application in new settings. *Journal of Applied Behavior Analysis, 24*(2), 251–264. doi:10.1901/jaba.1991.24-251 PMID:1890046

Durand, V. M., & Crimmins, D. B. (1988). Identifying the variables maintaining self-injurious behavior. *Journal of Autism and Developmental Disorders, 18*(1), 99–117. doi:10.1007/BF02211821 PMID:3372462

Durkin, M., Schupf, N., Stein, Z., & Susser, M. (2007). Mental retardation. Stamford, CT: Appleton & Lange.

Durkin, S., & Yeargin-Allsopp, M. (2018). *Socioeconomic status and pediatric neurologic disorders: current evidence.* Paper presented at the seminars in pediatric neurology. 10.1016/j.spen.2018.03.003

Dwyer, R. G., & Frierson, R. L. (2006). The presence of low IQ and mental retardation among murder defendants referred for pretrial evaluation. *Journal of Forensic Sciences, 51*(3), 678–682. doi:10.1111/j.1556-4029.2006.00115.x PMID:16696721

Dyer, W. J., McBride, B. A., & Jeans, L. M. (2009). A longitudinal examination of father involvement with children with developmental delays: Does timing of diagnosis matter? *Journal of Early Intervention, 31*(3), 265–281. doi:10.1177/0192513X09340386

Dyson, L. (1997). Fathers and mothers of school-age children with developmental disabilities: Parental stress, family functioning, and social support. *American Journal of Mental Retardation, 102*(3), 267–279. doi:10.1352/0895-8017(1997)102<0267:FAMOSC>2.0.CO;2 PMID:9394135

Dyson, L. (2010). Unanticipated effects of children with learning disabilities on their families. *Learning Disability Quarterly, 33*(1), 43–55. doi:10.1177/073194871003300104

Dyson, L. L. (1999). The psychosocial functioning of school-age children who have siblings with developmental disabilities: Change and stability over time. *Journal of Applied Developmental Psychology, 20*(2), 253–271. doi:10.1016/S0193-3973(99)00016-7

Eakes, G. G. (1995). Chronic sorrow: The lived experience of parents of chronically mentally ill individuals. *Archives of Psychiatric Nursing, 9*(2), 77–84. doi:10.1016/S0883-9417(95)80004-2 PMID:7755411

Eakes, G. G., Burke, M. L., & Hainsworth, M. A. (1998). Middle range theory of chronic sorrow. *Journal of Nursing Scholarship, 30*(2), 179–184. doi:10.1111/j.1547-5069.1998.tb01276.x PMID:9775562

Eapen, V. (2014). Developmental and mental health disorders: two sides of the same coin. *Asian Journal of Psychiatry, 8*, 7-11.

Eapen, V., & Jairam, R. (2009). Integration of child mental health services to primary care: challenges and opportunities. *Mental Health in Family Medicine, 6*(1), 43.

Eapen, V., Al-Gazali, L. I., Bin-Othman, S., & Pramathan, T. (1998). Learning disorders in school-going children–detection and diagnosis. *Journal of Tropical Pediatrics, 44*(4), 192-193.

Eastgate, G., Scheermeyer, E., van Driel, M., & Lennox, N. G. (2012). Intellectual disability, sexuality and sexual abuse prevention: A study of family members and support workers. *Disability, 41*(3), 135-139. Retrieved from https://www.racgp.org.au/afp/2012/march/intellectual-disability,-sexuality-and-sexual-abuse-prevention/

Eastgate, G. (2005). Sex, consent and intellectual disability. *Australian Family Physician, 34*(3), 163–166. PMID:15799666

Eastgate, G. (2011). Sex and intellectual disability: Dealing with sexual health issues. *Disability, 40*, 188–191. PMID:21597526

Ebuenyi, I. D., Rottenburg, E. S., Bunders-Aelen, J. F. G., & Regeer, B. J. (2018). Challenges of inclusion: A qualitative study exploring barriers and pathways to inclusion of persons with mental disabilities in technical and vocational education and training programmes in East Africa. *Disability and Rehabilitation, 6*, 1–9. doi:10.1080/09638288.2018.1503729 PMID:30398073

Edelstein, T. M., & Glenwick, D. S. (1977). Referral reasons for psychological services for adults with mental retardation. *Research in Developmental Disabilities, 18*(1), 45–59. doi:10.1016/S0891-4222(96)00037-6 PMID:9085429

Edwardraj, S., Mumtaj, K., Prasad, J. H., Kuruvilla, A., & Jacob, K. S. (2010). Perceptions about intellectual disability: A qualitative study from Vellore, South India. *Journal of Intellectual Disability Research, 54*(8), 736–748. doi:10.1111/j.1365-2788.2010.01301.x PMID:20633202

Egeland, B., Pianta, R., & O'brien, M. A. (1993). Maternal intrusiveness in infancy and child maladaptation in early school years. *Development and Psychopathology, 5*(3), 359–370. doi:10.1017/S0954579400004466

Einfeld, S. L., Ellis, L. A., & Emerson, E. (2011). Comorbidity of intellectual disability and mental disorder in children and adolescents: a systematic review. *Journal of Intellectual and Developmental Disability, 36*(2), 137-143.

Einfeld, L., Piccinin, A. M., Mackinnon, A., Hofer, S. M., Taffe, J., Gray, K. M., ... Tonge, B. J. (2006). Psychopathology in young people with intellectual disability. *Journal of the American Medical Association, 296*(16), 1981–1989. doi:10.1001/jama.296.16.1981 PMID:17062861

Einfeld, L., & Tonge, B. J. (1996a). Population prevalence of psychopathology in children and adolescents with intellectual disability: I rationale and methods. *Journal of Intellectual Disability Research, 40*(2), 91–98. doi:10.1111/j.1365-2788.1996.tb00610.x PMID:8731466

Einfeld, L., & Tonge, B. J. (1999). Observations on the use of the icd-10 guide for mental retardation. *Journal of Intellectual Disability Research, 43*(5), 408–412. doi:10.1046/j.1365-2788.1999.043005408.x PMID:10546965

Einfeld, S. L., Ellis, L. A., & Emerson, E. (2011). Comorbidity of intellectual disability and mental disorder in children and adolescents: A systematic review. *Journal of Intellectual & Developmental Disability, 36*(2), 137–143. doi:10.1080/13668250.2011.572548 PMID:21609299

Einfeld, S. L., & Tonge, B. J. (1996). Population prevalence of psychopathology in children and adolescents with intellectual disability: II epidemiological findings. *Journal of Intellectual Disability Research, 40*(2), 99–109. doi:10.1111/j.1365-2788.1996.tb00611.x PMID:8731467

Eisenhower, A. S., Baker, B. L., & Blacher, J. (2007). Early student–teacher relationships of children with and without intellectual disability: Contributions of behavioral, social, and self-regulatory competence. *Journal of School Psychology, 45*(4), 363–383. doi:10.1016/j.jsp.2006.10.002 PMID:21490876

Eisenhower, A., Blacher, J., & Baker, B. L. (2013). Mothers' perceived physical health during early and middle childhood: Relations with child developmental delay and behavior problems. *Research in Developmental Disabilities, 34*(3), 1059–1068. doi:10.1016/j.ridd.2012.12.002 PMID:23306002

Elliott, S. N., & Gresham, F. M. (1993). Social skills interventions for children. *Behavior Modification, 17*(3), 287–313. doi:10.1177/01454455930173004 PMID:8343100

Embregts, P. J. C. M., Heestermans, M., & Van den Bogaard, K. J. H. M. (2017). A Training Course for Psychologists: Learning to Assess (Alleged) Sexual Abuse Among Victims and Perpetrators Who Have Intellectual Disabilities. *Sexuality and Disability, 35*(1), 39–44. doi:10.100711195-017-9476-x PMID:28250542

Emerson, E. (2003). Prevalence of psychiatric disorders in children and adolescents with and without intellectual disability. *Journal of Intellectual Disability Research, 47*(1), 51-58.

Emerson, E. (2012). Deprivation, ethnicity and the prevalence of intellectual and developmental disabilities. *Journal of Epidemiology and Community Health, 66*(3), 218-224.

Emerson, E., & Hatton, C. (2007a). Contribution of socioeconomic position to health inequalities of british children and adolescents with intellectual disabilities. *Journal Information, 112*(2).

Emerson, E., & Hatton, C. (2007b). Mental health of children and adolescents with intellectual disabilities in Britain. *The British Journal of Psychiatry, 191*(6), 493-499.

Emerson, E. (2001). *Challenging behaviour: Analysis and intervention in people with severe learning disabilities* (2nd ed.). Cambridge, UK: Cambridge University Press. doi:10.1017/CBO9780511543739

Emerson, E. (2003). Prevalence of psychiatric disorders in children and adolescents with and without intellectual disability. *Journal of Intellectual Disability Research, 47*(1), 51–58. doi:10.1046/j.1365-2788.2003.00464.x PMID:12558695

Emerson, E. (2010). Self-reported exposure to disablism is associated with poorer self-reported health and well-being among adults with intellectual disabilities in England: A cross-sectional survey. *Public Health, 124*(12), 682–689. doi:10.1016/j.puhe.2010.08.020 PMID:21035153

Emerson, E., Blacher, J., Einfeld, S., Hatton, C., Robertson, J., & Stancliffe, R. J. (2014). Environmental risk factors associated with the persistence of conduct difficulties in children with intellectual disabilities and autistic spectrum disorders. *Research in Developmental Disabilities, 35*(12), 3508–3517. doi:10.1016/j.ridd.2014.08.039 PMID:25238636

Emerson, E., & Einfeld, S. (2011). *Challenging Behaviour*. Cambridge, UK: Cambridge University Press. doi:10.1017/CBO9780511861178

Emerson, E., & Hatton, C. (2007). Mental health of children and adolescents with intellectual disabilities in Britain. *The British Journal of Psychiatry, 191*(6), 493–499. doi:10.1192/bjp.bp.107.038729 PMID:18055952

Emerson, E., & Hatton, C. (2007). The socio-economic circumstances of children at risk of disability in Britain. *Disability & Society, 22*(6), 563–580. doi:10.1080/09687590701560154

Emerson, E., & Hatton, C. (2008). Poverty, socio-economic position, social capital and the health children with intellectual disability. *Journal of Intellectual Disability Research.*

Emerson, E., Kiernan, C., Alborz, A., Reeves, D., Mason, L., Mason, H., & Hatton, C. (2001). The prevalence of challenging behaviors: A total population study. *Research in Developmental Disabilities, 22*(1), 77–93. doi:10.1016/S0891-4222(00)00061-5 PMID:11263632

Employment of Persons with Disabilities in Public Sectors in India -Emerging Issues and Trends. (1995). *An Evaluation Study with Special Reference to Persons with Disabilities Act.* Commissioned by Planning Commission, Government of India.

Enoch, A., Mprah, W.K., Isaac, O., & Joseph, B. (2018). Role of Caregivers of Children with Intellectual Disabilities and Support Systems Available to them in Ghana. *Disability, CBR & Inclusive Development, 28*(4), 80-95. doi:. doi:10.5463/dcid.v28i4.645

Ericson, N. (2001). *Addressing the problem of juvenile bullying*. Washington, DC: U.S. Government Printing Office; doi:10.1037/e317892004-001

Eriksen, N., & Gerstel, N. (2002). A labor of love itself: Care work among adult brothers and sisters. *Journal of Family Issues, 23*, 836–856. doi:10.1177/019251302236597

Esbensen, A. J. (2011). Families of individuals with intellectual disability and comorbid mental health problems. *Journal of Mental Health Research in Intellectual Disabilities, 4*(3), 140–157. doi:10.1080/19315864.2011.597018

Esmail, S., Darry, K., Walter, A., & Knupp, H. (2010). Attitudes and perceptions towards disability and sexuality. *Journal Disability and Rehabilitation, 32*(14), 1148–1155. doi:10.3109/09638280903419277 PMID:20131952

Espelage, D. L., Low, S. K., & Jimerson, S. R. (2014). Understanding school climate, aggression, peer victimization, and bully perpetration: Contemporary science, practice, and policy. *School Psychology Quarterly, 29*(3), 233–237. doi:10.1037pq0000090 PMID:25198615

Espelage, D. L., & Swearer, S. M. (2003). Research on school bullying and victimization: What have we learned and where do we go from here? *School Psychology Review, 32*, 365–383.

Estell, D. B., Farmer, T. W., Irvin, M. J., Crowther, A., Akos, P., & Boudah, D. J. (2009). Students with exceptionalities and the peer group context of bullying and victimization in late elementary school. *Journal of Child and Family Studies, 18*(2), 136–150. doi:10.100710826-008-9214-1

European Agency for Development in Special Needs Education. (2011). *Mapping the implementation of policy for inclusive education - An exploration of challenges and opportunities for developing indicators*. Retrieved from http://www.european-agency.org/publications/flyers/mipie /MIPIE-summary-of-proposalsEN.pdf/view

Evans, D. R. (1994). Enhancing quality of life in the population at large. *Social Indicators Research, 33*(1-3), 47–88. doi:10.1007/BF01078958

Everington, C., & Fulero, S. M. (1999). Competence to confess: Measuring understanding and suggestibility of defendants with mental retardation. *Mental Retardation, 37*(3), 212–220. doi:10.1352/0047-6765(1999)037<0212:CTCMU A>2.0.CO;2 PMID:10473340

Eyberg, S. M., Boggs, S. R., & Algina, J. (1995). Parent–child interaction therapy: A psychosocial model for the treatment of young children with conduct problem behavior and their families. *Psychopharmacology Bulletin, 31*(1), 83–91. PMID:7675994

Fabes, R. A., Eisenberg, N., Karbon, M., Troyer, D., & Switzer, G. (1994). The relations of children's emotion regulation to their vicarious emotional responses and comforting behaviors. *Child Development, 65*(6), 1687–1693. doi:10.2307/1131287 PMID:7859549

Fabian, E. S. (1991). Using quality-of-life indicators in rehabilitation program evaluation. *Rehabilitation Counseling Bulletin, 34*(4), 344–356.

Fabrega, H. Jr. (1991). Psychiatric stigma in non-Western societies. *Comprehensive Psychiatry, 32*(6), 534–551. doi:10.1016/0010-440X(91)90033-9 PMID:1778081

Fairthorne, J., Jacoby, P., Bourke, J., de Klerk, N., & Leonard, H. (2015). Onset of maternal psychiatric disorders after the birth of a child with intellectual disability: A retrospective cohort study. *Journal of Psychiatric Research*, *61*, 223–230. doi:10.1016/j.jpsychires.2014.11.011 PMID:25499469

Farber, B., & Kirk, S. A. (1959). Effects of a severely retarded child on family integration. *Monographs of the Society for Research in Child Development*, *24*(2), 1–112. doi:10.2307/1165597

Farmer, T. W., Irvin, M. J., Motoca, L. M., Leung, M., Hutchins, B. C., Brooks, D. S., & Hall, C. M. (2015). Externalizing and internalizing behavior problems, peer affiliations, and bullying involvement across the transition to middle school. *Journal of Emotional and Behavioral Disorders*, *23*(1), 3–16. doi:10.1177/1063426613491286

Farmer, T. W., Petrin, R., Brooks, D. S., Hamm, J. V., Lambert, K., & Gravelle, M. (2012). Bullying involvement and the school adjustment of rural students with and without disabilities. *Journal of Emotional and Behavioral Disorders*, *20*(1), 19–37. doi:10.1177/1063426610392039

Fatima, M. (2012). *The effectiveness of computer –assisted exercise on certain cognitive variables among dyslexic children*. Retrieved from www.sodhgangainflibnet.ac.in

Fazel, S., Xenitidis, K., & Powell, J. (2008). The prevalence of intellectual disabilities among 12000 prisoners - A systematic review. *International Journal of Law and Psychiatry*, *31*(4), 369–373. doi:10.1016/j.ijlp.2008.06.001 PMID:18644624

Feeley, K., & Jones, E. (2006). Addressing challenging behaviour in children with Down syndrome: The use of applied behaviour analysis for assessment and intervention. *Down's Syndrome: Research and Practice*, *11*(2), 64–77. doi:10.3104/perspectives.316 PMID:17048800

Feil, N. (1993). *The validation breakthrough*. Sydney: McLennan & Petty.

Felce, D., & Perry, J. (1996). Exploring current conceptions of quality of life. In R. Renwick, I. Brown, & M. Nagler (Eds.), *Quality of life in health promotion and rehabilitation: Conceptual approaches, issues, and applications* (pp. 51–62). Thousand Oaks, CA: Sage Publications.

Feldman, A., & Werner, S. E. (2002). Collateral effects of behavioral parent training on families of children with developmental disabilities and behavior disorders. *Behavioral Interventions*, *17*(2), 75–83. doi:10.1002/bin.111

Feldman, M., Varhese, J., Ramsay, J., & Rajska, D. (2002). Relationships between social support, stress and mother–child interactions in mothers with intellectual disabilities. *Journal of Applied Research in Intellectual Disabilities*, *15*(4), 314–323. doi:10.1046/j.1468-3148.2002.00132.x

Feniger-Schaal, R., & Oppenheim, D. (2013). Resolution of the diagnosis and maternal sensitivity among mothers of children with Intellectual Disability. *Research in Developmental Disabilities*, *34*(1), 306–313. doi:10.1016/j.ridd.2012.08.007 PMID:22983017

Fenning, R. M. B., Baker, J. K., & Crnic, B. L. (2014). Parent-child interaction over time in families of young children with borderline intellectual functioning. *Journal of Family Psychology*, *28*(3), 326–335. doi:10.1037/a0036537 PMID:24707801

Fenning, R. M., Baker, J. K., Baker, B. L., & Crnic, K. A. (2007). Parenting children with borderline intellectual functioning: A unique risk population. *American Journal of Mental Retardation*, *112*(2), 107–121. doi:10.1352/0895-8017(2007)112[107:PCWBIF]2.0.CO;2 PMID:17295551

Fiese, B., Tomcho, T., Douglas, M., Josephs, K., Poltrock, S., & Baker, T. (2002). A review of 50 years of research on naturally occurring family routines and rituals: Cause for celebration? *Journal of Family Psychology*, *16*(4), 381–390. doi:10.1037/0893-3200.16.4.381 PMID:12561283

Fisher, C., Cea, C., Davidson, P., & Fried, A. (2006). Capacity of persons with mental retardation to consent to participate in randomized clinical trials. *The American Journal of Psychiatry*, *163*(10), 1813–1820. doi:10.1176/ajp.2006.163.10.1813 PMID:17012694

Fisher, W. W., Adelinis, J. D., Thompson, R. H., Worsdell, A. S., & Zarcone, J. R. (1998). Functional analysis and treatment of destructive behavior maintained by termination of "don't" (and symmetrical "do") requests. *Journal of Applied Behavior Analysis*, *31*(3), 339–356. doi:10.1901/jaba.1998.31-339 PMID:9757579

Fisher, W. W., Kuhn, D. E., & Thompson, R. H. (1998). Establishing discriminative control of responding using functional and alternative reinforcers during functional communication training. *Journal of Applied Behavior Analysis*, *31*(4), 543–560. doi:10.1901/jaba.1998.31-543 PMID:9891393

Flander, G. B., Stimac, D., Bagaric, E. S., & Vinscak, M. (2014). Patterns of and copying with cyberbullying in Croatia. *International Journal of Person Centered Medicine.*

Fletcher, I., Leadbetter, P., Curran, A., & O'Sullivan, H. (2009). A pilot study assessing emotional intelligence training and communication skills with 3rd year medical students. *Patient Education and Counselling*, *76*(3), 376-9.

Fletcher, J., Loschen, E., Stavrakaki, C., & First, M. (2007). *Diagnostic manual-intellectual disability: A textbook of diagnosis of mental disorders in persons with intellectual disability*. Kingston, NY: NADD.

Flippin, M., & Crais, E. R. (2011). The need for more effective father involvement in early autism intervention: A systematic review and recommendations. *Journal of Early Intervention*, *33*(1), 24–50. doi:10.1177/1053815111400415

Floyd, F. J., & Gallagher, E. M. (1997). Parental stress, care demands, and use of support services for school-age children with disabilities and behavior problems. *Family Relations*, *46*(4), 359–371. doi:10.2307/585096

Floyd, F. J., Greenberg, J. S., Hong, J., Pettee, Y., & Seltzer, M. M. (2001). Life course impacts of parenting a child with a disability. *American Journal of Mental Retardation*, *106*(3), 265–286. doi:10.1352/0895-8017(2001)106<0265:LCIOPA>2.0.CO;2 PMID:11389667

Floyd, F. J., & Zmich, D. E. (1991). Marriage and the parenting partnership: Perceptions and interactions of parents with mentally retarded and typically developing children. *Child Development*, *62*(6), 1434–1448. doi:10.2307/1130817 PMID:1786726

Flynt, S. W., & Morton, R. C. (2007). Bullying prevention and students with disabilities. *National Forum of Special Education Journal, 19*(1), 1-6.

Fogden, B. C., Thomas, S. D., Daffern, M., & Ogloff, J. R. (2016). Crime and victimisation in people with intellectual disability: A case linkage study. *BMC Psychiatry*, *16*(1), 170. doi:10.118612888-016-0869-7 PMID:27234810

Forlin, C., Loreman, T., Sharma, U., & Earle, C. (2009). Demographic differences in changing pre-service teachers' attitudes, sentiments and concerns about inclusive education. *International Journal of Inclusive Education*, *13*(2), 195–209. doi:10.1080/13603110701365356

Fox, C. L. (1989). Peer acceptance of learning disabled children in the regular classroom. *Exceptional Children*, *56*(1), 50–59. doi:10.1177/001440298905600108

Frey, G. C., & Temple, V. A. (2008). Health promotions for Latin Americans with intellectual disabilities. *Salud Pública de México*, *2*, 167–177. doi:10.1590/S0036-36342008000800010 PMID:18470345

Friedman, D., Holmbeck, G. N., Jandasek, B., Zukerman, J., & Abad, M. (2004). Parent functioning in families of preadolescents with spina bifida: Longitudinal implications for child adjustment. *Journal of Family Psychology*, *18*(4), 609–619. doi:10.1037/0893-3200.18.4.609 PMID:15598166

Fulcher, G. (1989). Disability: A social construction. In G. Lupton & J. Najman (Eds.), *Sociology of health and illness: Australian readings*. Melbourne: Macmillan.

Fulero, S. M., & Everington, C. (1995). Assessing competency to waive Miranda rights in defendants with mental retardation. *Law and Human Behavior*, *19*(5), 533–543. doi:10.1007/BF01499342

Fuller, T.E. (1997). Deinstitutionalization: A Psychiatric "Titanic". In *Out of the Shadows: Confronting America's Mental Illness Crisis*. John Wiley & Sons.

Gabel, S. (2004). South Asian Indian cultural orientations toward mental retardation. *Journal Information*, *42*(1), 12–25. PMID:14720098

Galil, A., Bachner, Y. G., Merrick, J., Flusser, H., Lubetzky, H., Heiman, N., & Carmel, S. (2006). Physician-parent communication as predictor of parent satisfaction with child development services. *Research in Developmental Disabilities*, *27*(3), 233–242. doi:10.1016/j.ridd.2005.03.004 PMID:15998579

Gallagher, S., & Hannigan, A. (2014). Depression and chronic health conditions in parents of children with and without developmental disabilities: The growing up in Ireland cohort study. *Research in Developmental Disabilities*, *35*(2), 448–454. doi:10.1016/j.ridd.2013.11.029 PMID:24361813

Gallagher, S., Phillips, A. C., Oliver, C., & Carroll, D. (2008). Predictors of psychological morbidity in parents of children with intellectual disabilities. *Journal of Pediatric Psychology*, *33*(10), 1129–1136. doi:10.1093/jpepsy/jsn040 PMID:18430761

Gardiner, E., Miller, A. R., & Lach, L. M. (2018). Family impact of childhood neurodevelopmental disability: Considering adaptive and maladaptive behaviour. *Journal of Intellectual Disability Research*, *62*(10), 888–899. doi:10.1111/jir.12547 PMID:30230656

Gath, A., & Gumley, D. (1987). Retarded children and their siblings. *Journal of Child Psychology and Psychiatry, and Allied Disciplines*, *28*(5), 715–730. doi:10.1111/j.1469-7610.1987.tb01554.x PMID:2959672

Gauthier-Boudreault, C., Gallagher, F., & Couture, M. (2017). Specific needs of families of young adults with profound intellectual disability during and after transition to adulthood: What are we missing? *Research in Developmental Disabilities*, *66*, 16–26. doi:10.1016/j.ridd.2017.05.001 PMID:28577424

Gavidia-Payne, S., Richdale, A., Francis, A., & Cotton, S. (1997). *The parenting hassles scale: measuring stress in parents of children with disabilities.* Paper presented at the 121st annual meeting of the american association on mental retardation, New York, NY.

Gavidia-Payne, S., & Hudson, A. (2002). Behavioural supports for parents of children with an intellectual disability and problem behaviours: An overview of the literature. *Journal of Intellectual & Developmental Disability*, *27*(1), 31–55. doi:10.1080/13668250120119626

Gavidia-Payne, S., & Stoneman, Z. (2006). Marital adjustment in families of young children with disabilities: Associations with daily hassles and problem-focused coping. *American Journal of Mental Retardation*, *111*(1), 1–14. doi:10.1352/0895-8017(2006)111[1:MAIFOY]2.0.CO;2 PMID:16332152

Gebeyehu, F., Sahile, A., & Ayalew, M. (2019). Burden, Social Support, and Life Satisfaction Among Caregivers of Children With Intellectual Disability: The Case of Felege Abay and Shembt Primary Schools, Bahir Dar, Ethiopia. *International Quarterly of Community Health Education*, *39*(3), 147–153. doi:10.1177/0272684X18819974 PMID:30602336

Genesi, D. (2000). *Disability Discrimination against students in the classroom.* Retrieved from http://www.cedarville.edu/academics/education/classes/edsp202/examples/literature_review_genesi.htm

Geng-qing, C., & Qu, H. (2003). Integrating persons with disabilities into the workforce: A study on employment of people with disabilities in foodservice industry. *International Journal of Hospitality & Tourism Administration*, *4*, 59–83. doi:10.1300/J149v04n04_04

Gerstein, E. D., Crnic, K. A., Blacher, J., & Baker, B. L. (2009). Resilience and the course of daily parenting stress in families of young children with intellectual disabilities. *Journal of Intellectual Disability Research*, *53*(12), 981–997. doi:10.1111/j.1365-2788.2009.01220.x PMID:19874449

Ghai, A. (2002). Disabled Women: An excluded agenda of Indian feminism. *Hypatia*, *17*(3), 49–66. doi:10.1111/j.1527-2001.2002.tb00941.x

Giallo, R., Seymour, M., Matthews, J., Gavidia-Payne, S., Hudson, A., & Cameron, C. (2015). Risk factors associated with the mental health of fathers of children with an intellectual disability in Australia. *Journal of Intellectual Disability Research, 59*(3), 193-207.

Giannouli, V. (2014). What do Greeks believe about elders and mental? *Agora International Journal of Juridical Sciences*, *8*(3), 1–5.

Giannouli, V. (2016). Crime and legal issues among intellectually disabled individuals. In R. T. Gopalan (Ed.), *Handbook of research on diagnosing, treating, and managing intellectual disabilities* (pp. 346–369). IGI Global. doi:10.4018/978-1-5225-0089-6.ch018

Giannouli, V. (2018a). Elder abuse and consent capacity: Our collective nemesis? In R. T. Gopalan (Ed.), *Social, psychological, and forensic perspectives on sexual abuse* (pp. 207–221). IGI Global. doi:10.4018/978-1-5225-3958-2.ch015

Giannouli, V. (2018b). On the importance of focusing on family and parent factors in multilevel analyses regarding psychopathology of adolescents with an intellectual disability who present to general hospital services. *Australasian Psychiatry*, *26*(3), 325–326. doi:10.1177/1039856217749055 PMID:29873561

Giannouli, V., Stamovlasis, D., & Tsolaki, M. (2018). Exploring the role of cognitive factors in a new instrument for elders' financial capacity assessment. *Journal of Alzheimer's Disease*, *62*(4), 1579–1594. doi:10.3233/JAD-170812 PMID:29504530

Giannouli, V., & Syrmos, N. (2017). Exploring attitudes towards endocrine diseases in Greece. *Endocrine*, *55*(2), 655–657. doi:10.100712020-016-1164-6 PMID:27822671

Giannouli, V., & Tsolaki, M. (2011). Competency and dementia: A challenge of today. [in Greek]. *Neurology*, *20*(6), 12–19.

Giannouli, V., & Tsolaki, M. (2014). Legal capacity of the elderly in Greece. *Hellenic Journal of Nuclear Medicine*, *17*, 2–6. PMID:24392459

Giannouli, V., & Tsolaki, M. (2015). A neglected drama for elders: Discrepancy between self-perception and objective performance regarding financial capacity in patients with cognitive deficits. *Psychological Thought*, *8*(2), 142–147. doi:10.5964/psyct.v8i2.130

Giannouli, V., & Tsolaki, M. (2016). Questions about Dementia with Lewy Bodies, personal beliefs and real performance for financial capacity tasks. *European Psychiatry Medicine*, *33*, 582.

Giannouli, V., & Tsolaki, M. (2019). Are left angular gyrus and amygdala volumes important for financial capacity in mild cognitive impairment? *Hellenic Journal of Nuclear Medicine*, *22*, 160–164. PMID:30877733

Gillberg, C., Persson, E., Grufman, M., & Themner, U. (1986). Psychiatric disorders in mildly and severely mentally retarded urban children and adolescents: Epidemiological aspects. *The British Journal of Psychiatry*, *149*(1), 68–74. doi:10.1192/bjp.149.1.68 PMID:2946351

Gil-Llario, M. D., Morell-Mengual, V., Ballester-Arnal, R., & Díaz-Rodríguez, I. (2018). The experience of sexuality in adults with intellectual disability. *Journal of Intellectual Disability Research*, *62*(1), 72–80. doi:10.1111/jir.12455 PMID:29159891

Gilmore, L., & Cuskelly, M. (2014). Vulnerability to loneliness in people with intellectual disability: An explanatory model. *Journal of Policy and Practice in Intellectual Disabilities*, *11*(3), 192–199. doi:10.1111/jppi.12089

Gilson, M., Davis, E., Johnson, S., Gains, J., Reddihough, D., & Williams, K. (2018). Mental health care needs and preferences for mothers of children with a disability. *Child: Care, Health and Development*, *44*(3), 384–391. doi:10.1111/cch.12556 PMID:29430692

Girimaji, S., Zahman, S., Wijetunja, P. M., Pejarasangharn, U., & Nagpal, J. (2001). *Mental Retardation: From Knowledge to Action*. Retrieved June 24, 2005 from http://whqlibdoc.who.int/searo/2001/SEA_Ment_119.pdf

Girimaji, S. C., & Pradeep, A. J. (2018). Intellectual disability in international classification of Diseases-11: A developmental perspective. Indian. *Journal of Social Psychiatry*, *34*(Suppl S1), 68–74.

Glaser, W., & Deane, K. (1999). Normalisation in an abnormal world: A study of prisoners with an intellectual disability. *International Journal of Offender Therapy and Comparative Criminology*, *43*(3), 338–356. doi:10.1177/0306624X99433007

Gleeson, B. (1995). Disability: A state of mind? *The Australian Journal of Social Issues*, *30*(1), 10–23. doi:10.1002/j.1839-4655.1995.tb01023.x

Glumbic, N., Kaljaca, S., & Brojcin, B. (2004). The attitude of future special educators towards inclusive education of children with mild intellectual disability. *Journal of Intellectual Disability Research*, *48*, 505–505.

Glumbic, N., & Zunic-Pavlovic, V. (2010). Bullying behavior in children with intellectual disability. *Procedia: Social and Behavioral Sciences*, *2*(2), 2784–2788. doi:10.1016/j.sbspro.2010.03.415

Goddard, H. H. (1912). *The Kallikak family: A study in the heredity of feeble-mindedness*. New York: Macmillan. doi:10.1037/10949-000

Goertzel, B. (2013). *The Wechsler Preschool and Primary Scale of Intelligence (WPPSI): A Brief Overview*. Retrieved from: http://goertzel.org/Preschool_IQ_Test_Overview.pdf

Gohel, M., Mukherjee, S., & Choudhary, S. K. (2011). Psychosocial impact on the parents of mentally retarded children in Anand District. *Healthline (Bhavnagar)*, *2*(2), 62–66.

Gold, M. W. (1972). stimulus factors in skill training of retarded adolescents on a complex assembly task: Acquisition, transfer, and relation. *American Journal of Mental Deficiency*, *76*, 517–526. PMID:5012132

Goode, D. A. (1994). *A world without words: The social construction of children born deaf and blind*. Philadelphia, PA: Temple University Press.

Goode, D. A., & Hogg, J. (1994). Towards an understanding of holistic quality of life in people with profound intellectual and multiple disabilities. In D. Goode (Ed.), *Quality of life for persons with disabilities: International perspectives and issues* (pp. 197–207). Cambridge, MA: Brookline Books.

Goodley, D. (2016). *Disability studies: An interdisciplinary introduction*. London: Sage.

Gopalan, R. T., Sharma, R., & Unnikrishnan, M. P. (2014). Socio-Demographic and Clinical Features of Children with Intellectual Disability and Their Parents-an Indian Study. *International Neuropsychiatric Disease Journal*, *2*(6), 289–302. doi:10.9734/INDJ/2014/10610

Gordon, B. O., & Rosenblum, K. E. (2001). Bringing Disability into the Sociological Frame: A comparison of disability with race, sex, and sexual orientation statuses. *Disability & Society*, *16*(1), 23–44.

Gostason, R. (1985). Psychiatric illness among the mentally retarded. *Acta Psychiat. Scand, 318*(suppl 71), 1-117.

Goudie, A., Narcisse, M. R., Hall, D. E., & Kuo, D. Z. (2014). Financial and psychological stressors associated with caring for children with disability. *Families, Systems & Health*, *32*(3), 280–290. doi:10.1037/fsh0000027 PMID:24707826

Govender, N. (2002). *Attitudes of Parents towards their Mentally Retarded Children: A Rural area Examination.* Academic Press.

Grace, N. C., Thompson, R., & Fisher, W. W. (1996). The treatment of covert self-injury through contingencies on response products. *Journal of Applied Behavior Analysis*, *29*(2), 239–242. doi:10.1901/jaba.1996.29-239 PMID:8682739

Graham, S., Bellmore, A. D., & Mize, J. (2006). Peer victimization, aggression, and their co-occurrence in middle school: Pathways to adjustment problems. *Journal of Abnormal Child Psychology*, *34*(3), 363–378. doi:10.100710802-006-9030-2 PMID:16648999

Granic, I., & Patterson, G. R. (2006). Toward a comprehensive model of antisocial development: A dynamic systems approach. *Psychological Review*, *113*(1), 101–131. doi:10.1037/0033-295X.113.1.101 PMID:16478303

Gratz, K. L., & Roemer, L. (2004). Multidimensional assessment of emotion regulation and deregulation Development, factor structure, and initial validation of the difficulties in emotion regulation scale. *Journal of Psychopathology and Behavioral Assessment*, *26*(1), 41–54. doi:10.1023/B:JOBA.0000007455.08539.94

Graves, T. B., Collins, B. C., Schuster, J. W., & Kleinert, H. (2005). Using video prompting to teach cooking skills to secondary students with moderate disabilities. *Education and Training in Developmental Disabilities*, *40*, 34–46.

Gray, E., Beech, A., & Rose, J. (2019). Using biofeedback to improve emotion regulation in sexual offenders with intellectual disability: A feasibility study. *International Journal of Developmental Disabilities*, 1–10.

Gray, K. M., Piccinin, A. M., Hofer, S. M., Mackinnon, A., Bontempo, D. E., Einfeld, S. L., ... Tonge, B. J. (2011). The longitudinal relationship between behavior and emotional disturbance in young people with intellectual disability and maternal mental health. *Research in Developmental Disabilities*, *32*(3), 1194–1204. doi:10.1016/j.ridd.2010.12.044 PMID:21295442

Grebler, A. M. (1952). Parental attitudes towards mentally retarded children. *American Journal of Mental Deficiency*, *56*, 475–483. PMID:14902885

Greef, A. P., & van der Walt, K. J. (2010). Resilience in families with an autistic child. *Education and Training in Autism and Developmental Disabilities*, *45*(3), 347–355.

Greene, J. G., Fox, N. A., & Lewis, M. (1983). The relationship between neonatal characteristics and three-month mother-infant interaction in high-risk infants. *Child Development*, *54*(5), 1286–1296. doi:10.2307/1129682 PMID:6354634

Green, S., & Bake, B. (2011). Parents emotion expression as a predictor of child's social competence: Children with or without intellectual disability. *Journal of Intellectual Disability Research*, *55*(3), 324–338. doi:10.1111/j.1365-2788.2010.01363.x PMID:21241394

Griffiths, D., & Unger, D. (1994). Views about planning for the future among parents and siblings of adults with mental retardation. *Family Relations*, *43*(2), 221–227. doi:10.2307/585326

Groce, N., & McGeown, J. (2013). *Witchcraft, Wealth and Disability: Reinterpretation of a folk belief in contemporary urban Africa* (Working Paper Series: No. 30). Leonard Cheshire Disability and Inclusive Development Centre, UCL.

Groce, N., Gazizova, D., & Hassiotis, P. (2014). Forced Marriage among Persons with Intellectual Disability. *Journal of Intellectual Disabilities.*

Gross, G. (1985). *Activities of the developmental disabilities adult offender project.* Olympia, WA: Washington State Developmental Disability Planning Council.

Gross, J. J. (2007). Preface. In J. J. Gross (Ed.), *Handbook of emotion regulation* (pp. xi–xiv). New York: Guilford Press.

Gross, J. J., & Muñoz, R. F. (1995). Emotion regulation and mental health. *Clinical Psychology: Science and Practice, 2*(2), 151–164. doi:10.1111/j.1468-2850.1995.tb00036.x

Gross, J. J., & Thompson, R. A. (2007). Emotion regulation: Conceptual foundations. In J. J. Gross (Ed.), *Handbook of emotion regulation* (pp. 3–24). New York: Guilford Press.

Gudjonsson, G. H., & Henry, L. (2003). Child and adult witnesses with intellectual disability: The importance of suggestibility. *Legal and Criminological Psychology, 8*(2), 241–252. doi:10.1348/135532503322363013

Gudjonsson, G. H., Murphy, G. H., & Clare, I. C. H. (2000). Assessing the capacity of people with intellectual disabilities to be witnesses in court. *Psychological Medicine, 30*(2), 307–314. doi:10.1017/S003329179900149X PMID:10824651

Gulati, G., Murphy, V., Clarke, A., Delcellier, K., Meagher, D., Kennedy, H., ... Dunne, C. P. (2018). Intellectual disability in Irish prisoners: Systematic review of prevalence. *International Journal of Prisoner Health, 14*(3), 188–196. doi:10.1108/IJPH-01-2017-0003 PMID:30274556

Gupta, V.B., Mehrotra, P. & Mehrotra, N (2012). *Parental Stress in Raising a Child with Disabilities in India*. Academic Press.

Gupta, A., & Singhal, N. (2004). Positive Perceptions in Parents of Children with Disabilities. *Asia Pacific Disability Rehabilitation Journal, 15*(1). Retrieved from http://english.aifo.it/disability/apdrj/apdrj104/positive-perceptions.pdf

Gupta, R. K., & Harpreet, K. (2010). Stress among parents of children with intellectual disability. *Asia Pacific Disability Rehabilitation Journal*, 21.

Gur, A., & Stein, M. A. (2019). Social worker attitudes toward parents with intellectual disabilities in Israel. *Disability and Rehabilitation, 7*, 1–11. doi:10.1080/09638288.2018.1537382 PMID:30616429

Guralnick, J. (1997). Effectiveness of early intervention for vulnerable children: A developmental perspective. *American Journal of Mental Retardation, 102*(4), 319–345. doi:10.1352/0895-8017(1998)102<0319:EOEIFV>2.0.CO;2 PMID:9475942

Guralnick, M. J. (1977). Peer social networks of young boys with developmental delays. *American Journal of Mental Retardation, 101*, 595–612. PMID:9152475

Guralnick, M. J. (1999). Family and child influences on the peer-related social competence of young children with developmental delays. *Mental Retardation and Developmental Disabilities Research Reviews, 5*(1), 21–29. doi:10.1002/(SICI)1098-2779(1999)5:1<21::AID-MRDD3>3.0.CO;2-O

Guralnick, M. J., Hammond, M. A., Connor, R. T., & Neville, B. (2006). Stability, change, and correlates of the peer relationships of young children with mild developmental delays. *Child Development, 77*(2), 312–324. doi:10.1111/j.1467-8624.2006.00872.x PMID:16611174

Gustafsson, C. (2003). *Intellectual disability and mental health problems: Evaluation of two clinical assessment instruments, occurrence of mental health problems and psychiatric care utilization.* Retrieved from: https://uu.divaportal.org/smash/get/diva2:163146

Gustiatas, R., & Young, E. W. D. (1986). *A time to be born, a time to die: Conflicts and ethics in an intensive care nursery*. Reading, MA: Addison-Wesley.

Hackman, A., Farah, M. J., & Meaney, M. J. (2010). Socioeconomic status and the brain: Mechanistic insights from human and animal research. *Nature Reviews. Neuroscience*, *11*(9), 651–659. doi:10.1038/nrn2897 PMID:20725096

Hagopian, L. P., Wilson, D. M., & Wilder, D. A. (2001). Assessment and treatment of problem behavior maintained by escape from attention and access to tangible items. *Journal of Applied Behavior Analysis*, *34*(2), 229–232. doi:10.1901/jaba.2001.34-229 PMID:11421317

Hagopian, L., Fisher, W., Sullivan, M., Acquisto, J., & LeBlanc, L. (1998). Effectiveness of functional communication training with and without extinction and punishment: A summary of 21 inpatient cases. *Journal of Applied Behavior Analysis*, *30*, 229–237. PMID:9652101

Haley, W., & Perkins, E. (2004). Current status and future directions in family caregiving and aging people with intellectual disabilities. *Journal of Policy and Practice in Intellectual Disabilities*, *1*(1), 24–30. doi:10.1111/j.1741-1130.2004.04004.x

Hall, A. M., Neuharth-Pritchett, S., & Belfiore, P. J. (1997). Reduction of aggressive behaviors with changes in activity: Linking descriptive and experimental analysis. *Education and Training in Mental Retardation and Developmental Disabilities*, *32*, 331–339.

Hall, S., Oliver, C., & Murphy, G. (2001). Early development of self-injurious behavior: An empirical study. *American Journal of Mental Retardation*, *106*(2), 189–199. doi:10.1352/0895-8017(2001)106<0189:EDOSIB>2.0.CO;2 PMID:11321609

Hallum, A. (1995). Disability and the transition to adulthood:Issues for the disabled child, the family, and the pediatrician. *Current Problems in Pediatrics*, *25*(1), 12–50. doi:10.1016/S0045-9380(06)80013-7 PMID:7720408

Hamdani, S., Atif, N., Tariq, M., Minhas, F., Iqbal, Z., & Rahman, A. (2014). Family networks to improve outcomes in children with intellectual and developmental disorders: A qualitative study. *International Journal of Mental Health Systems*, *8*(1), 7. doi:10.1186/1752-4458-8-7 PMID:24485093

Handen, B. L., & Gilchrist, R. (2006). Practitioner review: Psychopharmacology in children and adolescents with mental retardation. *Journal of Child Psychology and Psychiatry, and Allied Disciplines*, *47*(9), 871–882. doi:10.1111/j.1469-7610.2006.01588.x PMID:16930381

Hanley, G. P. (2012). Functional assessment of problem behavior: Dispelling myths, overcoming implementation obstacles, and developing new lore. *Behavior Analysis in Practice*, *5*(1), 54–72. doi:10.1007/BF03391818 PMID:23326630

Hanley, G. P., Iwata, B. A., & McCord, B. E. (2003). Functional analysis of problem behavior: A review. *Journal of Applied Behavior Analysis*, *36*(2), 147–185. doi:10.1901/jaba.2003.36-147 PMID:12858983

Hanley, G. P., Piazza, C. C., & Fisher, W. W. (1997). Noncontingent presentation of attention and alternative stimuli in the treatment of attention-maintained destructive behavior. *Journal of Applied Behavior Analysis*, *30*(2), 229–237. doi:10.1901/jaba.1997.30-229 PMID:9210303

Hannam, C. (1975). *Parents and Mentally Handicapped Children*. London: Penguin.

Harbour, C. K., & Maulik, P. K. (2010). History of Intellectual Disability. *International Encyclopedia of Rehabilitation*. Retrieved from http://cirrie.buffalo.edu/encyclopedia/en/article/143/

Harris, J. C. (2006). *Intellectual disability: Understanding its development, causes, classification, evaluation, and treatment*. Oxford University Press.

Harris, J. C. (2006). *Intellectual Disability: Understanding Its Development, Causes, Classification, Evaluation, and Treatment*. New York: Oxford University Press.

Harris, J. C. (2013). New Terminology for Mental Retardation in DSM-5 and ICD-11. *Current Opinion in Psychiatry, 26*(3), 260–262. doi:10.1097/YCO.0b013e32835fd6fb PMID:23507999

Harris, J. E. (2019). Legal capacity at a crossroad: Mental disability and family law. *Family Court Review, 57*(1), 14–20. doi:10.1111/fcre.12394

Hasani, G., & Tedadi, Y. (2011). The relationship between emotional intelligence and interpersonal problems. *Research in Health Psychology, 2*(4).

Hassall, R., Rose, J., & McDonald, J. (2005). Parenting stress in mothers of children with an intellectual disability: the effects of parental cognitions in relation to child characteristics and family support. *Journal of Intellectual Disability Research, 49*(6), 405-418.

Hassall, R., Rose, J., & McDonald, J. (2015). Parenting stress in mothers of children with an intellectual disability: The effects of parental cognitions in relation to child characteristics and family support. *Journal of Intellectual Disabilities, 49*(6), 405–418. doi:10.1111/j.1365-2788.2005.00673.x PMID:15882391

Hastings, P. (2002). Parental stress and behaviour problems of children with developmental disability. *Journal of Intellectual & Developmental Disability, 27*(3), 149–160. doi:10.1080/1366825021000008657

Hastings, P., & Beck, A. (2004). Practitioner review: Stress intervention for parents of children with intellectual disabilities. *Journal of Child Psychology and Psychiatry, and Allied Disciplines, 45*(8), 1338–1349. doi:10.1111/j.1469-7610.2004.00357.x PMID:15482495

Hastings, R. P. (2003). Child behaviour problems and partner mental health as correlates of stress in mothers and fathers of children with autism. *Journal of Intellectual Disability Research, 47*(4-5), 231–237. doi:10.1046/j.1365-2788.2003.00485.x PMID:12787155

Hastings, R. P., Daley, D., Burns, C., & Beck, A. (2006). Maternal distress and expressed emotion: Cross-sectional and longitudinal relationships with behavior problems of children with intellectual disabilities. *American Journal of Mental Retardation, 111*(1), 48–61. doi:10.1352/0895-8017(2006)111[48:MDAEEC]2.0.CO;2 PMID:16332156

Hastings, R. P., & Lloyd, T. (2007). Expressed emotion in families of children and adults with intellectual disabilities. *Mental Retardation and Developmental Disabilities Research Reviews, 13*(4), 339–345. doi:10.1002/mrdd.20173 PMID:17979206

Hatton, C. (2002). Psychosocial interventions for adults with intellectual disabilities and mental health problems: a review. *Journal of Mental Health, 11*(4), 357-374.

Hatton, C., & Emerson, E. (2003). Families with a person with intellectual disabilities: Stress and impact. *Current Opinion in Psychiatry, 16*(5), 497–501. doi:10.1097/00001504-200309000-00002

Hauser-Cram, P., Warfield, M. E., & Shonkoff, J. P. (2001). Children with disabilities: A longitudinal study of child development and parent wellbeing. *Monographs of the Society for Research in Child Development, 66*, 1–131. PMID:11677873

Hauser-Cram, P., Warfield, M. E., Shonkoff, J. P., Krauss, M. W., Upshur, C. C., & Sayer, A. (1999). Family influences on adaptive development in young children with Down syndrome. *Child Development, 70*(4), 979–989. doi:10.1111/1467-8624.00071 PMID:10446730

Hawker, D. S., & Boulton, M. J. (2000). Twenty years' research on peer victimization and psychosocial maladjustment: A meta-analytic review of cross sectional studies. *Journal of Child Psychology and Psychiatry, and Allied Disciplines, 41*(4), 441–455. doi:10.1111/1469-7610.00629 PMID:10836674

Hayashi, M., Arakida, M., & Ohashi, K. (2011). The effectiveness of a sex education program facilitating social skills for people with intellectual disability in Japan. *Journal of Intellectual & Developmental Disability, 36*(1), 11–19. doi:10.3109/13668250.2010.549463 PMID:21284415

Hayes, S. (1996). Recent research on offenders with learning disabilities. *Tizard Learning Disability Review, 1*(3), 7–15. doi:10.1108/13595474199600003

Hayes, S. C., Wilson, K. G., Gifford, E. V., Follette, V. M., & Strosahl, K. (1996). Experiential avoidance and behavioral disorders: A functional dimensional approach to diagnosis and treatment. *Journal of Consulting and Clinical Psychology, 64*(6), 1152–1168. doi:10.1037/0022-006X.64.6.1152 PMID:8991302

Hazarika, M., Das, S., & Choudhury, S. (2017). Parents' attitude towards children and adolescents with intellectual developmental disorder. International journal of child development and mental health, 5(1), 11–21.

Hazarika, M., Das, S., & Choudhury, S. (2017). Parents' attitude towards children and adolescents with intellectual developmental disorder. *International Journal of Child Development and Mental Health, 5*(1), 11.

Headey, B., & Wearing, A. (1992). *Understanding happiness: A theory of subjective well-being.* Melbourne: Longman Cheshire.

Health Commission of New South Wales. (1981). *Circular 81/8.* Sydney: Health Commission of New South Wales.

Heather, S. (2013). Fighting the stigma caused by mental disorders: past perspectives, present activities, and future directions. World Psychiatric Association.

Heifetz, M., Brown, H. K., Chacra, M. A., Tint, A., Vigod, S., Bluestein, D., & Lunsky, Y. (2019). Mental health challenges and resilience among mothers with intellectual and developmental disabilities. *Disability and Health Journal, 19*, 30107–4. doi:10.1016/j.dhjo.2019.06.006 PMID:31235446

Heikura, U., Taanila, A., Hartikainen, A. L., Olsen, P., Linna, S. L., Von, W. L., & Järvelin, M. R. (2006). Intellectual disability: A prospective longitudinal population-based study. *Intellectual Disability Research, 50*(4), 259–268. doi:10.1111/j.1365-2788.2005.00792.x PMID:16507030

Heilbronner, R. (2004). A status report on the practice of forensic neuropsychology. *The Clinical Neuropsychologist, 18*(2), 312–326. doi:10.1080/13854040490501574 PMID:15587677

Heiman, T. (2002). Parents of Children with Disabilities: Resilience, Coping, and Future Expectations. *Journal of Developmental and Physical Disabilities, 14*(2), 159–171. doi:10.1023/A:1015219514621

Heller, T. (2010). Age-related Health Issues in People with Intellectual Disability. *Impact, 23*(1).

Heller, T., & Caldwell, J. (2006). Supporting aging caregivers and adults with developmental disabilities in future planning. *Mental Retardation, 44*(3), 189–202. doi:10.1352/0047-6765(2006)44[189:SACAAW]2.0.CO;2 PMID:16677064

Heller, T., Miller, A., & Factor, A. (1997). Adults with mental retardation as supports to their parents: Effects on parental caregiving appraisal. *Mental Retardation, 35*(5), 338–346. doi:10.1352/0047-6765(1997)035<0338:AWMRAS>2.0.CO;2 PMID:9339062

Hemphill, S. A., Tollit, M., Kotevski, A., & Florent, A. (2015). Bullying in schools: Rates, correlates and impact on mental health. In J. Lindert & I. Itzhak (Eds.), *Violence and mental health: Its manifold faces* (pp. 185–205). Springer.

Henny, M. J., Schrojenstein, L. V., & Walsh, P. N. (2008). Managing Health Problems in People with Intellectual Disabilities. *British Medical Journal, 337*, 1408–1412. PMID:19064601

Herring, S., Gray, K., Taffe, J., Tonge, B., Sweeney, D., & Einfeld, S. (2006). Behaviour and emotional problems in toddlers with pervasive developmental disorders and developmental delay: Associations with parental mental health and family functioning. *Journal of Intellectual Disability Research, 50*(Pt 12), 874–882. doi:10.1111/j.1365-2788.2006.00904.x PMID:17100948

Hertz, M. F., Donato, I., & Wright, J. (2013). Bullying and suicide: A public health approach. *The Journal of Adolescent Health, 53*(1), S1–S3. doi:10.1016/j.jadohealth.2013.05.002 PMID:23790194

Hewstone, M. (2003). Inter-group contact: Panacea for prejudice? *The Psychologist, 12*(7), 352–355.

Hirisave, U., Oommen, A., & Kapur, M. (2002). Psychological assessment of children in the clinicalsetting - Introduction. In Psychological assessment of children in the clinical setting (pp. 1-5) Bangalore: NIMHANS.

Hockley, O. J., & Langdon, P. E. (2015). Men with intellectual disabilities with a history of sexual offending: Empathy for victims of sexual and non-sexual crimes. *Journal of Intellectual Disability Research, 59*(4), 332–341. doi:10.1111/jir.12137 PMID:24761788

Hodapp, R. M. (2002). Parenting children with mental retardation. In M. H. Bornstein (Ed.), Handbook of Parenting (pp. 355–381). London: Lawrence Erlbaum Associates.

Hodgins, S. (1992). Mental disorder, intellectual deficiency, and crime: Evidence from a birth cohort. *Archives of General Psychiatry, 49*(6), 476–483. doi:10.1001/archpsyc.1992.01820060056009 PMID:1599373

Hodgins, S., Mednick, S. A., Brennan, P. A., Schulsinger, F., & Engberg, M. (1996). Mental disorder and crime: Evidence from a Danish birth cohort. *Archives of General Psychiatry, 53*(6), 489–496. doi:10.1001/archpsyc.1996.01830060031004 PMID:8639031

Hogg, J., Lucchino, R., Wang, K., Janicki, M. P., & Group, W. (2000). *Healthy Ageing: Adults with Intellectual Disabilities: Ageing & Social Policy*. Geneva: World Health Organization.

Hogg, J., & Sebba, J. (1987). Profound retardation and multiple impairment: Vol. 1. *Development and learning*. Rockville, MD: Aspen Publishers.

Höglund, B., & Larsson, M. (2019). Midwives' work and attitudes towards contraceptive counselling and contraception among women with intellectual disability: Focus group interviews in Sweden. *The European Journal of Contraception & Reproductive Health Care, 24*(1), 39–44. doi:10.1080/13625187.2018.1555640 PMID:30633574

Holland, T., Clare, I. C. H., & Mukhopadhyay, T. (2002). Prevalence of 'criminal offending' by men and women with intellectual disability and the characteristics of 'offenders': Implications for research and service development. *Journal of Intellectual Disability Research, 46*(s1), 6–20. doi:10.1046/j.1365-2788.2002.00001.x PMID:12061335

Holroyd, J. (1974). The Questionnaire on Resources and Stress: An instrument to measure family response to a handicapped family member. *Journal of Community Psychology, 2*(1), 92–94. doi:10.1002/1520-6629(197401)2:1<92::AID-JCOP2290020133>3.0.CO;2-A

Holroyd, J., & McArthur, D. (1976). Mental retardation and stress on the parents: A contrast between Down's syndrome and childhood autism. *American Journal of Mental Deficiency, 80*, 431–436. PMID:129006

Holth, P. (2003). Generalized imitation and generalized matching to sample. *The Behavior Analyst, 26*(1), 155-158.

Hong, J. S., Davis, J. P., Sterzing, P. R., Yoon, J., Choi, S., & Smith, D. C. (2014). A conceptual framework for understanding the association between school bullying victimization and substance misuse. *The American Journal of Orthopsychiatry*, *84*(6), 696–710. doi:10.1037/ort0000036 PMID:25545436

Hong, J. S., Peguero, A. A., Choi, S., Lanesskog, D., Espelage, D. L., & Lee, N. Y. (2014). Social ecology of bullying and peer victimization of Latino and Asian youth in the United States: A review of the literature. *Journal of School Violence*, *13*(3), 315–338. doi:10.1080/15388220.2013.856013

Ho, P., Downs, J., Bulsara, C., Patman, S., & Hill, A. M. (2018). Addressing challenges in gaining informed consent for a research study investigating falls in people with intellectual disability. *British Journal of Learning Disabilities*, *46*(2), 92–100. doi:10.1111/bld.12217

Hopkins, H. L., & Smith, H. D. (1993). *Willard and Spackman's Occupational Therapy* (8th ed.). Philadelphia: J.B. Lippincott. Retrieved from http://www.sgh.org.sa/Portals/0/Articles/International%20Handbook%20of%20Occupational%20 Thera py%20Interventions.pdf

Horner, R. H., Day, H. M., Sprague, J. R., O'Brien, M., & Heathfield, L. T. (1991). Interspersed requests: A nonaversive procedure for reducing aggression and self-injury during instruction. *Journal of Applied Behavior Analysis*, *24*(2), 265–278. doi:10.1901/jaba.1991.24-265 PMID:1890047

Horrell, S.C.V., MacLean, W.E., & Conley, V.M. (2006) Patient and parent/guardian perspectives on the health care of adults with mental retardation. *Mental Retardation, 44*(4), 239-248.

Hosseinkhanzadeh, A. A., & Yeganeh, T. (2013). A study of the siblings relationships in families with mentally disable children. *Procedia: Social and Behavioral Sciences*, *84*, 864–868. doi:10.1016/j.sbspro.2013.06.663

Hounsome, J., Whittington, R., Brown, A., Greenhill, B., & McGuire, J. (2018). The structured assessment of violence risk in adults with intellectual disability: A systematic review. *Journal of Applied Research in Intellectual Disabilities*, *31*(1), e1–e17. doi:10.1111/jar.12295 PMID:27891723

Howell, A., Hauser-Cram, P., & Kersh, J. E. (2007). Setting the stage: Early child and family characteristics as predictors of later loneliness in children with developmental disabilities. *American Journal of Mental Retardation*, *112*(1), 18–30. doi:10.1352/0895-8017(2007)112[18:STSECA]2.0.CO;2 PMID:17181387

Howlett, S., Florio, T., Xu, H., & Trollor, J. (2015). Ambulatory mental health data demonstrates the high needs of people with an intellectual disability: results from the new south wales intellectual disability and mental health data linkage project. *Australian & New Zealand Journal of Psychiatry, 49*(2), 137-144.

Hsu, T. H., Huang, Y. T., Liu, Y. H., Ososkie, J., Fried, J., & Bezyak, J. (2015). Taiwanese attitudes and affective reactions toward individuals and coworkers who have intellectual disabilities. *American Journal on Intellectual and Developmental Disabilities*, *120*(2), 110–124. doi:10.1352/1944-7558-120.2.110 PMID:25715181

Hughes, K., Bellis, M. A., Jones, L., Wood, S., Bates, G., Eckley, L., ... Officer, A. (2005). Prevalence and risk of violence against adults with disabilities: A systematic review and meta-analysis of observational studies. *Lancet*, *379*(9826), 1621–1629. doi:10.1016/S0140-6736(11)61851-5 PMID:22377290

Hui, C. H., & Triandis, H. C. (1986). Individualism-Collectivism: A study of cross-cultural researchers. *Journal of Cross-Cultural Psychology*, *17*(2), 225–248. doi:10.1177/0022002186017002006

Hurley, D. (2006). Mood disorders in intellectual disability. *Current Opinion in Psychiatry*, *19*(5), 465–469. doi:10.1097/01.yco.0000238471.84206.0a PMID:16874117

Huxley, A., Dalton, M., Tsui, Y. Y., & Hayhurst, K. P. (2018). Prevalence of alcohol, smoking, and illicit drug use amongst people with intellectual disabilities. *Drugs Education Prevention & Policy*, 1–20. doi:10.1080/09687637.2018.1488949

Hymel, S., & Swearer, S. M. (2015). Four decades of research on school bullying. *The American Psychologist*, *70*(4), 293–299. doi:10.1037/a0038928 PMID:25961310

ICD 10. (1992). *Classification of mental and behavioural disorder: Diagnostic criteria for Research*. Author.

Ineland, J., & Hjelte, J. (2019). Knowing, being or doing? A comparative study on human service professionals' perceptions of quality in day-to-day encounters with clients and students with intellectual disabilities. *Journal of Intellectual Disabilities*, *22*(3), 246–261. doi:10.1177/1744629517694705 PMID:30134782

International Labour Office. (2003). *Employment of People with Disabilities: The impact of Legislation*. India Country Profile. Retrieved March, 17, 2005 from http://www.ilo.org/publi/english/employment/skills/disability/download/cpindia.pdf

Irazábal, M., Marsà, F., García, M., Gutiérrez-Recacha, P., Martorell, A., Salvador-Carulla, L., & Ochoa, S. (2012). Family burden related to clinical and functional variables of people with intellectual disability with and without a mental disorder. *Research In Developmental Disabilities, 33*(3), 796-803. doi:10.1016/j.ridd.2011.12.002

Irazábal, M., Marsà, F., & García, M. (2011). Family burden related to clinical and functional variables of people with intellectual disability with and without a mental disorder. *Research in Developmental Disabilities*, *32*, 796–803. PMID:22245729

Ivanova, D., & Giannouli, V. (2017). Lesch type III alcoholism in Bulgarian women: Implications and recommendations for psychotherapy. *International Journal of Caring Sciences*, *10*(3), 1569–1576.

Iverson, C., & Fox, R. A. (1989). Prevalence of psychopathology among mentally retarded adults. *Research in Developmental Disabilities*, *10*(1), 77–83. doi:10.1016/0891-4222(89)90030-9 PMID:2928581

Iwata, B. A., & DeLeon, I. (1996) The functional analysis screening tool. Gainesville, FL: The Florida Centre on Self-Injury, The University of Florida.

Iwata, B., Dorsey, M., Slifer, K., Bauman, K., & Richman, G. (1994). Toward a functional analysis of self-injury. *Journal of Applied Behavior Analysis, 27*, 197-209.

Iwata, B. A., & Dozier, C. L. (2008). Clinical application of functional analysis methodology. *Behavior Analysis in Practice*, *1*(1), 3–9. doi:10.1007/BF03391714 PMID:22477673

Iwata, B. A., Pace, G. M., Cowdery, G. E., & Miltenberger, R. G. (1994). What makes extinction work: An analysis of procedural form and function. *Journal of Applied Behavior Analysis*, *27*(1), 131–144. doi:10.1901/jaba.1994.27-131 PMID:8188555

Jacobson, J. W., Mulick, J. A., & Rojahn, J. (2007). Handbook of Intellectual and Developmental Disabilities. Academic Press. doi:10.1007/0-387-32931-5

Jahoda, A., Pert, C., Squire, J., & Trower, P. (1998). Facing stress and conflict: A comparison of the predicted responses and self-concepts of aggressive and non-aggressive people with intellectual disability. *Journal of Intellectual Disability Research*, *42*(5), 360–369. doi:10.1046/j.1365-2788.1998.00143.x PMID:9828067

Jahoda, A., Pert, C., & Trower, P. (2006a). Socioemotional understanding and frequent aggression in people with mild to moderate intellectual disabilities: Recognition of facial affect and role-taking abilities. *American Journal of Mental Retardation*, *111*(2), 77–89. doi:10.1352/0895-8017(2006)111[77:SUAFAI]2.0.CO;2 PMID:16466287

Jahoda, A., Pert, C., & Trower, P. (2006b). Frequent aggression and attribution of hostile intent in people with mild to moderate intellectual disabilities: An empirical investigation. *American Journal of Mental Retardation, 111*(2), 90–99. doi:10.1352/0895-8017(2006)111[90:FAAAOH]2.0.CO;2 PMID:16466288

Jakab, I. (1990). Neuropsychological evaluation and rehabilitation in mental retardation. *Neuropsychology Review, 1*(2), 137–164. doi:10.1007/BF01108715 PMID:2152529

James, H. (2004). Promoting effective working with parents with learning disabilities. *Child Abuse Review, 13*(1), 31–41. doi:10.1002/car.823

Jan, J.E., Owens, J.A., Weiss, M.D., Johnson, K.P., Wasdell, M.B., & Freeman, R.D. (2008). Sleep hygiene for children with neurodevelopmental disabilities. *Ipsiroglu O.S Pediatrics, 122*(6), 1343-50.

Jansen, S. L., van der Putten, A. A., & Vlaskamp, C. (2013). What parents find important in the support of a child with profound intellectual and multiple disabilities. *Child: Care, Health and Development, 39*(3), 432–441. doi:10.1111/j.1365-2214.2012.01381.x PMID:22515566

Jeevanandam, L. (2009). Perspectives of intellectual disability in Asia: Epidemiology, policy, and services for children and adults. *Current Opinion in Psychiatry, 22*(5), 462–468. doi:10.1097/YCO.0b013e32832ec056 PMID:19625968

Jencks, C., & Phillips, M. (1998). The Black-White Test Scope Gap: Why It Persists and What Can Be Done. *The Brookings Review, 16*(2), 24–27. doi:10.2307/20080778

Jenkins, R., & Angrosino, M. V. (1998). *Questions of competence: Culture, classification and intellectual disability.* Cambridge, UK: Cambridge University Press.

Jessop, D. J., Riessman, C. K., & Stein, R. E. (1998). Chronic childhood illness and maternal mental health. *Journal of Developmental and Behavioral Pediatrics, 9*, 147–156. PMID:3403730

Jobling, A., Moni, K., & Nolan, A. (2000). Understanding friendship: Young adults with Down syndrome explore relationships. *Journal of Intellectual & Developmental Disability, 25*(3), 235–245. doi:10.1080/13269780050144299

John, A. (2012). Stress among mothers of children with intellectual disabilities in urban India: Role of gender and maternal coping. *Journal of Applied Research in Intellectual Disabilities, 25*(4), 372–382. doi:10.1111/j.1468-3148.2011.00672.x PMID:22711485

Jokinen, N., Gomiero, T., Watchman, K., Janicki, M. P., Hogan, M., Larsen, F., ... Crowe, J. (2018). Perspectives on family caregiving of people aging with intellectual disability affected by dementia: Commentary from the International Summit on Intellectual Disability and Dementia. Journal. *Journal of Gerontological Social Work, 61*(4), 411–431. doi: 10.1080/01634372.2018.1454563 PMID:29583104

Jones, K. M., Drew, H. A., & Weber, N. L. (2000). Noncontingent peer attention as treatment for disruptive classroom behavior. *Journal of Applied Behavior Analysis, 33*(3), 343-346. doi:10.1901/jaba.2000.33-343

Jones, J. (2007). Persons with intellectual disabilities in the criminal justice system: Review of issues. *International Journal of Offender Therapy and Comparative Criminology, 51*(6), 723–733. doi:10.1177/0306624X07299343 PMID:17636203

Jones, J., & Passey, J. (2005). Family adaptation, coping, and resources: Parents of children with developmental disabilities and behaviour problems. *Journal on Developmental Disabilities, 11*(1), 31–46.

Jones, K. L., & Smith, D. W. (1997). *Smith's recognizable patterns of human malformation* (5th ed.). Philadelphia: Saunders.

Jones, L., Bellis, M. A., Wood, S., Hughes, K., McCoy, E., Eckley, L., ... Officer, A. (2012). Prevalence and risk of violence against children with disabilities: A systematic review and meta-analysis of observational studies. *Lancet*, *380*(9845), 899–907. doi:10.1016/S0140-6736(12)60692-8 PMID:22795511

Joseph, L., & Ittyerah, M. (2015). Recognition and understanding of emotions in persons with mild to moderate mental retardation. *Journal of Psychosocial Rehabilitation and Mental Health*, *2*(1), 59-66.

Joseph, J. (2005). The 1942 'euthanasia' debate in the American Journal of Psychiatry. *History of Psychiatry*, *16*(2), 171–179. doi:10.1177/0957154X05047004 PMID:16013119

Kabra, M., & Gulati, S. (2003). Mental retardation. *Indian Journal of Pediatrics*, *70*(2), 153–158. doi:10.1007/BF02723745 PMID:12661811

Kagohara, D. M., van der Meer, L., Ramdoss, S., O'Reilly, M. F., Lancioni, G. E., Davis, T. N., ... Sigafoos, J. (2013). Using iPods® and iPads® in teaching programs for individuals with developmental disabilities: A systematic review. *Research in Developmental Disabilities*, *34*(1), 147–156. doi:10.1016/j.ridd.2012.07.027 PMID:22940168

Kahng, S., Iwata, B. A., Fischer, S. M., Page, T. J., Treadwell, K. R., Williams, D. E., & Smith, R. G. (1998). Temporal distributions of problem behavior based on scatter plot analysis. *Journal of Applied Behavior Analysis*, *31*(4), 593–604. doi:10.1901/jaba.1998.31-593 PMID:9891396

Kahng, S., Iwata, B. A., & Lewin, A. B. (2002). Behavioral treatment of self-injury, 1964 to 2000. *American Journal of Mental Retardation*, *107*(3), 212–221. doi:10.1352/0895-8017(2002)107<0212:BTOSIT>2.0.CO;2 PMID:11966334

Kaltiala-Heino, R., Rimpela, M., Marttunen, M., Rimpela, A., & Rantanen, P. (1999). Bullying, depression, and suicidal ideation in Finnish adolescents: School survey. *British Medical Journal*, *319*(7206), 438–451. doi:10.1136/bmj.319.7206.348 PMID:10435954

Kandel, I., Morad, M., Vardi, G., & Merrick, J. (2005). Intellectual disability and parenthood. *The Scientific World Journal*, *5*, 50–57. doi:10.1100/tsw.2005.12 PMID:15674450

Karam, S. M., Barros, A. J. D., Matijasevich, A., dos Santos, I. S., Anselmi, L., Barros, F., ... Black, M. M. (2016). Intellectual Disability in a Birth Cohort: Prevalence, Etiology, and Determinants at the Age of 4 Years. *Public Health Genomics*, *19*(5), 290–297. doi:10.1159/000448912 PMID:27595410

Karl, R., McGuigan, D., Withiam-Leitch, M. L., Akl, E. A., & Symons, A. B. (2013). Reflective impressions of a precepted clinical experience caring for people with disabilities. *Intellectual and Developmental Disabilities*, *51*(4), 237–245. doi:10.1352/1934-9556-51.4.237 PMID:23909585

Katz, G., & Lazcano-Ponce, E. (2008). Intellectual disability: Definition, etiological factors, classification, diagnosis, treatment and prognosis. *Salud Pública de México*, *50*(2), 132–141. PMID:18470340

Katz, G., & Lazcano-Ponce, E. (2008). Sexuality in subjects with intellectual disability: An educational intervention proposal for parents and counsellors in developing countries. *Salud Pública de México*, *2*, 239–254. doi:10.1590/S0036-36342008000800018

Kavale, K. A., & Forness, S. R. (1995). Social skill deficits and training: A meta-analysis of the research in learning disabilities. *Advances in Learning and Behavioral Disabilities*, *9*, 119–160.

Kavale, K. A., & Forness, S. R. (1996). Social skill deficits and learning disabilities: A meta-analysis. *Journal of Learning Disabilities*, *29*(3), 226–237. doi:10.1177/002221949602900301 PMID:8732884

Kazak, A. E., & Marvin, R. S. (1984). Differences, difficulties and adaptation: Stress and social networks in families with a handicapped child. *Family Relations*, *33*(1), 67–77. doi:10.2307/584591

Kazdin, A. E. (2012). *Behavior modification in applied settings*. Waveland Press.

Kebbell, M. R., & Hatton, C. (1999). People with mental retardation as witnesses in court: A review. *Mental Retardation*, *37*(3), 179–187. doi:10.1352/0047-6765(1999)037<0179:PWMRAW>2.0.CO;2 PMID:10473337

Kebbell, M. R., Hatton, C., & Johnson, S. D. (2004). Witnesses with intellectual disabilities in court: What questions are asked and what influence do they have? *Legal and Criminological Psychology*, *9*(1), 23–35. doi:10.1348/135532504322776834

Keenan, B. (1992). *An evil cradling*. London: Vintage Press.

Keen, D., Brannigan, K. L., & Cuskelly, M. (2007). Toilet training for children with autism: The effects of video modeling. *Journal of Developmental and Physical Disabilities*, *19*(4), 291–303. doi:10.100710882-007-9044-x

Keith, K. D., & Bonham, G. S. (2005). The use of quality of life data at the organization and systems level. *Journal of Intellectual Disability Research*, *49*(part 10), 799–805. doi:10.1111/j.1365-2788.2005.00755.x PMID:16162131

Kellems, R. O., & Edwards, S. (2015). Using Video Modeling and Video Prompting to Teach Core Academic Content to Students With Learning Disabilities. *Preventing School Failure*, 1–8.

Keller, F. S., & Schoenfeld, W. N. (1950). *Principles of psychology: A systematic text in the science of behavior*. New York: Appleton-Century-Crofts. doi:10.1037/11293-000

Kelly, E. V., Newton, N. C., Stapinski, L. A., Slade, T., Barrett, E. L., Conrod, P. J., & Teesson, M. (2015). Suicidality, internalizing problems and externalizing problems among adolescent bullies, victims and bully-victims. *Preventive Medicine*, *73*, 100–105. doi:10.1016/j.ypmed.2015.01.020 PMID:25657168

Kelly, G., Crowley, H., & Hamilton, C. (2009). Rights, sexuality, and relationships in Ireland: "It'd be nice to be kind of trusted. *British Journal of Learning Disabilities*, *37*(4), 308–315. doi:10.1111/j.1468-3156.2009.00587.x

Kelly, G., & Parry, A. (2008). Managing Challenging Behaviour of People with Acquired Brain Injury in Community Settings: The first 7 years of specialist clinical service. *Brain Impairment*, *9*(3), 293–304. doi:10.1375/brim.9.3.293

Kemp, C., & Carter, M. (2002). The social skills and social status of mainstreamed students with intellectual disabilities. *Educational Psychology*, *22*(4), 391–411. doi:10.1080/01443410220000003097

Kempton, W., & Gochros, J. (1986). The developmentally disabled. In H. L. Gochros, J. S. Gochros, & J. Fisher (Eds.), *Helping the sexually oppressed* (pp. 224–237). Englewood Cliffs, NJ: Prentice-Hall.

Kennedy, C. H. (1994). Manipulating antecedent conditions to alter the stimulus control of problem behavior. *Journal of Applied Behavior Analysis*, *27*(1), 161–170. doi:10.1901/jaba.1994.27-161 PMID:8188556

Kern, L., Choutka, C. M., & Sokol, N. G. (2002). Assessment-based interventions used in natural settings to reduce challenging behaviors: A review of the literature. *Education & Treatment of Children*, *25*, 113–134.

Kersh, J., Hedvat, T. T., Hauser-Cram, P., & Warfield, M. E. (2006). The contribution of marital quality to the well-being of parents of children with developmental disabilities. *Journal of Intellectual Disability Research*, *50*(12), 883–893. doi:10.1111/j.1365-2788.2006.00906.x PMID:17100949

Khadi, P. B., & Hidangmayum, N. (2012). Parenting stress of normal and mentally challenged children. *Karnataka Journal of Agricultural Sciences*, *25*(2), 256–259.

Khandelwal, S. K., & Workneh, F. (1986). Perception of mental illness by medical students Indian. *Journal of Psychological Medicine*, *9*, 26–32.

Khare, S. (2015). Impact of quality of life in parents of mentally retarded children: Research findings in a regional centre. *Innovation Journal of Nursing and Healthcare, 1*(3), 171-178.

Kiani, R., & Miller, H. (2010). Sensory impairment and intellectual disability. *Advances in Psychiatric Treatment, 16*(3), 228–235. doi:10.1192/apt.bp.108.005736

Kijak, R. (2013). The Sexuality of Adults with Intellectual Disability in Poland. *Sexuality and Disability, 31*(2), 109–123. doi:10.100711195-013-9294-8 PMID:23704799

Kijak, R. J. (2011). Desire for love: Considerations on sexuality and sex education of people with intellectual disability in Poland. *Sexuality and Disability, 29*(1), 65–74. doi:10.100711195-010-9184-2 PMID:21423325

Kimura, M., & Yamazaki, Y. (2017). Having another child without intellectual disabilities: Comparing mothers of a single child with disability and mothers of multiple children with and without disability. *Journal of Intellectual Disabilities, 23*(2), 216–232. doi:10.1177/1744629517749129 PMID:29284333

King, T. L., Milner, A., Aitken, Z., Karahalios, A., Emerson, E., & Kavanagh, A. M. (2019). Mental health of adolescents: Variations by borderline intellectual functioning and disability. *European Child & Adolescent Psychiatry*, 1–10. PMID:30759281

Kirkham, A. (1993). Two-year follow-up of skills training with mothers of children with disabilities. *American Journal of Mental Retardation*. PMID:7681675

Kirkham, A., & Schilling, R. F. II. (1990). Life skills training with mothers of handicapped children. *Journal of Social Service Research, 13*(2), 67–87. doi:10.1300/J079v13n02_05

Kishore, M. T. (2011). Disability impact and coping in mothers of children with intellectual disabilities and multiple disabilities. *Journal of Intellectual Disabilities, 15*(4), 241–251. doi:10.1177/1744629511431659 PMID:22158461

Kishore, M. T., Nizamie, A., Nizamie, S. H., & Jahan, M. (2004). Psychiatric diagnosis in persons with intellectual disability in India. *Journal of Intellectual Disability Research, 48*(1), 19–24. doi:10.1111/j.1365-2788.2004.00579.x PMID:14675227

Kistner, J. A., & Gatlin, D. F. (1989). Sociometric differences between learning-disabled and nonhandicapped students: Effects of sex and race. *Journal of Educational Psychology, 81*(1), 118–120. doi:10.1037/0022-0663.81.1.118

Klimecki, M. R., Jenkinson, J., & Wilson, L. (1994). A study of recidivism among offenders with an intellectual disability. *Journal of Intellectual & Developmental Disability, 19*(3), 209–219.

Knox, M., & Bigby, C. (2007). Moving towards midlife careas negotiated family business: Accounts of people with intellectual disabilities and their families "Just getting along with their lives together". *International Journal of Disability Development and Education, 54*(3), 287–304. doi:10.1080/10349120701488749

Kohli, A., Mahotra, S., & Kehra, N. (2014). Neuropsychological Profile of Children with Hyperkinetic Disorder. Journal. *Indian Association Child Adolescent Mental Health, 10*(3), 167–193.

Kolevzon, A., Gross, R., & Reichenberg, A. (2007). Prenatal and Perinatal Risk Factors for Autism: A Review and Integration of Findings. *Archives of Pediatrics & Adolescent Medicine, 161*(4), 326–333. doi:10.1001/archpedi.161.4.326 PMID:17404128

Konstantareas, M. M., & Lunsky, Y. J. (1997). Socio-sexual knowledge, experience, attitudes, and interests of individuals with autistic disorder and developmental delay. *Journal of Autism and Developmental Disorders, 27*(4), 397–413. doi:10.1023/A:1025805405188 PMID:9261666

Kopecky, K. (2014). Cyberbullying and other risks of internet communication focused on university students. *Procedia: Social and Behavioral Sciences, 112*, 260–269. doi:10.1016/j.sbspro.2014.01.1163

Koskentausta, T., Iivanainen, M., & Almqvist, F. (2007). Risk factors for psychiatric disturbance in children with intellectual disability. *Journal of Intellectual Disability Research, 51*(1), 43–53. doi:10.1111/j.1365-2788.2006.00871.x PMID:17181602

Koslowski, N., Klein, K., Arnold, K., Koesters, M., Schuetzwohl, M., Salize, H. J., & Puschner, B. (2016). Effectiveness of interventions for adults with mild to moderate intellectual disabilities and mental health problems: systematic review and meta-analysis. *The British Journal of Psychiatry, 209*(6), 469-474.

Koul, R., & Clapsaddle, K. C. (2006). Effects of repeated listening experiences on the perception of synthetic speech by individuals with mild-to-moderate intellectual disabilities. *AAC: Augmentative & Alternative Communication, 22*, 112–122. PMID:17114169

Kozlowski, A. M., & Matson, J. L. (2012). Interview and observation methods in functional assessment. In J. L. Matson (Ed.), *Functional assessment for challenging behaviour* (pp. 105–124). New York, NY: Springer New York. doi:10.1007/978-1-4614-3037-7_7

Krauss, M. W. (1993). Child related and parenting stress: Similarities and differences between mothers and fathers of children with disabilities. *American Journal of Mental Retardation, 97*(4), 393–404. PMID:8427694

Kringelbach, M.L., & Berridge, K.C. (2010). The functional neuroanatomy of pleasure and happiness. *HHS Author Manuscripts, 9*(49), 579-587.

Kritsotakis, G., Galanis, P., Papastefanakis, E., Meidani, F., Philalithis, A. E., Kalokairinou, A., & Sourtzi, P. (2017). Attitudes towards people with physical or intellectual disabilities among nursing, social work and medical students. *Journal of Clinical Nursing, 26*(23-24), 4951–4963. doi:10.1111/jocn.13988 PMID:28771877

Krutchzer, S., Deluca, J., & Caplan, B. (2012). Encyclopedia of neuropsychology. Academic Press.

Kucuk, S., Platin, N., & Erdem, E. (2017). Increasing awareness of protection from sexual abuse in children with mild intellectualdisabilities: An education study. *Applied Nursing Research, 38*, 153–158. doi:10.1016/j.apnr.2017.10.016 PMID:29241509

Kumar, A. (2013). Normalization: Guiding Principle of Equal Opportunities in Education for Children with Disabilities in India. *American Journal of Epidemiology, 167*, 169–177.

Kumpulainen, K., Rasanen, E., & Puura, K. (2001). Psychiatric disorders and the use of mental health services among children involved in bullying. *Aggressive Behavior, 27*(2), 102–110. doi:10.1002/ab.3

Kuo, S. H. (1993). Forensic psychiatry in Taiwan. *International Journal of Law and Psychiatry, 6*(3-4), 457–472. doi:10.1016/0160-2527(83)90032-8 PMID:6679535

Kurth, J. A. (2014). Educational placement of students with autism: The impact of state of residence. *Focus on Autism and Other Developmental Disabilities.*

Kurtz, P. F., Boelter, E. W., Jarmolowicz, D. P., Chin, M. D., & Hagopian, L. P. (2011). An analysis of functional communication training as an empirically supported treatment for problem behavior displayed by individuals with intellectual disabilities. *Research in Developmental Disabilities, 32*(6), 2935–2942. doi:10.1016/j.ridd.2011.05.009 PMID:21696917

Lagerheim, B. (1986). Preparing disabled children for coping with adolescent stress. *International Journal of Adolescent Medicine and Health, 2*(4), 309–316.

Lakhan, R., & Sharma, M. (2010). A study of Knowledge, Attitudes and Practices (KAP) Survey of Families towards their Children with Intellectual Disability in Barwani, India. *Asia Pacific Disability Rehabilitation Journal*, 21.

Lalli, J. S., Browder, D. M., Mace, F. C., & Brown, D. K. (1993). Teacher use of descriptive analysis data to implement interventions to decrease students' problem behaviors. *Journal of Applied Behavior Analysis*, *26*(2), 227–238. doi:10.1901/jaba.1993.26-227 PMID:8331019

Lalli, J. S., Casey, S. D., & Kates, K. (1997). noncontingent reinforcement as treatment for severe problem behavior: Some procedural variations. *Journal of Applied Behavior Analysis*, *30*(1), 127–137. doi:10.1901/jaba.1997.30-127 PMID:9103988

Lambrick, F., & Glaser, W. (2004). Sex offenders with an intellectual disability. *Sexual Abuse*, *16*(4), 381–392. doi:10.1177/107906320401600409 PMID:15560418

Lamont, A., & Bromfield, L. (2009). Parental intellectual disability and child protection: Key issues. National Child Protection Clearing house. *Issues (Chicago, Ill.)*, *31*. Retrieved from http://www.aifs. gov

Landry, S. H., Smith, K. E., Swank, P. R., & Guttentag, C. (2008). A responsive parenting intervention: The optimal timing across early childhood for impacting maternal behaviors and child outcomes. *Developmental Psychology*, *44*(5), 1335–1353. doi:10.1037/a0013030 PMID:18793067

Lane, R. D., Reiman, E. M., Ahem, G. L., Schwartz, G. E., & Davidson, R. J. (1997). Neuroanatomical correlates of happiness, sadness and disgust. *The American Journal of Psychiatry*, *154*(7), 926–933. doi:10.1176/ajp.154.7.926 PMID:9210742

Langdon, P. E., Clare, I. C., & Murphy, G. H. (2011). Moral reasoning theory and illegal behaviour by adults with intellectual disabilities. *Psychology, Crime & Law*, *17*(2), 101–115. doi:10.1080/10683160903392384

Lanovaz, M. J., Argumedes, M., Roy, D., Duquette, J. R., & Watkins, N. (2013). Using ABC narrative recording to identify the function of problem behavior: A pilot study. *Research in Developmental Disabilities*, *34*(9), 2734–2742. doi:10.1016/j.ridd.2013.05.038 PMID:23787117

Lapidot-Lefler, N., & Dolev-Cohen, M. (2015). Comparing cyberbullying and school bullying among school students: Prevalence, gender, and grade level differences. *Social Psychology of Education*, *18*(1), 1–16. doi:10.100711218-014-9280-8

Larkin, P., Jahoda, A., MacMahon, K., & Pert, C. (2012). Interpersonal sources of conflict in young people with and without mild to moderate intellectual disabilities at transition from adolescent to adulthood. *Journal of Applied Research in Intellectual Disabilities*, *25*(1), 29–38. doi:10.1111/j.1468-3148.2011.00652.x PMID:22473946

Larrabee, G. J. (2005). *Forensic neuropsychology: A scientific approach*. New York: Oxford University Press.

Laurvick, C. L., Msall, M. E., Silburn, S., Bower, C., Klerk, N., & Leonard, H. (2006). Physical and mental health of mothers caring for a child with Rett syndrome. *Pediatrics*, *118*(4), e1152–e1164. doi:10.1542/peds.2006-0439 PMID:16966392

LaVigna, G. W., & Willis, T. J. (2012). The efficacy of positive behavioural support with the most challenging behaviour: The evidence and its implications. *Journal of Intellectual & Developmental Disability*, *37*(3), 185–195. doi:10.3109/13668250.2012.696597 PMID:22774760

Lee, J. (2013). Maternal stress, well-being, and impaired sleep in mothers of children with developmental disabilities: A literature review. *Research in Developmental Disabilities*, *34*(11), 4255–4273. doi:10.1016/j.ridd.2013.09.008 PMID:24080069

Lee, R. L. T., Brown, M., Leung, C., Chen, H., Louie, L., Chen, J. L., & Lee, P. H. (2019). Family carers' experiences of participating in a weight management programme for overweight children and adolescents with intellectual disabilities: An exploratory study. *Journal of Advanced Nursing*, *75*(2), 388–399. Epub2018Oct8. doi:10.1111/jan.13845 PMID:30187576

Lemay, J. F., Herbert, A. R., Dewey, D. M., & Micheil, A. I. (2003). A rational approach to the child with mental retardation for the paediatrician. *Journal of Paediatrics and Child Health*, *8*(6), 345–356. doi:10.1093/pch/8.6.345 PMID:20052328

Leonard, H., & Wen, X. (2002). The epidemiology of mental retardation: challenges and opportunities in the new millennium. *Mental Retardation and Developmental Disabilities Research Reviews, 8*(3), 117-134.

Leonard, H., Glasson, E., Nassar, N., Whitehouse, A., Bebbington, A., Bourke, J., . . . Bower, C. (2011). Autism and intellectual disability are differentially related to sociodemographic background at birth. *PloS One, 6*(3), e17875.

Leonard, H., Petterson, B., De Klerk, N., Zubrick, S. R., Glasson, E., Sanders, R., & Bower, C. (2005). Association of sociodemographic characteristics of children with intellectual disability in Western Australia. *Social Science & Medicine, 60*(7), 1499-1513.

Lerman, D., & Iwata, B. (1996). Developing a technology for the use of operant extinction in clinical settings: An examination of basic and applied research. *Journal of Applied Behavior Analysis*, *29*(3), 345–382. doi:10.1901/jaba.1996.29-345 PMID:8926226

Lerner, J. (2003). *Learning disabilities: Theories, diagnosis, and teaching practices* (9th ed.). Boston, MA: Houghton Mifflin Company.

Levine, K. A., Proulx, J., & Schwartz, K. (2018). Disconnected lives: Women with intellectual disabilities in conflict with the law. *Journal of Applied Research in Intellectual Disabilities*, *31*(2), 249–258. doi:10.1111/jar.12387 PMID:28718998

Lewandowski, L. J., & Barlow, J. R. (2000). Social cognition and verbal learning disabilities. *Journal of Psychotherapy in Independent Practice*, *4*(4), 35–47. doi:10.1300/J288v01n04_04

Lewis, T., Scott, T., & Sugai, G. (1994). The problem behaviour questionnaire: A teacher- long-term effects of functional communication training in home settings. *Journal of Applied Behavior Analysis*, *30*, 507–531.

Lindau, N., Amin, T., Zambon, A., & Scior, K. (2018). The effect of brief digital interventions on attitudes to intellectual disability: Results from a pilot study. *Journal of Applied Research in Intellectual Disabilities*, *31*(1), 106–113. doi:10.1111/jar.12366 PMID:28503872

Lindfors, P. J., Kaltiala-Heino, R., & Rimpela, A. H. (2012). Cyberbullying among Finnish adolescents – a population-based study. *BMC Public Health*, *12*(1), 1027. doi:10.1186/1471-2458-12-1027 PMID:23176715

Lindsay, S., & McPherson, A. C. (2012). Strategies for improving disability awareness and social inclusion of children and young people with cerebral palsy. *Child: Care, Health and Development*, *38*(6), 809–816. doi:10.1111/j.1365-2214.2011.01308.x PMID:21880056

Lindsay, W. R. (2002). Integration of recent reviews on offenders with intellectual disabilities. *Journal of Applied Research in Intellectual Disabilities*, *15*(2), 111–119. doi:10.1046/j.1468-3148.2002.00112.x

Lindsay, W. R., Allan, R., Parry, C., Macleod, F., Cottrell, J., Overend, H., & Smith, A. H. W. (2004). Anger and aggression in people with intellectual disabilities: Treatment and follow-up of consecutive referrals and a waiting list comparison. *Clinical Psychology & Psychotherapy*, *11*(4), 255–264. doi:10.1002/cpp.415

Lindsay, W. R., Carson, D., Holland, A. J., Taylor, J. L., O'Brien, G., Wheeler, J. R., & Steptoe, L. (2013). Alcohol and its relationship to offence variables in a cohort of offenders with intellectual disability. *Journal of Intellectual & Developmental Disability*, *38*(4), 325–331. doi:10.3109/13668250.2013.837154 PMID:24279785

Lindsay, W. R., Law, J., Quinn, K., Smart, N., & Smith, A. H. (2001). A comparison of physical and sexual abuse: Histories of sexual and non-sexual offenders with intellectual disability. *Child Abuse & Neglect*, *25*(7), 989–995. doi:10.1016/S0145-2134(01)00251-4 PMID:11523873

Lindsay, W. R., Michie, A. M., Baty, F. J., Smith, A. H. W., & Miller, S. (1994). The consistency of reports about feelings and emotions from people with intellectual disability. *Journal of Intellectual Disability Research*, *38*(1), 61–66. doi:10.1111/j.1365-2788.1994.tb00348.x PMID:8173224

Lindsay, W. R., Smith, A. H., Quinn, K., Anderson, A., Smith, A., Allan, R., & Law, J. (2004). Women with intellectual disability who have offended: Characteristics and outcome. *Journal of Intellectual Disability Research*, *48*(6), 580–590. doi:10.1111/j.1365-2788.2004.00627.x PMID:15312059

Lindsay, W. R., Taylor, J. L., & Sturmey, P. (Eds.). (2004). *Offenders with developmental disabilities*. Chichester, UK: John Wiley & Sons. doi:10.1002/9780470713440

Lindsay, W. R., Tinsley, S., & Emara, M. (2012). Alcohol use and offending in people with intellectual disability. *Alcohol-Related Violence. Prevention & Treatment*, 285–302.

Linehan, M. M. (1993). *Cognitive-behavioral treatment of borderline personality disorder*. New York: Guilford.

Linehan, M. M. (1993a). *Cognitive behavioral treatment for borderline personality disorder*. New York, NY: Guilford Press.

Linehan, M. M. (1993b). *Skills training manual for treating borderline personality disorder*. New York, NY: Guilford Press.

Lin, L. Y., Orsmond, G. I., & Seltzer, M. M. (2007). Mothers of adolescents and adults with autism: Parenting multiple children with disabilities. *Intellectual and Developmental Disabilities*, *45*(4), 257–270. doi:10.1352/1934-9556(2007)45[257:MOAAAW]2.0.CO;2 PMID:17627373

Lin, L.-P., Hsu, S.-W., Kuo, M.-T., Wu, J.-L., Chu, C., & Lin, J.-D. (2014). Onset aging conditions of adults with an intellectual disability associated with primary caregiver depression. *Research in Developmental Disabilities*, *35*(3), 632–638. doi:10.1016/j.ridd.2013.12.013 PMID:24467811

Llewellyn, A. (2000). Perceptions of mainstreaming: A systems approach. *Developmental Medicine and Child Neurology*, *42*(2), 106–115. doi:10.1017/S0012162200000219 PMID:10698328

Lobato, J. (2002). Integrated sibling-parent group intervention to improve sibling knowledge and adjustment to chronic illness and disability. *Journal of Pediatric Psychology*, *27*(8), 711–716. doi:10.1093/jpepsy/27.8.711 PMID:12403861

Lobato, J., & Kao, B. T. (2005). Brief report: Family-based group intervention for young siblings of children with chronic illness and developmental disability. *Journal of Pediatric Psychology*, *30*(8), 678–682. doi:10.1093/jpepsy/jsi054 PMID:16260437

Loewy, J., Hallan, C., Friedman, E., & Martinez, C. (2006). Sleep/sedation in children undergoing EEG testing: A comparison of chloral hydrate and music therapy. *American Journal of Electroneurodiagnostic Technology*, *46*(4), 343–355. doi:10.1080/1086508X.2006.11079593 PMID:17285817

Longo, D. C., & Bond, B. (1984). Families of the handicapped child: Research and practice. *Family Relations*, *33*(1), 57–65. doi:10.2307/584590

Lopez, V., Clifford, T., & Minnes, P. (2008). Parental stress and coping in families of children with and without developmental delays. *Journal on Developmental Disabilities*, *14*, 99–103.

Lopez, V., Clifford, T., Minnes, P., & Kuntz, H. O. (2008). Parental stress and coping in families of children with and without developmental delays. *Journal on Developmental Disabilities*, *14*(2).

Lorenzo, L. A. (1991). Societal prejudice reflected in our courts: The unfavorable treatment of the mentally retarded. *Seton Hall Const. LJ*, *2*, 771.

Louhiala. (2004). *Preventing intellectual disability. Ethical and clinical issues.* Cambridge, UK: Cambridge University Press.

Low, L.P., Chien, W.T, Lam, L.W., & Wong, K.K. (2017). A qualitative study protocol of ageing carers' caregiving experiences and their planning for continuation of care for their immediate family members with intellectual disability. *BMC Geriatrics, 17*(1), 81. doi:10.118612877-017-0473-9

Luckasson, R., Borthwick-Duffy, S., Buntinx, W. H. E., Coulter, D. L., Craig, E. M., Reeve, A., ... Tasse´, M. J. (2002). *Mental retardation:Definition, classification, and systems of supports* (10th ed.). Washington, DC: American Association on Mental Retardation.

Lund, J. (1985). The prevalence of psychiatric morbidity in mentally retarded adults. *Acta Psychiatrica Scandinavica, 72*(6), 563-570.

Lund, J. (1990). Mentally retarded criminal offenders in Denmark. *The British Journal of Psychiatry*, *156*(5), 726–731. doi:10.1192/bjp.156.5.726 PMID:2095951

Lunsky, Y., Bradley, E. A., Gracey, C. D., Durbin, J., & Koegl, C. (2009). Gender differences in psychiatric diagnoses among inpatients with and without intellectual disabilities. *Journal Information*, *114*(1). PMID:19143463

Luukkonen, A. H., Riala, K., Hakko, H., & Rasanen, P. (2010). Bullying behavior and substance abuse among underage psychiatric inpatient adolescents. *European Psychiatry*, *25*(7), 382–389. doi:10.1016/j.eurpsy.2009.12.002 PMID:20435448

Lyall, I., Holland, A. J., & Collins, S. (1995). Offending by adults with learning disabilities and the attitudes of staff to offending behaviour: Implications for service development. *Journal of Intellectual Disability Research*, *39*(6), 501–508. doi:10.1111/j.1365-2788.1995.tb00570.x PMID:8746737

Maccoby, E. E., & Martin, J. A. (1983). *Socialization in the context of the family: Parent-child interaction.* New York: Wiley.

MacDonald, E. E., & Hastings, R. P. (2010). *Fathers of children with developmental disabilities*. John Wiley & Sons.

Macinnes, M. D. (2008). One's enough of now: Children, disability, and subsequent childbearing of mothers. *Journal of Marriage and the Family*, *70*(3), 758–771. doi:10.1111/j.1741-3737.2008.00519.x PMID:23946550

Maclean, M. J., Sims, S., Bower, C., Leonard, H., Stanley, F. J., & O'Donnell, M. (2017). Maltreatment risk among children with disabilities. *Pediatrics*, *139*(4), e20161817. doi:10.1542/peds.2016-1817 PMID:28264988

MacLean, W. E. Jr, Tervo, R. C., Hoch, J., Tervo, M., & Symons, F. J. (2010). Self-Injury among a community cohort of young children at risk for intellectual and developmental disabilities. *The Journal of Pediatrics*, *157*(6), 979–983. doi:10.1016/j.jpeds.2010.05.052 PMID:20630541

Mactavish, J. B., & Schleien, S. J. (2004). Re-injecting spontaneity and balance in family life: Parents' perspectives on recreation in families that include children with developmental disability. *Journal of Intellectual Disability Research*, *48*(2), 123–141. doi:10.1111/j.1365-2788.2004.00502.x PMID:14723655

Madhavan, T., Kalyan, M., Naidu, S., Pashwarla, R., & Narayan, J. (1999). *Mental retardation- a manual for psychologists.* Secunderabad, India: National Institute for the Mentally Handicapped.

Madhavan, T., Menon, D. K., & Kalyan, M. (1988). *Mental Retardation: A Manual for Village Rehabilitation Workers.* National Institute for the Mentally Handicapped.

Maes, B., Broekman, T. G., Došen, A., & Nauts, J. (2003). Caregiving burden of families looking after persons with intellectual disability and behavioural or psychiatric problems. *Journal of Intellectual Disability Research, 47*(6), 447-455. doi:10.1046/j.1365-2788.2003.00513.x

Mafifei-Almodovar, L., & Sturmey, P. (2012). Evidence-based practice and crisis intervention. In D. D. Reed, R. F. D. DiGennaro, & J. K. Luiselli (Eds.), *Handbook of crisis intervention for individuals with developmental disabilities*. New York: Springer.

Maggi, S., Irwin, L. J., Siddiqi, A., & Hertzman, C. (2010). The social determinants of early child development: an overview. *Journal of Paediatrics and Child Health, 46*(11), 627-635.

Mak, W. S., & Ho, S. M. (2007). Care giving perceptions of Chinese mothers of children with intellectual disability in Hong Kong. *Journal of Applied Research in Intellectual Disabilities, 20*(2), 145–156. doi:10.1111/j.1468-3148.2006.00309.x

Malin, A. J. (1949). Manual of Malin's Intelligence Scale for Indian Children. Lucknow: Indian Psychological Corporation.

Man, J., & Kangas, M. (2019). Service satisfaction and helpfulness ratings, mental health literacy and help seeking barriers of carers of individuals with dual disabilities. *Journal of Applied Research in Intellectual Disabilities, 32*(1), 184-193. doi:10.1111/jar.12520

Mandleco, B., Olsen, S. F., Dyches, T., & Marshall, E. (2003). The relationship between family and sibling functioning in families raising a child with a disability. *Journal of Family Nursing, 9*(4), 365–396. doi:10.1177/1074840703258329

Manion, M. L., & Bersani, H. A. (1987). Mental retardation as a Western sociological construct: A cross-cultural analysis. *Disability, Handicap & Society, 2*(3), 231–245. doi:10.1080/02674648766780301

March, R. E., Horner, R. H., Lewis-Palmer, T., Brown, D., Crone, D., Todd, A. W., & … . (2000). *Functional Assessment Checklist: Teachers and Staff (FACTS)*. Eugene, OR: Educational and Community Supports.

Marini, Z. A., Dane, A. V., Bosacki, S. L., & Cura, Y. (2006). Direct and indirect bully-victims: Differential psychosocial risk factors associated with adolescents involvement in bullying and victimization. *Aggressive Behavior, 32*(6), 551–569. doi:10.1002/ab.20155

Marmot, M. G., Allen, J., Goldblatt, P., Boyce, T., McNeish, D., Grady, M., & Geddes, I. (2010). *Fair society, healthy lives: strategic review of health inequalities in England post-2010*. Academic Press.

Martell, D. A. (1992). Forensic neuropsychology and the criminal law. *Law and Human Behavior, 16*(3), 313–336. doi:10.1007/BF01044772

Martlew, M., & Hodson, J. (1991). Children with mild learning difficulties in an integrated and in a special school: Comparisons of behavior, teasing and teachers' attitudes. *The British Journal of Educational Psychology, 61*(3), 355–372. doi:10.1111/j.2044-8279.1991.tb00992.x PMID:1786214

Martorell, A., Gutiérrez-Recacha, P., Irazábal, M., Marsà, F., & García, M. (2011). Family impact in intellectual disability, severe mental health disorders and mental healthdisorders in ID. A comparison. *Research in Developmental Disabilities, 32*(6), 2847–2852. doi:10.1016/j.ridd.2011.05.021 PMID:21641769

Marvin, R.S., & Pianta, R.C. (1996). Mothers' reactions to their child's diagnosis: Relations with security of attachment. *Journal of Clinical Child Psychology, 25*(4), 436-445.

Maryland Coalition for Inclusive Education. (2011). *Quality indicators for inclusive building based practices*. Retrieved from: http://www.mcie.org/usermedia/application/8/quality-indicators---buildingbased-practices-(2011).pdf

Mary, N. L. (1990). Reactions of black, hispanic, and white mothers to having a child with handicaps. *Mental Retardation, 28*(1), 1–5. PMID:2308509

Masi, G. (1998). Psychiatric illness in mentally retarded adolescents: Clinical features. *Adolescence, 33*(130), 425–434. PMID:9706328

Mason, J., & Scior, K. (2004). 'Diagnostic overshadowing' amongst clinicians working with people with intellectual disabilities in the UK. *Journal of Applied Research in Intellectual Disabilities, 17*(2), 85-90.

Mather, N., & Goldstein, S. (2015). *Behaviour Modification in the classroom.* Retrieved from http://www.ldonline.org/article/6030/

Matheson, C., Olsen, R. J., & Weisner, T. (2007). A good friend is hard to find: Friendship among adolescents with disabilities. *American Journal of Mental Retardation, 112*(5), 319–329. doi:10.1352/0895-8017(2007)112[0319:AGFIHT]2.0.CO;2 PMID:17676957

Matheson, E., & Jahoda, A. (2005). Emotional understanding in aggressive and nonaggressive individuals with mild or moderate mental retardation. *American Journal of Mental Retardation, 110*(1), 57–67. doi:10.1352/0895-8017(2005)110<57:EUIAAN>2.0.CO;2 PMID:15568967

Matson, J. L. (2012). Functional assessment for challenging behaviors. New York, NY: Springer. doi:10.1007/978-1-4614-3037-7

Matson, J. L., & Coe, D. A. (1992). Applied Behaviour Analysis: Its impact on the treatment of mentally retarded emotionally disturbed people. *Research in Developmental Disabilities, 13*(2), 171–189. doi:10.1016/0891-4222(92)90023-Y PMID:1574625

Matson, J. L., Horovitz, M., Kozlowski, A. M., Sipes, M., Worley, J. A., & Shoemaker, M. E. (2011). Person characteristics of individuals in functional assessment research. *Research in Developmental Disabilities, 32*(2), 621–624. doi:10.1016/j.ridd.2010.12.012 PMID:21211941

Matson, J. L., & Vollmer, T. R. (1995). *User's guide: Questions About Behavioral Function (QABF).* Baron Rouge, LA: Scientific Publishers, Inc.

Maulik, P. K., & Harbour, C. K. (2010). Epidemiology of intellectual disability. *International Encyclopaedia of Rehabilitation.*

Maulik, P. K., & Harbour, C. K. (2010). Epidemiology of intellectual disability. *International Encyclopedia of Rehabilitation, 2.*

Maulik, P. K., Mascarenhas, M. N., Mathers, C. D., Dua, T., & Saxena, S. (2011). Prevalence of intellectual disability: A meta-analysis of population-based studies. *Research in Developmental Disabilities, 32*(2), 419–436. doi:10.1016/j.ridd.2010.12.018 PMID:21236634

Mayer, G. R., Sulzer-Azaroff, B., & Wallace, M. (2014). *Behavior analysis for lasting change* (3rd ed.). Cornwall-on-Hudson, NY: Sloan Publishing.

Mazzucchelli, T. G., & Sanders, M. R. (2011). Preventing behavioural and emotional problems in children who have a developmental disability: A public health approach. *Research in Developmental Disabilities, 32*(6), 2148–2156. doi:10.1016/j.ridd.2011.07.022 PMID:21831592

McAfee, J. K., Cockram, J., & Wolfe, P. S. (2001). Police reactions to crimes involving people with mental retardation: A cross-cultural experimental study. *Education and Training in Mental Retardation and Developmental Disabilities*, 160–171.

McCabe, M. P. (1999). Sexual knowledge, experience, and feelings among people with disability. *Sexuality and Disability, 17*(2), 157–170. doi:10.1023/A:1021476418440

McCarron, M., Lombard-Vance, R., Murphy, E., May, P., Webb, N., Sheaf, G., … O'Donovan, M.A. (2019). Effect of deinstitutionalisation on quality of life for adults with intellectual disabilities: a systematic review. *BMJ Open, 9*(4). doi: . doi:10.1136/bmjopen-2018-025735

McCarthy, J., & Boyd, J. (2002). Mental health services and young people with intellectual disability: is it time to do better? *Journal of Intellectual Disability Research, 46*(3), 250-256.

McCarthy, A., Cuskelly, M., van Kraayenoord, C. E., & Cohen, J. (2006). Predictors of stress in mothers and fathers of children with fragile X syndrome. *Research in Developmental Disabilities, 27*(6), 688–704. doi:10.1016/j.ridd.2005.10.002 PMID:16361079

McCarthy, M., Bates, C., Triantafyllopoulou, P., Hunt, S., & Milne Skillman, K. (2019). "Put bluntly, they are targeted by the worst creeps society has to offer": Police and professionals' views and actions relating to domestic violence and women with intellectual disabilities. *Journal of Applied Research in Intellectual Disabilities, 32*(1), 71–81. doi:10.1111/jar.12503 PMID:29992718

McClure, K. S., Halpern, J., Wolper, P. A., & Donahue, J. J. (2009). Emotional regulation and intellectual disability. *Journal of Developmental Disabilities.* Retrieved from http://www.researchgate.net/publication/263763300

McConachie, H. (1986). *Parents & Young mentally handicapped children: a review of research issues.* London: Croom Helm.

McConkey, R., Kahonde, C., & McKenzie, J. (2016). Tackling Stigma in Developing Countries: The Key Role of Families. In K. Scior & S. Werner (Eds.), *Intellectual Disability and Stigma: Stepping Out from the Margins.* Palgrave Macmillan. doi:10.1057/978-1-137-52499-7_12

McConkey, R., Truesdale-Kennedy, M., Chang, M.-Y., Jarrah, S., & Shukri, R. (2008). The impact on mothers of bringing up a child with intellectual disabilities: A cross-cultural study. *International Journal of Nursing Studies, 45*(1), 65–74. doi:10.1016/j.ijnurstu.2006.08.007 PMID:17022985

McConnel, D., & Llewllyn, G. (2002). Stereotypes, parents with intellectual disability and child protection. *Journal of Social Welfare and Family, 24*(3), 297–317. doi:10.1080/09649060210161294

McConnel, D., & Savage, A. (2015). Stress and resilience among families caring for children with disability: Expanding the research agenda. *Current Developmental Disorders Reports, 2*(2), 100–109. doi:10.100740474-015-0040-z

McConnell, D., Savage, A., & Breitkreuz, R. (2014). Resilience in families raising children with disabilities and behavior problems. *Research in Developmental Disabilities, 35*(4), 833–848. doi:10.1016/j.ridd.2014.01.015 PMID:24491480

McCubbin, H. I. (1993). Families coping with illness: The resiliency model of family stress, adjustment, and adaptation. In Families, Health & Illness: Perspectives on coping and intervention. Winstead & Fry.

McDonagh, P., Goodey, C. F., & Stainton, T. (Eds.). (2018). *Intellectual disability: A conceptual history, 1200-1900.* Oxford, UK: Oxford University Press.

McDonald, K. E., Keys, C. B., & Balcazar, F. E. (2007). Disability, race/ethnicity and gender: Themes of cultural oppression, acts of individual resistance. *American Journal of Community Psychology, 39*(1-2), 145–161. doi:10.100710464-007-9094-3 PMID:17294120

McGillivray, J. A., Gaskin, C. J., Newton, D. C., & Richardson, B. A. (2016). Substance use, offending, and participation in alcohol and drug treatment programmes: A comparison of prisoners with and without Intellectual Disabilities. *Journal of Applied Research in Intellectual Disabilities*, *29*(3), 289–294. doi:10.1111/jar.12175 PMID:25754684

McGillivray, J. A., & Moore, M. R. (2001). Substance use by offenders with mild intellectual disability. *Journal of Intellectual & Developmental Disability*, *26*(4), 297–310. doi:10.1080/13668250120087317

McGrail, J. P., & Rieger, A. (2013). Coping humor and family functioning in parents of children with disabilities. *Rehabilitation Psychology*, *58*(1), 89–97. doi:10.1037/a0031556 PMID:23438005

McHale, S. M., & Gamble, W. C. (1987). Sibling relationships and adjustment of children with disabled brothers and sisters. In F. Fuchs Schachter & R. K. Stine (Eds.), Practical concerns about siblings: Bridging the research-practice gap (pp. 131-158). New York: Haworth Press.

McHale, S. M., & Gamble, W. C. (1989). Sibling relationships of children with disabled and nondisabled brothers and sisters. *Developmental Psychology*, *25*(3), 421–429. doi:10.1037/0012-1649.25.3.421

McIntyre, L. L. (2008). Adapting Webster-Stratton's incredible years parent training for children with developmental delay: Findings from a treatment group only study. *Journal of Intellectual Disability Research*, *52*(12), 1176–1192. doi:10.1111/j.1365-2788.2008.01108.x PMID:18671808

Mcintyre, L. L., Blacher, J., & Baker, B. L. (2006). The transition to school: Adaptation in young children with and without developmental delays. *Journal of Intellectual Disability Research*, *50*(5), 349–361. doi:10.1111/j.1365-2788.2006.00783.x PMID:16629928

Mcintyre, L., Blacher, J., & Baker, B. L. (2002). Behaviour/mental health problems in young adults with intellectual disability: The impact on families. *Journal of Intellectual Disability Research*, *46*(3), 239–249. doi:10.1046/j.1365-2788.2002.00371.x PMID:11896809

McKenzie, K., Milton, M., Smith, G., & Ouellette-Kuntz, H. (2016). Systematic review of the prevalence and incidence of intellectual disabilities: current trends and issues. *Current Developmental Disorders Reports, 3*(2), 104-115.

McKenzie, K., Milton, M., Smith, G., & Ouellette-Kuntz, H. (2016). Systematic Review of the Prevalence and Incidence of Intellectual Disabilities: Current Trends and Issues. *Current Developmental Disorders Reports*, *3*(2), 104–115. doi:10.100740474-016-0085-7

McKinlay & McGowan. (2003). Forensic issues in neuropsychology. In P. W. Halligan, U. Kischka, & J. C. Marshall (Eds.), *Handbook of clinical neuropsychology* (pp. 676–693). New York: Oxford University Press.

McLean, L. K., Brady, N. C., & McLean, J. E. (1996). Reported communication abilities of individuals with severe mental retardation. *American Journal of Mental Retardation, 100*, 580–589. PMID:8735572

McLean, L. K., Brady, N. C., McLean, J. E., & Behrens, G. A. (1999). Communication forms and functions of children and adults with severe mental retardation in community and institutional settings. *Journal of Speech, Language, and Hearing Research: JSLHR*, *42*(1), 231–240. doi:10.1044/jslhr.4201.231 PMID:10025557

McLeod, S. A. (2008). *Erik Erikson/Psychological Stages*. Retrieved from www.simplypsychology.org/Erik-Erikson.html

McLoyd, V. C. (1990). The impact of economic hardship on Black families and children: Psychological distress, parenting, and socioemotional development. *Child Development*, *61*(2), 311–346. doi:10.2307/1131096 PMID:2188806

McLoyd, V. C., & Wilson, L. (1990). Maternal behavior, social support, and economic conditions as predictors of distress in children. *New Directions for Child and Adolescent Development*, *1990*(46), 49–69. doi:10.1002/cd.23219904605 PMID:2348935

McNamara, J. K., Willoughby, T., & Chalmers, H. (2005). Psychosocial status of adolescents with learning disabilities with and without comorbid attention deficit hyperactivity disorder. *Learning Disabilities Research & Practice*, *20*(4), 234–244. doi:10.1111/j.1540-5826.2005.00139.x

McNulty, C., Kissi-Deborah, R., & Newsom-Davies, I. (1995). Police involvement with clients having intellectual disabilities: A pilot study in South London. *Mental Handicap Research*, *8*(2), 129–136. doi:10.1111/j.1468-3148.1995.tb00150.x

Mechling, L. C., Gast, D. L., & Barthold, S. (2003). Multimedia computer-based instruction to teach students with moderate intellectual disabilities to use a debit card to make purchases. *Exceptionality*, *11*(4), 239–254. doi:10.1207/S15327035EX1104_4

Meltzer, H., Gatward, R., Goodman, R., & Ford, T. (2000). *Mental health of children and adolescents in Great Britain*. London: The Stationery Office.

Mencap. (2007). *Death by indifference*. Mencap.

Mental Disability Rights International (MDRI). (2007). *Ruined Lives: Segregation from Society in Argentina's Psychiatric Asylums*. Washington, DC: Mental Disability Rights International.

Meppelder, M., Hodes, M., Kef, S., & Schuengel, C. (2015). Parenting stress and child behaviour problems among parents with intellectual disabilities: The buffering role of resources. *Journal of Intellectual Disability Research*, *59*(7), 664–677. doi:10.1111/jir.12170 PMID:25472805

Merrill, E. C., & Mar, H. H. (1987). Differences between mentally retarded and nonretarded persons' efficiency of auditory sentence processing. *American Journal of Mental Deficiency*, *91*, 406–414. PMID:3812610

Mesibov, G. B., Shea, V., & Schopler, E. (2004). *The TEACCH approach to autism spectrum disorders*. Springer Science & Business Media. doi:10.1007/978-0-306-48647-0

Meyer, K. A., Ingersoll, B., & Hambrick, D. Z. (2011). Factors influencing adjustment in siblings of children with autism spectrum disorders. *Research in Autism Spectrum Disorders*, *5*(4), 1413–1420. doi:10.1016/j.rasd.2011.01.027

Michael, J. (1982). Distinguishing between discriminative and motivational functions of stimuli. *Journal of the Experimental Analysis of Behavior*, *37*(1), 149–155. doi:10.1901/jeab.1982.37-149 PMID:7057126

Michael, J. (2000). Implications and refinements of the establishing operation concept. *Journal of Applied Behavior Analysis*, *33*(4), 401–410. doi:10.1901/jaba.2000.33-401 PMID:11214018

Miclea, D. L., Cuzmici, Z., & Pop, I. V. (2015). Genetic testing in patients with global developmental delay / intellectual disabilities. *A review Med.*, *88*(3), 288–292. PMID:26609258

Milani, D., Ronzoni, L., & Esposito, S. (2015). Genetic Advances in Intellectual Disability. *Journal of Pediatric Genetics*, *4*(3), 125–127. doi:10.1055-0035-1564438 PMID:27617122

Mindell, J. A., Kuhn, B., Lewin, D. S., Meltzer, L. J., & Sadeh, A. (2006). Behavioral treatment of bedtime problems and night wakings in infants and young children. *American Academy of Sleep Medicine Sleep.*, *29*(10), 1263–1276. PMID:17068979

Minnes, P. M. (1988). Family stress associated with a developmentally handicapped child: A multi-dimensional perspective. In N. W. Bray (Ed.), *International Review of Research in Mental Retardation* (pp. 195–226). Birmingham, AL: University of Alabama.

Miodrag, N., & Hodapp, R. M. (2010). Chronic stress and health among parents of children with intellectual and developmental disabilities. *Current Opinion in Psychiatry, 23*(5), 407-411.

Mishna, F. (2003). Learning disabilities and bullying: Double jeopardy. *Journal of Learning Disabilities*, *36*(4), 336–347. doi:10.1177/00222194030360040501 PMID:15490906

Mishna, F., Khoury-Kassabri, M., Gadalla, T., & Daciuk, J. (2012). Risk factors for involvement in cyber bullying: Victims, bullies, and bully-victims. *Children and Youth Services Review*, *32*(1), 63–70. doi:10.1016/j.childyouth.2011.08.032

Mitchell, C., McLanahan, S., Brooks-Gunn, J., Garfinkel, I., Hobcraft, J., & Notterman, D. (2013). Genetic differential sensitivity to social environments: implications for research. *American Journal of Public Health, 103*(s1), s102-s110.

Mitchell, D. B., & Hauser-Cram, P. (2008). The well-being of mothers of adolescents with developmental disabilities in relation to medical care utilization and satisfaction with health care. *Research in Developmental Disabilities*, *29*(2), 97–112. doi:10.1016/j.ridd.2006.12.002 PMID:17267176

Moeschler, J. B., & Shevell, M. (2006). Clinical genetic evaluation of the child with mental retardation or developmental delays. *Pediatrics*, *117*(6), 2304–2316. doi:10.1542/peds.2006-1006 PMID:16740881

Mohapatra, S., & Mohanty, M. (2004). *Abuse and activity limitation: A study on domestic violence against disabled women in Orissa, India.* Bhubaneswar, Orissa: Swabhiman.

Mohapatra, S., & Mohanty, M. (2004). Abuse and Activity Limitation: A Study on Domestic Violence Against Disabled Women in Orissa, India. *Indian. The Journal of Educational Research*, *2*, 56–67.

Molteno, G., Molteno, C. D., Finchilescu, G., & Dawes, A. R. L. (2001). Behavioural and emotional problems in children with intellectual disability attending special schools in Cape Town, South Africa. *Journal of Intellectual Disability Research, 45*(6), 515-520.

Molteno, G., Molteno, C. D., Finchilescu, G., & Dawes, A. R. L. (2001). Behavioural and emotional problems in children with intellectual disability attending special schools in Cape Town, South Africa. *Journal of Intellectual Disability Research*, *45*(6), 515–520. doi:10.1046/j.1365-2788.2001.00368.x PMID:11737538

Mondal, A., & Mete, J. (2011). *Education of Children with Disabilities in India: Concern and Policy Perspective.* Academic Press.

Moore, D. G. (2001). Reassessing emotion recognition performance in people with mental retardation: A review.bn. *American Journal of Mental Retardation*, *106*(6), 481–502. doi:10.1352/0895-8017(2001)106<0481:RERPIP>2.0.CO;2 PMID:11708935

Moran, G., Pederson, D. R., Pettit, P., & Krupka, A. (1922). Maternal sensitivity and infant-mother attachment in a developmentally delayed sample. *Journal of Infant Behavior and Development*, *15*(4), 427–442. doi:10.1016/0163-6383(92)80011-I

Morgan, H. (1992). An analysis of Gardner's Theory of Multiple Intelligence. *Roeper Review*, *18*(4), 263–269. doi:10.1080/02783199609553756

Mori, Y., Downs, J., Wong, K., & Leonard, H. (2019). Longitudinal effects of caregiving on parental well-being: the example of Rett syndrome, a severe neurological disorder. *European Child and Adolescent Psychiatry, 28*(4), 505-520. doi:10.100700787-018-1214-0

Morin, D., Rivard, M., Boursier, C. P., Crocker, A. G., & Caron, J. (2015). Norms of the Attitudes Toward Intellectual Disability Questionnaire. *Journal of Intellectual Disability Research*, *59*(5), 462–467. doi:10.1111/jir.12146 PMID:25041088

Morin, D., Rivard, M., Crocker, A. G., Boursier, C. P., & Caron, J. (2013). Public attitudes towards intellectual disability: A multidimensional perspective. *Journal of Intellectual Disability Research*, *57*(3), 279–292. doi:10.1111/jir.12008 PMID:23279318

Morin, D., Valois, P., Crocker, A. G., Robitaille, C., & Lopes, T. (2018). Attitudes of health care professionals toward people with intellectual disability: A comparison with the general population. *Journal of Intellectual Disability Research*, *62*(9), 746–758. doi:10.1111/jir.12510 PMID:29968307

Morisse, F., Vandemaele, E., Claes, C., Claes, L., & Vandevelde, S. (2013). Quality of Life in Persons with Intellectual Disabilities and Mental Health Problems: An Explorative Study. *The Scientific World Journal*, 8.

Morris, C. D., Niederbuhl, J. M., & Mahr, J. M. (1993). Determining the capability of individuals with mental retardation to give informed consent. *American Journal of Mental Retardation*, *98*(2), 263–272. PMID:8398085

Morris, J. (2005). *Citizenship and disabled People, Disability Rights Commission*. London: DRC.

Morrison, G. M., Furlong, M. J., & Smith, G. (1994). Factors associated with the experience of school violence among general education, leadership class, opportunity class, and special day class pupils. *Journal of Education and Treatment of Children*, *17*, 356–369.

Morrissey, E., Wandersman, A., Seybolt, D., Nation, M., Crusto, C., & Davino, K. (1997). Toward a framework for bridging the gap between science and practice in prevention: A focus on evaluator and practitioner perspectives. *Evaluation and Program Planning*, *20*(3), 367–377. doi:10.1016/S0149-7189(97)00016-5

Moss, S., Emerson, E., Kiernan, C., Turner, S., Hatton, C., & Alborz, A. (2000). Psychiatric symptoms in adults with learning disability and challenging behaviour. *The British Journal of Psychiatry*, *177*(5), 452–456. doi:10.1192/bjp.177.5.452 PMID:11060000

Mulder, E., Tudor, M. E., & Walsh, C. E. (2013). Predictors of parent stress in a sample of children with ASD: Pain, problem behaviour, and parental coping. *Research in Autism Spectrum Disorders*, *7*(2), 256–264. doi:10.1016/j.rasd.2012.08.010

Mullineaux, P. Y., Deater-Deckard, K., Petrill, S. A., & Thompson, L. A. (2009). Parenting and child behaviour problems: A longitudinal analysis of non-shared environment. *Infant and Child Development: An International Journal of Research and Practice*, *18*(2), 133–148. doi:10.1002/icd.593 PMID:19436771

Munir, M. (2016). The co-occurrence of mental disorders in children and adolescents with intellectual disability/intellectual developmental disorder. *Current Opinion in Psychiatry*, *29*(2), 95–102. doi:10.1097/YCO.0000000000000236 PMID:26779862

Murch, A. J., Choudhury, T., Wilson, M., Collerton, E., Patel, M., & Scior, K. (2018). Explicit and implicit attitudes towards people with intellectual disabilities: The role of contact and participant demographics. *Journal of Applied Research in Intellectual Disabilities*, *31*(5), 778–784. doi:10.1111/jar.12429 PMID:29168267

Murphy, B. (2000). Australian WHOQoL instruments: User's manual and interpretation guide. Melbourne, Australia: Australian WHOQoL Field Study Centre.

Murphy, G., & Mason, J. (2014). Forensic and offending behaviours. In E. Tsakanikos & J. McCarthy (Eds.), Handbook of psychopathology in intellectual disability (pp. 281-303). New York: Springer. doi:10.1007/978-1-4614-8250-5_18

Murphy, C., Lincoln, S., Meredith, S., Cross, E. M., & Rintell, D. (2016). Sex Education and Intellectual Disability: Practices and Insight from Pediatric Genetic Counselors. *Journal of Genetic Counseling*, *25*(3), 552–560. doi:10.100710897-015-9909-6 PMID:26581379

Murphy, W., Coleman, E., & Haynes, M. (1983). Treatment and evaluation issues with the mentally retarded sex offender. In J. G. Greer & I. R. Stuart (Eds.), *The sexual aggressor: Current perspectives on treatment* (pp. 22–41). New York: Van Nostrand Reinhold.

Murthy, R. S. (2010). *Mental Health Care in India –Past*. Present and Future.

Myers, J. S. (1962). Education and Rehabilitation. *Journal of Education, 145*, 1, 3–34.

Myrbakk, E., & von Tetzchner, S. (2008). Psychiatric disorders and behaviour problems in people with intellectual disability. *Research in Developmental Disabilities, 29*(4), 316–332. doi:10.1016/j.ridd.2007.06.002 PMID:17616450

N'dri, L., Ross, M., Castillo, W. C., Reeves, G., & Butler, b. (2019). Care management for youth with co-morbid developmental and mental health conditions: A discrete choice experiment pilot study. *Academic Pediatrics*. PMID:31128382

Nabuzoka, D. (2003). Teacher ratings and peer nominations of bullying and other behavior of children with and without learning difficulties. *Educational Psychology, 23*(3), 307–321. doi:10.1080/0144341032000060147

Nabuzoka, D., & Smith, P. K. (1993). Sociometric status and social behaviour of children with and without learning difficulties. *Journal of Child Psychology and Psychiatry, and Allied Disciplines, 34*(8), 1435–1448. doi:10.1111/j.1469-7610.1993.tb02101.x PMID:8294529

Nadeau, L., & Tessier, R. (2006). Social adjustment of children with cerebral palsy in mainstream classes: Peer perception. *Developmental Medicine and Child Neurology, 48*(05), 331–336. doi:10.1017/S0012162206000739 PMID:16608539

Nambi, S. (2005). Marriage, Mental health and the Indian legislation. *Indian Journal of Psychiatry, 47*(1), 3–14. doi:10.4103/0019-5545.46067

Nam, S. J., & Park, E. Y. (2017). Relationship between caregiving burden and depression in caregivers of individuals with intellectual disabilities in Korea. *Journal of Mental Health (Abingdon, England), 26*(1), 50–56. doi:10.1080/09638237.2016.1276538 PMID:28084102

Nankervis, K. (1997). *Keynote Address*. Paper presented at the Annual Conference, Australian Society for the Study of Intellectual Disability, Hobart, Australia.

Nansel, T. R., Overpeck, M., Pilla, R. S., Ruan, W. J., Simons-Morton, B., & Scheidt, P. (2001). Bullying behaviors among US youth: Prevalence and association with psychosocial adjustment. *Journal of the American Medical Association, 285*(16), 2094–2100. doi:10.1001/jama.285.16.2094 PMID:11311098

Narayan, J., & Kurani, D.R. (1990). *Vocational training and employment of persons with mental retardation*. Academic Press.

Naskar, S., & Nath, K. (2016). A clinical study on intellectual disability in northeastern India: Insight into the sociodemographic risk factors of a developing country. *International Journal of Medical Science and Public Health, 5*(9), 1789–1797. doi:10.5455/ijmsph.2016.23122015323

National Legal Services Authority. (2010). *Legal services to the mentally ill persons and persons with mental disabilities: Scheme Sheet*. Author.

Navas, P., Verdugo, M. A., Gómez, L. E., & Schalock, R. L. (2012). The concept of quality of life and its role in enhancing human rights in the field of intellectual disability. *Journal of Intellectual Disability Research, 56*(11), 1036–1045. doi:10.1111/j.1365-2788.2012.01585.x PMID:22672317

Neece, C. L. (2014). Mindfulness-based stress reduction for parents of young children with developmental delays: Implications for parental mental health and child behaviour problems. *Journal of Applied Research in Intellectual Disabilities, 27*(2), 174–186. doi:10.1111/jar.12064 PMID:23813562

Neece, C., & Baker, B. L. (2008). Predicting maternal parenting stress in middle childhood: The roles of child intellectual status, behavior problems and social skills. *Journal of Intellectual Disability Research, 52*(12), 1114–1128. doi:10.1111/j.1365-2788.2008.01071.x PMID:18513339

Neely, L., Rispoli, M., Camargo, S., Davis, H., & Boles, M. (2013). The effect of instructional use of an iPad on challenging behavior and academic engagement for two students with autism. *Research in Autism Spectrum Disorders*, *7*(4), 509–516. doi:10.1016/j.rasd.2012.12.004

Neuwirth, G. S., Heisler, P. A., & Goldrich, K. S. (1974). Capacity, competence, consent: Voluntary sterilization of the mentally retarded. *Columbia Human Rights Law Review*, *6*, 447. PMID:11663600

New South Wales. Law Reform Commission. (1994). *People with an intellectual disability and the criminal justice system: Courts and sentencing issues* (Vol. 35). The Commission.

Ng, C. H. (1997). The stigma of mental illness in Asian cultures. *The Australian and New Zealand Journal of Psychiatry*, *31*(3), 382–390. doi:10.3109/00048679709073848 PMID:9226084

Nihira, K., Mink, I. T., & Meyers, C. E. (1985). Home environment and development of slow-learning adolescents: Reciprocal relations. *Developmental Psychology*, *21*(5), 784–794. doi:10.1037/0012-1649.21.5.784

Nimbalkar, S., Raithatha, S., & Shah, R. (2014). *A qualitative study of psychosocial problems among parents of children with cerebral palsy attending two tertiary care hospitals in Western India.* ISRN Family Medicine. doi:10.1155/2014/769619

Nishina, A., Juvonen, J., & Witkow, M. (2005). Sticks and stones may break my bones, but names will make me sick: The consequences of peer harassment. *Journal of Clinical Child and Adolescent Psychology*, *34*, 37–48. doi:10.120715374424jccp3401_4 PMID:15677279

Noorden, T. H. J., Haselager, G. J. T., Cillessen, A. H. N., & Bukowski, W. M. (2015). Empathy and involvement in bullying in children and adolescents: A systematic review. *Journal of Youth and Adolescence*, *44*(3), 637–657. doi:10.100710964-014-0135-6 PMID:24894581

Norins-Bardon, Matsumoto, & Siperstein. (2005). *US students attitudes to students with intellectual disabilities.* Global Youth Summit, Nagano, Japan. Available at www.specialolympics.org

Norlin, D., Axberg, U., & Broberg, M. (2014). Predictors of harsh parenting practices in parents of children with disabilities. *Early Child Development and Care*, *184*(9-10), 1472–1484. doi:10.1080/03004430.2013.845562

Norman, J. M., Collins, B. C., & Schuster, J. W. (2001). Using an instructional package including video technology to teach self-help skills to elementary students with mental deficiency. *Journal of Special Education Technology*, *16*(3), 5–18. doi:10.1177/016264340101600301

Norrgard, K. (2008). Human testing, the eugenics movement, and IRBs. *Nature Education*, *1*(1), 170.

Norwich, B., & Kelly, N. (2004). Pupils' views on inclusion: Moderate learning difficulties and bullying in mainstream and special schools. *British Educational Research Journal*, *30*(1), 43–65. doi:10.1080/01411920310001629965

Novaco, R. W., & Taylor, J. L. (2004). Assessment of anger and aggression among male offenders with developmental disabilities. *Psychological Assessment*, *16*(1), 42–50. doi:10.1037/1040-3590.16.1.42 PMID:15023091

Nowicki, E. A. (2006). A cross-sectional multivariate analysis of children's attitudes towards disability. *Journal of Intellectual Disability Research*, *50*(5), 335–348. doi:10.1111/j.1365-2788.2005.00781.x PMID:16629927

NSW Ministry of Health. (2015). *NSW school-link strategy and action plan 2014-2017*. Sydney, Australia: NSW Ministry of Health.

Ntombela, T. (1991). *The family of a mentally retarded child* (Vol. 1). Social Work Practise.

Nunes, F. R. P., Neves, F. A. D., Geraldes, F. D. P. B., & Lopes, A. M. F. R. (2017). Contraception in adolescents with intellectual disability. *The European Journal of Contraception & Reproductive Health Care*, *22*(6), 401–406. doi:10.1080/13625187.2017.1402875 PMID:29188744

O'Brennan, L. M., Bradshaw, C. P., & Sawyer, A. L. (2009). Examining development differences in the social-emotional problems among frequent bullies, victims, and bully/victims. *Psychology in the Schools*, *46*(2), 100–115. doi:10.1002/pits.20357

O'Callaghan, A. C., & Murphy, G. H. (2007). Sexual relationships in adults with intellectual disabilities: Understanding the law. *Journal of Intellectual Disability Research*, *51*(3), 197–206. doi:10.1111/j.1365-2788.2006.00857.x PMID:17300415

O'Dwyer, C., McCallion, P., Henman, M., McCarron, M., O'Leary, E., Burke, E., . . . O'Dwyer, M. (2019). Prevalence and patterns of antipsychotic use and their associations with mental health and problem behaviours among older adults with intellectual disabilities. *Journal of Applied Research in Intellectual Disabilities*. PMID:31038275

O'Neill, R., Horner, R., & Albin, R. (1997). *Functional Assessment and Programme Development for Problem Behaviour: A Practical Handbook*. Brooks/Cole Publishing.

O'Neill, R. E., Horner, R. H., Albin, R. W., Sprague, J. R., Storey, K., & Newton, J. S. (1997). *Functional Assessment and Program Development for Problem Behavior* (2nd ed.). Pacific Grove, CA: Brooks/Cole.

O'Neill, R. E., Horner, R. H., Albin, R. W., Storey, K., & Sprague, J. R. (1990). Functional Analysis of Problem Behavior: A Practical Assessment Guide. *Sycamore Publishing, Sycamore, IL.* of challenging behaviours in individuals with mild mental retardation: meta-analysis of single- subject research. *American Journal of Mental Retardation*, *111*, 290–298.

O'Brien, G., Barnard, L., Pearson, J., & Rippon, L. (2002). Physical health and clinical phenotypes. *Physical Health of Adults With Intellectual Disabilities*, 35-62.

Oliver, A., Revuelto, L., Fernández, I., Simó-Algado, S., & Galiana, L. (2019). An integrative model of the subjective well-being of staff working in intellectual disabilityservices. *Research in Developmental Disabilities*, *87*, 1–8. doi:10.1016/j.ridd.2019.01.007 PMID:30685682

Oliver, M. (1996). *Understanding disability: From theory to practice*. London: Macmillan Press. doi:10.1007/978-1-349-24269-6

Olsson, B., & Hwang, C. P. (2001). Depression in mothers and fathers of children with intellectual disability. *Journal of Intellectual Disability Research*, *45*(6), 535–543. doi:10.1046/j.1365-2788.2001.00372.x PMID:11737541

Olthof, T., & Goossens, F. A. (2008). Bullying and the need to belong: Early adolescents' bullying-related behavior and the acceptance they desire and receive from particular classmates. *Social Development*, *17*(1), 24–46.

Olvera, D. R., Dever, R. B., & Earnest, M. A. (2000). Mental retardation and sentences for murder: Comparison of two recent court cases. *Mental Retardation*, *38*(3), 228–233. doi:10.1352/0047-6765(2000)038<0228:MRASFM>2.0.CO;2 PMID:10900930

Olweus, D. (1978). *Aggression in the schools: Bullies and whipping boys*. Washington, DC: Hemisphere Press.

Olweus, D. (1993). *Bullying at school: What we know and what we can do*. Blackwell Publishing.

Orchard, A. (2013). *The burning issue: Why do people with intellectual disability commit arson?* (MSc dissertation). University of Portsmouth.

Orsmond, G. I., Seltzer, M. M., Krauss, M. W., & Hong, J. (2003). Behavior problems in adults with mental retardation and maternal well being: Examination of the direction of effects. *American Journal of Mental Retardation, 108*(4), 257–271. doi:10.1352/0895-8017(2003)108<257:BPIAWM>2.0.CO;2 PMID:12780337

Osborn, R., Roberts, L., & Kneebone, I. (2019). Barriers to accessing mental health treatment for parents of children with intellectual disabilities: A preliminary study. *Disability and Rehabilitation*, 1-7.

Osborn, F. (1937). Development of a Eugenic Philosophy. *American Sociological Review, 2*(3), 389–397. doi:10.2307/2084871

Oti-Boadi, M. (2017). Exploring the Lived Experiences of Mothers of Children With Intellectual Disability in Ghana. *SAGE Open, 7*(4), 1–12. doi:10.1177/2158244017745578

Ou, J.-J., Shi, L.-J., Xun, G.-L., Chen, C., Wu, R.-R., Luo, X.-R., ... Zhao, J.-P. (2015). Employment and financial burden of families with preschool children diagnosed with autism spectrum disorders in urban China: Results from a descriptive study. *BMC Psychiatry, 15*(1), 42–57. doi:10.118612888-015-0382-4 PMID:25608486

Ouyang, L., Grosse, S. D., Riley, C., Bolen, J., Bishop, E., Raspa, M., & Bailey, D. B. Jr. (2014). A comparison of family financial and employment impacts of fragile X syndrome, autism spectrum disorders, and intellectual disability. *Research in Developmental Disabilities, 35*(7), 1518–1527. doi:10.1016/j.ridd.2014.04.009 PMID:24755230

Owen, A., Browning, M., & Jones, R. P. (2001). Emotion recognition in adults with mild moderate learning disabilities. *Journal of Learning Disabilities, 5*(3), 267–281. doi:10.1177/146900470100500309

Ozdemir, M., & Stattin, H. (2011). Bullies, victims, and bully-victims: A longitudinal examination of the effects of bullying-victimization experiences on youth well-being. *Journal of Aggression, Conflict and Peace Research, 3*(2), 97–102. doi:10.1108/17596591111132918

Pancsofar, N., & Vernon-Feagans, L. (2010). Fathers' early contributions to children's language development in families from low-income rural communities. *Early Childhood Research Quarterly, 25*(4), 50–463. doi:10.1016/j.ecresq.2010.02.001 PMID:21057648

Panksepp, J., Asma, S., Curran, G., Gabriel, R., & Greif, T. (2010). The philosophical implications of affective neuroscience. *Journal of Consciousness Studies, 19*(3-4), 6–48.

Paransky, O., & Zurawin, R. (2003). Management of menstrual problems and contraception in adolescents with mental retardation: A medical, legal and ethical review with new suggested guidelines. *Journal of Pediatric and Adolescent Gynecology, 16*(4), 223–235. doi:10.1016/S1083-3188(03)00125-6 PMID:14550386

Pardellar, S., Frajo-Apor, B., Kemmler, G., & Hofer, A. (2017). Emotional Intelligence and cognitive abilities - association and sex difference. *Psychology Health and Medicine, 22*(8), 1001–1010. doi:10.1080/13548506.2016.1255766

Parish, L., Seltzer, M. M., Greenberg, J. S., & Floyd, F. (2004). Economic implications of caregiving at midlife: Comparing parents with and without children who have developmental disabilities. *Mental Retardation, 42*(6), 413–426. doi:10.1352/0047-6765(2004)42<413:EIOCAM>2.0.CO;2 PMID:15516174

Parmenter, R., Einfeld, S. L., Tonge, B. J., & Dempster, J. A. (1998). Behavioural and emotional problems in the classroom of children and adolescents with intellectual disability. *Journal of Intellectual & Developmental Disability, 23*(1), 71–77. doi:10.1080/13668259800033591

Parmenter, T. R. (2008). The present, past and future of the study of intellectual disability: Challenges in developing countries. *Salud Pública de México, 50*, s124–s131. doi:10.1590/S0036-36342008000800004 PMID:18470339

Parry, J., & Drogin, E. Y. (2007). *Mental disability law, evidence, and testimony: A comprehensive reference manual for lawyers, judges, and mental disability professionals*. American Bar Association.

Passey, J., & Feldman, M. (2004). Descriptive analysis of parent–child interactions in young children with or at risk for developmental delay. *Behavioral Interventions*, *19*(4), 233–246. doi:10.1002/bin.164

Patel, M., & Rose, J. (2014). Students' attitudes towards individuals with an intellectual disability. *Journal of Intellectual Disabilities*, *18*(1), 90–103. doi:10.1177/1744629513511355 PMID:24196840

Patton, A., Ware, R., McPherson, L., Emerson, E., & Lennox, N. (2018). Parent-related stress of male and female carers of adolescents with intellectual disabilities and carers of children within the general population: A cross-sectional comparison. *Journal of Applied Research in Intellectual Disabilities*, *31*(1), 51–61. doi:10.1111/jar.12292 PMID:27704663

Pearl, R., & Bay, M. (1999). Psychosocial correlates of learning disabilities. In V. L. Schwean & D. H. Saklofske (Eds.), *Handbook of psychosocial characteristics of exceptional children* (pp. 443–470). New York, NY: Kluwer Academic / Plenum Publishers. doi:10.1007/978-1-4757-5375-2_17

Pelleboer-Gunnink, H. A., Oorsouw, V., Weeghel, V. J., & Embregts, P. J. C. M. (2017). Mainstream health professionals' stigmatising attitudes towards people with intellectualdisabilities: A systematic review. *Journal of Intellectual Disability Research*, *61*(5), 411–434. doi:10.1111/jir.12353 PMID:28198094

Pereira, C.M.G., & Faria, S.M.M. (2013). Emotional development in children intellectual disability - A comparative approach with "normal" children. *Journal of Modern Education Review*, *2*(2), 120-135.

Perkins, E. A. (2009). Caregivers of adults with intellectual disabilities: The relationship of compound caregiving and reciprocity to quality of life. *Graduate Theses and Dissertations*. Retrieved from https://scholarcommons.usf.edu/etd/2140

Perren, S., Dooley, J., Shaw, T., & Cross, T. (2010). Bullying in school and cyberspace: Associations with depressive symptoms in Swiss and Australian adolescents. *Child and Adolescent Psychiatry and Mental Health*, *23*(4), 28. doi:10.1186/1753-2000-4-28 PMID:21092266

Perry, J., & Felce, D. (2005). Factors associated with outcomes in community group homes. *American Journal of Mental Retardation*, *110*(2), 121–135. doi:10.1352/0895-8017(2005)110<121:FAWOIC>2.0.CO;2 PMID:15762822

Persha, A., Arya, S., & Nagar, R. K. (2007). Biological and Psychological Predictors of Developmental Delay in Persons with Intellectual Disability: Retrospective Case- File Study. *Asia Pacific Disability Rehabilitation Journal*, *18*(1), 93–100.

Perske, R. (1991). *Unequal justice? What can happen when persons with retardation or other developmental disabilities encounter the criminal justice system*. Nashville, TN: Abingdon Press.

Perske, R. (2005). Search for persons with intellectual disabilities who confessed to serious crimes they did not commit. *Journal Information*, *43*(1), 58–65. PMID:15628935

Perske, R. (2008). False confessions from 53 persons with intellectual disabilities: The list keeps growing. *Intellectual and Developmental Disabilities*, *46*(6), 468–479. doi:10.1352/2008.46:468-479 PMID:19006433

Perske, R. (2011). Perske's list: False confessions from 75 persons with intellectual disability. *Intellectual and Developmental Disabilities*, *49*(5), 365–373. doi:10.1352/1934-9556-49.5.365 PMID:21905830

Peshawaria, R., Menon, D. K., Ganguly, R., Roy, S., Pillay, R.P.R.S., & Gupta, A. (1995). *Understanding the Indian Families Having Persons with Mental Retardation*. NIMH. Retrieved from http://nimhindia.gov.in/Understanding%20 Indian%20Families.pdf

Peshawaria, R., Menon, D.K., Ganguly, R., Roy, S., Rajan Pillay, P.R.S., Gupta, A., Kumar V, Giri, R.S., & Ayub, L. (1995). *Understanding Indian Families, having persons with mental retardation.* Academic Press.

Peshawaria, R., Menon,, D.K., Ganguly, R., & Roy, S., RajanPillay, P.R.S., & Gupta, A. (1998). A study offacilitators and inhibitors that affect coping in parents of children with mental retardation in India. *Asia Pacific Disability Rehabilitation Journal*, *9*(1).

Petalas, M. A., Hastings, R. P., Nash, S., Hall, L. M., Joannidi, H., & Dowey, A. (2012). Psychological adjustment and sibling relationships in siblings of children with Autism Spectrum Disorders: Environmental stressors and the Broad Autism Phenotype. *Research in Autism Spectrum Disorders*, *6*(1), 546–555. doi:10.1016/j.rasd.2011.07.015

Pettigrew, T. F., & Tropp, L. R. (2000). Reducing prejudice and discrimination. *The Claremont Symposium on Applied Social Psychology*, 93-114.

Petty, J. L., Bacarese-Hamilton, M., Davies, L. E., & Oliver, C. (2014). Correlates of self-injurious, aggressive and destructive behaviour in children under five who are at risk of developmental delay. *Research in Developmental Disabilities*, *35*(1), 36–45. doi:10.1016/j.ridd.2013.10.019 PMID:24216345

Phan, K. L., Wager, T., Taylor, S. F., & Liberzon, L. (2002). Functional neuroanatomy of emotion: A meta-analysis of emotion activation studies in PET and fMRI. *Journal of Neuroimage*, *16*(2), 331–348. doi:10.1006/nimg.2002.1087 PMID:12030820

Piaget, J. (1997). The essential Piaget. In R. E. Gruber & J. J. Voneche (Eds.), *The language and thought of the child* (p. 85). New York: Basic Books, Inc. Publishers.

Pianta, R. C., Marvin, R. S., Britner, P. A., & Borowitz, K. C. (1996). Mothers' resolution of their children's diagnosis: Organized patterns of caregiving representations. *Infant Mental Health Journal*, *17*(3), 239–256. doi:10.1002/(SICI)1097-0355(199623)17:3<239::AID-IMHJ4>3.0.CO;2-J

Piazza, C. C., Hanley, G. P., & Fisher, W. W. (1996). Functional analysis and treatment of cigarette pica. *Journal of Applied Behavior Analysis*, *29*(4), 437–450. doi:10.1901/jaba.1996.29-437 PMID:8995829

Piecuch, R. E., Leonard, C. H., Cooper, B. A., & Sehring, S. A. (1997). Outcome of extremely low birth weight infants (500 to 999 grams) over a 12-year period. *Pediatrics*, *100*(4), 633–639. doi:10.1542/peds.100.4.633 PMID:9310517

Pisula, E. (2011). Parenting stress in mothers and fathers of children with autism spectrum disorders In A Comprehensive Book on Autism Spectrum Disorders. InTech. doi:10.5772/18507

Plant, A., McDermott, E., Chester, V., & Alexander, R. T. (2011). Substance misuse among offenders in a forensic intellectual disability service. *Journal of Learning Disabilities and Offending Behaviour*, *2*(3), 127–135. doi:10.1108/20420921111186589

Plant, K. M., & Sanders, M. R. (2007). Predictors of care-giver stress in families of preschool-aged children with developmental disabilities. *Journal of Intellectual Disability Research*, *51*(2), 109–124. doi:10.1111/j.1365-2788.2006.00829.x PMID:17217475

Plant, K. M., & Sanders, M. R. (2007). Reducing problem behavior during care-giving in families of preschool-aged children with developmental disabilities. *Research in Developmental Disabilities*, *28*(4), 362–385. doi:10.1016/j.ridd.2006.02.009 PMID:16781115

Polder, J. J., Meerding, W. J., Bonneux, L., & van der Maas, P. J. (2002). Healthcare costs of intellectual disability in the netherlands: a cost-of-illness perspective. *Journal of Intellectual Disability Research, 46*(2), 168-178.

Polloway, E. A. (2015). *The death penalty and intellectual disability*. Washington, DC: American Association on Intellectual and Developmental Disabilities.

Polloway, E. A., & Lubin, J. (2009). Feeblemindedness. Encyclopedia of American Disability History of children and adolescents with intellectual disabilities in Britain: A replication. *Journal of Intellectual Disability Research*, *51*, 866–874.

Popa, B., Guillet, L., & Mullet, E. (2014). Cultural differences in the appraisal of stress. *Psicológica (Valencia)*, *35*, 745–760.

Poppes, P., van der Putten, A. J. J., & Vlaskamp, C. (2010). Frequency and severity of challenging behaviour in people with profound intellectual and multiple disabilities. *Research in Developmental Disabilities*, *31*(6), 1269–1275. doi:10.1016/j.ridd.2010.07.017 PMID:20728304

Population Census. (2011). Retrieved from: www.census2011.co.in/disability.php1802-2019

Powell, T. H., & Ogle, P. A. (1985). *Brothers & sisters: A special part of exceptional families*. Baltimore, MD: Paul H. Brookes Publishing.

Pownall, J. D., Jahoda, A., & Hastings, R. P. (2012). Sexuality and sex education of adolescents with intellectual disability: Mothers' attitudes, experiences, and support needs. *Journal of Intellectual & Developmental Disability*, *50*(2), 140–154. doi:10.1352/1934-9556-50.2.140 PMID:22642968

Prasher, V. P., & Routhu, S. K. (2003). Epidemiology of learning(intellectual) disability and comorbid conditions. *Psychiatry*, *2*, 8.

Prevalence and types of aggressive behaviour among adults with intellectual disabilities. (n.d.). *Journal of Intellectual Disability Research*, *50*(9), 652-661. doi:10.1111/j.1365-2788.2006.00815.x

Psalti, A. (2012). Bullies, victims, and bully-victims in Greek schools: Research data and implications of practice. *Hellenic Journal of Psychology*, *9*(2), 132–157.

Quality of life of young people with an intellect disability in Ireland: Interim Report. (2003). Retrieved from: https://www.fedvol.ie

Quesenberry, A., Ostrosky, M. M., & Corso, R. (2007). Skilled and knowledgeable caregivers: The role of fathers in supporting young children's development. *Young Exceptional Children*, *10*(4), 11–19. doi:10.1177/109625060701000402

Rademakers, J., Mouthaan, I., & de Neef, M. (2005). Diversity in sexual health: Problems and dilemmas. *The European Journal of Contraception & Reproductive Health Care*, *10*(4), 207–211. doi:10.1080/13625180500279847 PMID:16448946

Radford, J. P. (1991). Sterilization versus segregation: Control of the 'feebleminded', 1900-1938. *Social Science & Medicine*, *33*(4), 449–458. doi:10.1016/0277-9536(91)90327-9 PMID:1948159

Radliff, K. M., Wheaton, J. E., Robinson, K., & Morris, J. (2012). Illuminating the relationship between bullying and substance use among middle and high school youths. *Addictive Behaviors*, *37*(4), 569–572. doi:10.1016/j.addbeh.2012.01.001 PMID:22277772

Raina, P., & Lunsky, Y. (2010). A comparison study of adults with intellectual disability and psychiatric disorder with and without forensic involvement. *Research in Developmental Disabilities*, *31*(1), 218–223. doi:10.1016/j.ridd.2009.09.008 PMID:19854026

Rao, L., Govinda, & Sivakumar, T. C. (2003). Vocational Training of the mentally retarded. *EDUTRACTS*, *2*(10).

Ravindranadan, V., & Raju, S. (2007). Adjustment and attitude of parents of children with mental retardation. *Journal of the Indian Academy of Applied Psychology*, *33*(1), 137–141.

Ravindranodan, S., & Raju, V. (2007). Attitudes of parents of children with mental retardation. *Journal of the Indian Academy of Applied Psychology*, *1*, 137–141.

Rawlins, R. C. A. (1983). *Attitudes to Mental retardation: a cross cultural study* (MA Counseling Psychology Thesis). Pietermaritzburg: University of Natal.

Reardon, T. C., Gray, K. M., & Melvin, G. A. (2015). Anxiety disorders in children and adolescents with intellectual disability: Prevalence and assessment. *Research in Developmental Disabilities*, *36*, 175–190. doi:10.1016/j.ridd.2014.10.007 PMID:25462478

Reder, P., & Lucey, C. (1995). *Assessment of parenting: Psychiatric and psychological contributions*. Hove, NY: Brunner-Routledge, Taylor and Francis Group.

Reed, E. J. (1997). Criminal law and the capacity of mentally retarded persons to consent to sexual activity. *Virginia Law Review*, *83*(4), 799–827. doi:10.2307/1073749

Rehfeldt, R. A., Dahman, D., Young, A., Cherry, H., & Davis, P. (2003). Teaching a simple meal preparation skill to adults with moderate and severe mental retardation using video modeling. *Behavioral Interventions*, *18*(3), 209–218. doi:10.1002/bin.139

Reid, M. J., Webster-Stratton, C., & Hammond, M. (2007). Enhancing a classroom social competence and problem-solving curriculum by offering parent training to families of moderate-to-high-risk elementary school children. *Journal of Clinical Child and Adolescent Psychology*, *36*(4), 605–620. doi:10.1080/15374410701662741 PMID:18088218

Reilly, P. R. (1987). Involuntary sterilization in the United States: A surgical solution. *The Quarterly Review of Biology*, *62*(2), 153–170. doi:10.1086/415404 PMID:3299450

Reiter, S., Bryen, D., & Shachar, I. (2007). Adolescents with intellectual disabilities as victims of abuse. *Journal of Intellectual Disabilities*, *11*(4), 371–387. doi:10.1177/1744629507084602 PMID:18029413

Reiter, S., & Lapidot-Leflet, N. (2007). Bullying among special education students with intellectual disabilities: Differences in social adjustment and social skills. *Journal of Intellectual & Developmental Disability*, *45*(3), 174–181. doi:10.1352/1934-9556(2007)45[174:BASESW]2.0.CO;2 PMID:17472426

Remington, B. (1998). Applied behaviour analysis and intellectual disability: A long-term relationship?1. *Journal of Intellectual & Developmental Disability*, *23*(2), 121–135. doi:10.1080/13668259800033631

Repp, A. C., & Karsh, D. (1994). A hypothesis-based interventions for tantrum behavior of person with developmental disabilities in school settings. *Journal of Applied Behavior Analysis*, *27*(1), 21–31. doi:10.1901/jaba.1994.27-21 PMID:8188561

Reschly, D. J. (1996). Identification and Assessment of Students with Disabilities. *The Future of Children Special Education for Students With Disabilities*, *6*(1). Retrieved from https://www.princeton.edu/futureofchildren/publications/docs/06_01_02.pdf

Rethink autism provides distance BCBA supervision to candidates seeking certification in behavior analysis . (2010). PR Newswire.

Review of Vineland Adaptive Behavior Scales-Second Edition (Vineland-II). (2012). *Early Childhood Measurement and Evaluation*. Retrieved from www.cup.ualberta.ca

Reynolds, T. B. A., Zupanick, C. E., & Dombeck, M. (2013). *Intellectual Diasability, Mentalhelp.Net. An American Addiction center resources*. Retrieved on 14 February 2019.Retrived from http://www.mentalhelp.net/articles/intellectual-functioning-mental-abilities/

Reynolds, Zupanick, & Dombeck. (2013). *Intellectual Disability and Severity Codes*. Retrieved from https://www.mentalhelp.net/articles/intellectual-disability-and-severity-codes/

Reynolds, T., Zupanick, C. E., & Dombeck, M. (2013). *Historical and Contemporary Perspectives on Intellectual Disabilities*. Intellectual Disabilities.

Ricciardelli, L. A., & Jaskyte, K. (2019). A value-critical policy analysis of Georgia's beyond a reasonable doubt standard of proof of Intellectual Disability. *Journal of Disability Policy Studies*.

Richardson, S. O. (1996). Coping with dyslexia in the regular classroom: Inclusion or exclusion. *Annals of Dyslexia*, *46*(1), 37–48. doi:10.1007/BF02648170 PMID:24234266

Richdale, A., & Wiggs, L. (2005). Behavioural approaches to the treatment of sleep problems in children with developmental disorders. What is state of the art? *International Journal of Behavioral and Consultation Therapy*, *1*(3), 165–187. doi:10.1037/h0100743

Ridley, A. M., Gabbert, F., & La Rooy, D. J. (2012). *Suggestibility in legal contexts: psychological research and forensic implications*. Chichester, UK: John Wiley & Sons.

Rigby, K., & Cox, I. K. (1996). The contributions of bullying and low self-esteem to acts of delinquency among Australian teenagers. *Personality and Individual Differences*, *21*(4), 609–612. doi:10.1016/0191-8869(96)00105-5

Rigby, K., & Slee, P. T. (1991). Bullying among Australian school children: Reported behaviour and attitudes to victims. *The Journal of Social Psychology*, *131*(5), 615–622. doi:10.1080/00224545.1991.9924646 PMID:1798296

Rimmerman, A. (1998). Factors relating to attitudes of Israeli corporate executives towards the employability of persons with intellectual disability. *Journal of Intellectual & Developmental Disability*, *23*(3), 245–254. doi:10.1080/13668259800033731

Ritzema, A.M., & Sladeczek, I.E. (2011). Stress in parents of children with developmental disabilities over time. *Journal of Developmental Disabilities, 17*, 21-34.

Roberts, C., Mazzucchelli, T., Studman, L. J., & Sanders, M. R. (2006). Behavioral family intervention for children with developmental disabilities and behavioral problems. *Journal of Clinical Child and Adolescent Psychology, 35*(2), 180-193.

Roberts, C. M., & Smith, P. R. (1999). Attitudes and behavior of children towards peers with disabilities. *International Journal of Disability Development and Education*, *46*(1), 35–50. doi:10.1080/103491299100713

Robertson, J., Emerson, E., Baines, S., & Hatton, C. (2018). Self-reported smoking, alcohol and drug use among adolescents and young adults with and without mild to moderate intellectual disability. *Journal of Intellectual & Developmental Disability*, 1–11. doi:10.3109/13668250.2018.1440773

Robinson, M., & Neece, C. L. (2015). Marital satisfaction, parental stress, and child behavior problems among parents of young children with developmental delays. *Journal of Mental Health Research in Intellectual Disabilities*, *8*(1), 23–46. doi:10.1080/19315864.2014.994247

Rodrigue, J. R., Morgan, S. B., & Geffken, G. R. (1992). Psychosocial adaptation of fathers of children with autism, Down syndrome, and normal development. *Journal of Autism and Developmental Disorders*, *22*(2), 249–263. doi:10.1007/BF01058154 PMID:1385591

Rogers, S. J., Hepburn, S. L., Stackhouse, T., & Wehner, E. (2003). Imitation performance in toddlers with autism and those with other developmental disorders. *Journal of Child Psychology and Psychiatry, and Allied Disciplines*, *44*(5), 763–781. doi:10.1111/1469-7610.00162 PMID:12831120

Rohwerder, B. (2018). *Disability stigma in developing countries*. Institute of Development Studies.

Roos, P. (1977). Parents of mentally retarded people. *International Journal of Mental Health, 6*(1), 96–119. doi:10.1080/00207411.1977.11448758

Rose, J., West, C., & Clifford, D. (2000). Group interventions for anger in people with intellectual disabilities. *Research in Developmental Disabilities, 21*(3), 171-181. doi:10.10160891-4222(00)00032-9

Rose, C. A., & Espelage, D. L. (2012). Risk and protective factors associated with the bullying involvement of students with emotional and behavioral disorders. *Behavioral Disorders, 37*(3), 133–148. doi:10.1177/019874291203700302

Rose, C. A., Espelage, D. L., & Monda-Amaya, L. E. (2009). Bullying and victimization rates among students in general and special education: A comparative analysis. *Educational Psychology, 29*(7), 761–776. doi:10.1080/01443410903254864

Rose, C. A., Forber-Pratt, A. J., Espelage, D. L., & Aragon, S. R. (2013). The influence of psychosocial factors on bullying involvement of students with disabilities. *Theory into Practice, 52*(4), 272–279. doi:10.1080/00405841.2013.829730

Rose, C. A., Monda-Amaya, L. E., & Espelage, D. L. (2011). Bullying perpetration and victimization in special education: A review of the literature. *Remedial and Special Education, 32*(2), 114–130. doi:10.1177/0741932510361247

Rose, J., & West, C. (1999). Assessment of anger in people with intellectual disabilities. *Journal of Applied Research in Intellectual Disabilities, 12*(3), 211–224. doi:10.1111/j.1468-3148.1999.tb00078.x

Rose, J., West, C., & Clifford, D. (2000). Group intervention for anger in people with intellectual disabilities. *Research in Developmental Disabilities, 21*(3), 171–181. doi:10.1016/S0891-4222(00)00032-9 PMID:10939316

Rossiter, L., & Sharpe, D. (2001). The siblings of individuals with mental retardation: a quantitative integration of the literature. *Journal of Child and Family Studies, 10*(1), 65-84.

Roux, G., Sofronoff, K., & Sanders, M. R. (2013). A Randomized Controlled Trial of Group Stepping Stones Triple P: A Mixed-Disability Trial. *Family Process, 52*(3), 411–424. doi:10.1111/famp.12016 PMID:24033239

Ruff, C. F., Templer, D. I., & Ayers, J. L. (1976). The intelligence of rapists. *Archives of Sexual Behavior, 5*(4), 327–329. doi:10.1007/BF01542085 PMID:952615

Ruggeri-Stevens, G., & Goodwin, S. (2007). "Learning to work" in small businesses: Learning and training for young adults with learning disabilities. *Education + Training, 49*(8/9), 745–755. doi:10.1108/00400910710834139

Rush, A. J., & Frances, A. T. (2000). The expert consensus guidelines: Treatment of psychiatric and behavioral problems in mental retardation. *American Journal of Mental Retardation, 105*, 159–1228.

Rutledge, M. S., & Scott, M. H. (1997). Students' attitudes towards people with mental retardation. *Academic Medicine, 72*(4).

Rutter, M., Graham, J., & Yule, W. (1970). *A neuropsychiatric study in childhood.* London: Heinemann Medical Books.

Ryan, T. A., & Scior, K. (2014). Medical students' attitudes towards people with intellectual disabilities: A literature review. *Research in Developmental Disabilities, 35*(10), 2316–2328. doi:10.1016/j.ridd.2014.05.019 PMID:24952372

Ryckman, D. B., & Henderson, R. S. (1965). The meaning of a retarded child for his parents—A focus for counsellors. *Journal of Mental Retardation., 3*(4). PMID:14342622

Rydin-Orwin, T., Drake, J., & Bratt, A. (1999). The effects of training on emotion recognition skills for adults with an intellectual disability. *Journal of Applied Research in Intellectual Disabilities, 12*(3), 253–262. doi:10.1111/j.1468-3148.1999.tb00081.x

Ryoo, J. H., Wang, C., & Swearer, S. M. (2015). Examination of the change in latent statuses in bullying behaviors across time. *School Psychology Quarterly*, *30*(1), 105–122. doi:10.1037pq0000082 PMID:25111466

Saarni, C. (2011). Emotional development in childhood. *Encyclopedia on early childhood development*, 24-29.

Sacks, O. (1995). *An anthropologist on Mars*. Sydney: Pan Macmillan Australia.

Sailor, W., Wolf, N., Choi, H., & Roger, B. (2009). Sustaining positive behavior support in a context of comprehensive school reform. In W. Sailor, G. Dunlop, G. Sugai, & R. Horner (Eds.), *Handbook of positive behavior support* (pp. 633–669). New York: Springer Publishing. doi:10.1007/978-0-387-09632-2_26

Sakamoto, M., Ando, H., & Tsutou, A. (2013). Comparing the effects of different individualized music interventions for elderly individuals with severe dementia. *International Psychogeriatrics*, *25*(5), 775–784. doi:10.1017/S1041610212002256 PMID:23298693

Salavert, J., Clarabuch, A., Fernández-Gómez, M. J., Barrau, V., Giráldez, M. P., & Borràs, J. (2018). Substance use disorders in patients with intellectual disability admitted to psychiatric hospitalisation. *Journal of Intellectual Disability Research*, *62*(11), 923–930. doi:10.1111/jir.12514 PMID:29961996

Salekin, K. L., Olley, J. G., & Hedge, K. A. (2010). Offenders with intellectual disability: Characteristics, prevalence, and issues in forensic assessment. *Journal of Mental Health Research in Intellectual Disabilities*, *3*(2), 97–116. doi:10.1080/19315861003695769

Salend, S. J., & Duhaney, L. M. G. (1999). The impact of inclusion on students with and without disabilities and their educators. *Remedial and Special Education*, *20*(2), 114–126. doi:10.1177/074193259902000209

Salkind, N. J. (2002). *Child development*. New York: Macmillan Reference USA.

Saloviita, T., Itälinna, M., & Leinonen, E. (2003). Explaining the parental stress of fathers and mothers caring for a child with intellectual disability: A double abcx model. *Journal of Intellectual Disability Research, 47*(4-5), 300-312.

Sameroff, A. E. (2009). *The transactional model of development: how children and contexts shape each other*. American Psychological Association.

Sameroff, J., & Seifer, R. (1983). Familial risk and child competence. *Child Development*, *54*(5), 1254–1268. doi:10.2307/1129680 PMID:6354632

Sandberg, N. M., & Ahlström, G. (2015). Prevalence of older people with intellectual disability in Sweden: A spatial epidemiological analysis. *Journal of Intellectual Disability Research*, *59*(12), 1155–1167. doi:10.1111/jir.12219 PMID:26306552

Sanders, M. R., Mazzecchelli, T. G., & Studman, L. J. (2003). *Practitioner's manual for standard stepping stones triple p: for families with a child who has a disability*. Brisbane, Australia: Triple P International.

Sanders, M. R., Mazzucchelli, T. G., & Studman, L. J. (2003). *Practitioner's manual for standard Stepping Stones Triple P*. Brisbane: Triple P International Pty. Ltd.

Sanders, M. R., Mazzucchelli, T. G., & Studman, L. J. (2004). Stepping Stones Triple P: The theoretical basis and development of an evidence-based positive parenting program for families with a child who has a disability. *Journal of Intellectual & Developmental Disability*, *29*(3), 265–283. doi:10.1080/13668250412331285127

Sansone, R. A., & Sansone, L. A. (2008). Bully victims: Psychological and somatic aftermaths. *Psychiatry*, *5*(6), 62–64. PMID:19727287

Sappock, T., Budczies, J., Bohe, S., Dziobek, K.I., Dosen, A., & Diefenbacher, A. (2013). Emotional development in adults with autism and intellectual disabilities: A retrospective clinical analysis. *Journal Plus One.*. doi:10.1371/journal.pone.0074036

Satchidanand, N., Gunukula, S. K., Lam, W. Y., McGuigan, D., New, I., Symons, A. B., ... Akl, E. A. (2012). Attitudes of healthcare students and professionals toward patients with physical disability: A systematic review. *American Journal of Physical Medicine & Rehabilitation*, *91*(6), 533–545. doi:10.1097/PHM.0b013e3182555ea4 PMID:22596075

Savage, S., & Bailey, S. (2004). The impact of caring on caregivers' mental health: A review of the literature. *Australian Health Review*, *27*(1), 103–109. doi:10.1071/AH042710111 PMID:15362303

Scelles, R. (1997). The impact of a person's disability on his or her sibling. *International Journal of Rehabilitation Research. Internationale Zeitschrift fur Rehabilitationsforschung. Revue Internationale de Recherches de Readaptation*, *20*(2), 129–137. doi:10.1097/00004356-199706000-00002 PMID:9226496

Schaafsma, D., Kok, G., Stoffelen, J.M.T., & Curfs, L.M.G. (2015). Identifying Effective Methods for Teaching Sex Education to Individuals With Intellectual Disabilities: A Systematic Review. *The Journal of Sex Research*, *52*(4), 412–432. doi:10.1080/00224499.2014.919373

Schalock, R. L. (1999, September). *The application of the concept of quality of life: IASSID Quality of Life Consensus Document: Discussion draft.* Paper presented at the 35th National Conference of the Australian Society for the Study of Intellectual Disabilities, Sydney, Australia.

Schalock, R. L. (2002, June). The concept of quality of life: What we know and do not know. Paper presented at the Inaugural IASSID Europe Quadrennial Conference, University College, Dublin, Ireland.

Schalock, R. L. (1997). The concept of quality of life in 21st century disability programmes. In R. I. Brown (Ed.), *Quality of life for people with disabilities: Models, research and practice* (2nd ed.; pp. 327–340). Cheltenham, UK: Stanley Thornes.

Schalock, R. L. (2004). Quality of life: What we know and what we don't know. *Journal of Intellectual Disability Research*, *48*(3), 203–216. doi:10.1111/j.1365-2788.2003.00558.x PMID:15025663

Schalock, R. L. (Ed.). (1990). *Quality of Life: Perspectives and issues.* Washington, DC: American Association on Mental Retardation.

Schalock, R. L., Bonham, G. S., & Verdugo, M. A. (2008). The conceptualization and measurement of quality of life: Implications for program planning and evaluation in the field of intellectual disabilities. *Evaluation and Program Planning*, *31*(2), 181–190. doi:10.1016/j.evalprogplan.2008.02.001 PMID:18394704

Schalock, R. L., Borthwick-Duffy, S. A., Bradley, V. J., Buntinx, W. H., Coulter, D. L., & Craig, E. M. (2010). *Intellectual Disability: Definition, Classification, and Systems of Supports.* Washington, DC: ERIC.

Schalock, R. L., Gardner, J. F., & Bradley, V. J. (2007). *Quality of life for persons with intellectual and other developmental disabilities: Applications across individuals, organizations, communities, and systems.* Washington, DC: American Association on Intellectual and Developmental Disabilities.

Schalock, R. L., Luckasson, R. A., & Shogren, K. A. (2007). The renaming of mental retardation: Understanding the change to the term intellectual disability. *Journal Information*, *45*(2). PMID:17428134

Schalock, R. L., & Ruth, A. (2007). The Renaming of Mental Retardation: Understanding the Change to the Term Intellectual Disability. *Intellectual and Developmental Disabilities*, *45*(2), 116–124. doi:10.1352/1934-9556(2007)45[116:TROMRU]2.0.CO;2 PMID:17428134

Schalock, R. L., & Verdugo, M. A. (2002). *Handbook on quality of life for human services practitioners*. Washington, DC: American Association on Mental Retardation.

Schalock, R. L., Verdugo, M. A., Bonham, G. S., Fantova, F., & Van Loon, J. S. (2008). Enhancing personal outcomes: Organizational strategies, guidelines, and examples. *Journal of Policy and Practice in Intellectual Disabilities*, *5*(4), 276–285. doi:10.1111/j.1741-1130.2007.00135.x

Schatz, S. J. (2018). Interrogated with Intellectual Disabilities: The risks of false confession. *Stanford Law Review*, *70*, 643. PMID:29486553

Schlossar, S. (2004). *Opening Doors. Multicultural Disability Advocacy Association of NSW*. Retrieved on June. 13.2015 from http://www.mdaa.org.au/publications/ethnicity/indian/IndianOpenDoors.pdf

Schoenberg, M. R., & Scott, J. G. (2011). *The little black book of neuropsychology: a syndrome-based approach*. New York: Springer Science & Business Media. doi:10.1007/978-0-387-76978-3

Schor, D. P. (1987). Sex and sexual abuse in developmentally disabled adolescents. *Seminars in Adolescent Medicine*, *3*, 1–7. PMID:2955493

Schuengel, C., Rentinck, I. C. M., Stolk, J., Voorman, J. M., Loots, G. M. P., Ketelaar, M., ... Becher, J. G. (2009). Parents' reactions to the diagnosis of cerebral palsy: Associations between resolution, age and severity of disability. *Child: Care, Health and Development*, *35*(5), 673–680. doi:10.1111/j.1365-2214.2009.00951.x PMID:19320906

Schuiringa, H., van Nieuwenhuijzen, M., & de Castro, B. O. (2015). Parenting and the parent–child relationship in families of children with mild to borderline intellectual disabilities and externalizing behavior. *Research in Developmental Disabilities*, *32*, 1–12. doi:10.1016/j.ridd.2014.08.018 PMID:25262097

Scior, K. (2011). Public awareness, attitudes and beliefs regarding intellectual disability: A systematic review. *Research in Developmental Disabilities*, *32*(6), 2164–2182. doi:10.1016/j.ridd.2011.07.005 PMID:21798712

Scior, K., Kan, K. Y., McLoughlin, A., & Sheridan, J. (2010). Public attitudes toward people with intellectual disabilities: A cross-cultural study. *Intellectual and Developmental Disabilities*, *48*(4), 278–289. doi:10.1352/1934-9556-48.4.278 PMID:20722478

Scior, K., & Werner, S. (Eds.). (2016). *Intellectual disability and stigma: Stepping out from the margins*. London: Palgrave McMillan. doi:10.1057/978-1-137-52499-7

Scott, H. (1998). Helping clients in their sexual expression. *British Journal of Nursing (Mark Allen Publishing)*, *7*(10), 568. doi:10.12968/bjon.1998.7.10.5678 PMID:9775763

Scott, M. H., & Rutledge, C. M. (1997). Students' attitudes toward people with mental retardation. *Academic Medicine*, *72*(4), 246–247. doi:10.1097/00001888-199704000-00005 PMID:9125936

Scruggs, T. E., & Mastropieri, M. A. (1996). Teacher perceptions of inclusion/ mainstreaming, 1958-1995: A research synthesis. *Exceptional Children*, *1996*, 59–74. doi:10.1177/001440299606300106

Scully, J. L. (2018). Epistemic Exclusion, Injustice, and Disability. In D. T. Wasserman & A. Cureton (Eds.), *The Oxford Handbook of Philosophy and Disability*. Oxford, UK: Oxford University Press.

Segeren, M. W., Fassaert, T. J., Kea, R., de Wit, M. A., & Popma, A. (2018). Exploring differences in criminogenic risk factors and criminal behavior between young adult violent offenders with and without mild to borderline intellectual disability. *International Journal of Offender Therapy and Comparative Criminology*, *62*(4), 978–999. doi:10.1177/0306624X16674009 PMID:29409403

Serrata, C. A. (2012). Psychosocial aspects of parenting a child with autism. *Journal of Applied Rehabilitation Counseling, 43*(4), 29–35. doi:10.1891/0047-2220.43.4.29

Sevcik, R. A., & Romski, M. A. (Eds.). (2016). *Communication interventions for individuals with severe disabilities: Exploring research challenges and opportunities*. Baltimore, MD: Brookes.

Sexuality and Disability in the Indian Context. (2010). TARSHI.

Shannon, J. D., Tamis-LeMonda, C. S., London, K., & Cabrera, N. (2002). Beyond rough and tumble: Low-income fathers' interactions and children's cognitive development at 24 months. *Parenting, Science and Practice, 2*(2), 77–104. doi:10.1207/S15327922PAR0202_01

Sharma, A., & Chowhan, S. (2014). *The Neuropsychological Components of Visual Processing and Learning in High and Low Functioning Children Exhibiting Autism Spectrum Disorder: A Comparative Study*. Unpublished manuscript.

Sheard, C., Clegg, J., Standen, P., & Cromby, J. (2001). Bullying and people with severe intellectual disability. *Journal of Intellectual Disability Research, 45*(5), 407–415. doi:10.1046/j.1365-2788.2001.00349.x PMID:11679046

Shearn, J., & Todd, S. (2000). Maternal employment and family responsibilities: The perspectives of mothers of children with intellectual disabilities. *Journal of Applied Research in Intellectual Disabilities, 13*(3), 109–131. doi:10.1046/j.1468-3148.2000.00021.x

Sheeran, T., Marvin, R. S., & Pianta, R. C. (1997). Mothers' resolution of their child's diagnosis and self-reported measures of parenting stress, marital relations, and social support. *Journal of Pediatric Psychology, 22*(2), 197–212. doi:10.1093/jpepsy/22.2.197 PMID:9114643

Sheridan, J., & Scior, K. (2013). Attitudes towards people with intellectual disabilities: A comparison of young people from British South Asian and White British backgrounds. *Research in Developmental Disabilities, 34*(4), 1240–1247. doi:10.1016/j.ridd.2012.12.017 PMID:23417129

Sherman, B. R., & Cocozza, J. J. (1984). Stress in families of the developmentally disabled: A literature review of factors affecting the decision to seek out-of-home placements. *Family Relations, 33*(1), 95–103. doi:10.2307/584594

Sheydaei, M., Adibsereshki, N., & Movallali, G. (2015). The effectiveness of emotional intelligence training on communication skills in students with intellectual disabilities. *Iranian Rehabilitation Journal, 3*(3).

Shipley-Benamou, R., Lutzker, J. R., & Taubman, M. (2002). Teaching daily living skills to children with autism through instructional video modeling. *Journal of Positive Behavior Interventions, 4*(3), 165–175. doi:10.1177/109830070200 40030501

Shrivastava, S. P. (Ed.). (1970). Social Work and the Rehabilitation of the Physically Handicapped, The Journal of Rehabilitation in Asia, 11(1).

Siddiqi, A., Irwin, L. G., & Hertzman, C. (2007). *The total environment assessment model of early child development*. Evidence report for the world health organization's commission on the social determinants of health, oms.

Siebelink, E. M., de Jong, M. D. T., Taal, E., & Roelvink, L. (2006). Sexuality and people with intellectual disabilities: Assessment of knowledge, attitudes, experiences, and needs. *Mental Retardation, 44*(4), 283–294. doi:10.1352/0047-6765(2006)44[283:SAPWID]2.0.CO;2 PMID:16834465

Sieman, M. (1984). Siblings of the chronically ill or disabled child. *The Nursing Clinics of North America, 19*, 295–307. PMID:6233538

Silver, H. (1957). *The Physically Handicapped, Social Work Year Book*. Academic Press.

Simplican, S. C. (2019). Intellectual disability and stigma: Stepping out from the margins. *Disability & Society, 34*(2), 335-337.

Simpson, M. K., & Hogg, J. (2001). Patterns of offending among people with intellectual disability: A systematic review. Part I: Methodology and prevalence data. *Journal of Intellectual Disability Research, 45*(5), 384–396. doi:10.1046/j.1365-2788.2001.00345.x PMID:11679044

Singal, N. (2009). *Education of children with disabilities in India.* Retrieved from http://unesdoc.unesco.org/images/0018/001866/186611e.pdf

Singer, G. H. S., Marquis, J., Powers, L. K., Blanchard, L., Divenere, N., Santelli, B., . . . Sharp, M. (1999). A multi-site evaluation of parent to parent programs for parents of children with disabilities. *Journal of Early Intervention, 22*(3), 217–229. doi:10.1177/105381519902200305

Singer, G. H. S., Ethridge, B. L., & Aldana, S. I. (2007). Primary and secondary effects of parenting and stress management interventions for parents of children with developmental disabilities: A meta-analysis. *Mental Retardation and Developmental Disabilities Research Reviews, 13*(4), 357–367. doi:10.1002/mrdd.20175 PMID:17979202

Singer, G., & Todis, B. (1991). Stress and stress management in families with adopted children who have severe disabilities. *The Journal of the Association for Persons with Severe Handicaps, 16*(1), 3–13. doi:10.1177/154079699101600102

Singh, N. N., Lancioni, G. E., Winton, A. S. W., Adkins, A. D., Singh, J., & Singh, A. N. (2007). Mindfulness training assists individuals with moderate mental retardation to maintain their community placements. *Behavior Modification, 31*(6), 800–814. doi:10.1177/0145445507300925 PMID:17932236

Singh, N. N., Lancioni, G. E., Winton, A. S., Fisher, B. C., Wahler, R. G., Mcaleavey, K., ... Sabaawi, M. (2006). Mindful parenting decreases aggression, noncompliance, and self-injury in children with autism. *Journal of Emotional and Behavioral Disorders, 14*(3), 169–177. doi:10.1177/10634266060140030401

Singh, N. N., Lancioni, G. E., Winton, A. S., Karazsia, B. T., Myers, R. E., Latham, L. L., & Singh, J. (2014). Mindfulness-Based Positive Behavior Support (MBPBS) for mothers of adolescents with autism spectrum disorder: Effects on adolescents' behavior and parental stress. *Mindfulness, 5*(6), 646–657. doi:10.100712671-014-0321-3

Singh, N. N., Lancioni, G. E., Winton, A. S., Singh, J., Curtis, W. J., Wahler, R. G., & McAleavey, K. M. (2007). Mindful parenting decreases aggression and increases social behavior in children with developmental disabilities. *Behavior Modification, 31*(6), 749–771. doi:10.1177/0145445507300924 PMID:17932234

Singh, N. N., Lancioni, G. E., Winton, A. S., Singh, J., Singh, A. N., Adkins, A. D., & Wahler, R. G. (2010). Training in mindful caregiving transfers to parent–child interactions. *Journal of Child and Family Studies, 19*(2), 167–174. doi:10.100710826-009-9267-9

Siperstein, G. N., KeerthiSugumaran, D., Bardon, J.N., & Parker, R.C. (n.d.). *Attitudes of the Public in India towards People with Intellectual Disabilities.* Retrieved from: https://www.media.specialolympics.org

Siperstein, G. N., Sugumaran, K., Bardon, J. N., & Parker, R. S. (2001). *Attitudes of the Public in India towards People with Intellectual Disabilities.* Retrieved from www.specialolympics.org/uploadedfiles/.../india_full%20report.pdf

Siperstein, G. N. (2003). *Multinational study of attitudes towards individuals with intellectual disabilities: General findings and calls to action.* Special Olympics.

Siperstein, G. N., Hardman, M. L., Wappett, M. T., & Clary, L. (2001). *National Evaluation of the Special Olympics Unified Sports Program (Final Report for Special Olympics, Incorporated).* Boston: University of Massachusetts, Center for Social Development and Education.

SirlopuD.GonzalezR.BohnerG.SieblerF.OrdonnezG.MillarA., & De

Sivakumar, T. C., & Kumar, R. (2009). *Selection and Training to develop adult independent living skills in the Indian context across socio cultural and economic levels.* Report of the National Seminar - Planning for Comprehensive Rehabilitation of Individuals with mental retardation, Chennai, India.

Sjgafoos, J., Elkins, J., Kerr, M., & Attwood, T. (1994). A survey of aggressive behaviour among a population of persons with intellectual disability in Queensland. *Journal of Intellectual Disability Research, 38*(4), 369–381. doi:10.1111/j.1365-2788.1994.tb00417.x PMID:7949789

Skapinakis, P., Bellos, S., Gkatsa, T., Magklara, K., Lewish, G., Araya, R., & ... . (2011). The association between bullying and early stages of suicidal ideation in late adolescents in Greece. *BMC Psychiatry, 11*(1), 1–9. doi:10.1186/1471-244X-11-22 PMID:21303551

Smyer, M. A., McHale, S. M., Birkel, R., & Madle, R. A. (1988). Impairments, handicapping environments, and disability: A life-span perspective. In P. S. Van Hasselt, P. S. Dtrain, & M. Herson (Eds.), *Handbook of developmental and physical disabilities* (pp. 9–20). New York: Permagon.

Snell, M. E., Brady, N., McLean, L., Ogletree, B. T., Siegel, E., Sylvester, L., ... Sevcik, R. (2010). Twenty years of communication intervention research with individuals who have severe intellectual and developmental disabilities. *American Journal on Intellectual and Developmental Disabilities, 115*(5), 364–380. doi:10.1352/1944-7558-115-5.364 PMID:20687822

Sobsey, D. (1994). *Violence and abuse in the lives of people with disabilities: The end of silent acceptance?* Baltimore, MD: Paul H. Brookes Publishing Co.

Sobsey, D., & Mansell, S. (1990). The prevention of sexual abuse and assault: Sexual exploitation of people with disabilities. *Sexuality and Disability, 9*, 243–259. doi:10.1007/BF01102395

Söderholm, S., Meinander, M., & Alaranta, H. (2001). Augmentative and alternative communication methods in locked-in syndrome. Journal of Rehabilitation Medicine, 33, 235-239.

Sofair, A. N., & Kaldijian, L. C. (2000). Eugenic sterilization and a qualified Nazi analogy: The United States and Germany, 1930-1945. *Annals of Internal Medicine, 132*(4), 312–319. doi:10.7326/0003-4819-132-4-200002150-00010 PMID:10681287

Sofronoff, K., Jahnel, D., & Sanders, M. R. (2011). Stepping Stones Triple P seminars for parents of a child with a disability: A randomized controlled trial. *Research in Developmental Disabilities, 32*(6), 2253–2262. doi:10.1016/j.ridd.2011.07.046 PMID:21871779

Solomon, M., Ono, M., Timmer, S., & Goodlin-Jones, B. (2008). The effectiveness of parent–child interaction therapy for families of children on the autism spectrum. *Journal of Autism and Developmental Disorders, 38*(9), 1767–1776. doi:10.100710803-008-0567-5 PMID:18401693

Soltani, S., Khosravi, B., & Salehiniya, H. (2015). Prevalence of intellectual disability in Iran: Toward a new conceptual framework in data collection. *Journal of Research in Medical Sciences, 20*(7), 714–715. doi:10.4103/1735-1995.166234 PMID:26622264

Søndenaa, E., Rasmussen, K., & Nøttestad, J. A. (2008). Forensic issues in intellectual disability. *Current Opinion in Psychiatry, 21*(5), 449–453. doi:10.1097/YCO.0b013e328305e5e9 PMID:18650685

Søndenaa, E., Rasmussen, K., Palmstierna, T., & Nøttestad, J. A. (2008). The prevalence and nature of intellectual disability in Norwegian prisons. *Journal of Intellectual Disability Research, 52*(12), 1129–1137. doi:10.1111/j.1365-2788.2008.01072.x PMID:18498332

Son, E., Parish, S. L., & Peterson, N. A. (2012). National prevalence of peer victimization among young children with disabilities in the United States. *Children and Youth Services Review, 34*(8), 1540–1545. doi:10.1016/j.childyouth.2012.04.014

Sourander, A., Klomek, A. B., Ikonen, M., Lindroos, J., Luntamo, T., Koskelainen, M., & … . (2010). Psychosocial risk factors associated with cyberbullying among adolescents: A population based study. *Archives of General Psychiatry, 67*(7), 720–728. doi:10.1001/archgenpsychiatry.2010.79 PMID:20603453

Sovner, R., & Hurley, A. D. (1986). Four factors affecting the diagnosis of psychiatric disorders in mentally retarded persons. *Psychiatric Aspects of Mental Retardation Reviews, 5*(9), 45–49.

Special Olympics. (2004). *A Study of Youth Attitudes about Intellectual Disabilities.* Retrieved from http://www.specialolympics.org

Special Olympics. (2005). *Multinational Study of Attitudes towards Individuals with Intellectual Disabilities.* Retrieved from www.specialolympics.org/...Studies.../Multinational_Attitudes_Study.asp

Sprafkin, J., & Gadow, K. (1987). An observational study of emotionally disturbed and learning-disabled children in school settings. *Journal of Abnormal Child Psychology, 15*(3), 393–408. doi:10.1007/BF00916457 PMID:3668086

Srinath, S., & Girimaji, S. C. (1999). Epidemiology of child and adolescent mental health problems and mental retardation. *Nimhans Journal, 17*, 355–366.

Sroufe, L. A. (1979). The coherence of individual development. *The American Psychologist, 34*(10), 834–841. doi:10.1037/0003-066X.34.10.834

State of Nebraska Health and Human Services. (2006). *Nebraska developmental disabilities provider profiles.* Lincoln, NE: State of Nebraska Health and Human Services, Division of Developmental Disabilities.

Statistics, A. B. (2015). Disability, ageing and carers, Australia: Summary of findings. *Retrieved Januari, 18*, 2018.

Stavrakantonaki, M., & Johnson, T. P. (2018). Effects of Rosa's Law on Intellectual-Disability reporting. *Public Opinion Quarterly, 82*(3), 593–604. doi:10.1093/poq/nfy024

Steiner, C. (2003). *Emotional Literacy; Intelligence with a Heart.* Retrieved from Http://dgek.de/wp-content/uploads/2015/09/steiner-emotional-literacy.pdf

Stella, C. S. C., Forlin, C., & Lan, A. M. (2007). The influence of an inclusive education course on attitude change of pre-service secondary teachers in Hong Kong. *Asia-Pacific Journal of Teacher Education, 35*(2), 161–179. doi:10.1080/13598660701268585

Steptoe, L., Lindsay, W. R., Forrest, D., & Power, M. (2006). Quality of life and relationships in sex offenders with intellectual disability. *Journal of Intellectual and Developmental Disabilities, 31*(1), 13-19.

Sterzing, P. R., Shattuck, P. T., Narendrof, S. C., Wagner, M., & Cooper, B. P. (2012). Bullying involvement and autism spectrum disorders: Prevalence and correlates of bullying involvement among adolescents with an autism spectrum disorder. *Archives of Pediatrics & Adolescent Medicine, 166*(11), 1058–1064. doi:10.1001/archpediatrics.2012.790 PMID:22945284

Stevenson, M., & Crnic, K. (2013). Intrusive fathering, children's self-regulation and social skills: A mediation analysis. *Journal of Intellectual Disability Research, 57*(6), 500–512. doi:10.1111/j.1365-2788.2012.01549.x PMID:22458354

Stewart, C. A., & Singh, N. N. (1995). Enhancing the recognition and production of facial expressions of emotion by children with mental retardation. *Research in Developmental Disabilities*, *16*(5), 365–382. doi:10.1016/0891-4222(95)00024-H PMID:8532916

Stewart, R., Kozak, A., Tingley, L., Goddard, J., Blake, E., & Cassel, W. (2001). Adult sibling relationships: Validation of a typology. *Personal Relationships*, *8*(3), 299–324. doi:10.1111/j.1475-6811.2001.tb00042.x

Stoffelen, J. M. T., Schaafsma, D., Kok, G., & Curfs, L. M. G. (2018, September). Women Who Love: An Explorative Study on Experiences of Lesbian and Bisexual Women with a Mild Intellectual Disability in The Netherlands. *Sexuality and Disability*, *36*(3), 249–264. doi:10.100711195-018-9519-y PMID:30220750

Stokes, S. (1990). Restaurant supervisors: Don't discount the disabled. *The Cornell Hotel and Restaurant Administration Quarterly*, *30*(4), 14–17. doi:10.1177/001088049003000405

Stoyanova, S., & Giannouli, V. (2018). Bulgarian students' impulsivity differentiated by gender, age, and some scientific areas. *Psychological Thought*, *11*(2), 138–147. doi:10.5964/psyct.v11i2.250

Straus, M. A., & Stewart, J. H. (1999). Corporal punishment by American parents: National data on prevalence, chronicity, severity, and duration, in relation to child and family characteristics. *Clinical Child and Family Psychology Review*, *2*(2), 55–70. doi:10.1023/A:1021891529770 PMID:11225932

Straus, M. S., & Donnelly, D. A. (2001). *Beating the devil out of them. Corporal punishment in American families and its effects on children.* New Brunswick, NJ: Transaction Publishers.

Strnadová, I., Collings, S., Loblinzk, J., & Danker, J. (2019). Parents with intellectual disabilities and their perspective of peer support: "It depends on how they give it. *Journal of Applied Research in Intellectual Disabilities*, *32*(4), 879–889. doi:10.1111/jar.12579 PMID:30790398

Stromme, P., & Diseth, T. H. (2000). Prevalence of psychiatric diagnoses in children with mental retardation: data from a population-based study. *Developmental Medicine & Child Neurology, 42*(04), 266-270.

Stromme, P., & Magnus, P. (2000). Correlations between socioeconomic status, iq and aetiology in mental retardation: a population-based study of Norwegian children. *Social Psychiatry and Psychiatric Epidemiology, 1*(35).

Strømme, P., & Hagberg, G. (2007). Aetiology in severe and mild mental retardation: A population-based study of Norwegian children. *Developmental Medicine and Child Neurology*, *42*(2), 76–86. doi:10.1111/j.1469-8749.2000.tb00050.x PMID:10698323

Strømme, P., & Magnus, P. (2000). Correlations between socioeconomic status, IQ and aetiology in mental retardation: A population-based study of Norwegian children. *Social Psychiatry and Psychiatric Epidemiology*, *35*(1), 12–18. doi:10.1007001270050003 PMID:10741531

Strydom, A., Haveman, M., Heller, T., Lee, L., Maaskant, M., & Shooshtari, S. (n.d.). *Major Health Risks in Aging Persons With Intellectual Disabilities: An Overview of Recent Studies.* . doi:10.1111/j.1741-1130.2010.00248

Stuart, H. (2012). United nations convention on the rights of persons with disabilities: a roadmap for change. *Current Opinion in Psychiatry, 25*(5), 365-369.

Stuart, W., & Kingstone, M. (2018). The complexity of lifelong co morbidities with severe intellectual disability. *Journal of Intellectual and Developmental Disability.*

Sturmey, P. (1995). Dsm-iii-r and persons with dual diagnoses: conceptual issues and strategies for future research. *Journal of Intellectual Disability Research, 39*(5), 357-364.

Sturmey, P. (2007). Functional analysis in clinical treatment. Amsterdam: Academic Press.

Su, K. P., Yu, J. M., Yang, T. W., Tsai, S. Y., & Chen, C. C. (2000). Characteristics of mentally retarded criminal offenders in Northern Taiwan. *Journal of Forensic Sciences*, *45*(6), 1207–1209. doi:10.1520/JFS14869J PMID:11110172

Sullivan, P. M., & Knutson, J. F. (2000). Maltreatment and disabilities: A population-based epidemiological study. *Child Abuse & Neglect*, *24*(10), 1257–1273. doi:10.1016/S0145-2134(00)00190-3 PMID:11075694

Sultana, S. A. G., Lam-Po-Tang, T. R. L., Wright, F., Linderman, R., & Purvis-Smith, S. (1995). Fragile X mental retardation in an Indonesian family. *Medical Journal of Indonesia*, *4*, 17–17. doi:10.13181/mji.v4i1.885

Suto, W. M. I., Clare, I. C. H., Holland, A. J., & Watson, P. C. (2005). Capacity to make financial decisions among people with mild intellectual disabilities. *Journal of Intellectual Disability Research*, *49*(3), 199–209. doi:10.1111/j.1365-2788.2005.00635.x PMID:15713195

Swearer, S. M., Siebecker, A. B., Johnsen-Frerichs, L., & Wang, C. (2010). Assessment of bullying/victimization: The problem of comparability across studies and across methodologies. In S. R. Jimerson, S. M. Swearer, & D. L. Espelage (Eds.), *Handbook of bullying in schools: An international perspective* (pp. 305–327). New York, NY: Routledge.

Sweet, J. J., King, J. H., Malina, A. C., Bergman, M. A., & Simmons, A. (2002). Documenting the prominence of forensic neuropsychology at national meetings and in relevant professional journals from 1990 to 2000. *The Clinical Neuropsychologist*, *16*(4), 481–494. doi:10.1076/clin.16.4.481.13914 PMID:12822057

Tammy Reynolds, T., Zupanick, C. E., & Dombeck, M. (2013). *History Of Stigmatizing Names For Intellectual Disabilities Continued.* Retrieved from https://www.mentalhelp.net/articles/history-of-stigmatizing-names-for-intellectual-disabilities-continued/

Tarbox, J., Wallace, M. D., Tarbox, R. S. F., Landaburu, H. J., & Williams, W. L. (2004). Functional analysis and treatment of low rate problem behavior in individuals with developmental disabilities. *Behavioral Interventions*, *19*(3), 187–204. doi:10.1002/bin.158

Tassé, M. J., Schalock, R. L., Balboni, G., Bersani, H., & Sharon, A. (2012). The Construct of Adaptive Behavior: Its Conceptualization, Measurement, and Use in the Field of Intellectual Disability. *American Journal on Intellectual and Developmental Disabilities*, *117*(4), 291–303. doi:10.1352/1944-7558-117.4.291 PMID:22809075

Taylor, J. L. (2002). A review of the assessment and treatment of anger and aggression in offenders with intellectual disability. *Journal of Intellectual Disability Research*, *46*(s1), 57–73. doi:10.1046/j.1365-2788.2002.00005.x PMID:12031019

Taylor, L., Hatton, C., Dixon, L., & Douglas, C. (2004). Screening for psychiatric symptoms: Pas-add checklist norms for adults with intellectual disabilities. *Journal of Intellectual Disability Research*, *48*(1), 37–41. doi:10.1111/j.1365-2788.2004.00585.x PMID:14675229

Tellegen, C. L., & Sanders, M. R. (2013). Stepping Stones Triple P-Positive Parenting Program for children with disability: A systematic review and meta-analysis. *Research in Developmental Disabilities*, *34*(5), 1556–1571. doi:10.1016/j.ridd.2013.01.022 PMID:23475006

Tervo, R. C., Azuma, S., Palmer, G., & Redinius, P. (2002). Medical students' attitudes toward persons with disability: A comparative study. *Archives of Physical Medicine and Rehabilitation*, *83*(11), 1537–1542. doi:10.1053/apmr.2002.34620 PMID:12422321

Tezanos-Pinto, P., & … . (2008). Promoting positive attitudes toward people with Down syndrome: The benefit of school inclusion programs. *Journal of Applied Social Psychology*, *38*(11), 2710–2736. doi:10.1111/j.1559-1816.2008.00411.x

The Centre for Developmental Disability Health Victoria (CDDH). (2015). *Working with people with intellectual disabilities in healthcare settings: Fact Sheet*. Retrieved from: www.cddh.monash.org

Thomas, S. D., Nixon, M., Ogloff, J. R., & Daffern, M. (2019). Crime and victimization among people with intellectual disability with and without comorbid mental illness. *Journal of Applied Research in Intellectual Disabilities*, jar.12598. doi:10.1111/jar.12598 PMID:30990251

Thompson, R. J., & O'Quinn, A. N. (1979). Developmental disabilities: Etiologies, manifestations, diagnoses, and treatments. New York: Oxford.

Thompson, R. A. (1991). Emotional regulation and emotional development. *Educational Psychology Review*, *3*(4), 269–307. doi:10.1007/BF01319934

Thompson, R. H., & Iwata, B. A. (2007). A comparison of outcomes from descriptive and functional analyses of problem behavior. *Journal of Applied Behavior Analysis*, *40*(2), 333–338. doi:10.1901/jaba.2007.56-06 PMID:17624074

Thom, R. P., Grudzinskas, A. J. Jr, & Saleh, F. M. (2017). Sexual Behavior Among Persons With Cognitive Impairments. *Current Psychiatry Reports*, *19*(5), 25. doi:10.100711920-017-0777-7 PMID:28417268

Timms, S., & Goreczny, A. J. (2002). Adolescent sex offenders with mental retardation: Literature review and assessment considerations. *Aggression and Violent Behavior*, *7*(1), 1–19. doi:10.1016/S1359-1789(00)00031-8

Tiong, S. J., Blampied, N. M., & Le Grice, B. (1992). Training community-living, intellectually handicapped people in fire safety using video prompting. *Behaviour Change*, *9*(2), 65–72. doi:10.1017/S0813483900006379

To, T., Guttmann, A., Dick, P. T., Rosenfield, J. D., Parkin, P. C., Tassoudji, M., . . . Harris, J. K. (2004). Risk markers for poor developmental attainment in young children: results from a longitudinal national survey. *Archives of Pediatrics & Adolescent Medicine, 158*(7), 643-649.

Tolu, E.A., Temitayo, & Kofoworola, A. (2014). Exclusion of Children with Intellectual Disabilities from Regular Classroom: Nigeria Perspective. *African Journal for the Psychological Study of Social Issues*, *17*, 99-109. Retrieved from http://ajpssi.org/index.php/ajpssi/article/view/94/pdf_65

Tomasik, M. (2007). Effective inclusion activities for high school students with multiple disabilities. *Journal of Visual Impairment & Blindness*, *101*(10), 657–659. doi:10.1177/0145482X0710101012

Tonge, B., & Einfeld, S. (2000). The trajectory of psychiatric disorders in young people with intellectual disabilities. *Australian and New Zealand Journal of Psychiatry, 34*(1), 80-84.

Tonge, B., & Einfeld, S. L. (2003). Psychopathology and intellectual disability: the australian child to adult longitudinal study. *International Review of Research in Mental Retardation, 26*, 61-91.

Touchette, P. E., MacDonald, R. F., & Langer, S. N. (1985). A scatter plot for identifying stimulus control of problem behavior. *Journal of Applied Behavior Analysis*, *18*(4), 343–351. doi:10.1901/jaba.1985.18-343 PMID:4086416

Tower, C. (1989). *Understanding child abuse and neglect*. Boston: Allyn and Bacon.

Tracy, J., & McDonald, R. (2015). Health and Disability: Partnerships in Health care. *Journal of Applied Research in Intellectual Disabilities*, *28*(1), 22–32. doi:10.1111/jar.12135 PMID:25530571

Tremblay, K. N., Richer, L., Lachance, L., & Côté, A. (2010). Psychopathological manifestations of children with intellectual disabilities according to their cognitive and adaptive behavior profile. *Research in Developmental Disabilities*, *31*(1), 57–69. doi:10.1016/j.ridd.2009.07.016 PMID:19700260

Trute, B. (1990). Child and parent predictors of family adjustment in households containing young developmentally disabled children. *Family Relations, 39*(3), 292–297. doi:10.2307/584874

Turnbull, A. P., Brown, I., & Turnbull, R. H. (Eds.). (2004). *Families and people with mental retardation and quality of life: International perspectives.* Washington, DC: American Association on Mental Retardation.

Turner, G. W., & Crane, B. (2016). Pleasure is paramount: Adults with intellectual disabilities discuss sensuality and intimacy. *Sexualities, 19*(5–6), 677–697. doi:10.1177/1363460715620573

Turner, G. W., & Crane, B. (2016). Sexually silenced no more, adults with learning disabilities speak up: A call to action for social work to frame sexual voice as a social justice issue. *British Journal of Social Work, 46*(8), 2300–2317. doi:10.1093/bjsw/bcw133

Turner, W. J. (2018). Conceptualization of intellectual disability in medieval English law. In *Intellectual disability.* Manchester University Press.

U.S. Census Bureau. (2007). *American with disabilities act: July 26.* Author.

U.S. Census Bureau. (2011). *National intercensal estimates (2000-2010): Table 1 Intercensal estimates of the resident population by sex and age for the United States: April 1, 2000, to July 1, 2010.* Retrieved from www.census.gov/popest/data/intercensal/national/nat2010.html

U.S. Census Bureau. (2014). *Total population by child and adult populations.* Retrieved from http://datacenter.kidscount.org/data/tables/99-total-population-by-child-and-adult-populations?loc=1&loct=1#detailed/1/any/false/35,18,17,16,15/39,41/416,417

U.S. Census Bureau. (2015a). *Annual estimates of the resident population for selected age groups by sex for the United States, states, and counties, and Puerto Rico Commonwealth and municipios: April 1, 2010, to July 1, 2014.* Retrieved from http://factfinder.census.gov/faces/tableservices/jsf/pages/productview.xhtml?src=bkmk

U.S. Census Bureau. (2015b). *CPS table creator.* Retrieved from www.census.gov/cps/data/cpstablecreator.html

U.S. Department of Education. (2013). *Thirty-fifth annual report to Congress on the implementation of the Individuals with Disabilities Education Act, Parts B and C. 2013: Part B data descriptions and data files.* Retrieved from http://www2.ed.gov/about/reports/annual/osep/2013/parts-b-c/part-b-data/index.html

U.S. Department of Education. (2014). *2012 IDEA part B child count and educational environments.* Retrieved from https://inventory.data.gov/dataset/2012-idea-part-b-child-count-and-educationalenvironments/resource/a68a23f3-3981-47db-ac75-98a167b65259?inner_span=True

Underwood, M. K., Galen, B. R., & Paquette, J. A. (2001). Top ten challenges for understanding gender and aggression in children: Why can't we all just get along? *Social Development, 10*(2), 248–266. doi:10.1111/1467-9507.00162

United Nations Educational, Scientific and Cultural Organization. (1994). *The Salamanca Statement and framework for action on special needs education.* Paris: Author.

United Nations Educational, Scientific and Cultural Organization. (2008). *Defining an Inclusive Education agenda: Reflection around the 48th session the International Conference on Education.* Retrieved from www.ibe.unesco.org/.../48th.../Defining_Inclusive_Education_Agenda_2

United Nations Educational, Scientific and Cultural Organization. (2008). *Inclusive education: The way of the future.* 48th session of the International Conference on Education, Genova.

United Nations. (n.d.). Conventions on the Rights of the Persons with Disabilities. *Treaty Series, 2515*, 3. Retrieved November 17, 2015, from UN Treaty Collection website: https://treaties.un.org/Pages/ViewDetails.aspx?src=TREATY&mtdsg_no=IV-15&chapter=4&lang=en

University Legal Services. (2012). *The Work Option for Individuals with Intellectual Disabilities: The Obstacles and the Possibilities*. Retrieved from www.ulsdc.org/Employment%20Report_FINAL.pdf

UNNATI. (2004). *Understanding Disability: Attitude and Behaviour Change for Social Inclusion*. Retrieved from: http://www.unnati.org/pdfs/books/research-eng.pdf, 2.

Upadhyaya, G. R., & Havalappanavar, N. B. (2008). Coping in parents of the mentally challenged. *Journal of the Indian Academy of Applied Psychology*, *34*(2), 221–225.

Uysal, A., Albayrak, B., Koçulu, B., Kan, F., & Aydın, T. (2014). Attitudes of nursing students toward people with disabilities. *Nurse Education Today*, *34*(5), 878–884. doi:10.1016/j.nedt.2013.09.001 PMID:24080269

Van Cleave, J., & Davis, M. M. (2006). Bullying and peer victimization among children with special health care needs. *Pediatrics*, *118*(4), 1212–1219. doi:10.1542/peds.2005-3034 PMID:17015509

Van Dyke, D. E., Mc Brien, D. M., & Sherbondy, A. (1995). Issues of sexuality in Down Syndrome. *Down's Syndrome: Research and Practice*, *3*(2), 65–69. doi:10.3104/reviews.53

Van Houten, R., Axelrod, S., Bailey, J. S., Favell, J. E., Foxx, R. M., Iwata, B. A., & Lovaas, O. I. (1988). The right to effective behavioral treatment. *Journal of Applied Behavior Analysis*, *21*(4), 381–384. doi:10.1901/jaba.1988.21-381 PMID:3225255

Van Riper, M. (2000). Family variables associated with well-being in siblings of children with down syndrome. *Journal of Family Nursing*, *6*(3), 267–286. doi:10.1177/107484070000600305

Vandevelde, S., Broekaert, E., Schuyten, G., & Van Hove, G. (2005). Intellectual abilities and motivation toward substance abuse treatment in drug-involved offenders: A pilot study in the Belgian criminal justice system. *International Journal of Offender Therapy and Comparative Criminology*, *49*(3), 277–297. doi:10.1177/0306624X04270779 PMID:15851508

Vaughan, P. J., Pullen, N., & Kelly, M. (2000). Services for mentally disordered offenders in community psychiatry teams. *Journal of Forensic Psychiatry*, *11*(3), 571–586. doi:10.1080/09585180010004829

Veerman, J. W., & Van Yperen, T. A. (2007). Degrees of freedom and degrees of uncertainty:A developmental model for the establishment of evidence-based youth care. *Evaluation and Program Planning*, *30*(2), 212–221. doi:10.1016/j.evalprogplan.2007.01.011 PMID:17689326

Vera, H., Barnard, G. W., & Holzer, C. (1979). The intelligence of rapists: New data. *Archives of Sexual Behavior*, *8*(4), 375–377. doi:10.1007/BF01541880 PMID:475583

Verdugo, M. A., Bermejo, B. G., & Fuertes, J. (1995). The maltreatment of intellectually handicapped children and adolescents. *Child Abuse & Neglect*, *19*(2), 205–215. doi:10.1016/0145-2134(94)00117-D PMID:7780782

Vereenooghe, L., Flynn, S., Hastings, R. P., Adams, D., Chauhan, U., Cooper, S.-A., . . . Jahoda, A. (2018). Interventions for mental health problems in children and adults with severe intellectual disabilities: a systematic review. *BMJ Open, 8*(6), e021911.

Violence against Disabled Children: A summary report. (2005, July 28). UNICEF at the United Nations.

Vissers, L., Gilissen, C., & Joris, A. (2016). Genetic studies in intellectual disability and related disorders. *Nature Reviews. Genetics*, *17*(1), 9–18. doi:10.1038/nrg3999 PMID:26503795

Vollmer, T. R., Marcus, B. A., Ringdahl, J. E., & Roane, H. S. (1995). Progressing from brief assessments to extended experimental analyses in the evaluation of aberrant behavior. *Journal of Applied Behavior Analysis*, *28*(4), 561–576. doi:10.1901/jaba.1995.28-561 PMID:16795882

Vrijmoeth, C., Monbaliu, E., & Lagast, E. (2011). Behavioral problems in children with motor and intellectual disabilities: Prevalence and associations with maladaptive personality and marital relationship. *Research in Developmental Disabilities*, *32*, 1027–1038. PMID:22502827

Waasdorp, T. E., & Bradshaw, C. P. (2015). The overlap between cyberbullying and traditional bullying. *The Journal of Adolescent Health*, *56*(5), 483–488. doi:10.1016/j.jadohealth.2014.12.002 PMID:25631040

Waldman, H. B., Swerdloff, M., & Perlman, S. P. (1999). A "dirty secret": The abuse of children with disabilities. *ASDC Journal of Dentistry for Children*, *66*(3), 197–202. PMID:10476359

Walker-Hirsch, L. (2007). *The Facts of Life...and More Sexuality and Intimacy for People with Intellectual Disabilities*. Brookes Publishing Co.

Wallander, J.L., Dekker, M.C., & Koot, H.M. (1992). *Variations in prenatal sociodemographic factors associated with intellectual disability*. Academic Press.

Wallinius, M., Nordholm, J., Wagnström, F., & Billstedt, E. (2019). Cognitive functioning and aggressive antisocial behaviors in young violent offenders. *Psychiatry Research*, *272*, 572–580. doi:10.1016/j.psychres.2018.12.140 PMID:30616126

Walsbren, S. E. (1980). Parents' reactions after the birth of a developmentally disabled child. *American Journal of Mental Deficiency*, *84*(4), 345–351. PMID:6444494

Walter, J. (n.d.). From taboo to self-actualization–acceptance problems and learning processes in working with mentally handicapped patients. *Praxis der Kinderpsychologie und Kinderpsy*chiatrie, *51*(8), 587-597.

Wang, J., Iannotti, R. J., Luk, J. W., & Nansel, T. R. (2010). Co-occurrence of victimization from five subtypes of bullying: Physical, verbal, social exclusion, spreading rumors, and cyber. *Journal of Pediatric Psychology*, *35*(10), 1103–1112. doi:10.1093/jpepsy/jsq048 PMID:20488883

Ward, K., Trigler, J., & Pfeiffer, K. (2001). Community services, issues, and service gaps for individuals with developmental disabilities who exhibit inappropriate sexual behaviors. *Mental Retardation*, *39*(1), 11–19. doi:10.1352/0047-6765(2001)039<0011:CSIASG>2.0.CO;2 PMID:11270210

Ward, R. L., Nichols, A. D., & Freedman, R. I. (2010, November). Uncovering Health care Inequalities among adults with intellectual and developmental disabilities. *Health & Social Work*, *35*(4), 280–290. doi:10.1093/hsw/35.4.280 PMID:21171535

Warren, S. F., & Brady, N. C. (2007). The role of maternal responsivity in the development of children with intellectual disabilities. *Mental Retardation and Developmental Disabilities Research Reviews*, *13*(4), 330–338. doi:10.1002/mrdd.20177 PMID:17979201

Watson, L. S. Jr. (1968). Application of behaviour-shaping devices to training severely and profoundly mentally retarded children in an institutional setting. *Mental Retardation*, *6*, 21–23. PMID:5705586

Webster-Stratton, C. (2000). The Incredible Years Training series. Office of Juvenile Justice and Delinquency Prevention Bulletin Review, 1–24.

Webster-Stratton, C. (2001). *The Incredible Years: Parents, teachers, and children training series, leader's guide*. Seattle, WA: Author.

Weise, J., Fisher, K. R., & Trollor, J. N. (2018). What makes generalist mental health professionals effective when working with people with an intellectual disability? A family member and support person perspective. *Journal of Applied Research in Intellectual Disabilities, 31*(3), 413-422.

Wells, T., Sandefur, D., & Hogan, D. P. (2003). What happens after the high school years among young persons with disabilities? *Social Forces, 82*(2), 803–832. doi:10.1353of.2004.0029

Wenhua, L. (2005). Analysis of 294 cases of murder in forensic psychiatric expertise. *Journal of Clinical Psychosomatic Diseases, 4,* 25.

Werner, D. (2006). *Disabled Village Children: A Guide for Community Health Workers, Rehabilitation Workers, and Families*. Berkeley, CA: Hesperian Foundation.

Werner, S. (2019). Service use and perceptions of service effectiveness by parents of individuals with intellectualdisabilities: Comparing Jewish and Arab Israeli parental caregivers. *Journal of Intellectual Disability Research, 18*. doi:10.1111/jir.12611 PMID:30775831

Werner, S., Stern, I., Roth, D., & Tenenbaum, A. (2019). Help-Seeking by Parental Caregivers of Individuals with Intellectual Disabilities and Dual Diagnosis. *Administration and Policy in Mental Health, 46*(3), 321–333. doi:10.100710488-018-00915-w PMID:30604003

Wert, B. Y., & Neisworth, J. T. (2003). Effects of video self-modeling on spontaneous requesting in children with autism. *Journal of Positive Behavior Interventions, 5*(1), 30–34. doi:10.1177/10983007030050010501

Weschsler, D. (1950). Cognitive, Conative and Non-intellective Intelligence. *American Psychological Association, 5*(3), 78-83.

Whitaker, S. (2001). Anger control for people with learning disabilities: A critical review. *Behavioural and Cognitive Psychotherapy, 29*(3), 277–293. doi:10.1017/S1352465801003022

White, N., & Hastings, R. P. (2004). Social and professional support for parents of adolescents with severe intellectual disabilities. *Journal of Applied Research in Intellectual Disabilities, 17*(3), 181-190.

Whitehouse, J. O., Durkin, K., Jaquet, E., & Ziatas, K. (2009). Friendship, loneliness and depression in adolescents with asperger's syndrome. *Journal of Adolescence, 32*(2), 309–322. doi:10.1016/j.adolescence.2008.03.004 PMID:18692233

Whitehouse, J. O., Watt, H. J., Line, E. A., & Bishop, D. V. M. (2009). Adult psychosocial outcomes of children with specific language impairment, pragmatic language impairment and autism. *International Journal of Language & Communication Disorders, 44*(4), 511–528. doi:10.1080/13682820802708098 PMID:19340628

White, L., & Riedmann, A. (1992). Ties among adult siblings. *Social Forces, 71*(1), 85–102. doi:10.1093f/71.1.85

Whitney, I., Nabuzoka, D., & Smith, P. K. (1992). Bullying in schools: Mainstream and special needs. *Support for Learning, 7*(1), 3–7. doi:10.1111/j.1467-9604.1992.tb00445.x

Whitney, I., Smith, P. K., & Thompson, D. (1994). Bullying and children with special educational needs. In P. K. Smith & S. Sharp (Eds.), *School bullying: Insights and perspectives* (pp. 213–240). London: Routledge.

Whittingham, K., Sofronoff, K., Sheffield, J., & Sanders, M. R. (2009). Stepping Stones Triple P: An RCT of a parenting program with parents of a child diagnosed with an autism spectrum disorder. *Journal of Abnormal Child Psychology, 37*(4), 469–480. doi:10.100710802-008-9285-x PMID:19023654

Whittle, C., & Butler, C. (2018). Sexuality in the lives of people with intellectual disabilities: A meta-ethnographic synthesis of qualitative studies. *Research in Developmental Disabilities, 75*, 68–81. doi:10.1016/j.ridd.2018.02.008 PMID:29486384

Whittle, L., Fisher, K. R., Reppermund, S., Lenroot, R., & Trollor, J. (2018). Barriers and enablers to accessing mental health services for people with intellectual disability: A scoping review. *Journal of Mental Health Research in Intellectual Disabilities, 11*(1), 69–102. doi:10.1080/19315864.2017.1408724

Wiese, E. (2018). Improving the Quality of Life of Elderly with Intellectual Disability: A Literature Review on Environment and care. *Journal of Degenerative Intellectual and Development Disabilities, 1*(5).

Wikler, D. (1979). Paternalism and the mildly retarded. *Philosophy & Public Affairs*, 377–392.

Wikler, L. (1981). Chronic stresses of families of mentally retarded children. *Family Relations, 30*(2), 281–288. doi:10.2307/584142

Williams, F., Kouimtsidis, C., & Baldacchino, A. (2018). Alcohol use disorders in people with intellectual disability. *BJPsych Advances, 24*(4), 264–272. doi:10.1192/bja.2017.37

Williams, J. R., & Algozzine, B. (1979). Teachers' Attitudes toward Mainstreaming. *The Elementary School Journal, 80*(2), 63–67. doi:10.1086/461173

Willner, P., Brace, N., & Phillips, J. (2005). Assessment of anger coping skills in individuals with intellectual disabilities. *Journal of Intellectual Disability Research, 49*(5), 329–339. doi:10.1111/j.1365-2788.2005.00668.x PMID:15817050

Wilson, A. S. (2007). *Caregiver Attitude of Sexuality of the Intellectually Disabled Population*. Proquest Theses & Dissertation.

Wilson, M. C., & Scior, K. (2015). Implicit attitudes towards people with intellectual disabilities: Their relationship with explicit attitudes, social distance, emotions and contact. *PLoS One, 10*(9), e0137902. doi:10.1371/journal.pone.0137902 PMID:26366575

Wishart, J. G., Cebula, K. R., Willis, D. S., & Pitcairn, T. K. (2007). Understanding of facial expressions of emotion by children with intellectual disabilities of differing etiology. *Journal of Intellectual Disability Research, 51*(7), 551–563. doi:10.1111/j.1365-2788.2006.00947.x PMID:17537169

Wissink, I. B., Vugt, V. E., Moonen, X., Stams, G. J., & Hendriks, J. (2015). Sexual abuse involving children with an intellectual disability (ID): A narrative review. *Research in Developmental Disabilities, 36*, 20–35. doi:10.1016/j.ridd.2014.09.007 PMID:25310832

Witwera, A. N., & Lecavaliera, L. (2008). Psychopathology in children with intellectual disability: Risk markers and correlates. *Journal of Mental Health Research in Intellectual Disabilities, 1*(2), 75–96. doi:10.1080/19315860801988327

Wolfe, B., Song, J., Greenberg, J. S., & Mailick, M. R. (2014). Ripple effects of developmental disabilities and mental illness on nondisabled adult siblings. *Social Science & Medicine, 108*, 1–9. doi:10.1016/j.socscimed.2014.01.021 PMID:24607704

Wolfe, P. S. (1992). Challenges for service providers. In P. J. McLaughlin & P. Wejman (Eds.), *Developmental disabilities: A handbook for best practice* (pp. 124–141). Boston: Andover Medical.

Wolfgang, C. H. (2001). *Solving discipline and classroom management programs: Methods and models for today's teachers*. New York: John Wiley.

Wolf, M. M. (1978). Social validity: The case for subjective measurement or how applied behavior analysis is finding its heart. *Journal of Applied Behavior Analysis, 11*(2), 203–214. doi:10.1901/jaba.1978.11-203 PMID:16795590

Wong, J. G., Clare, I. C. H., Holland, A. J., Watson, P. C., & Gunn, M. (2000). The capacity of people with a 'mental disability' to make a health care decision. *Psychological Medicine, 30*(2), 295-306.

Woodman, A. C., Mawdsley, H. P., & Hauser-Cram, P. (2011). Parenting stress and child behavior problems within families of children with developmental disabilities: Transactional relations across 15 years. *Research in Developmental Disabilities, 32*, 264–276. PMID:25462487

Woolfenden, S., Goldfeld, S., Raman, S., Eapen, V., Kemp, L., & Williams, K. (2013). Inequity in child health: the importance of early childhood development. *Journal of Paediatrics and Child Health, 49*(9), e365-e369.

Woolfenden, S., Williams, K., Eapen, V., Mensah, F., Hayen, A., Siddiqi, A., & Kemp, L. (2014). Developmental vulnerability–don't investigate without a model in mind. *Child: Care, Health and Development.*

World Health Organisation. (2003). *Caring for children and adolescents with mental disorders*. WHO.

World Health Organisation. (2007). International Classification Diseases (10th ed.). Geneva: WHO.

World Health Organisation. (2009a). *Mental health aspects of women's reproductive health. A global review of literature*. WHO.

World Health Organisation. (2009b). *Promoting Sexual and Reproductive Health for People with Disabilities*. WHO.

World Health Organization (WHO). (2001). *The World Health Report 2001- Mental Health: New Understanding, New Hope*. Retrieved from: http://www.who.int/whr/2001/en/

World Health Organization (WHO). (2011). *World Report on Disability*. Retrieved from: http://www.who.int/whosis/whostat/2011/en/

World Health Organization. (1992) The ICD-10 classification of mental and behavioral disorders: Clinical descriptions and diagnostic guidelines. Geneva, Switzerland: WHO.

World Health Organization. (1992). *The ICD-10 classification of mental and behavioural disorders: Clinical descriptions and diagnostic guidelines*. Geneva: World Health Organization.

World Health Organization. (2000). Ageing and Intellectual Disabilities - Improving Longevity and Promoting Healthy Ageing: Summative Report. Geneva, Switzerland: WHO.

World Health Organization. (2007). *Atlas: global resources for persons with intellectual disabilities*. Geneva: World Health Organization. Retrieved from http://www.who.int/mental_health/evidence/atlas_id_2007.pdf

World Health Organization. (2011). *Rehabilitation. World report on disability*. WHO.

Yamaoka, Y., Tamiya, N., Moriyama, Y., Sandoval Garrido, F. A., Sumazaki, R., & Noguchi, H. (2015). Mental health of parents as caregivers of children with disabilities: Based on Japanese nationwide survey: E0145200. *PLoS One, 10*(12), e0145200. doi:10.1371/journal.pone.0145200 PMID:26692344

Yazbeck, M., McVilly, K., & Parmenter, T. R. (2004). Attitudes toward people with intellectual disabilities an Australian perspective. *Journal of Disability Policy Studies, 15*(2), 97–111. doi:10.1177/10442073040150020401

Yeargin-Allsopp, M., Drews, C. D., Decouflé, P., & Murphy, C. C. (1995). Mild mental retardation in black and white children in metropolitan Atlanta: A case-control study. *American Journal of Public Health, 85*(3), 324–328. doi:10.2105/AJPH.85.3.324 PMID:7892913

York, A. M., Ruediger, T., & Voltenburg, N. (2017). Doctor of physical therapy students' attitudes towards people with disabilities: A descriptive study. *Disability and Rehabilitation*, *39*(1), 91–97. doi:10.3109/09638288.2016.1140830 PMID:26883300

York, J., Vandercook, T., MacDonald, C., Heise-Neff, C., & Caughey, E. (1992). Feedback about integrating middle school students with severe disabilities in general education classes. *Exceptional Children*, *58*(3), 244–257. doi:10.1177/001440299105800307 PMID:1839896

Young-Southward, G., Cooper, S.-A., & Philo, C. (2017). Health and wellbeing during transition to adulthood for young people with intellectual disabilities: A qualitative study. *Research in Developmental Disabilities*, *70*, 94–103. doi:10.1016/j.ridd.2017.09.003 PMID:28918309

Zablotsky, B., Bradshaw, C. P., Anderson, C., & Law, P. A. (2013). The association between bullying and the psychological functioning of children with autism spectrum disorders. *Journal of Developmental and Behavioral Pediatrics*, *34*(1), 1–8. doi:10.1097/DBP.0b013e31827a7c3a PMID:23275052

Zapf, W., Glatzer, W., Noll, H. H., Habich, R., Berger-Schmitt, R., & Breuer, S. (1987). German social report: Living conditions and subjective well-being, 1978–1984. *Social Indicators Research*, *19*, 1.

Zeanah, H., Boris, N. W., & Larrieu, J. A. (1997). Infant development and developmental risk: A review of the past 10 years. *Journal of the American Academy of Child and Adolescent Psychiatry*, *36*(2), 165–178. doi:10.1097/00004583-199702000-00007 PMID:9031569

Zeedyk, S. M., Rodrigeuz, G., Tipton, L. A., Baker, B. L., & Blacher, J. (2014). Bullying of youth with autism spectrum disorder, intellectual disability, or typical development: Victim and parent perspectives. *Research in Autism Spectrum Disorders*, *8*(9), 1173–1183. doi:10.1016/j.rasd.2014.06.001 PMID:25285154

Zeitlin, S., & Williamson, G. (1990). Coping characteristics of disabled and nondisabled young children. *The American Journal of Orthopsychiatry*, *60*(3), 404–411. doi:10.1037/h0079183 PMID:2143354

Zisberg, A., Young, H., Schepp, K., & Zysberg, L. (2007). A concept analysis of routine: Relevance to nursing. *Journal of Advanced Nursing*, *57*(4), 442–453. doi:10.1111/j.1365-2648.2007.04103.x PMID:17291208

Zupanick, C. E. (2019, May 26). Support & Help for Families With Intellectually Disabled Children [Weblog post]. Retrieved from https://www.mentalhelp.net/articles/support-amp-help-for-families-with-intellectually-disabled-children/

About the Contributors

Rejani Thudalikunnil Gopalan is an Academician and registered Clinical Psychologist who has closer to two decades work experience in mental health area. Currently she is working as Professor and Head of Clinical Psychology in Mahatma Gandhi Medical College and Hospital. Jaipur, India. She has received many awards for her academic excellence and contribution to mental health area and research. Her specialized services extended to clinical consultation and therapeutic remedies for the group including adults and children with mental illness in Prison and juvenile homes along with court related disputes. Research Area: Traumas and abuses, especially sexual abuse; childhood mental health issues, school mental health, forensic, neuro psychological and mental health issues among convicted adult and juvenile offenders.

* * *

Prathibha Augustus Kurishinkal is a PhD research scholar at Institute of Behavioral Sciences, Gujarat Forensic Sciences University, Gujarat, India.

Norharlina Bahar received her MD and MMed (Psych) from Universiti Kebangsaan Malaysia in 1997 and 2005 respectively. She worked and trained in Melbourne for her subspecialty in Child and Adolescent Psychiatry. Her special interests are in the area of Infant Mental Health; Early Childhood Emotional Development; Parent-Child Relationship; and Internet Addiction. She is an international Board Member of the International Society of Internet Addiction. She is now heading the Child & Adolescent Psychiatry Unit in Hospital Selayang. She is active in several non-governmental organizations and schools to advocate the needs of children, adolescents and people with mental health issues.

Priyanka Behrani is working as an Assistant Professor in the department of life skills, Teamlease Skills University, Vadodara. She did her master's in psychology from Kanpur University, India in 1993 and Doctorate in 2000 in the area of Personality Psychology. She completed her certificate course in Disability specializing in Mental Retardation. She has attended National and International conferences, seminars, workshops in the area of Educational and Industrial Psychology. She has published papers and chapters in various books and journals.

Sandamita Choudhury is a licensed Clinical Psychologist (RCI) currently working in 151 Base Hospital, Basistha, Guwahati, Assam. After completion of M.Phil in Clinical Psychology in 2016 from Gujarat Forensic Sciences University, Gandhinagar, she had been involved in clinical work in her hometown Guwahati, Assam. She is a consultant in Indian Institute of Information technology, Guwahati (IIIT-G), MINDIndia Institute of positive research and mental health, Astitva. He has been associated as a Guest faculty in TISS, Guwahati, Composite regional centre for people with disabilities, Cotton University and various training and manpower building sessions for NIPCCD. She carried out researches among Homeless Youth, Domestic Violence among Men, HIV Pregnant women, intellectually disabled and their rehabilitation, Caregivers of Mentally ill and Adolescents.

Sumita Chowhan received her PhD degree from Andhra University, Vishakhapatnam, India. She is a doctoral guide and assistant professor in Jain University, Bangalore, India. She is EAP (Employee Assistant Programme) Affiliate (Psychologist) working with Workplace Options. Astute, result oriented with proven success in counselling, research, training (SPSS) and teaching. She has international exposure both in education and job in US and UK. She received Cognitive behavioural therapy diploma from UK. She has five plus years of experience in versatile fields like Research (SPSS) /Teaching/Counselling/ Training and HR. She also attended and presented papers in national/international conferences. She had published research articles and chapter in journals and Book. She is peer reviewer and board of editorial member of different journals. Her areas of interest are Education, clinical, child psychology and developmental, positive psychology (character strength), Neuropsychology and Industrial.

Anjali Daisy is a full-time research scholar in School of Management, SASTRA Deemed University. Her research area is in the field of emotional intelligence.

Dorothy Bhandari Deka received her Mphil from Gujarat Forensic Sciences University. She is presently working in a hospital in Guwahati as a Cynical Psychologist. She has done a diploma course in Clinical and Applied Hyposis. She also works with the Chemo therapy patients that includes psychological services to cancer patients.

Valsamma Eapen is Chair of Infant, Child and Adolescent Psychiatry at the University of New South Wales, and Head of the Academic Unit of Child Psychiatry South West Sydney (AUCS). After graduating in Medicine, she completed her postgraduate training in London. Starting her academic career at the University College London, her clinical and research interests since then have focussed on issues of early development and neurodevelopmental disorders including Tourette Syndrome and autism. She has authored around 300 scientific publications including five books and 27 book chapters and presented at over 135 conferences. She is a member of several international consortiums including Obsessive Compulsive Foundation Genetics Collaborative, Homozygosity Mapping Collaborative for Autism and Psychiatric Genomics Consortium. She is part of several collaborative initiatives and grants including from NHMRC, ARC, and she is Program 1 Director for Autism CRC. She is the Director of BestSTART System Transformation and Research translation Centre, South West Sydney and Stream Leader for the Clinical Academic Group on "Early Life Determinants of Health (ELDoH)" under the Sydney Partnership for Health Education Research and Enterprise (SPHERE), an NHMRC accredited Advanced Health Research and Translation Centre (AHRTC).

Jamila Firdaus is the Head counselor in Navrachana school wherein she looks after students with mental health issues. She also provides her expert guidance to junior counselors and teachers working in the school for managing common problems faced by students. She also extends her services to cater to the difficulties faced by the parents in managing these issues.

Vaitsa Giannouli received her PhD in Neuroscience from the School of Medicine, Aristotle University of Thessaloniki. She is a cognitive psychologist and neuropsychologist. She is currently a research fellow at Aristotle University of Thessaloniki (AUTh), Greece. She has received numerous accolades and scholarships for her work as an undergraduate and graduate student. She is working as a research assistant and is involved in several cross-cultural research projects focusing on issues of cognition and lifespan development.

Aili Hanim Hashim is a Consultant Psychiatrist for Child, Adolescent and Adult Mental Health. She is currently an academic staff at the Department of Psychological Medicine, Faculty of Medicine, University Malaya, Kuala Lumpur. As a consultant child and adolescent psychiatrist, Dr. Aili has had extensive experience in both working with schools, educators, children and families, support group and both government and non-government agencies. Her work involved around recognition, assessment and treatment of mental health difficulties in children and adult. Her main interest includes understanding and recognizing mental health difficulties in both children and adults, with an emphasis on early intervention. The emphasis is extended in her teaching of both undergraduates and postgraduates highlighting the role of mental health professionals and the use of talking therapy (CBT and psychotherapy) in assessment and treatment of children and adult with mental health difficulties.

Mythili Hazarika is an Associate Professor of Clinical Psychology at the Gauhati Medical College & Hospital (GMCH) in Guwahati, India and has multiple accreditations.

Mansi Jadeja has completed her specialization in Clinical Psychology and hold a M.Phil degree. She has been practicing and making her contribution to academics since last 3 years. She is an Assistant Professor in the University and is also in-charge of the Department's Counseling cell wherein her job profile includes administration and training for clinical work.

Manveen Kaur, a Child and Adolescent Psychiatrist, works at the Department of Psychological Medicine, University Malaya. She is a Senior Lecturer, whose clinical duties at the PAC Unit (Child & Adolescent Psychiatry Unit), involve treating children and adolescents with mental health difficulties. In addition to this, she is active in research and teaching postgraduates in the field of both General and Child Psychiatry. An integral part of her work involves reaching out to the Community, where educating the public, and working with teachers and councilors, in order to better support children.

Tanay Maiti (MBBS, DPM, DNB Psych) is a young enthusiastic psychiatrist and mental health professional, with more than half a decade experience as a trainee, learner and later as a full time professional in the field, though his inquisitive nature and exploring mind hasn't come to a pause ever! He has done his MBBS from the prestigious Medical College Hospital, Kolkata and DPM from Christian Medical College, Vellore, DNB from Vidyasagar Institute of Mental Health, Neuro and Allied sciences, Delhi. He worked as senior resident at child and adolescent unit in CMC Vellore and also in All India

Institute of Medical Sciences, Bhubaneswar. He has multiple national and international publications to his credits, and has won multiple awards for his paper/posters as well. He has also been chosen for the prestigious fellowship from 'Dr. Ramachandra N Moorthy Foundation' at 6th Leadership and Professional Skills course for Early Career Psychiatrist' at NIMHANS, Feb 2018 (one among the sixteen from the entire SAARC region) and also been recognized amongst the promising young psychiatrists and won a fellowship from World Psychiatric Association(one of the thirty seven winners from the entire globe)for the same at recently conducted 'World Congress of Psychiatry' September 2018 at Mexico City, Mexico. With direct experience to work and learn from the three of the premier institutes in country(VIMHANS, New Delhi; Christian Medical College, Vellore and AIIMS, Bhubaneswar) Dr. Tanay is currently focusing his work on extensive research and both undergraduate and post graduate training(writing books and book chapters for them), along with regular clinical works and managing difficult patients and clinical scenarios. Dr. Maiti's primary interest of work and research lies upon child and adolescent psychiatry, developmental psychology, and adolescent substance abuse.

Nisha Mathew, after completing a Bachelor of Psychology (Hons) at the University of New South Wales, Sydney, is now undertaking a PhD at the University of New South Wales School of Women's and Children's Health focusing on the medical comorbidities, immune and microbiotic biomarkers in children with Autism Spectrum Disorders.

Jahirul Mullick has educational research experience for more than a decade with a demonstrated history of working in higher education industry both in research and teaching capacity. He earned his doctoral degree in Leadership practices and inclusive education from Monash University. He was recipient of Monash Graduate Scholarship (MGS) and Monash International Postgraduate Research Scholarship (MIPRS). He is Sessional Lecturer in teacher education programs in the Faculty of Education at Monash University, Australia. He teaches Inclusive education, Learning, and Positive Behaviour Development. He has a strong interest in the theory and practice of applied behaviour analysis (ABA) and positive behaviour support (PBS) in a wide range of settings such as schools, clinics, homes, residential facilities, etc. He has expertise in contextualising behavioural principles to meet the learning and behaviour support needs of children and adults. He has authored several academic articles and book chapters that focus on leadership practice, inclusive and special education and teacher development.

Jyoti Mishra Pandey received her M.Phil in medical and social psychology (M.M&SP) from Central Institute of Psychiatry (CIP), Ranchi in 2011. She has been awarded as a first rank holder in her M.Phil (M&SP). She has completed her Ph.D from Ranchi Institute of Neuro-Psychiatry and Allied Sciences (RINPAS), Ranchi. She has also worked as assistant professor in the department of clinical psychology at central institute of psychiatry (CIP). She has also worked as a clinical psychologist in the department of psychiatry and pediatric at Bharati Vidyapeeth Medical College and Hospital, Pune. Professional member of IACP & registered in RCI. She has various publications and has presented papers on national conference. She has two chapters in an international index books and also two chapters are in process of publication. She has delivered lectures and conducted workshops on the academic level. Currently, she is working as a clinical psychologist at GMCH, Deptt of psychiatry, Chandigarh.

Plabita Patowary has completed her M.Phil. in Clinical Psychology from Gujarat Forensic Sciences University in 2016. She is currently associated as a Clinical Psychologist at Happy Minds, Kolkata, India. Her field of experience includes conducting psychometric assessments for diagnosis and therapeutic purposes and is well-versed in different categories of psychotherapy. Adolescent and adult population are her areas of interest. She has attended and presented papers in National and International conferences and published research articles in various journals.

K. Santhosh is Assistant Professor of the Department of Psychology at Christ University (Bangalore, Karnataka) in India, since 2016. His Ph.D. is in the area of Rorschach based Cognitive-motivational-personality factors that have a relationship with resilience in young adults, from the Department of Psychology at Bharathiar University (Coimbatore, Tamil Nadu) in India. His research interests span Strength-based research, solution focused thinking, resilience, and pratixas. Dr. Santhosh has authored 23 publications (one book, seven chapters, and 16 journal articles). He is currently the primary investigator of the major research project (funded by Centre for Research-Projects, Christ University), collaborating in a Japanese project (funded by JSPS with Tokoha University, Japan) and has been awarded two research grants for a short-term project by European Brief Therapy Association. He is a) member of International Positive Psychology Association, b) professionally associated with Association of Solution Focused Practices-India, and c) voluntarily involved in the community extension activities supporting AMMAPSYCDAC Society for Mental Health (Palakkad, Kerala) in India.

Rajesh (Jay) Sharma, BCBA, has an extensive professional experience in special education, psychology practice, and applied behaviour analysis (ABA) in a variety of settings including schools, psychiatric & drug de-addiction facilities, department of education, and NGO sector. Jay has keen interest in developing innovative interventions to treat maladaptive & problematic behaviours and help people improve their quality of life. He is a clinical director at Sunrise Behavioural Health Pty Ltd. Jay practises applied behaviour analysis (ABA) and teach special education at Torrens University Australia in Melbourne.

Palak Upadhyay works as an Assistant Professor at Dayanand medical college and hospital (DMC&H), Department of Psychiatry, Ludhiana (Punjab). She has received her M.Phil in clinical psychology from a very renowned mental health Institutes in India, Ranchi Institute of Neuro-Psychiatry and Allied Sciences (RINPAS), Ranchi.. She is a professional member of Indian Association of Clinical Psychology (IACP) and also registered in RCI. She has done various research publications and has presented research papers on national and international conferences and also conducted various workshops.

Amelia Walter, DClinPsych/MSc, BA (Hons, Psych), is a child and adolescent Clinical Psychologist who holds a part-time position as a Research Officer within SWSLHD and a Conjoint Lectureship within the School of Psychiatry, UNSW. Amelia has experience in conducting large-scale research projects implementing and evaluating intervention programs for infants, children and adolescents with mental health concerns and developmental disabilities. She has a particular research interest in the early detection of and intervention for Autism Spectrum Disorder (ASD), and holds several publications in this area. Amelia works closely with CI-Eapen and has existing working collaborations with many of the CIs in this application. Amelia will provide consultation and assistance to this project, particularly with regard to the administration and scoring of gold-standard developmental assessments, as well as data management and analysis.

Wan Salwina Wan Ismail is a Consultant Psychiatrist for Child, Adolescent and Adult Mental Health She obtained her medical degree from the University of Adelaide, South Australia, in 1994. After completing her internship, she worked as a medical officer in a psychiatric institution in Ulu Kinta, Perak. She completed Masters in Psychiatry, from Universiti Kebangsaan Malaysia, in 2003. In 2006, she furthered her study in Advanced Masters in Child and Adolescent Psychiatry, Universiti Kebangsaan Malaysia, and had been working with children and adolescents since. She is currently a lecturer, Child and Adolescent Psychiatrist, and Head of Child and Adolescent Psychiatry Unit, Department of Psychiatry, Faculty of Medicine, Universiti Kebangsaan Malaysia.

Michelle F. Wright, Ph.D., is a Research Associate at The Pennsylvania State University and a research fellow at Masaryk University in Brno, the Czech Republic. Her research focus is on the contextual factors which influence children's, adolescents', and young adults' involvement in aggressive behaviors, with a special interest in social goals, peer status, and cultural values. She has published on these topics, with her most recent work focused on culture and anonymity, and their role in cyberbullying among adolescents.

Index

www.ingramcontent.com/pod-product-compliance
Lightning Source LLC
LaVergne TN
LVHW062112300926
849161LV00010B/2446